ESSENTIALS OF
LEWIS'S
CHILD AND
ADOLESCENT
PSYCHIATRY

ESSENTIALS OF
LEWIS'S
CHILD AND
ADOLESCENT
PSYCHIATRY

Fred R. Volkmar, MD
Irving Harris Professor of Child Psychiatry,
 Psychology and Pediatrics
Director, Child Study Center
Yale University School of Medicine
New Haven, Connecticut

Andrés Martin, MD, MPH
Riva Ariella Ritvo Professor
Yale University School of Medicine
New Haven, Connecticut

Wolters Kluwer | Lippincott Williams & Wilkins
Health
Philadelphia · Baltimore · New York · London
Buenos Aires · Hong Kong · Sydney · Tokyo

Acquisitions Editor: Charles Mitchell
Product Manager: Tom Gibbons
Vendor Manager: Alicia Jackson
Senior Manufacturing Manager: Benjamin Rivera
Marketing Manager: Brian Freiland
Design Coordinator: Holly McLaughlin
Production Services: Aptara, Inc.

Printed in China

Library of Congress Cataloging-in-Publication Data

Volkmar, Fred R.
    Essentials of Lewis's child and adolescent psychiatry / Fred R. Volkmar, Andrés Martin.
    p. ; cm.
    Lewis's child and adolescent psychiatry
    Companion guide to: Lewis's child and adolescent psychiatry / editors, Andres Martin, Fred R. Volkmar. 4th ed. c2007.
    Includes bibliographical references and index.
    Summary: "This body of work draws on various, sometimes distinctive and sometimes overlapping, historical and professional traditions, including the expanding knowledge about both normative child development and developmental processes as well as about the origins, expression, and treatment of psychopathology. Parts of the field have their origins in the social welfare movement and the concern for better approaches to juvenile justice"–Provided by publisher.
    ISBN-13: 978-0-7817-7502-1 (pbk. : alk. paper)
    ISBN-10: 0-7817-7502-7 (pbk. : alk. paper)
    1. Child development.   2. Sick children–Psychology.   3. Child psychiatry.   I. Martin, Andrés.
II. Lewis, Melvin, 1926–2007.   III. Lewis's child and adolescent psychiatry.   IV. Title.   V. Title: Lewis's child and adolescent psychiatry.
    [DNLM: 1. Mental Disorders.   2. Adolescent.   3. Child.   4. Infant. WS 350]
    RJ131.L42 2011
    618.92'89—dc22

                                                                                    2011006401

10 9 8 7 6 5 4 3 2 1

RRS1103

To our wives, Lisa and Rebecca;
to our children, Lucy and Emily; Max, Ariela,
Gabriela, and Jacob Donald; and to the memory of
our dear mentor and colleague, Melvin Lewis.

■ PREFACE

Mark Twain once apologized to a correspondent for sending him a long letter, as he did not have time to write a shorter one. We have been mindful of this comment in our effort to distill the essence of *Lewis's Child and Adolescent Psychiatry: A Comprehensive Textbook, Fourth Edition* into a concise introduction to the topic.

Before he undertook the task of editing the first edition of his comprehensive textbook, our colleague, the late Melvin Lewis, had published shorter books highlighting clinical aspects of child development as relevant to medical students, house staff, and others in training. Even before his untimely passing, we had begun to talk with him about an introductory version of "the big book," which would convey the "essentials" of the topic.

In the process of this distillation, we have faced difficult choices in terms of range and depth of coverage but have attempted to keep the focus relevant to students, house staff, and other trainees with an emphasis on the most practical and salient information. As with the parent volume, we have adopted an organizational approach that provides a short introduction to the field and an overview of child development research. This is followed by a series of chapters focused on specific disorders and syndromes, concluding with chapters on treatment and areas of interface, such as pediatrics and the law. Whenever possible, we have tried to retain tables and figures from the parent volume and encourage interested readers to consult that resource for more detailed information; reading lists are also provided at the end of each chapter. This shorter companion book also includes a number of new case vignettes intended to make the material as clinically relevant and applicable as possible.

We are very grateful to Tom Gibbons and Charley Mitchell for their editorial guidance for both this and the parent volume. We also thank the many colleagues who have kindly granted us permission for use of materials, and specially thank Lori Klein, Emily Deegan Hau, and Rosemary Serra for their help with manuscript preparation.

Fred R. Volkmar, MD
Andrés Martin, MD, MPH
New Haven, CT

■ CONTENTS

CHAPTER 1 ▪ AN INTRODUCTION TO CHILD PSYCHIATRY: HISTORY, THEORY, AND METHODS

HISTORICAL PERSPECTIVES

The field of child mental health in general and child psychiatry in particular is a relatively recent one. Work in the area increased dramatically in the 20th century with an explosion of knowledge over the past several decades in particular. This body of work draws on various, sometimes distinctive and sometimes overlapping, historical and professional traditions, including the expanding knowledge about both normative child development and developmental processes as well as about the origins, expression, and treatment of psychopathology. Parts of the field have their origins in the social welfare movement and the concern for better approaches to juvenile justice. Another contribution stems from long-standing concerns for children with significant intellectual deficiency (mental retardation). All of these efforts had their origins in an interest in children and their development that had begun in the 1700s and was fueled by concerns for the education of future citizens and decreasing rates of child mortality.

Interest in understanding children's development can be traced to ancient times. Several different models of development were proposed. The prefomationists included individuals such as Hippocrates who assumed that body structured in the embryo were formed simultaneously. Others, such as Aristotle, suggested that development was more dynamic with the embryo formed by a series of transformations and differentiations (Hunt, 1961). Preformationist thought continued well into the 1600s when, with the development of the microscope, small humans were initially seen in views of human sperm (Figure 1.1)!

The period referred to as the Enlightenment in the 18th century had a major impact on changes in many areas, including an increased interest in education of citizens in the newly independent United States. The Enlightenment was not a single movement, and indeed, many of the philosophers central in it had divergent and sometimes contradictory views. For example John Locke, the Scottish physician and philosopher, was interested in education and psychological development. He suggested that babies are born with a mind that is a blank slate ("tabula rasa") upon which experience and growing conscious awareness shape the developing child. For him, education was therefore essential. Although agreeing with Locke on the importance of education, in contrast, the philosopher Jean-Jacques Rousseau believed that children were innately good and that a corrupt society contributed to their difficulties.

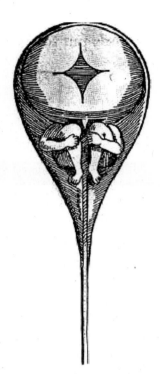

FIGURE 1.1. Hartoseker's drawing of a human sperm (1694) reflected "preformationist" ideas about embryologic development. The increased awareness of the complexity of development during the embryonic period paralleled an increased interest in the ways in which children's psychological development changed and reorganized over time. (From *Nicholas Hartsoeker, 1656–1725, Essay de dioptrique.* Paris: Jean Anisson 1694. Courtesy of Cushing/Whitney Medical Library, Yale University School of Medicine.)

In the 19th century, the growing emphasis on education, attempts to reform child labor laws (as well as concerns about slavery), and an expanding interest in women's rights (including the right to an education) had a major impact. Darwin's work on evolution revolutionized psychology as well as biology. Darwin was interested in psychological development in men and animals (and published a book on facial expressions in man and animals) to clarify potential biological relationships. His interest in children also reflected an awareness that, to some extent, children's development has important similarities, particularly at the embryologic level, to evolutionary development. Darwin also kept a detailed diary of one of his children's development. His work inspired subsequent psychologists, including Freud as well as individuals such as G. Stanley Hall, who tried to understand child development in an evolutionary context.

Reduced rates of infant and child mortality also meant that more children survived to need educational and other services. Beginning in the 19th century, several factors contributed to reducing mortality rates. These included better nutrition; housing; sanitation; various public health efforts (e.g., the mechanisms of disease pathogenesis became clear); the development of immunizations to prevent frequent, serious childhood infections; and, finally, the development of antibiotics. Before the 1800s, child mortality in general and infant mortality in particular were high, with considerable fluctuation reflecting epidemics, famine, conflict, and other factors. Probably at least one-third of infants succumbed to illness on average.

Pediatrics began to develop as a specialty with the growing awareness of differences in medical care in younger patients reflecting differences in physiology and drug metabolism. Hospitals for the care of sick children began to be established in Europe and the United States. These physicians were also increasingly concerned with fostering children's development and providing practical guidance to parents.

Interest in intellectual deficiency and mental retardation also contributed to the development of the various child mental health specialists. Although recognized since antiquity, scientific interest increased as attempts were made to understand the underlying brain basis of severe cognitive impairment. For example, the English anatomist Thomas Willis related intellectual deficiency to small brain size, and by 1866 John Down suggested that the syndrome that now carries his name (trisomy 21) reflected an evolutionary throwback in development. Inspired by Darwin, individuals in the Eugenics movement suggested the idea of improving society through selective breeding (see Gould, 1996).

A different, and more optimistic, approach to the care of mentally retarded individuals arose in France where work by Itard on the so-called feral child Victor (Figure 1.2) stimulated his interest in the remediation of significant developmental difficulty. He inspired the French physician Édouard Séguin, leading to a new approach in classifications and attempts to improve functional outcome. Sequin immigrated to the United States and had a profound influence on the development of intervention programs. In the United States, a series of special institutions, originally focused on rehabilitation of developmentally disabled children, developed. Other such institutions were established to care for children with blindness or deafness. A professional organization was established in 1876 that became what is today the American Association on Mental Retardation. The development of the first reliable tests of intelligence by Binet and Simon (see Chapters 3 and 5) also contributed to earlier identification of less

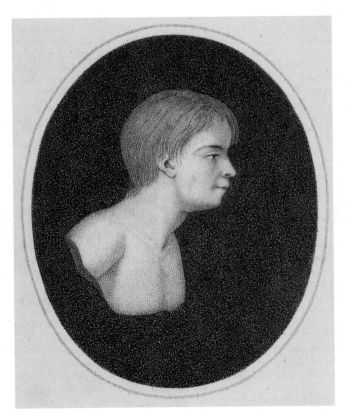

FIGURE 1.2. Victor the "wild boy" of Aveyron was reported to be a feral child who had lived alone in the words prior to his eventual capture. Although reports of wild or "feral" children abound in mythology, usually such reports relate either to children raised in profound isolation (but NOT by animals) or with serious developmental problems like autism. (From Itard, E. M. (1802). *An Historical Account of the Discovery and Éducation of a Savage Man, or of the First Developments and Moral, of the Young Savage Caught in the Woods Near Aveyron, in the Year 1798.* London: Richard Phillips.) Courtesy of the Cushing/Whitney Medical Library, Yale University School of Medicine.

severely impaired children with developmental delays. Clinics for the care of children with developmental difficulties began to be established in the late 19th century. Although the development of institutions and better approaches to assessment were positively intended, both led to abuses. Intelligence tests were used, sometimes highly inappropriately, to bolster the efforts of the Eugenics movement and, over time, the many negative effects of institutionalization also became apparent In the United States, G. Stanley Hall, a pioneer psychologist and educator, began to use new approaches to studying normative development. He used questionnaires to assess what children had learned and to document their interests and activities. He used this information to help teachers understand development. The growing child study movement led to the establishment in the early 20th century of a number of research centers across the country. Around this time, the length of children's years of education began to increase as increase in technology required a more educated workforce. Hall's work influenced many of the next generation of researchers, including Arnold Gesell and Gesell's student, Benjamin Spock.

Children who had difficulties with the law became a focus of increased concern. In the early 1900s, Healy established a clinic that advised the juvenile court regarding children. Healy's psychologically informed approach proved influential. He collaborated with a number of individuals, including Jane Adams, whose work at Hull House in Chicago served as a base for the development of social work as a discipline. Healy eventually moved to Boston, where he and a colleague founded the clinic supported by the Judge Baker Foundation. Around the same time, Arnold Gesell, one of the first PhDs in developmental psychology, moved to Yale, where he completed medical and pediatric training and founded what would become the Yale Child Study Center. In contrast to Healey's work, that of Gesell strongly emphasized the recognition of innate factors in development. Gesell conducted innovative work in charting normal development in infants and younger children using techniques such as still frame movie cameras to examine more precisely the aspects of infant motor development. His work had a profound influence on pediatrics, education, and childrearing practices. The contrasting views of various individuals, each emphasizing either biological or environmental factors, paralleled an earlier debate on the relative contributions of nature versus nurture (see Chapter 2). These tensions continued theoretically (e.g., in the tensions among theories of development grounded in behaviorism and psychoanalysis).

The increased interest in children with developmental, mental health, and legal issues led to the establishment of the American Orthopsychiatric Association in the 1920s. This organization strongly supported the importance of interdisciplinary collaboration in child mental health work. The interface of mental health issues with pediatrics led to the formal establishment of child psychiatry as a discipline. Although psychiatrists such as Maudsely in the 1800s had recognized the childhood onset of major psychiatric difficulties, it was only in 1930 that Leo Kanner was recruited to Johns Hopkins to serve as a liaison between pediatrics and psychiatry there. Kanner had strong connections to both departments and wrote the first textbook of child psychiatry. Among his many accomplishments was his pioneering work in pediatric consultation-liaison psychiatry (see Chapter 26) and the recognition of autism as distinctive conditions (see Chapter 4). Before World War II, pediatricians were beginning to spend time training in child psychiatry as fellows in various sites across the country. At that time, psychoanalytic influences also became strong and were further strengthened by an influx of European psychoanalysts before and after the war. Shortly after the war, the federal government established the first training grants. As the Child Guidance clinics increased, so did the need for psychiatrists with specialized pediatric training. The American Academy of Child Psychiatry was established in 1953, and by 1957, the field was recognized as a subspecialty of psychiatry with standards for training and board examinations and its own journal.

THEORIES OF DEVELOPMENT

Over the past century, a number of attempts have been made to provide broad, overarching theories of development. Typically, these approaches draw on one or more perspectives in their attempt to account for the complex interplay of biological and experiential or psychological factors that play a role as children grow and develop. These approaches vary in a number of respects. Some focus more on one aspect of development (emotional or cognitive), and others are more concerned with mechanisms (e.g., of learning). Although many early theories, such as Freud's, were concerned with early development, subsequent work has often extended these theories to other aspects of the life cycle (e.g., Erik Ericson was inspired by psychoanalytic theory and provided an overarching model for development from infancy to old age).

An increased awareness of the complexity of both genetic and experiential mechanisms and their interaction has also clarified important issues in development. For example, genes may change in their function over time. Specific environmental factors may have more effects at some points than at others. For example, early exposure may predispose some children to develop allergic responses. Another complexity arises because some traits, behaviors, and features may reflect a stronger genetic or psychological component. Environmental factors, including both endogenous and exogenous ones, may contribute, in varying degrees, to development. The idea of experience-dependent plasticity has been used when there are strong effects of experience at certain points in development. A child deprived of vision early in life may later have trouble, if sight is restored, in coordinated use of the eyes and perception of depth and three dimensions. Finally, of course, development occurs in family–societal contact. The environment that children experience is itself partly shaped by the parents' experience and endowment.

All theories of development face several important challenges. How is the interplay between endowment (nature) and experience (nurture) to be understood (see Chapter 2)? How and why does change happen? Is development continuous or discontinuous? For example, for a theorist such as Piaget who proposes rather major changes in cognitive functioning over childhood, what accounts for these changes? Relating theories to age and normative expectations presents another challenge. Early studies of child development were initially concerned with documenting normative processes. It became possible to describe typical behavior of a 1-year-old child simply by evoking age as an explanation. Given major changes and developmental accomplishments, it is typical for presentations on children's development to be constructed around intervals that are roughly age defined (e.g., infancy, toddler, preschool, school age, adolescent). Although understandable, this type of exposition tends to perpetuate the notion that somehow developmental change is caused by age alone. Over time, the field has moved from an initial focus on simple measures and age-related correlation to more sophisticated approaches. Although many broad theories of development have been postulated, a recent trend has been the focus on very specific aspects of development. In this chapter, we briefly summarize three major theories of development that have had a major impact on the field—psychoanalysis, Piaget's cognitive theory, and learning theory.

Psychoanalytic Theory

This approach to understanding children's development is based on the work of Sigmund Freud and others. Trained as a neurologist but also with a strong interest in embryology and Darwinian thought, Freud actually developed several different, often overlapping, theories. His work includes a general theory attempting to understand the mind and behavior as well as mental illness. He had a strong interest in child development and had a profound influence on the development of early psychotherapeutic work with children and adults (see Chapter 22). Freud's early work focused on distinctions between conscious and unconscious thinking and the impact of trauma in causing mental illness. His early work with women who had hysteria led him to assume, based on their reports, that trauma, particularly of a sexual nature, contributed to their difficulties. Although his subsequent theoretical model continued to emphasize the importance of sexual factors (including from very early in life), he became aware that the early reports could not be taken at face value and rather reflected the complicated interaction of wishes; cultural values and norms; and difficulties in coping with sexual thoughts, impulses, and feelings. His work led him to speculate that a significant contribution came from factors that were in the unconscious part of the mind. This, in turn, led him to think about other processes such as dreams, slips of the tongues, and mistakes of various types as having psychological meaning. His theory developed a distinction between the conscious and unconscious mind, the latter being characterized by what he termed the "primary process" whose contents could be inferred from dreams; behavior; slips; and, eventually, through his method of treatment called free association.

Freud's initial "topographic" model posited that the mind was divided into conscious, preconscious, and unconscious systems of thought. His growing interest in sexuality and gender identity led him to development a model with a very developmental focus. He proposed this model in 1905 in his book *Three Essays on the Theory of Sexuality*, in which he described various phases of psychosexual development: an oral phase (from birth to early toddlerhood), an anal phases (roughly ages 2 to years 4 or so), and the oedipal phase (after the anal phase up to about age 5 years). After the oedipal phase, he suggested there was a period of psychosexual latency (roughly school age) that lasted until puberty, when sexual feelings strongly resurfaced. In his view, fixations (developmental arrests) could occur at these various phases and result in characteristic psychiatric problems.

Over time, Freud became increasingly concerned with understanding phenomena such as depression, suicide, and the effects of trauma, and his thinking began to include an emphasis on understanding aggressive as well as sexual feelings. By 1923, he proposed revised model in which he postulated the existence of an id, ego, and superego. The id is presumed to be the place where basic impulses and instincts arise with little organization and outside immediate awareness. The ego is the part of the mind that develops as the infants struggles as she or he operates in the world, and the basis impulses of the id must cope with the various reality constraints all of us experience. In contrast to the id (which operates on the pleasure principle), the ego operations based on the reality principle. In Freud's model, the superego is that part of the ego that develops a capacity for self-reflection and judgment. Although the id is outside consciousness, both the ego and the superego have conscious as well as partly conscious aspects. He also focused on ways that these structures coped with anxiety (defense mechanisms, i.e., defending again the experience of anxiety).

One of the most famous of Freud's ideas was the importance of what he termed the Oedipus complex in children's development. This idea refers to the mechanisms, early in life, in which the child's sexual feelings for the opposite-sex parents become transformed into an identification with the same-sex parent, resulting in a consolidation of gender identity formation.

Although he did not directly treat children himself, he did publish early work on a childhood phobia (the treatment actually conducted by the child's father). After his death, Freud's daughter Anna made important contributions to child development and more general psychoanalytic theory, particularly around understanding the work of the conscious mind and defense mechanisms. This work was also carried on in the United States by a group of psychoanalysts who focused on what was termed "ego psychology." Developmental considerations continued to be highly important theoretically and clinically.

Another prominent British psychoanalyst, Melanie Klein, focused more on the interpersonal aspects of development and the ways people developed representations of themselves or others. This approach, termed *object relations theory*, is also highly developmentally but, if anything, moved critical issues and conflicts to very early in life. This model attracted a number of proponents in Great Britain and has been applied in the study of more severe psychiatric disturbances in children and adults.

Other aspects of psychoanalysis were incorporated in theories, including attachment theory. Many of the current "talking therapies" owe a great deal to Freud's attempt to understand human behavior and help patients struggling with psychiatric difficulties. Although classical psychoanalysis is now less common, an increasing body of work has attempted to clarify the situations in which it is useful (see Chapter 22).

Freud's influence also had a profound impact on a number of students, some of whom developed their own approaches to understanding development. For example, Erik Erickson was a teacher who enrolled in the Vienna Psychoanalytic Institute and relocated to Boston and then to New Haven. He was interested in understanding cultural influences on development and worked with children of the Sioux. After some years in California, he returned to Massachusetts to work at the Austin Riggs Center. He developed a lifetime model of development characterized by a series of stages, not just limited to the first years of life. His approach focused around a series of tensions (e.g. initially over trust vs. mistrust). Erikson also made major contributions to the growing field of ego psychology. His interest in cultural factors in a lifespan approach was also reflected in a series of psychologically informed biographies of Martin Luther and Gandhi. His interest in continued development, particularly adolescence, also contributed to renewed interest in clinical work with this age group.

Piaget's Theory

In contrast to Freud, the Swiss psychologist Jean Piaget (1896–1980) was more concerned with children's cognitive development. He had an early interest in teaching, worked briefly on the early tests of intelligence, and became intrigued by the issue of why children made certain kinds of mistakes. Eventually, he developed a comprehensive model for cognitive development that was not, however, widely appreciated in the United States until the 1960s, in large part because his methods (direction discussion with children, including his own children) was so antithetical to the research approach used in American psychological research. In addition, he wrote in French, and his language was somewhat difficult to translate. Despite the early lack of interest, his work has now become widely appreciated.

Piaget was interested in both the content and process of children's thinking and problem solving. Similar to Freud, he made various modifications in this theory over time. He noticed early on in his career that in talking with children, over development they moved from a highly self-centered, egocentric world view to one that was much more able to appreciate other people and their views. His method started with a set of standard questions, and he would then ask other questions, remaining very alert to the meaning of children's answers, including their mistakes and indeed finding those as intriguing as successes. He began his consideration of development by believing that the ways in which children think and learn are an important extension of biological adaptation. He developed several key concepts regarding this process: assimilation, accommodation, and schemas.

A **schema** is a way of relating to the world (e.g., an infant exploring an object with his or her mouth). In **assimilation,** the child uses an existing **schema,** (e.g., the baby who has been breastfeeding discovers she can also suck her thumb). On the other hand, if the new experience, material, or event is so different that it cannot be assimilated, the child is then forced to **accommodate** or modify the schema. For example, if you are learning a new language, you initially will try to pronounce words using the patterns you are familiar with in your native language. If the new language has very different sounds, you will, over time, accommodate so that you hear can differences not heard before. Similarly, a child learning a new word such as "horsie" may initially apply that label to all animals, but over time, the concept will be refined and much more specific.

In Piaget's view, some of the early reflexive behaviors, such as sucking, become modified over time by this process so that, for example, the infant moves away from exploring things with his or her mouth, taste, and smell and more to visual inspection. It is important to emphasize that Piaget's theory is not simply one of innate maturation; rather, he saw it as an active process depending on the individual child and his or her environment. As he considered children's development using this idea and with a strong awareness of some of the unusual aspects of children's thinking, he developed a model with a series of progressive stages that elaborate children's growing appreciation of reality and increasingly sophisticated cognitive ability. Toward the end of his life, he also became interested in other processes such as perception and memory.

The **sensorimotor period** lasts from birth to roughly 18 months to 2 years of age. Initially, the infant has reflexes, but his or her behavior is poorly coordinated. The initial phase of this period (what Piaget termed the **stage of simple reflexes**) involves baby's use of basic reflexes in relating to the world. As the processes of assimilation and accommodation occur, the infant begins to coordinate processes. Between the first and fourth months (roughly), the infant develops progressively more motor control and also is able to experience pleasure and can discover ways to maintain this (e.g., by repeating an activity). This repetition is what Piaget termed a **primary circular reaction** (the name for this phase) (Piaget, 1952) and underscores the importance of both sensation and motor coordination at this point in development. The third stage (of **secondary circular reactions**) typically occurs between the fourth and eighth months. During this time, the infant becomes more oriented to the world and objects and may, for example, discover that shaking a rattle produces a noise and that this action can be repeated. This phase is followed by a period of **coordination of secondary circular reactions** (roughly 8 months to 1 year) when intentionality becomes more obvious. Behavior is now more goal directed (e.g., use of a tool to get a desired object). At this time, objects start to acquire meaning, and the child will search for objects that have vanished from sight (**object permanence**). As Piaget noted, this implies a capacity for symbolic thinking that, for humans, becomes critical for language and subsequent cognitive development. For the first time, the baby realizes things exist even if they are not visible. The fifth period is one of **active experimentation** on the part of the infant. During this phase (of what Piaget termed "tertiary circular reactions," roughly 12 to 18 months), there is a strong interest in new objects and a willingness to try new things. During the final phase of the sensorimotor period (internalization of schemas period, roughly 18 to 24 months), symbolic thinking begins to dominate as mental representations begin to endure. The child now starts to develop a whole new way of viewing the world.

The **preoperational stage** (roughly ages 2 to 6 or 7 years) is heralded by this shift to more symbolic modes of thinking. During this, time the child is able to engage in verbal reasoning, and the beginnings of make-believe play are observed. On the other hand, the child's view of the world continues to be constrained in some ways so that, for example, inanimate objects are believed to have feeling or life (animism). Similarly, the child's perception of life and death has to do with movement or whether something has come something that is alive (e.g., a potential complication in toileting if the child assumes that his or her feces are alive—only to see them flushed away!). Similarly, a fall over a toy may result in the child's being angry at the toy for tripping him! Temporal or spatial relationships may be assumed to reflect some aspect of causality. Although the child has great capacities for symbolic thinking, these are not yet as flexible as they will be somewhat later. Animistic thinking is common; Piaget noted that children may exhibit animism in describing the movement of the sun or moon.

During this time, language has an increasingly important role in mediating experience, and the child's behavior and thought become more complex and less focused on concrete goals. During this time, however, thought remains limited in important ways. Perception tends to dominate, and even here the child has difficulty if he or she needs to attend to more than one perceptual dimension at a time. Thought remains very egocentric, and the child has trouble differentiating thoughts and feelings and objective reality (one of the reasons dreams and nightmares at this period can be very frightening). Nonlogical relationships are assumed based continuity in space or time rather than on cause and effect, and the child is relatively unconcerned about the inconsistencies that emerge from this point of view. This is also often reflected in children's drawing various parts of an object while being unaware of important interrelationships.

These difficulties are also reflected in ways children at this age deal with concepts such as number. If, for example, you arrange a row of candies in front of a 4-year-old child and then arrange a second row with exactly the same number of candies behind the first but make it longer, the child may say that there are more candies in the longer row. Thus, the child focuses on the length of the row rather than number. Piaget termed this difficulty *static representation*. He also noted that thought remained egocentric at this age (e.g., a child might use a made-up word, not realizing that others might not understand it).

By around age 4 years or so, another fundamental shift in cognitive development takes place. This stage of the preoperational period is often referred to as the **period of decentration** when children begin to increasingly see the world from the point of view of other people. This shift reflects increased cognitive and communicative capabilities and the increasing degree of social engagement with other children as well as with adults. The child discovers that his or her thoughts, feelings, and reactions may not be the same as those of others. Although children continue, in some respects, to be constrained in their thinking, there is an increased accommodation to reality. Concepts of justice and moral development remain somewhat simplistic (immanent justice, an "eye for an eye" approach is favored), and the child cannot yet make allowances for special situations or instances in which important rules can, and should, be violated. Perception continues to have major importance in children's construction or reality. Often, children can attend only to one aspect or dimension of a situation at a time. Similarly, although children are aware of familiar routines and sequences, temporal understanding remains limited. There can also be difficulties in differentiating between fantasy and reality, but the advent of more truly imaginative play contributes to a refinement of the child's thinking.

In the **concrete operational phase** (roughly ages 7 to 11 or 12 years), thought becomes increasingly sophisticated but remains, in important ways, constrained by concrete reality (i.e., actual problems or issues rather than more hypothetical problems). During this time, children acquire several important abilities. They have a more detailed understanding of transitivity (e.g., if Jim is bigger than Sally and Sally is bigger than Pete, then Jim is bigger than Peter). Children at this age also begin to understand classification of objects, of sorting objects by and along any number of characteristic features. They also understand reversibility (e.g., of mathematical operations) and can start to take into account multiple issues in solving a problem. They also have a firm knowledge of conservation (e.g., changing the length of a piece of clay does not actually change its mass). Socially, the increased ability to "decenter" gives children strong social-cognitive capacities to anticipate based on other people's knowledge and to make predictions.

The **period of formal operations** (roughly coinciding with adolescence at ages 11 to 12 and older) is the final period of cognitive development in Piaget's view. The major difference from the previous phase is the ability to increasingly grasp abstract problems. Conclusions can be drawn logically without the need for actual demonstration. Children becomes capable of highly abstract thought and can see the world not only as it is but how it might be (presumably accounting for much of the youthful ardor for change). Adolescents have an ability to solve hypothetical problems and no longer need to rely on trial and error but can use deduction and hypothetical reasoning. Adolescents also have a more sophisticated approach to issues of judgment, issues of long-term planning, and increasingly sophisticated social skills. Adolescents' increased self-awareness can also result in both increased self-consciousness, an awareness of their personal uniqueness, and self-awareness.

Piaget's account of development has been highly influential. Initial interest in his theory lagged, particularly in the United States, because his approach was so foreign to American developmental psychology. His work has had important implications for understanding many areas of development in addition to cognition. It has inspired several lines of work (e.g., on moral development in children) that have become major areas of study in their own right, and his work underscores, for health professionals dealing with children, the importance of considering the level of the child's understanding in dealing with clinical problems. This can be reflected in phenomena as diverse as toddlers' difficulties with toileting, children's understanding of death as an irreversible phenomena and of seeing illness as a punishment for their transgressions, and even in adolescents for difficulties in dealing with chronic health problems.

Some important objections to aspects of Piaget's theory have also been raised. As he himself noted, the issue of how change or transition occurs from one stage to another remains an issue. His focus is very much on cognitive development with lesser emphasis in other areas and very little concern for emotional or sexual development or, for that matter, for the role of family and culture. Other psychologists have advocated different approaches to children's understanding of domain specific knowledge and for understanding the role of language in development.

Learning Theory

This body of work has developed in a more collaborative way over the past century and is grounded in a large body of work on how children (and others) learn and remember. Starting with Pavlov's description of classical condition and then extended into many other types of learning, this theory is much more concerned with overt behavior rather than underlying psychological constructs. Although lacking, in some ways, the grand theoretical vision of Freud or Piaget this body has work has great applicability (e.g., in teaching children with learning problems such as autism; see Chapter 4) and, increasingly, in clinical psychology in which cognitive behavior therapy (see Chapter 22) relies heavily on learning-based approaches in treatment. Learning theory focuses on overt behavior and its antecedents and consequences. This functional perspective helps us understand how behaviors are maintained over time and what factors in the environment contribute to behavior maintenance and change.

Pavlov's study of classical condition represented the earliest approaches to the scientific study of learning. In his model, a stimulus such as food (unconditioned stimulus) that elicited a reflexive response such as salivation in his dog (unconditioned response) was paired with a stimulus such as the sound of a bell (conditioned stimulus) that otherwise would not elicit a response. But with repeated learning, the bell comes to elicit the response without a need for the unconditional stimulus. It should be noted that in this case, the association is new, but the response itself, salivation, is not a new one. Pavlov's work was extended to clinical work (and children) by Jones and Watson, who showed that this phenomenon could be used to account for phobia. They, and others subsequently, have noted that the avoidance behavior induced by a phobia prevents extinction from occurring, thus helping the phobia to be maintained.

Classical conditioning has also been used in models of other conditions such as depression and mood problems, addictive phenomena, and psychosomatic problems. Therapy methods based on aspects of classical condition include desensitization, exposure training, and counterconditioning, among others (see Chapter 22). Operant conditioning focuses on acquisition of new behaviors and relies heavily on the work of B.F. Skinner, whose work elegantly demonstrated how new behaviors could be acquired and shaped through the use of systematic reinforcement. The fundamental notion is straightforward in that responses are shaped by consequences. Whereas positive reinforcement is any consequence that is rewarding, negative reinforcement involves removal of a negative experience. Punishment is a consequence that decreases the probability of a behavior. Skinner's work and that of many others have also shown the importance of the timing or "schedule" of reinforcement. It can, for example, be continuous (every time a button is pressed, a reward is dispensed) or intermittent (e.g., every third time the button is pressed, the happy event happen). The timing of the reinforcement can also be systematically varied. Often, in initially producing or "shaping" a behavior, more frequent reinforcement is used, but over time, it is shifted to a variable model; the latter is particularly effective in maintaining behavior.

Similar principles apply to the elimination of a behavior (i.e., extinction). For extinction to occur, a previous reinforcement is withheld or decreased (often this is initially associated with an early increase in the behavior, a phenomenon called *extinction burst*). Elimination of a problem behavior also may be facilitated by simultaneous work on the acquisition (and systematic reinforcement of) a new behavior—one that is incompatible with the problem behavior. Other work conducted within the learning theory perspective has focused on observational learning (e.g., the ability of children to learn simply through observation) as well as on aversive conditioning. In actual work with patients, therapy using behavioral principles focuses on an analysis of the entire behavior (antecedents and consequences). A number of treatment approaches are available, including applied behavior analysis and parent management training (see Chapter 23).

METHODS OF RESEARCH

As a field, child psychiatry has drawn on multiple sources of information and the perspectives of many different disciplines in its attempt to understand children's development and psychopathology. Although integrating these diverse perspectives sometimes presents practical challenges, it has also stimulated considerable interdisciplinary and cross-disciplinary work, which adds to the intellectual excitement of work in this field. Over the past several decades, research accomplishments in a number of different areas have translated into innovations in treatments and have advanced our knowledge base. In this concluding section of this opening chapter, we will highlight some of this work; the Selected Readings at the end of the chapter provides resources for readers seeking additional information.

Advances in statistical methods and epidemiologic research have been made on several fronts. Solid normative data continue to help frame the broad (and sometimes narrow) range of normative development and contribute to better measure of maladaptive behaviors and psychiatric disorders. This work has helped clarify the role of risk factors and their significance in child psychopathology. At the global level, such surveys have also drawn attention to the focus on global aspects of child mental health problems. These data are important in terms of service planning and, unfortunately, often underscore the availability of appropriate supports and the need for new models of care. Epidemiologic data have also underscored the frequent onset of adult disorders in childhood and adolescence. Epidemiologic work is also strongly related to advances in measurement, assessment, and statistics (e.g., with development of more reliable and valid screeners and assessment instruments) (Fombonne, 2007). Statistical approaches have also become much more sophisticated with advances that allow for more rigorous experimental control and examination of new models of statistical analysis. The increased sophistication of epidemiologic and statistical methods has also been reflected in the growing body of work on evidence-based treatments (Hamilton, 2005). For child psychiatry, this is a particularly challenge because research data may be sparse, and results from the many different research traditions may not always fit easily in the more traditional model of evidence-based medicine. Despite these concerns, this is a clearly growing body of expertise (Reichow et al., 2010) that will have increasing importance in the coming decade.

Neurobiological work has also drawn on multiple disciplines and research traditions, including genetics, neuroimaging, neurochemistry, and other branches of neuroscience. Within genetics, it has become increasingly clear that multiple genes interact with environmental factors and, possibly, epigenetic influences in the expression of clinical disorder (Fernandez & State, 2005). This makes the identification of disease-related genes somewhat difficult. Accordingly, a number of strategies have been used, including linkage, association, and molecular cytogenetic approaches. These have used both common and rare variation approaches. Particularly over the past several years, significant progress in the identification of risk alleles has been made, such as for Tourette's disorder (see Chapter 13) and autism (see Chapter 4). Advances in genetic technology and the increased available of large, well-characterized samples likely will only accelerate the productivity of this work. The potential for exploring ways that genes can be expressed in individuals' brains and behavior (e.g., in animal models) are also likely to prove a landmark in the field (Lombroso & Leckman, 2005). Although the possibility of gene therapy remains in the future, advances in our genetic understanding, particularly for the single-gene disorders, makes this no longer seem impossible.

Advances in neurobiology and psychopharmacology have helped expand our understanding of brain mechanisms and now hold the promise of better and more effective and targeted treatments. These advances have been, in part, based on the knowledge gained in genetics, particularly (at least so far) for the single-gene disorders such as Rett's and fragile X syndromes. But now, and certainly in the future, this understanding may be extended to the more complex disorders such as autism, mood and anxiety, and attention-deficit disorders. Work in these areas has proceeded at several areas. One line has focused on neuronal circuitry, neural transmission, and intracellular signaling. Both the short- and long-term effects of pharmacologic intervention on brain function and structures have been investigated and have often reminded us of the complex ways in which various risk factors interact.

Although it has faced some significant challenges, pediatric neuroimaging work has also blossomed over the past decade (MRI Unit, 2005). The practical challenges include, particularly for functional imaging methods, the difficulties that even normal children have in remaining still—difficulties that become much more formidable when the child's neurodevelopmental problems entail issues in attention, engagement, and activity level. A body of work on approaches to coping with these problems through teaching, desensitization, and advance preparation has yielded impressive results in terms of our ability to engage children in a range of scanning procedures. For very young children, scanning during sleep is another possibility. Other challenges come with the understandable limitations that research design and ethical issues raise (e.g., for positron emission tomography scanning in children). Still others come from the potential methodologic and conceptual issues that complicate the interpretation of imaging data, which typically tell us more about macroscopic brain structure and activity rather than finer structures.

In neuroimaging, one major challenge arises with regard to distinguishing cause from aftereffect (e.g., presumably, chronic illness itself leads to brain adaption and change). This is a particular issue when cross-sectional designs are used, and such studies are among the most common. Thus, larger volume of a specific brain region might represent compensation effects. To some extent, this issue can be dealt with by including analyses of other measures (e.g., symptom severity). Developmental issues are also important, making longitudinal studies particularly important. Finally, the frequent comorbidity of disorders (see Chapter 3) also presents specific challenges for neuroimaging studies

Selected Readings

Candland, D. K. (1993). *Feral Children and Clever Animals: Reflections on Human Nature*. New York: Oxford University Press.

Darwin, C. (1877). A biographical sketch of an infant. *Mind*, 2, 285–294.

Erikson, E. (1997). The Life Cycle Completed. New York: W.W. Norton & Co.

Fernandez, T., & State, M. W. (2007). Assessing risk: Gene discovery. In A. Martin & F. Volkmar (Eds.). *Lewis's Child and Adolescent Psychiatry*, 4th edition. Philadelphia: Lippincott Williams & Wilkins, pp. 189–199.

Fombonne, E. (2007). Epidemiology. In A. Martin & F. Volkmar (Eds.). *Lewis's Child and Adolescent Psychiatry*, 4th edition. Philadelphia: Lippincott Williams & Wilkins, pp. 150–170.

Freud, A. (1936). *The Ego and the Mechanisms of Defense* (Vol II, 1966 edition). New York: International Universities Press.

Freud, A. (1946). *The Psycho-analytical Treatment of Children*. London: Imago Publishing.

Freud, S. (1955). Analysis of a phobia in a five-year-old boy. In J. E. Strachey (Ed.). *The Standard Edition of the Complete Psychological Works of Sigmund Freud* (Vol X). London: Hogarth Press, pp. 3–149.

Freud, S. (1962). *Three Essays on the Theory of Sexuality* (trans., James Strachey). New York: Basic Books. (1996). *Drei Abhandlungen zur Sexualtheorie* [reprint of the 1905 edition]. Fischer: Frankfurt am Main.

Gould, S. J. (1996). *The Mismeasure of Man*. New York: W.W. Norton & Co.

Hale, N. G. (1971). *Freud and the Americans: The Beginning of Psychoanalysis in the United States, 1876–1917*. New York: Oxford University Press.

Hamilton, J. (2007). Evidence-based practice as a conceptual framework. In A. Martin & F. Volkmar (Eds.). *Lewis's Child and Adolescent Psychiatry*, 4th edition. Philadelphia: Lippincott Williams & Wilkins, pp. 124–139.

Hogan, J. D. (2000). Developmental psychology: History of the field. In A. E. Kazdin (Ed.). *Encyclopedia of Psychology*. Washington, DC: American Psychological Association.

Hunt, J. McV. (1961). *Intelligence and Experience*. New York: The Ronald Press Company.

Jones, M. C. (1924). A laboratory study of fear: The case of Peter. *Pedagogical Seminary*, 31, 308–315.

Kanner, L. (1935). *Child Psychiatry*. Springfield, IL: Charles C. Thomas.

Kazdin, A. E. (2000). Developing a research agenda for child and adolescent psychotherapy. *Archives of General Psychiatry*, 57, 829–835.

Klein, M. (1932). *The Psychoanalysis of Children*. London: Hogarth Press. In A. Martin & F. Volkmar (Eds.). *Lewis's Child and Adolescent Psychiatry*, 4th edition. Philadelphia: Lippincott Williams & Wilkins, pp. 214–233.

Lombroso, P. J., & Leckman, J.F. (2007). Molecular basis of select childhood psychiatric disorders. In A. Martin & F. Volkmar (Eds.). *Lewis's Child and Adolescent Psychiatry*, 4th edition. Philadelphia: Lippincott Williams & Wilkins, pp. 200–213.

Musto, D. F. (2007). Prevailing and shifting paradigms: A historical perspective. In A. Martin & F. Volkmar (Eds.). *Lewis's Child and Adolescent Psychiatry*, 4th edition. Philadelphia: Lippincott Williams & Wilkins, pp. 11–16.

Piaget, J. (1932). *The Moral Judgment of the Child*. London: Kegan Paul, Trench.

Piaget, J. (1952). *The Origins of Intelligence in Children*. New York: International University Press. [Original work published 1936.]

Piaget, J. (1955). *The Child's Construction of Reality*. London: Routledge and Kegan Paul.

Piaget, J. (1962). *Play, Dreams and Imitation in Childhood*. New York: Norton.

Reichow, B., Doehring, P., Cicchetti, D., & Volkmar, F. (Eds.) (2010). *Evidence-Based Practices and Treatments for Children with Autism*. New York: Springer.

Robbins, S. J., Schwartz, B., & Wasserman, E. A. (2001). *Psychology of Learning and behavior*, 5th edition. New York: W. W. Norton & Company

Salkind, N. J. (2004). *An Introduction to Theories of Human Development*. Thousand Oaks, CA: Sage Publications.

Sears, R. R. (1975). *Your Ancients Revisited: A History of Child Development*. Chicago: University of Chicago Press.

Singer, D. G., & Revenson, T. A. (1996). *A Piaget Primer: How a Child Thinks* (Revised). New York: Edition Plume (Penguin Books).

Strachey, J. (1965/1933). *Introductory Lectures on Psycho-Analysis*. New York: W.W. Norton & Co.

Volkmar, F. R. (2005). Neuroimaging methods in the study of childhood psychiatric disorders. Charles Darwin (1809–1882). *American Journal of Psychiatry*, 162, 249.

CHAPTER 2 ■ NORMAL CHILD DEVELOPMENT

Development occurs throughout the life cycle, and although we frequently focus on some particular aspect of development (cognitive, motor, and so on), in reality, developmental processes are fundamentally interrelated. The term *maturation* is often used to describe the sequential pattern of growth, but both experience (nurture) and endowment (nature) interact in complex ways. As described in Chapter 1, various approaches, methods, and theories have been used to understand development. For many investigators, the development of embryos and fetuses has served as a model for subsequent development with the various processes interacting reciprocally. One of the observations consistent with this view is the awareness that early development of motor skills moves in top-down (cephalocaudal or head to tail) and center-out (proximodistal) fashion so that, for example, head control is achieved before trunk control and before leg control, and arm control is achieved before hand control.

Clearly, although the human genome both gives considerable developmental potential, it also sets certain limits. Depending on the particular skill being studied, the relative dominance of genetic or experiential factors may shift so that even if a baby has good genetic potential, his or her placement in a severely depriving environment will result in developmental delays. Conversely, a child born having experienced the effects of some insult in utero such as fetal alcohol exposure may not be able to achieve normative levels of functioning no matter what environment is provided, although even here, optimal development would be more likely in a supportive environment. It is appropriate to begin any consideration of development with a discussion of development before birth.

PRENATAL DEVELOPMENT

Development starts at conception as the zygote begins to develop actively when the egg is fertilized. Within a few days, it will have reached the uterus and implanted and may be 0.1 inches in length. With 2 weeks, the menstrual period may be missed and may alert the mother to the pregnancy. Over the next 6 weeks, major organs and structures develop primarily following the cephalocaudal and proximodistal pattern. By about 8 weeks, the embryo is recognizably human. After this time, the fetus grows rapidly with increased differentiation. The head initially grows more actively than other parts of the body and gradually slows during fetal life so that at birth, the head is about one-fourth the length of the entire body, but in adulthood, it is only about one-sixth. Conversely, at birth, the legs are about one-third of body length, but this increases to half by adulthood.

By about the third month in utero, fetuses can swallow, make a fist, and wiggle his or her toes. By the fourth month, fetuses can respond to light, and by the fifth month, loud sounds may elicit movement. Similarly, more organized behaviors, such as the sucking reflex, develop before birth; this is also a time when processes such as breathing, body temperature regulation, and swallowing are sufficiently organized to make life possible outside the uterus (problems that must be dealt with in supporting very early premature infants). By around 8 months, fetal fat stores accumulate rapidly. Antibodies from the mother help prevent infection postpartum.

Even before the child is born, the parents begin to experience the child and are impacted by him or her. This happens in various ways. For the mother, the experience of fetal movement ("quickening") provokes a series of responses as mother observes that the child may be soothed by her speech or movement. Similarly, the mother's impact on the child begins as soon as fertilization has occurred. Although intrauterine life is relatively homeostatic, it can be influenced by the mother's health (both physical and psychological) as well as by other factors. Mothers typically gain 25 to 30 lb, and this weight gain is important for fetal growth. Mothers who fail to gain appropriate weight or who are undernourished may increase the likelihood that their baby will be small. Other factors that may adversely impact the development of the child in utero include exposure to radiation, maternal infection, and exposure to drugs.

The effects of teratogens depend on several factors. These include the timing of the exposure (e.g., in some cases, these may even antedate the pregnancy). The first weeks after conception are particularly sensitive as this is a time major organs form; subsequent exposure may impact growth in utero. The dose also is important depending on the agent, with effects ranging from minimal to maximal. The route of the teratogen may also be important. The effects of teratogens can be more generalized or more specific (e.g., thalidomide exposure is associated with limb defects, and alcohol exposure in utero produces a range of problems).

The adverse effects of alcohol on developing fetuses have been recognized since ancient times. Although reports on potential adverse effects on fetuses began to appear in the medical literature in the 1700s, Jones and Smith in 1973 brought new attention to the significant teratogenic effects of alcohol exposure in utero. Fetal alcohol syndrome (FAS) is associated with growth deficiency, usually mild intellectual deficiency, a characteristic "flattened" face, motor problems, and other morphologic features. A number of learning difficulties are noted as are language difficulties and continued growth problems. In the United States, alcohol continues to be the most frequently used teratogens and is one of the more common causes of intellectual deficiency. The current recommendation is to avoid alcohol entirely during pregnancy. Chronic alcohol abuse is associated with greater risk, and unfortunately, these are also mothers who are likely to smoke, giving even greater risk to the developing fetus.

A wide range of other common agent have potential deleterious effects. Maternal smoking, for example, clearly impacts birth weight, early delivery, increases rates of placenta previa, and placental abruption as well as still birth. Cigarette smoking contributes to low birth weight and increased risk for sudden infant death syndrome (SIDS). Stopping smoking at any point in the pregnancy is beneficial but is particularly so in the first trimester. Similarly, the potentially adverse role of prescription and street drugs has been recognized. The effects of these agents vary. Phenytoin is associated with increased risk for heart defects, and tetracycline can cause staining of teeth and interfere with bone growth. Similarly, streptomycin can be associated with hearing loss, and DES can cause genital abnormalities as well as vaginal and cervical cancer in adolescent girls. Use of many of the commonly available street drugs such as cocaine and crack is associated with increased newborn irritability and sometimes with growth retardation. Agents such as heroin and methadone can result in a withdrawal syndrome in the infant and an increased risk for sudden death.

Maternal Infections can be associated with various adverse effects. Congenital rubella can lead to severe mental retardation, visual and sensory problems, and cardiac difficulties. AIDS is associated with a number of congenital malformations, although fortunately, work on prevention has advanced dramatically in the more developed countries. Similarly, cytomegalovirus and toxoplasmosis may be associated with significant learning difficulties, intellectual deficiency, and a range of other problems.

Heavy metals and other environmental toxins can be have teratogenic effects as can exposure to radiation. Other risks arise with increased both very young (teenage) or comparatively older (>35 years) maternal age. For older mothers, the risk for Down syndrome begin to increase substantially. Similarly, malnutrition in the mother can be faced with growth retardation and behavioral difficulties in the newborn. Other maternal health issues (e.g., diabetes) can be associated with risk.

Perinatal Variables

Prematurity is an important risk factor for subsequent developmental problems. Premature infants also present challenges for parenting and are more likely to be abused or neglected. Preterm babies (born before the 37th week of pregnancy) or babies with low birth weight (born at or near term but who are small for gestational age) both have increased risk. Although babies born as early as 24 weeks now survive, the lack of development of important organ systems, particularly the respiratory system, presents major challenges. Although we made strides have been made in supporting preterm infants, prevention continues to be a significant public health challenge.

Premature preterm infants are at increased risk for various problems, including neurologic problems, retinopathy, and developmental disabilities. Cardiovascular and respiratory problems are also common. Risks increase with the degree of prematurity. Even when babies are born on time as many as 3% of all infants exhibit significant malformations or birth defects, and another 7% or so may exhibit less serious problems. Babies born with severe developmental difficulties often have difficulties that started even before labor and delivery, although sometimes a traumatic birth can result in major neurologic damage.

Parents of premature babies and babies with birth defects are associated with significant challenges. All parents worry about their babies before birth, but the experience of having a baby with a problem can bring up a host of unpleasant feelings, including anger, anxiety, and even revulsion (if the child has an obvious facial disfigurement as in cleft palate). The sense of loss of the anticipated perfect baby can be a shock and a source of depression. The child's continued presence serves as a constant reminder of the loss of the idealized infant.

The reactions of the parents are a function of their own histories and personality as well as the visibility and location of the birth defect. For example, hypospadias may require multiple surgical correction and impact the parents' feelings and attitudes toward the child's gender. Cleft palate is highly visible and may complicate feeding of the infant, but fortunately, it is usually quite correctable. Congenital heart problems may be noted at birth or sometime later and range considerably in severity. Congenital sensory impairments present special problems. Infants with congenital blindness can show unusual motor mannerisms and have delays in development. Sometimes the parental response is one that tends to isolate the baby—at a time when even more sensory stimulation is called for. On the other hand, visually impaired babies will begin to smile at the sound of the parent's voice and, with support, can do very well. Although often congenital blindness is thought of as a greater disability, congenital deafness is actually more frequently associated with developmental disturbance and psychiatric problems, presumably reflecting the central importance of language in human development. Intellectual disability is usually diagnosed in infants only when an obvious syndromal condition is present or when the degree of delay is likely to be severe or profound. This condition presents special challenges for parents who must cope with accepting a severely delayed child, their own feelings about the loss of the desired baby, and often associated medical problems.

Responses of Parents and Family of the Newborn

Various factors shape the parents' attitude towards the fetus and neonate. The first is their relationships with their own parents. There are several views of the ways pregnancy is experienced;

these range from the idea that pregnancy is inherently a crisis to the other extreme, which views pregnancy as a normal part of development. With advances in technology, mothers (and often fathers) are aware of the pregnancy at a very early stage. Often, the first picture of the fetus during ultrasonography concretizes this knowledge. The mother may find herself increasingly preoccupied with herself and then, with the detection of movement in the fetus, she has an independent physical confirmation of the person within her. Although the process goes well for most mothers, sometimes the process is associated with feelings of ambivalence that can precede depression.

Fathers sometime experience some of the symptoms of pregnancy along with their partners (in some culture, fathers may experience feelings at the time of childbirth, couvade). Some fathers will sense, and resent, the preoccupation of the mother with the pregnancy. As with mothers, the father's experience of being parented can play a major role, although even fathers who have had difficult parental experiences can be loving and affectionate. Sometimes a prospective father becomes more anxious because of a sense of greater responsibility or unresolved issues with his own father. Sometimes the couple's expectations of each other are changed by the pregnancy. Having a warm and supportive father–child relationship is a clear advantage for the child.

In addition to the parents, other members of the family also play important roles. Around the world, probably the bulk of childrearing (apart from breastfeeding) is done by other children, usually siblings. In developed countries, grandparents, aunts, and uncles often play major roles. Parents may find this helpful or intrusive. Preparation of a sibling for the arrival of a new brother or sister varies depending on the child's age. Significant siblings conflict or sibling rivalry is more likely in the context of a problematic parent–child relationship, particularly as the mother's attendance to the older child decreases.

INFANCY AND TODDLERHOOD

In the first weeks after birth, infants quickly become active in learning about the world. They begin to explore the environment through multiple modalities, can track moving objects, screen out invariant stimuli, and become active players in the "social game." For a typically developing infant, the face or voice of the parent is the most engaging thing in the environment, and this early social interest sets the stage for many subsequent skills in multiple areas. Tables 2.1 and 2.2 summarize some of the landmarks of development in the first year of life.

After about 1 month of age, infants' ability to engage in voluntary motor movement begins to increase. Infants also begin to produce more sounds and become increasingly differentiated in their affective responses. Between two and 7 months, there is increased social interaction along with an increased awareness of the nonsocial world and greater coordination of sensation and motor action. By about 4 months, imitation becomes more striking (and further consolidates social interest and attachment). Shortly thereafter, the earliest aspects of object permanence are seen so that things exist to the baby even when not visible; at around this time, infants' awareness of cause-and-effect relationships also increases (see Chapter 1 for a discussion of Piaget's model of cognitive development in infancy). Both discoveries are important building blocks in social-cognitive development (i.e., as infants appreciate their own ability to impact the world and the stability of people in that world). Object permanence is an important foundation for symbolic thinking and language development, and the appreciation of cause and effect helps infants gain a new appreciation of intentionality. Socially, these skills are reflected in games such as peek-a-boo.

Between 7 and 9 months of age, infants develop an awareness that they can be understood by others (i.e., that their mothers or fathers can understand their feelings, wishes, and desires, a phenomenon termed *intersubjectivity*). Infants' behavior also becomes more goal directed. Around this time, infants develop more sophisticated strategies for obtaining desired ends by grouping behaviors together in a sequence. These phenomena also serve as a basis for communicative gesturing (e.g., pointing at or reaching for an object while looking at the mother or father to request help in getting it). Advances in object permanence and in social

TABLE 2.1

SELECTED SOCIAL, COMMUNICATIVE AND COGNITIVE MILESTONES: BIRTH TO 1 YEAR OF AGE

Age (weeks)	Social-Affective	Communicative	Cognitive-Adaptive
0–4	Looks at face of caregiver	Makes small, throaty noises	Responds to sounds
4–8	Social smile	Babbles spontaneously	Facial response to sounds
8–12	Recognizes mother visually	Single vowels	Glances at rattle in hand
12–16	Smiles at mirror image	Coos or chuckles	Anticipatory excitement
16–20	Aware of novel situations	Laughs, vocalizes excitement	Takes rattle to mouth
20–24	Shows displeasure over loss of toy	Spontaneous social vocalization	Visual dropped object pursuit of
24–28	Plays simple interaction games	Attends to music or singing	Bangs objects on tabletop
28–32	Shows anxiety to strangers	Makes polysyllabic vowel sounds	Shakes rattle
32–36	Imitates simple adult movements	Says single syllables ("da," "ba," "ka")	Plays with two toys at the same time
36–40	Waves bye-bye	Says "dada," "mama" (nonspecific)	Uncovers toy hidden by cloth
40–44	Inhibits activity on command	Says "dada," "mama" (specific)	Combines toys in play
44–48	"Gives" toy to mirror image	Says one word besides "mama" and "dada"	Preference for certain toys over others
48–52	Initiates games with adult	Says two words beside "mama" and "dada"	Uses crayon to "dot" imitatively

Adapted from Volkmar, F. R. (1995). Normal development. In H. Kaplan and B. Sadock (Eds.), *Comprehensive Textbook of Psychiatry*, 6th edition, pp. 2:2154–2160. Baltimore: Williams & Wilkins.

TABLE 2.2

SELECTED MOTOR AND SELF-CARE MILESTONES: BIRTH TO 1 YEAR OF AGE

Age (weeks)	Motor	Personal and Self-Care
0–4	Asymmetrical posture	Quiets when picked up
4–8	Sometimes holds head erect	Reacts to feeding position
8–12	Rolls partway to side	Anticipates lifting
12–16	Actively holds rattle	Regards own hand
16–20	Hands engage in midline	Anticipates feeding on sight
20–24	Holds head erect and steady	Pats or fingers bottle or breast
24–28	Rolls to prone position	Drinks from cup with assistance
28–32	Transfers objects between hands	Holds objects voluntarily
32–36	Pivots while in prone position	Feeds self cracker or cookie
36–40	Sits alone with no support	Responds to "pick up" gesture
40–44	Uses index finger to secure object	Cooperates in social games
44–48	Rolls ball while sitting	Gives toy to others without release
48–52	Takes two steps independently	Releases toys to others

Adapted from Volkmar, F. R. (1995). Normal development. In H. Kaplan and B. Sadock (Eds.), *Comprehensive Textbook of Psychiatry*, 6th edition, pp. 2:2154–2160. Baltimore: Williams & Wilkins.

skills development also help infants develop a strong sense of attachment to their caregivers. This is expressed in various ways, including phenomena such as separation anxiety (often starting between 6 to 8 months and peaking sometime after the first birthday) and in the related phenomenon of stranger anxiety (often beginning around 8 months and peaking around age 2 years). Both phenomena speak to infants' strong awareness of essential caregivers and the ability to differentiate them from strangers.

Several new milestones are usually achieved by, or shortly after, the first birthday and mark major changes in the life of the infant and family. Motor and motor coordination skills advance (Table 2.1) so that typically by about 12 months, infants begin to be able to walk independently.

Attachment

Although the importance of emotional connections between infants and caregivers has been known (and discussed) for centuries, only starting in the 20th century was much attention paid to the centrality of these connections for normal child development. The idea of attachment (in the sense of psychological connectedness) has come to encompass many aspects of this process. Psychological attachment is the emotional connection one person has to another (over space and time). Attachments are very specific and can be of varying degrees of strength and typically are strongly positive.

From the first moments of life, the adult and infant are embarked an emotionally intense social interaction that has strong biological and psychological aspects. In some animals (birds and mammals), particularly those that can move and walk shortly after birth, the phenomenon of "imprinting" is observed (i.e., the young animal begins to follow around the apparent parental object, whether it is a mother goose or an ethologist such as Konrad Lorenz). For other species (including humans) in which a long period of care is required before the young can move away independently, a complex series of processes occurs and is referred to by the concept of attachment.

The awareness of this phenomenon in infants came through many individuals but particularly the British psychiatrist and psychoanalyst John Bowlby, who noted the major difficulties children had when separated from their parents because of the child's illness. He was aware of the many emerging studies on the negative effects of inappropriate early care (e.g., as in orphanages) and was not satisfied with earlier psychoanalytic views of parent–child relationships. In a very influential monograph for the World Health Organization, Bowlby suggested the critical important of a supportive mother–child relationship, and his work and that of his student and colleague Mary Ainsworth stimulated considerable research on the topic over the next decades. Bowlby's work extended into many areas, including ethology, developmental psychology, and evolutionary biology (among others). Workers such as Harry Harlow demonstrated the importance of a soft, cloth mother substitute for developing rhesus monkeys, and Ainsworth developed a specific psychological paradigm (the "strange situation") that involved brief separations of young children and their mothers and observations of reunion behavior to estimate the quality of the attachment present. Bowlby's work and that of others led to closing congregate care settings for young children in the developed world.

Attachment processes are strongly developmental but are also lifelong. Various patterns of attachments in infants and toddlers have been identified along with many of the behavioral and developmental correlates of this process. Attachment can be disrupted by various factors, including a lack of an appropriate parent or parent substitute or unavailability of the parent (e.g., because of severe maternal depression). Children who have been abused may still form attachments, although the quality of the attachment may be unusual.

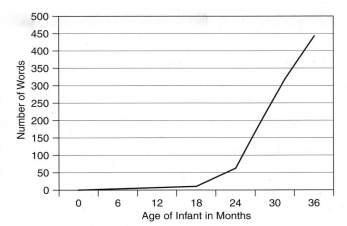

FIGURE 2.1. Typical rate of increase in expressive vocabulary of infants. Reprinted from L. Mayes, W. Gilliam, & L. Sosinsky (2005). The infant and toddler. In A. Martin and F. Volkmar (Eds), *Lewis's Child and Adolescent Psychiatry*, 4th edition. Philadelphia: Lippincott Williams & Wilkins, p. 258.

Similarly, with the onset of language (usually also around this time) and greater symbolic capacities, infants are able to hold multiple bits of information in mind and to appreciate new ways to solve problems using trial and error. Important foundations for language are well established by age 1 year and include the ability to engage in reciprocal interaction, differentiated babbling, and use of sounds and intonation (prosody) typical of their native tongue. When language acquisition starts, knowledge of words usually dramatically increases (Figure 2.1). Usually by age 2 years, toddlers' expressive vocabulary is between 50 and 75 words and increases over the next several months so that by age 3 years, is between 500 and 100 words. By this age, typical toddlers also use sentences of three to four words (Figure 2.2). Increased ability to use language and think symbolically gives the potential for advance planning rather than trial and error.

The increased ability to use symbols also makes for a major reorganization of cognitive development after age 18 months. Increased cognitive abilities are also reflected in phenomena such as deferred (i.e., remembered) imitation. Infants begin to use symbols in play, and play begins to shift from simple functional use of materials to more abstract levels.

Various problems can negatively impact normative development. These are summarized in Table 2.3 and include problems in self-regulation (eating, sleeping, impulse control, aggression,

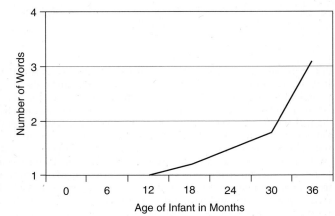

FIGURE 2.2. Typical rate of increase in number of words per sentence in infants. Reprinted from L. Mayes, W. Gilliam, & L. Sosinsky (2005). The infant and toddler. In A. Martin and F. Volkmar (Eds), *Lewis's Child and Adolescent Psychiatry*, 4th edition. Philadelphia: Lippincott Williams & Wilkins, p. 258.

TABLE 2.3

FORCES THAT MAY COMPROMISE NORMATIVE DEVELOPMENTAL PROCESSES

1. **Regulatory disturbances**
   A. Sleep disturbances (e.g., frequent waking)
   B. Excessive crying or irritability
   C. Eating difficulties (e.g., finicky eating or food refusal)
   D. Low frustration tolerance
   E. Self-stimulatory or unusual movements (e.g., rocking, head banging, excessive finger sucking)
2. **Social or environmental disturbances**
   A. Failure to discriminate caregiver
   B. Apathetic, withdrawn, no expression of affect or interest in social interaction
   C. Excessive negativism
   D. No interest in objects or play
   E. Abuse, neglect, or multiple placements or caregivers
   F. Repeated or prolonged separations from caregivers
3. **Psychophysiological disturbances**
   A. Non-organic failure to thrive
   B. Recurrent vomiting or chronic diarrhea
   C. Recurrent dermatitis
   D. Recurrent wheezing
4. **Developmental delays**
   A. Specific delays (e.g., gross motor, language)
   B. General delays or arrested development
5. **Genetic and metabolic disorders with known neurodevelopmental sequelae**
   A. Down syndrome
   B. Fragile X syndrome
   C. Inborn errors of metabolism
6. **Exposure to toxins**
   A. Fetal alcohol syndrome
   B. Lead poisoning
7. **Central nervous system damage**
   A. Traumatic brain injuries
   B. Intraventricular hemorrhages
8. **Prematurity and serious illnesses early in life**

Reprinted from L. Mayes, W. Gilliam, & L. Stout Sosinsky. (2005) The infant and toddler. In A. Martin & F. Volkmar (Eds.), *Lewis's Child and Adolescent Psychiatry: A Comprehensive Textbook*, 4th edition, p. 258. Philadelphia: Lippincott Williams & Wilkins.

and mood or anxiety difficulties). Given the centrality of social factors in early development, disturbances in relatedness are particularly important; these can arise as a result of environmental stress, deprivation, or with disorders such as autism. Maternal or parental deprivation can arise because of problems in the parent or life circumstance. Risks arise because of repeated changes in the primary caregiver as well as because of abuse and neglect (see Chapter 20). In some respects, the intersection of mental health and physical problems can be seen most dramatically at this age, and disentangling cause-and-effect and relationship or individual issues can be difficult. These can take the form of eating problems (see Chapter 14).

Developmental delays can occur in isolation or across multiple areas. Problems in some areas (e.g., language) may be reflected in other areas as well. Risk is increased by factors such as prematurity and parental substance abuse or nonavailability. Various models of early intervention have been developed and can be helpful. Typically, mild cognitive delays are not noted until later, but more severe delays, often associated with specific genetic and metabolic disorders, can be seen in infants. These include conditions such as Down syndrome, fragile X syndrome, and Prader-Willi syndrome.

THE PRESCHOOL PERIOD

As emphasized by Piaget, major changes in cognitive, communicative, and social-affective development occur between 2 and 5 years of age. These capacities are intrinsically and fundamentally interrelated so that greater cognitive capacities are reflected in new and more complex language as well as in increasingly sophisticated and nuanced social relationships. Children become more capable of understanding and reflecting on their own feelings and responses and can be highly verbal in indicating their wants and desires.

This time often marks the exposure to other children (e.g., in childcare or early preschool programs). This is also a time when siblings are commonly born. Although medical providers continue to play a central role in giving parents information, others, including teachers, day care providers, and parents, also become important resources. These individuals may also be the first to notice problems in a child. Frequent behavioral-developmental difficulties in this age group can include problems with peers (particularly if the child is aggressive), anxiety problems (often around separation), and developmental delays of all types (but particularly speech-language delays). An increased awareness of the earliest manifestations of problems that come to later be diagnosed as disorder (e.g., anxiety and mood problems) has stimulated interest in the diagnosis and epidemiology of developmental and mental health problems in this age group (Egger, 2009). At the same time, there is also awareness of the potential for short-term (or longer term) stresses to be reflected in behavioral and developmental change.

The growth of language that begins with the explosion of word acquisition by age 2 years continues during the preschool period. During this time, children may learn about nine words each day. By the end of this time, children will have extensive vocabularies and a good sense of many aspects of correct language use, including morphology, grammar, and syntax. Children at this age also have a marked capacity for learning other languages (an ability that begins to diminish, at least in terms of its ease, after about age 6 years). Some of the relevant milestones in development in the preschool period are summarized in Tables 2.4 and 2.5.

The ability to think more abstractly and symbolically is expressed in many ways. Children begin to use drawings to represent the world (Figure 2.3). During this period, young children also have a growing ability to organize and engage in forward planning (executive functions) that become important later for school success. There is a strong desire to learn, and children often take great pride in their learning and have a desire to "show off" as well as a sense of invulnerability (the latter can contribute to poor judgment and accidents). As children are exposed to peers, they become more adept at accurate self-appraisal. A major focus of early educational program is in the support of children's interest in learning and exploration. Sensitive programs (and parents) are careful to arrange opportunities for learning that are mildly challenging as well as stimulating, thus helping children be involved in a continuous process of learning. Self-care and other "adaptive" skills also increase. Games provide important insights into the idea of rules as well as some basic abilities in recognition and manipulation of symbols that will become relevant to later school performance.

By ages 4 to 5 years, children will, for the most part, have achieved an awareness of the thoughts, feelings, and beliefs of others. This accomplishment, often termed the acquisition of a "theory of mind," helps children advance dramatically in the social world and opens a range of new possibilities to children, including an increased sense of self. It also is reflected in new capacities for even more sophisticated play. Play and play activities are important sources of growth for preschool children. Rough and tumble play is common in toddlers (and indeed in many animal species) but as children become a bit older, play becomes increasingly dominated by capacities for symbolic thought, language, and social issues. Children can play with language and integrate language into their play. As they develop the capacity for symbolic thinking, pretend play activities are no longer constrained by the actual object (i.e., it can be used as a "stand in" for anything real or imagined). Pretense becomes increasingly complex

TABLE 2.4

SELECTED SOCIAL, COMMUNICATIVE AND COGNITIVE MILESTONES: 1 TO 6 YEARS OF AGE

Age (years)	Social-Affective	Communicative	Cognitive-Adaptive
1.25	Shows desire to please parents	Combines words and gesture	Builds tower of two blocks
1.5	Hugs or feeds doll	Speaks in sentences	Draws imitative stroke
1.75	Shares toys or possessions	Says 50 or more words	Uses tool to attain object out of reach
2	Simple make-believe play	Jargon discarded, speech mostly intelligible	Makes simple generalizations
2.5	Identifies own mirror image	States first and last names	Matches simple shapes
3	Labels affects in self	Uses past tense, knows some songs or nursery rhymes	Designates action in pictures, copies circle
3.5	Cooperative play, games with rules	Uses adjectives and adverbs	Copies square, compares sizes
4	Assumes specific role in play	Participates in conversations appropriately	Draws person with two parts, counts three objects
4.5	Elaborate, dramatic play	Uses compound sentences	Names missing parts, counts four objects
5	Understands rules of games	Defines words, names coins	Knows days of week, counts 10 objects
6	Has "best friend"	Prints words from memory, reads simple stories	Draws person with head, neck, hands

Adapted from Volkmar, F. R. (1995). Normal development. In H. Kaplan and B. Sadock (Eds.), *Comprehensive Textbook of Psychiatry*, 6th edition, pp. 2:2154–2160. Baltimore: Williams & Wilkins.

TABLE 2.5

SELECTED MOTOR AND SELF-CARE MILESTONES: AGE 1 TO 6 YEARS

Age (years)	Motor	Personal and Self-Care
1.25	Runs well with little falling	Points to one body part
1.5	Turns knobs	Understands the meaning of "hot"
1.75	Kicks ball	Uses spoon well
2	Turns pages of book, walks up and down stairs	Pulls on simple clothing
2.5	Holds crayon with fingers	Toilet trained during the day
3	Rides tricycle	Helps put things away
3.5	Does complex block constructions	Does simple chores
4	Hops	Apologizes for unintentional mistakes
4.5	Bounces ball	Orders food in restaurant
5	Throws ball, skips well	Dresses and undresses mostly independently
6	Rides bicycle	Chooses activities independently

Adapted from Volkmar, F. R. (1995). Normal development. In H. Kaplan and B. Sadock (Eds.), *Comprehensive Textbook of Psychiatry*, 6th edition, pp. 2:2154–2160. Baltimore: Williams & Wilkins.

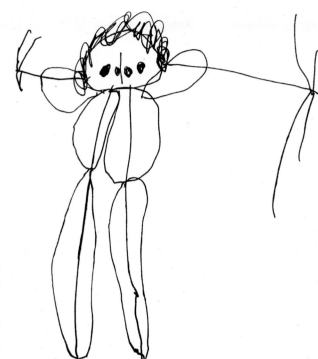

FIGURE 2.3. A 4-year-old child's drawing of her father. Note the presence of a body, head, arms, legs, and a few facial features. Children's ability to draw the human form reflects their cognitive, social, and visual-motor development and is strongly related to developmental level. (Courtesy of Emily Volkmar.)

Drawing Abilities

Children's ability to draw has a strong developmental component as does their ability to draw one of their favorite subjects—other people. Children who are 18 to 24 months old start to scribble and, over the next several months, begin to use circular strokes so that by or shortly after age 2 years, the child is able to copy a circle in reasonable fashion. The circle becomes the prototype for most drawing. Children who are 2 and 3 years old begin to label their drawings, and by 3 to 4 years of age, they start to produce rudimentary people, often with the circle as the body and stick arms and legs added on along with a smaller circle for the head. By age 3 years, children can typically copy a cross. Visual motor coordination continues to advance so that by age 5 years, children can make a reasonable copy of a square (this is also an age when hand dominance is firmly established). By age 5 to 6 years, children progressively add more detail, including to the background of the image. Subsequent changes reflect increased cognitive ability as well as improved graphomotor skills so that by 9 or 10 years, children typically desire highly realistic and detailed drawings. Children may accurately depict physical disabilities or areas of somatic concern in their drawing (e.g., a child whose mother exhibits an atrophied limb might consistently portray this in his or her drawings). The strong developmental correlates of drawing ability are reflected in the use of activities that involve person drawing as simple proxies for overall cognitive ability.

Temperament

As parents (particularly parents of more than one child) are aware, noteworthy individual differences are apparent in children from birth. The term *temperament* has been used to denote these relatively stable individual differences in affective "tone," responsivity, and motivation. The term has some relation to the idea of personality type as it used later in life.

The work of Thomas and Chess in their longitudinal study of infants in the 1950s noted the importance of infant temperament as an enduring characteristic impacting child behavior and parent–child interaction from early in life but having some persistence throughout childhood. In thinking about temperament, they looked at features such as levels of activity, intensity of affective reactions, attention, sensitivity to the environment, and so forth. They also developed the notion of "goodness of fit" to summarize the degree to which child characteristics met parental expectations. A difficult child might, then, be one who, for one set of parents, would not be challenging but, for another, would be very challenging.

Subsequently, others have modified the concept. For example, Jerome Kagan and colleagues have focused on issues of reactivity and inhibition. Differences have been noted in long-term outcome, particularly for children who are more inhibited.

The concept can be very helpful for parents in understanding the sometimes surprising aspects of their children's individuality and responding to it appropriately. Recognition of their own temperaments and their impact on their children and their responses to their children is also helpful.

and flexible. As play becomes more social and less "parallel" in nature (i.e., when children play independently but near each other), toys and activities are shared and become more elaborate. By around age 4 years, play tends to take on more complex themes and often takes the form of a story with a goal, plot, characters, and so forth.

Having solid and secure attachments to adults facilitates play and social competence. Temperament can also be important in this regard so that excessively shy and inhibited children (and those who are overly active and disinhibited) can have problems with play and peer relationships. Increased abilities to play also provide the potential for great insight into children's worries, concerns, and inner experience, a phenomenon than be used in play interviews with younger children (Chapter 3). For some children, play can also be used as a therapeutic tool.

If is fairly common for preschool children to have imaginary friends and companions. Children may firmly insist on the reality of these individuals. This occasionally presents some challenges for parents (and mental health professionals) but usually is harmless. It is important to keep in mind that distinctions about reality and fantasy are not well appreciated until later. Issues of independence and separation can become prominent in this age group.

Transitions can present special challenges for toddlers and preschoolers, and some may use transitional objects to help them deal with these transitions. These difficulties can sometimes be exacerbated by stresses common in this age group (parental relocation, birth of a sibling). It is important for parents (and caregivers) to appreciate the difficulties separations can cause given the limited coping skills of this age group. Preschool children may repeatedly question their parents or caregivers about separation (e.g., why the parents are leaving, where they are going); this reflects the lack of fully developed capacities for internalization and memory. Transitional objects may help in this regard, and so can use of a picture or some other "token" left by the parent to remind the child that the parents will return. These difficulties can also be reflected (to some degree) around issues of transitions to new teachers, day care workers, baby sitters, and so forth. Issues of separation loom large particularly when divorce or parental separation

Transitional Objects

Often, by the end of the first year, typically developing children have developed a strong attachment for a "transitional object." This phenomenon was described by the British pediatrician and psychoanalyst Donald Winnicott, who noted several key features: the object is usually soft (a blanket, pillow, or stuffed animal), the child is very attached to the object and wants it with him or her, and the object helps with transitions (e.g., at bedtime). The presence of the actual object (not a substitute) is critically important. In his view, the object helped in the development of a sense of self (apart from the mother) and was a unique "me/not me" possession that he also saw as one aspect of a range of transitional phenomena. The child uses the object to help with separations, and the smell and feel of the object are often important. The child invariably leaves the object in various places, resulting in parental panic that it has been lost. Interestingly, children with autism often have hard rather than soft objects, and it is the class of object (e.g., any magazine, bundle of twigs) that is important for them.

becomes a fact of the child's life. As much as possible, the principle of continuity of care should be paramount. Although courts are sometimes asked to adjudicate custody disputes (which can drag on for years and sadly become a vehicle for continued parental contact and discord), it is increasingly the case the joint custody arrangement and mutually acceptable arrangements are worked out by the parents to ensure constancy and continuity of care as much as possible. Sensible consistency, structure, and predictability are helpful.

A range of anxieties, not just around separation, often become more striking between ages 2 and 4 years. This increase in fearfulness is normative (and to some extent adaptive) and tends to happen just as stranger anxiety and separation anxiety start to diminish. Children who are well attached to their parents look to them for support and reassurance and may be more cautious than children who are abused or neglected. Common sources of fear include issues of bedtime and are often associated with changes in routine. In some ways, children's greater capacity for symbolic thinking also contributes (i.e., children can now imagine a range of adverse outcomes). Other issues arise given children's difficulties in sorting out differences between dreams and nightmares and reality. Children in this age group often manage to feel both quite powerful but also rather helpless. Even though their language skills have increased, preschoolers may have difficulty giving voice to their fears and concerns. Some children may exhibit anxiety by withdrawal or avoidance, but others become disorganized and overly active.

The mastery of aggressive impulses is a major accomplishment for most children during the preschool years. Difficulties with the modulation of aggression is a frequent source of mental health referral in this age group. Such behavior can complicate children's placement in day care or an educational setting. Many factors contribute to difficulties with aggression, including past experience, endowment, and cognitive and language abilities. Having an ability to "use your words" gives children much more socially acceptable alternatives to aggressive behavior; not surprisingly, children whose language is delayed have more difficulty. The presence of important models of aggressive behavior (violent television and games, older siblings, and adults) can also exacerbate this problem. On the other hand, some degree of independence is desirable and normative. Toddlers make frequent use of words and phrases such as "Mine!" and "Me do!"; temper tantrums may erupt when children are frustrated. For some children, aggressive thoughts or feelings may be expressed more in fantasy and play than in behavior.

Preschoolers who are overly aggressive are at increased risk for a range of problems, both short and longer term. A thoughtful evaluation includes an assessment of the antecedents, behavior, and consequences of the behavior (i.e., what situations elicit it, what happens as a result). This assessment should also address the potential for anxiety to contribute to the behavioral difficulties. Physical aggression usually diminishes after age 3 years as verbal aggression begins to increase. The focus of aggression also shifts with younger children being more concerned with needs and aggression in children in school often having a more social context. Fortunately, most aggressive 3-year-old children do not become aggressive 6-year-old children. Helping children learn better approaches to dealing with angry (and anxious) feelings, modeling appropriate behavior (not aggression), and encouraging verbal expression are important.

It is increasingly common for preschoolers to be enrolled in child care and early education programs. Given this increase, it is increasingly common for younger children to be referred for developmental and behavioral difficulties. Efforts have been made to bring services more directly into programs, and the availability of supports and consultants also has some advantages for mental health professionals who can see children in more natural settings. Other models of consultation focus primarily on the classroom or behaviors that are problematic on a more general basis. Unfortunately, poor reimbursement and limited training for child care and teaching staff are continuing problems. Problems in care providers, such as depression, may impact their experience of (and reactions to) children with difficulties.

SCHOOL-AGE CHILDREN

In the developed world, this period of development is defined by the experience of school. Peers come to be a major influence rivaling, or surpassing, that of parents and siblings. Although Freud referred to this as the "latency period" (presuming that sexual drives are relatively dormant until adolescence), this is an oversimplification. In some ways, Erickson, with his characterization of "industry versus inferiority" as the central developmental task, more accurately captured the challenge for this age group. School success and progress are essential for self-esteem, peer relations, and subsequent academic development. In addition to the important role of peers, effects of culture (including from media and social media) as well as societal and economic factors have more impact. Table 2.6 summarizes the considerable growth that occurs over this time.

By age 5 years, the brain has reached about 90% of its adult volume. The rate then slows until puberty. Modification of structures continue, and myelinization is almost complete by age 7 years, when the brain reaches about adult size. Other ongoing changes include synaptic pruning in the prefrontal cortex. Some gender differences are observed with boys having, on average, brains that are about 10% larger; other differences are observed in structures such as the basal ganglia. Growth in the frontal lobe helps children be able to engage in inhibition and thus focus and process information more successfully. Differences in the timing of the neurochemical systems in the brain are also observed. At the psychological level, these advances are reflected in greater coordination of motor skills, increased capacities for self-regulation, speed of information processing, and increased ability to attend. These gains are also manifest in a growing ability to read (a process that is typically well in place by the second grade).

The process of puberty has its earliest beginning during this time as sex hormones begin to increase. Sexual interest can be reflected in sex play (solitary or group) and for many children with homosexual orientations in adulthood, it is during this period that an awareness of their sexual orientation becomes apparent. During this time, children begin to function more in same-sex peer groups with some degree of avoidance of the opposite sex; this begins to change in pre-adolescents when, for many children, an attraction to a movie or rock star may be a sign of growing interest in the opposite sex. For girls, the onset of puberty may begin between the ages of 9 to 11 years as breast growth accelerates.

Other gender differences noted at this time include the tendency for girls to have greater academic achievement in verbally mediated skills; boys often do better in math and science. These generalizations reflect complex effects of expectation and socialization as well as intrinsic ability. These differences have, however, likely been involved in perpetuating some notions of gender that may disadvantage girls in academic work.

TABLE 2.6

CHARACTERISTICS OF SCHOOL-AGED CHILDREN

	Child Entering First Grade (5–6 Years Old)	Completing Fifth Grade (10–11 Years Old)
Motor	Hops, skips, jumps, throws, catches, kicks a ball Reasonable balance, able to stand still and hold arms steady; stand on one foot, left and right General sense of left and right, not always consistent Able to do rapid alternating movements Mild synkinesis on fine finger movements	Hops, skips, jumps, throws, catches, and kicks a ball with ease Elaborates (e.g., dance steps; throwing behind back or tricking the receiver) Balance is good; tandem walking with ease Accurate distinction of left and right No synkinesis
Writing and drawing	Able to name and copy circle, square, triangle, and cross easily Some copy diamond and asterisk Five-pointed star is possible if child has been exposed to this in kindergarten Draws person with body, arms, and legs; can put detailed features but often leaves them out; can draw house and tree as well	Circle, square, triangle, diamond, asterisk, five-pointed star; cube can be accomplished but often only after shown how to draw it Draws more detailed person with hands, feet, and action figures; girls draw more decorative detail and boys draw more action detail
Stories	About drawings, persons are largely self-referential; even if a figure has a different name, the life circumstances are usually identical to the child's	May draw someone who is not self and can have a story about another, even made up family; creates complex plots using well-developed descriptive language
Fund of knowledge (depends on exposure)	Recites alphabet; counts beyond 20, writes first and last name; recognizes printed letters and numbers (not cursive); writes most letters and numbers; may have some reversals	Reads aloud and to self with comprehension; performs doubledigit addition and subtraction in head; multiplies, divides, and does fractions on paper; knows details about historical figures, geography, natural phenomena, body systems
Cognitive	Egocentric; idiosyncratic definitions of "scientific" observations; centration, defining by only one dimension; beginning concrete operations: conservation and classification	Conservation of number, weight, and volume; flexibility of operational skills, including reversibility
Moral	Defines right and wrong in terms of punishment and pain or other personal and idiosyncratic rationales Interested in how the world works, including life and death, religion; uses magical thinking	Defines right and wrong through internal principles Has empathy and can weigh issues from another's position

(continued)

TABLE 2.6

(CONTINUED)

	Child Entering First Grade (5–6 Years Old)	Completing Fifth Grade (10–11 Years Old)
Social	Enjoys the company of other children; names several friends Interactional play with rules, often externally determined Creative play is imitative Peers judged by whether they are nice to child Games of individual prowess; may play on team but cooperates based on rules rather than complex strategizing	Likely to have a best friend and a close circle of friends Activities with peers are increasingly independent of parental supervision Able to create games and make up rules; consideration for others, particularly with girls Increasing self-reliance and responsibility Peers judged by their qualities Teamwork
Self-view	Dependent on others' descriptions	Dependent on view of success, competence, and evaluation by internal standards, as well as comparison with peers and social pressures Selects from multiple available models to define standard for "cool" for self and select friends
Sex	Interested in sexual differences; pleasure from touching oneself; generally play with same-sex friends but comfortable with organized co-ed activities	Secondary sexual changes from Tanner stages II–V with girls usually 2 years ahead of boys; prefers same-sex friends. Some awkwardness about growth (slouching, embarrassment about breast development and foot size) Wide range of pubertal onset in peer group may create challenges to individual self-esteem Some admiration of individual members of the opposite sex versus thinking others are "yucky" Interest expressed through teasing, messages sent through others
Family	Identification with parents or siblings, primarily same-sex ones Participates in family rituals and routines around meals and bedtimes	Compares parents with other adults, including teachers and other children's parents More independent of family rituals and routines More responsibility for household tasks, own self-care, and homework

Reprinted from L. Combrinck-Graham, & G. Fox. (2005). Development of school age children. In A. Martin & F. Volkmar (Eds.), *Lewis's Child and Adolescent Psychiatry: A Comprehensive Textbook*, 4th edition, p. 269. Philadelphia: Lippincott Williams & Wilkins.

As noted in Chapter 1, Piaget's view of cognitive development emphasizes the move from what he termed "preoperational thinking" to more complex "operational" thought. This is reflected in greater conceptual ability and recognizing notions such as conservation of number or mass (i.e., changing the shape does not change the mass of materials). Children can think of alternatives; understand hierarchies, categories, and series; and master new concepts such as reversibility, sequencing, and so forth. Children can also now see the world from points of view other than their own ("decentration") and can engage in more sophisticated cognitive and social operations, including advanced games and group activities. These new cognitive abilities also help children gain new understandings of biological processes, including death, which is now understood to be irreversible.

The gains are also seen in the increased sophistication of conversation. Often, there is a desire for order and ritual, and many school-age children develop a need for symmetry and order as well as some ritualistic behaviors. This is a time when collecting things (insects, stamps, rocks, coins) is prominent, and the collection and its ordering and reordering becomes a focus of interest.

Attention and "executive function" skills also increase in children of school age. Children are able to develop plans for action and can use private speech as well as a series of strategies to memorize, order, rehearse, and plan. The capacity for increased self-regulation is important in setting the stage for adolescence.

The topic of moral development in school-age children has been the focus of much attention, starting with Piaget (see Chapter 1), who emphasized that morality at this age focused very much on "the rules" and their interpretation. Other subsequent investigations, such as by Kohlberg, talked about this as a time of "conventional morality"; this concept includes an aspect of a desire to please authority figures (parents and teachers) and the importance of rules in guiding behavior. Gender differences in moral judgment at this age are noted and may reflect some of the differences in play (with more emphasis on social interaction and empathy in girls).

For school-age children, emotional development at this age centers on competence and the social-community environment. Competence is expected in many areas (e.g., in self-care, academic, social, and physical). In the view of Erickson (see Chapter 1), the major risk for the child at this age has to do with feelings of inferiority, although, at least to some extent, failures in one area can be compensated for by success in another. By the middle school years, individual children often have a strong sense of areas of strength and weakness, and these perceptions are often quite persistent. The nature of anxiety and fear changes somewhat as children enter school age. Given their greater exposure to the world and events, they often become more worried about catastrophic events, death, and so forth. Children who struggle with issues of competence may be particularly likely to be at risk for emotional difficulties.

Baumrind (1996) has described the authoritative style of parenting that is both highly responsive and sets high expectations while allowing some degree of autonomy. Issues of "goodness of fit" often arise and can arise in different ways at different points in development. A growing body of work has revealed the importance of genetic influences on parent–child interaction. As children spend more time in school, teachers and peers assume more importance. Particularly as more parents have worked, children often spend time in after-school or other programs. As a result, children become more aware of (and point out to their parents) differences in childrearing practices and rules in other families. They may also question parental practices or beliefs. Changes arise as the family itself becomes more involved in activities at school or with sports, clubs, and so forth. Parents can meet new friends who themselves can provide, for parents as well as for children, new opportunities for learning and modifications of parental style.

Effects of Media, Peers, and School

The role of media, broadly defined, has been exploding in recent years. For decades, there has been considerable debate about the effects (or ill effects) of television and more recently of video games, social networking, and the Internet. These activities can isolate children from interaction with family members and peers, may model inappropriate behaviors, and may provide a highly unrealistic view of the world. In addition, they are usually rather sedentary activities and may contribute to growing rates of obesity and lack of physical fitness in children. On the other hand, such media may be a source of comfort to some children and help consolidate their connections to peers.

The peer culture has an important role in fostering socialization experiences and children's strivings for acceptance and competency within their peer group. There issues are also very relevant to children's sense of self and self-concept.

Peer relationships have their own characteristic pattern of development beginning in preschool and developing, during the primary school years, into more cooperative and truly dyadic partnerships and then on to more intimate peer relationships (best friends) just before adolescence. Same-sex peers become increasingly important as children become older. Gender differences are noted with girls preferring patterns that involved greater intimacy than boys. During this transition, the kinds of games children engage in develop more group process features, more rules, and greater complexities. As in the family, modulation of angry and aggressive impulses become an important issue in dealing with peers. Children who are, or remain, more overtly aggressive are more likely to be isolated and rejected; they may form their own peer groups, but social isolation and aggression are important risk factors for subsequent development problems.

Enrollment in school for the vast majority of school-age children is a relatively new historical phenomenon. Children arrive at school with many different experiences and perspectives. Dramatic sociocultural differences are observed. Many middle and upper class families have children who have attended preschool, have witnessed the value of more "academic" skills in the lives of their parents, and have a strong interest in books and reading. These opportunities may be less available to children from poor, minority, and inner-city families. In other situations (e.g., children of immigrants), children may not yet have a functional understanding of English. Children who live in poverty may also have had very different experiences involving assuming responsibilities in the household or translating for their parents if the latter are immigrants. Parental background is highly related to school achievement. Children with secure attachments to their parents, who have grown in a supportive environment, and whose parents emphasize academic expectations and values are less likely to have difficulty adjusting to the demands of school. For some children, the availability of model preschool programs or Head Start may provide an important facilitation for school entry.

One of the central tasks of the early school years is gaining the ability to read. This is a complex process with both content and relational and interactional aspects (see Chapter 6). Skills needed in preparation for reading include both the content and structure of books and other written materials. Children who lack a foundation of basic skills are more likely to have difficulties in learning to read. Academic material is ideally constructed in such a way to be just at the point of "proximal development" for children (i.e., a bit—but only a bit—further than they presently are in terms of their skills set). Both the ability of the child and the knowledge of the teacher are important in ensuring successful learning. Peer learning is also important, with specific methods such as "cooperative learning" used to help children learn together and work as a group. Sensitive teachers are also aware of each child's strengths and weaknesses and learning style as well as their readiness and motivation to learn. Even when curricula are appropriate to grade level, some children will be advanced or behind.

Parental involvement is also essential, and for schools to be effective, they must also function as communities, meaning, at least for large schools, that ways must be found to foster engagement in smaller groups. One of the major effects of the No Child Left Behind legislation has been a great focus on performance, sometimes at the risk of losing sight of the bigger picture of fostering a community focused on learning. Progress in school can be limited by factors in the child as well, including developmental and learning difficulties. Other problems arise for children and families that must cope with chronic medical illness. In these cases, a focus on helping the child learn as effectively as possible and helping the child establish a positive view of him- or herself is a major goal. Children who experience repeated failure are at risk for a variety of difficulties, including depression, social isolation, and further academic difficulties. Externalizing behavior disorders can also develop and may severely impact children.

It is important to note that although schooling is the norm within the United States and more developed countries in the first world, most (90%) children in Africa and Asia are involved in work, live in extreme poverty, and have limited opportunities for education.

ADOLESCENCE

Adolescence is a time of transition defined by the intersection of several factors. Children transition from people with some but minimal responsibility to adults with the entire set of responsibilities typical of adulthood. This is a time of recurrent paradox. Youngsters vary at very different rates in their development but typically acquire physical maturity well before they have reached their adult levels of social-emotional and intellectual maturity. Over the past century, adolescence has begun earlier, often between the ages of 9 and 12 years; for some individuals, this means they reach sexual maturity by the time they are 13 or so years of age. The increasing societal demands for education have resulted in an opposing trend that lengths the process of education. In contrast to the situation a century ago, employment before age 16 years is typically prohibited and school attendance required. Financial independence is usually only achieved well after high school and can continue through college and beyond. Legal issues also impact independence. Legal status represents a complicated mix of laws and regulation; younger adolescents may drive farm equipment (or even an airplane) but not a car. Similarly, a 17-year-old adolescent might be in the Army when she or he cannot yet vote. Regulations vary from state to state and may impact things such as rights to independent medical care.

Even though adolescents are not yet financially independent, the youth market represents a substantial economic force. Adolescents are specifically targeted in television and other programming and in ads, which are often dominated by sex and aggression. As King (2005) points out, although theories of development have tended to focus on the task of achieving independence, it is actually more accurate to discuss *interdependence*, that is, an ability to develop supportive relationships outside the immediate family. Adolescence must also be viewed in the context of cultural, family, school, and community factors. All of these factors interact so that the adolescent is both influenced by the family while also influencing it. In considering adolescent development, the truly very broad range of experience and diversity that adolescents experience should be acknowledged. This increasingly includes nontraditional family structures, differences in sexual orientation, experience of poverty, and so forth. In other cultures, different patterns emerge. For example, in some cultures, issues of autonomy are less central in adolescence; adolescents growing up in pre-industrial societies may experience less of the turmoil and parental conflict more typical in industrialized countries. Over the past century, different factors have impacted adolescence with a move of families from farms to cities, better health care and longer life spans, smaller families and longer periods of financial dependence on parents, and the increasing importance of social media and other information resources.

Puberty refers to the physical and physiological changes that note the transition from childhood to adulthood. Physical changes include the development of primary and secondary sexual characteristics. The adrenal glands' production of androgens begins to increase even as early as 6 to 8 years of age and leads to both increased skeletal growth and the beginning of body hair even before puberty proper. The latter is marked by pulsatile release of gonadal hormones (testosterone in boys and estrogen in girls) along with the increased release of growth hormone. As a result, the pubertal growth spurt begins. Puberty typically takes about 4 to 5 years in total. Girls, at least in the more developed countries, often start this process about 2 years before boys to (typically, ages 9 to 11 years for girls and 11 to 13 years for boys). Tanner has classified the various changes in the development of secondary sex characteristics into five stages (Table 2.7). Pubertal staging can be accomplished by physical examination or self-report (although the former is more accurate). Typically, the first sign that puberty is beginning is accelerated height; this can be as great as 10 cm in a given year. The "gangling" appearance of early adolescents precedes the development of increased muscle mass and strength that is associated with later stages of puberty.

TABLE 2.7

TANNER'S STAGES OF PUBERTY

Stage	Boys	Girls
1	Preadolescent	Preadolescent
2	Slight amount of pubic hair, slight enlargement of penis and scrotum	Sparse pubic hair, breasts begin to develop
3	Increased pubic hair, penis longer, testes bigger	Increased pubic hair, breasts enlarged
4	Pubic hair pattern resembles adult pattern but still sparser than in adults	Abundant pubic hair (less than in adults), nipples become more prominent
5	Adult male distribution of pubic hair, adult size testes and penis	Adult female pattern of pubic hair, breasts of mature adult

Adapted from Tanner, J. M. (1962). *Growth at Adolescence,* 2nd edition. Oxford, England: Blackwell and Daniel, W. A. (1977). *Adolescents in Health and Disease.* St. Louis: Mosby.

For girls, menarche is the major marker of puberty. Initially, periods may be irregular, and fertility may take up to 2 years to develop. For menarche to occur, a critical body weight and fat-to-muscle ratio must be met. For some girls who train intensively (or have anorexia; see Chapter 14), menarche can be delayed. The average age of menarche is progressively decreasing, with some racial differences noted; in developing countries, the age is later than in developed countries.

For boys, the growth of the genitalia and spermatogenesis in early and middle adolescence are associated with ejaculation (either spontaneously at night or because of masturbation). Unlike menarche, which is a frequent topic of conversation among early adolescent girls, boys typically are rather private in discussing this issue, at least in Western cultures.

A large body of research has focused on the impact of early versus late maturation in boys and girls. Briefly summarized, the result of this work is that for boys, early maturation leads to greater popularity, feelings of self-esteem, and greater academic and intellectual success, although possibly also incurring some risk for conduct and behavior problems perhaps related to older peer group influences. For girls, the issues are more complicated. In general, it appears that early-maturing girls may have more problems with self-image and greater risk for mood and anxiety problems. They may also be at risk for eating problems and risk taking (including sexual risk taking). Other issues impact this, including culture, social class, peers, and so on. Although popular culture frequently refers to the "raging hormones" of adolescence, evidence for an association between gonadal hormonal levels and behavioral or mental health problems is rather weak.

Other changes that come with puberty include an increased appetite and changes in sleep patterns. Unlike 10- to 12-year-olds, who sleep slightly more than 9 hours a night on average, for high school students, the typical night's sleep is about 7 hours, with many adolescents sleeping even less. Chronic sleep deprivation is common.

In Piaget's view, the period of formal operations in adolescence marks the ability to consider issues of propositional logic, deductive reasoning, hypothesis testing, and so on. Put another way, adolescents are no longer constrained simply by their observations of the world; rather, an appreciation of what "might be" is now possibly, leading partly to adolescents' enthusiasms and idealism. Although the specifics of many aspects of Piaget's theory have been debated, there is agreement that cognitive abilities significantly increase in complexity at this stage and include the ability to consider multiple problem solutions and outcomes and to more effectively and quickly process information. These cognitive changes also contribute to more sophisticated social-cognitive and moral development. Adolescents can see problems from multiple points of view and aspects and can appreciate subtle moral reasoning. Despite these gains, adolescents do not, however, always make wise decisions, and their judgment can be clouded by strong emotions, peer pressure, and substance use or abuse.

TABLE 2.8

GROWTH TASKS BY DEVELOPMENTAL PHASE

The normative psychological tasks of adolescence are:
- Developing a satisfactory and realistic body image
- Developing increased independence from parents and adequate capacities for self-care and regulation
- Developing satisfying relationships outside the family
- Developing appropriate control and expression of increased sexual and aggressive drives
- Identity consolidation, including a personal moral code and at least provisional plans for a vocation and economic self-sufficiency

Reprinted from R. King, (2005) Adolescence. In A. Martin & F. Volkmar (Eds.), *Lewis's Child and Adolescent Psychiatry: A Comprehensive Textbook*, 4th edition, p. 282. Philadelphia: Lippincott Williams & Wilkins.

The physical, neurobiological, and cognitive changes experienced herald dramatic shifts in adolescents' relationship to their own body, to their parents, to their peers, and for self-image. Adolescence brings a number of psychological challenges, which are summarized in Table 2.8.

One of the greatest challenges comes from these major physical changes that come with adolescence. Sexual development presents opportunities for gratification and embarrassment. Adolescents are typically very aware of similar changes in peers and evaluate themselves carefully in reference to them. The wide variation of development can pose significant issues in this regard. Girls are often particularly preoccupied with the ideal (and unrealistic) body image presented in the media. Obesity can be a problem for adolescents of both genders, although significant racial and ethnic differences are noted. Eating disorders in girls are particularly common, and girls are more likely than boys to engage in measures designed to help them lose weight (e.g., laxatives, vomiting). Changes in the body also pose issues for self-representation. Teenagers of both genders spend considerable amounts of their discretionary income on products designed to improve their appearance or reach some ideal body or appearance. This can include use of supplements, exercise programs, and even anabolic steroids in boys and endless "makeovers" in girls. Other options include tattoos and piercing. In other cases, the preoccupation with a changed body and dissatisfaction can result in other behaviors (e.g., cutting).

Other challenges come from major changes in relationships with parents and siblings. During adolescence, children spend less time with their parents and much more time with their peers. Increases in cognitive capacities and concerns about the future also typically result in some de-idealization of parents. Desires for continued closeness with parents compete with other desires for autonomy. These competing interests result in considerable ambivalence (as conveyed in books for parents of teens such as *Get Out of My Life, but First Could You Drive Me and Cheryl to the Mall?*). Despite these issues, for most adolescents, parents remain the primary sources of support and assistance. Even though this is true, the subjective changes in the relationship have major importance.

Conflicts with parents become more frequent with disputes about rules and chores and then continue over time with new topics such as curfews, dating, and so forth. These disputes often seem to peak in mid-adolescence and then decrease. Mother–daughter pairs are at particular risk in terms of frequency of disputes, although father–son pairs often have more intense disputes. Mental health issues (e.g., depression) or other problems (e.g., substance abuse) can exacerbate these tensions, which take a toll on the parents as well as on the child. The apparent focus on disputes is often trivial (e.g., over hairstyle, clothes, chores); however, these disputes are symbolic of other issues and have considerable additional psychological meaning. For most parents, a combination of warmth and engagement coupled with a firm expectation-based approach works best (what is often referred to as an authoritative parenting style).

Fortunately, by the time adolescents finish high school and enter college, they can be more autonomous and engaged in a new and more mature way with parents and family members.

Although most adolescents are healthy, their lifestyles can contribute to lifelong habits that impact their health through diet, exercise, driving, sexual behaviors, and so forth. On the other hand, for some teenagers, an awareness of chronic illness may significantly impact the adolescent' experience and have important implications for health care. The sense of invulnerability in adolescence, coupled with a desire to fit in, may lead to noncompliance with medical treatments (see Chapter 26). For example, many teenagers with diabetes may be noncompliant with treatment. Children with other illnesses may stop or "forget" medications. Unfortunately, the attempt to avoid or deny the reality of medical needs can further compound this problem.

Adolescence brings the new experiences of sexual desire and attraction. These can take infinite forms and are the focus of considerable research and debate in the extensive literature on this topic. Although obvious sexual behaviors are minimal before adolescence, they typically increase around age 10 years and may initially focus on same-sex peers. In some cultures, various ceremonies and rites of passage begin as early as age 10 or 11 years. The ability to combine feelings of sexual interest with emotional intimacy is a major challenge for adolescents. Early in adolescence, sexual feelings of boys may focus on television, movie, or other media figures; for girls, the focus is on real or fantasized romantic relationships and perpetual discussion of who is "going out" with whom. Over the course of adolescence, masturbation and heterosexual activities increase dramatically. Homosexual experiences are more frequent in early adolescence (slightly more than a quarter of 13-year-old boys report such experience). Sexual fantasies (often initially during masturbation) are highly personal and can play an important part in the development of each adolescent's unique sexuality. As adolescence progresses, a major challenge is the combination of erotic longings into relationships. Social and ethnic factors can have a major impact on this process. Gender differences are noteworthy. For girls, the relationship element of the encounter is critical, but for boys, sexual gratification may be more important (but this is only a generalization, and many variations on these themes are noted). The ability to fall in love is an important aspect of sexuality for adolescents as they mature, and conflicts with parents often develop around or over issues that involve some aspect of the child's growing sexuality (e.g., appearance, dating, curfews).

Beginning with the work of Erikson, there has been more attention to the centrality of adolescents' self-concept. More recently, the emphasis has been on self-concept and "identity" as reflected in any number of areas, including social, academic, physical or athletic, and so forth. The increased cognitive abilities of adolescents give them the capacity to view all of these issues from new perspectives, including a moral perspective, and over time, result in each individual's achieving a unique view of him- or herself. Special issues arise for children coming from minority communities or where ethnic issues or concerns are strong. Other issues arise around differences in sexual orientation. In all of these cases, the adolescent must develop a sense of him- or herself relative both to the general culture and his or her specific group.

Mental Health Issues in Adolescents

About one in five adolescents has a specific clinical disorder. However, a much larger number experiences mood issues or problems with parents or engages in significant risk-taking behaviors. Depression and mood problems increase during adolescence, particularly in girls. It remains unclear to what extent the emotional liability and negative emotions frequent in adolescence contribute to this problem, but more than one-third of adolescents report issues related to depressed mood. This is more common in girls than boys, possibly reflecting endocrinologic factors. Various issues, including increased academic, social, and cognitive demands, may contribute as can the high rates of adolescent mood variability.

Accidents and injuries associated with risk taking present another challenge for adolescents. Even though cognitive capacities increase in adolescence, this process is a long and complex one, and brain mechanisms that involve forward planning and inhibition are often not yet fully established. About three-fourths of deaths in individuals ages 10 to 24 years can be attributed to activities with a significant element of risk taking (car accidents, homicide, and suicide). High rates of risk tasking are reported in national samples, including drinking while driving, not wearing seat belts, carrying weapons, and unprotected sexual encounters.

Becoming an Adult

Although the onset of adolescence is relatively clearly marked, its close is not. In earlier times, some specific event, such as getting married, getting a job, or entering the military, served to close adolescence. Today, many factors blur this transition because many students move from high school to college remaining highly dependent on their parents for financial support. Marriage and employment can be postponed until after college or graduate school. Arnett (1999) has proposed the term "emerging adulthood" to describe this new phenomenon. Adolescence today often is followed by a relative long period of semi-autonomy with fully independence from parents being achieved only in the late 20s and early 30s.

SUMMARY

Development is a dynamic process in which experience and endowment interact to varying degrees and in complex ways. Major transitions and shifts in functioning occur over time. Tasks of infancy include establishment of essential social-affective bonds and acquisition of cognitive abilities such as object permanence. For toddlers, issues of autonomy, language development, and behavior modulation become more prominent. As children enter the preschool and school age period, issues of peer relationships become more essential as children gain increasing cognitive, motor, linguistic, and social skills. For adolescents, there is a fundamental, and enduring, tension in the various forces both encouraging and inhibiting development and independence. Considerable cognitive capacities give adolescents greater awareness of the world both as it is and should be. In Western cultures, this period has become increasingly prolonged even as sexual maturity often comes earlier.

In thinking about the individual child, it is important to keep in mind that a "normal" child does not, as such, exist. Rather, a "normative" child is typically described in chapters of this kind, and astute clinicians will be aware both of what is normative but also what is within the broad range of normal.

Selected Readings

Aber, J. L., Jones, S. M., & Cohen, J. (2000). The impact of poverty on the mental health and development of very young children. In Zeanah CH (Ed.),*Handbook of Infant Mental Health*. New York: The Guilford Press; 2000.

Arnett, J. (1999). Adolescent storm and stress, reconsidered. *The American Psychologist, 54*, 317–326.

Baumrind, D. (1996). The discipline controversy revisited. *Family Relations, 45*, 405–414.

Briggs-Gowan, M. J., Carter, A. S., Bosson-Heenan, J., Guyer, A. E., & Horwitz, S. M. (2006). Are infant-toddler social-emotional and behavioral problems transient? *Journal of the American Academy of Child & Adolescent Psychiatry, 45*, 849–858.

Brooks-Gunn, J., & Duncan, G. J. (1997). The effects of poverty on children. *Future of Children, 7*(2), 55–71.

Bronfenbrenner, U. (1986). Ecology of the family as a context for human development: Research perspectives. *Developmental Psychology, 22*, 723–742.

Cameron, J. L. (2004). Interrelationships between hormones, behavior, and affect during adolescence: understanding hormonal, physical, and brain changes occurring in association with pubertal activation of the reproductive axis. *Annals of the New York Academy of Sciences, 1021*, 110–123.

Carter, A. S., Briggs-Gowan, M. J., & Davis, N. O. (2004). Assessment of young children's social-emotional development and psychopathology: Recent advances and recommendations for practice. *Journal of Child Psychology & Psychiatry & Allied Disciplines, 45*, 109–134.

Centers for Disease Control and Prevention (2006). Youth risk behavior surveillance—United States. *Morbidity and Mortality Weekly Report, 55*(SS-5), 1–108.

Centers for Disease Control and Prevention. (2010). Youth risk behavior surveillance—United States. *Morbidity and Mortality Weekly Report, 59*(SS-5), 1–142.

Chess, S., & Thomas, A. (1986). *Temperament in Clinical Practice*. New York: Guilford Press.

Cicchetti, D., Rogosch, F. A., & Toth, S. L. (1998). Maternal depressive disorder and contextual risk: Contributions to the development of attachment insecurity and behavior problems in toddlerhood. *Development and Psychopathology,10*(2), 283–300.

Collins, W. A., & Steinberg, L. (2006). Adolescent development in interpersonal context. In W. Damon & R. M. Lerner (Eds.), *Handbook of Child Psychology*, vol 3, 6th edition, pp. 1003–1067. Hoboken, NJ: John Wiley & Sons.

Cronbrink-Grahan, L., Fox, G. S., & Mayes, L. C. (2005). Development of school-age children. In A. Martin & F. Volkmar (Eds.), *Lewis's Child and Adolescent Psychiatry: A Comprehensive Textbook*, 4th edition, pp. 267–278. Philadelphia: Wolters Kluwer.

Egger, H. L. (2009). Psychiatric assessment of young children. *Child and Adolescent Psychiatric Clinics of North America*, 18(3), 559–580.

Erikson, E. H. (1963). *Childhood and Society*, 2nd (revised) edition. New York: Norton.

Erikson, E. H. (1994). *Identity and the Life Cycle*. New York: Norton.

Gilligan, C. (1982). *In a Different Voice: Psychological Theory and Women's Development*. Cambridge, MA: Harvard University Press.

Hart, B., & Risley, T. R. (1995). *Meaningful Differences in the Everyday Experience of Young American Children*. Baltimore: Paul H Brookes Publishing.

Kagan, J., Reznik, R. J., Clarke, C., Snidman, N., & Garcia-Coll, C. (1984). Behavioral inhibition to the unfamiliar.*Child Development, 55,* 2212–2225.

Kagan, J., & Snidman, N. (2009). *The Long Shadow of Temperament*. Cambridge, MA: Harvard University Press.

King, R. A. (2007). Adolescence. In A. Martin & F. Volkmar (Eds.), *Lewis's Child and Adolescent Psychiatry: A Comprehensive Textbook*, 4th edition, pp. 279–290. Philadelphia: Wolters Kluwer.

Kohlberg, L. (1969). Stage and sequence: The cognitive-development approach to socialization. In Goslin DA (Ed.),*Handbook of Socialization Theory and Research*. Chicago: Rand-McNally.

Lerner, R., & Steinberg, L. (2004). *Handbook of Adolescent Psychology*, 2nd edition, pp. 45–84. Hoboken, NJ: Wiley.

Mayes, L. C., Gilliam, W. S., & Stout Sosinsky, L. (2007). The infant and toddler. In A. Martin & F. Volkmar (Eds.), *Lewis's Child and Adolescent Psychiatry: A Comprehensive Textbook*, 4th edition, pp. 252–260. Philadelphia: Lippincott Williams & Wilkins.

Mayes, L. C., Gilliam, W. S. & Stout Sosinsky, L. (2007). The preschool child. In A. Martin & F. Volkmar (Eds.), *Lewis's Child and Adolescent Psychiatry: A Comprehensive Textbook*, 4th edition, pp. 261–266. Philadelphia: Lippincott Williams & Wilkins.

Mayes, L. C. (1995). The assessment and treatment of the psychiatric needs of medically compromised infants: Consultation with preterm infants and their families. *Child and Adolescent Psychiatric Clinics of North America, 4*(3), 555–569.

Offer, D., Ostrov, E., Howard, K. l., & Atkinson, R. (1988). *The Teenage World: Adolescents' Self-Image in Ten Countries*. New York: Plenum Medical.

Petrill, S. A., Plomin, R., Defries, J. C., & Hewitt, J. K. (2003). *Nature, Nurture and the Transition to Early Adolescence*. New York: Oxford University Press.

Reiss, D., Plomin, R., Neiderhiser, J. M., & Hetherington, E. M. (2003). *The Relationship Code: Deciphering Genetic and Social Influences on Adolescent Development (Adolescent Lives)*. Cambridge, MA: Harvard University Press.

Rutter, M. (1982). *Fifteen Thousand Hours: Secondary Schools and Their Effects on Children*. Cambridge, MA: Harvard University Press.

Sameroff, A. J. (1987). The social context of development. In Eisenberg N (Ed.), *Contemporary Topics in Development*. New York: Wiley.

Shaw, P., Greenstein, D., Lerch, J., Clasen, L., Lenroot, R., Gogtay, N., Evans, A., Rapoport J., & Giedd, J. (2006). Intellectual ability and cortical development in children and adolescents. *Nature, 440*(7084), 676–679.

Shonkoff, J. P., & Phillips, D. A. (2000). *From Neurons to Neighborhoods: The Science of Early Childhood Development*. Washington, DC: National Academy Press.

Sosinsky, L. S., & Gilliam, W. S. (2007). Child care: How pediatricians can support children and families. In R. M. Kliegman, R. E. Behrman, H. B. Jenson, & B. F. Stanton (Eds.), *Nelson Textbook of Pediatrics*, 18th edition. Philadelphia: Elsevier. pages 81–86.

Sroufe, L., & Rutter, M. (1984). The domain of developmental psychopathology. *Child Development,55*(1), 17–29.

Steinberg, L. (2004). Risk taking in adolescence: What changes, and why? *Annals of the New York Academy of Sciences, 1021,* 51–58.

Stout Sosinskuy, L., Gilliam, W. S., & Mayes, L. C. (2005). The preschool child. In A. Martin & F. Volkmar (Eds.), *Lewis's Child and Adolescent Psychiatry: A Comprehensive Textbook*, 4th edition, pp. 261–266. Philadelphia: Lippincott Williams & Wilkins.

Vygotsky L. (1978). Tool and symbol in child development and internalization of higher psychological functions. In M. Cole, V. John-Steiner, S. Scribner, & E. Souberman (Eds.), *Mind in Society*, p. 20. Cambridge, MA: Harvard University Press.

Wolf, A. E. (1991). *Get Out of My Life, but First Could You Drive Me and Cheryl to the Mall?: A Parent's Guide to the New Teenager*. New York: Noonday Press.

CHAPTER 3 ■ CLASSIFICATION AND ASSESSMENT

PRINCIPLES OF CLASSIFICATION

Classification helps us be better observers and formulate hypotheses and principles. Shared approaches to classification help us communicate more effectively and develop better theories. In psychiatry, and indeed in medicine in general, the process of giving a label may be associated with some sense of relief on the part of the patient or the patient's parents; unfortunately, this often reflects a mistaken belief that having a label implies having an explanation. Like all human constructions, classification schemes can be abused or ill-used. There is no single "right" way to classify disorders in childhood. Systems vary, depending on the purpose of classification and what is being classified. Official diagnostic systems, such as the World Health Organization's International Classification of Diseases (ICD-10) and the American Psychiatric Association's *Diagnostic and Statistical Manual* (DSM-IV-TR), are generally categorically oriented, but dimensional approaches can be quite useful as well for clinical purposes. To be useful, classification schemes must be used readily and reliably, must provide adequate descriptions of disorders (so they can be reliability differentiated from each other), and must be useful across the range of age and severity. Deviant behavior itself does not necessarily constitute a disorder unless it is a manifestation of dysfunction within the individual person (e.g., conflicts over political beliefs do not constitute a mental disorder). Although it is often assumed that mental disorders must have a biological basis, this need not be the case; for example, maladaptive, enduring personality patterns can readily be classified as disorders. As with any classification, the approach chosen inevitably involves certain tradeoffs. Whereas the ICD-10 approach provides separate guidelines for research and clinical work, the DSM-IV approach provides one set of guidelines for both purposes.

Models of Classification

Various approaches to classification can be used (Table 3.1), These are not necessarily incompatible with each other. For example, a continuous variable such as IQ or blood pressure can be used to define levels of severity (e.g., of mental retardation) or disorder (hypertension).

The issue of which model works best depends on the specific situation. For example, structured rating scales and diagnostic interviews have been developed for many disorders. In addition a series of well-designed, psychometrically sound structured interviews "keyed" to

TABLE 3.1
APPROACHES TO CLASSIFICATION

Categorical approaches	Presence or absence of disorder Examples: autism, appendicitis

Dimensional approaches	Assess dimensions of function
	  or dysfunction
	Examples: intelligence,
	  hypertension

Ideographic approaches	Focus on the individual person Examples: individualized education plan

DSM-IV diagnostic concepts has been developed; these are particularly use for epidemiologic studies and screening purposes (see Angold, Costello, & Egger, 2007) for a review. Another approach has focused on more global assessments of psychopathology with derivation of more basic "factors" (e.g., internalizing vs. externalizing disorders on the Child Behavior Checklist; Achenbach, 1991). Such instruments have both research and clinical utility and may have importance for screening but do not usually translate straightforwardly into DSM-type diagnoses. As discussed later, there are major issues depending on the nature of the instrument and the informant—parents, teachers, peers, and the children themselves can, and often do, exhibit sometimes radically different perspectives.

Developmental issues are of great importance in classifying disorders in children and adolescents (and occasionally adults). Disorders such as autism and mental retardation have their origin during specific times of development, and other disorders, such as Tourette's disorder, may be preceded by other developmental problems. In other cases, preexisting disorders may complicate the diagnosis of other conditions (e.g., a child with mental retardation who goes on to develop schizophrenia in adolescence). For some conditions, diagnostic guidelines have a strong developmental orientation, but for others, the deviant nature of the symptoms predominates.

Theoretically based classification systems tended to be more common in the past. For example, Anna Freud had a model of classification based on her psychoanalytically informed understanding of child development. Theoretically based classification systems tend to be most useful for clinicians working with that specific theoretical framework; they may be much less useful for clinicians who do not share the same orientation. For several decades, the official classification systems have focused less on such theories and more on a theoretical, phonologically based approach. The latter approach is based on clinical experience, and concepts derived in this way have proven enduring even when the theory they originally were based on proved wrong (e.g., Langdon Down provided an enduring description of the condition we now understand is caused by trisomy of chromosome 21, but his original theory for this, which was based on racial stereotypes, did not).

It is often assumed that classification systems are developed to approximate some ideal diagnostic system in which the cause could be directly related to clinical condition. This is not, in fact, the case, in that no single ideal system is waiting to be discovered and that cause need not be included in classification systems. Different etiologic factors may result in rather similar conditions, and the same etiologic factor may be associated with a range of clinical conditions. Aspects of intervention may be more directly related to the clinical condition than to the cause. Remedial services for children with mental retardation are, for example, much more likely to be oriented around aspects of developmental level than around the precise origin of the specific mental retardation syndrome. With a few exceptions (e.g., reactive attachment or posttraumatic stress disorders in the DSM-IV), etiologic factors are not generally included in official diagnostic systems.

Clearly, contextual factors are particularly important in understanding childhood psychopathology. Thus, variables such as family, school, or cultural setting can serve as major modifiers of clinical presentation. For example, a child who had attentional difficulties because of an inappropriate school placement should not have a diagnosis of attention-deficit disorder. Contextual variables are particularly problematic in disorders of infancy and early childhood in which child and parent variables often interact with each other. Cultural differences may also be important and may interact in complex ways with child vulnerability and family variables.

Finally, it is important to emphasize that *disorders*, not children, are classified. This may seem a subtle point, but it is not. There are potential negative effects (and positive ones) related to labeling. Clearly, it is children, and not labels, who need help, and it is not appropriate to equate people with their problems (e.g., the use of the word "autistics" to describe children with autism is just as inappropriate as would be the term "pneumatics" to refer to individuals with pneumonia). Labels can have some social stigma or other untoward effects or may be associated with more realistic expectations on the part of parents and teachers and provision of potentially more appropriate services.

Research Issues

As official classification systems have become more complex and sophisticated, issues of reliability and validity have assumed increasing importance. For example, both the DSM-IV and the ICD-10 use results of large national or international field trials in providing definitions of disorders. Categorical and dimensional approaches to classification share certain statistical concerns including validity and reliability. *Validity* refers to the extent to which the diagnostic category captures the phenomena it purports to (e.g., does the diagnostic category have some meaning relative to course and treatment or family history or associated conditions?). *Reliability* refers to the ability of different individuals to use the diagnostic approach in the same way. As with validity, various kinds of reliability are identified, and these are impacted by various factors such as the theoretical bias of the clinician. In providing diagnostic criteria and descriptions, there is often a trade-off between the level of detail of a definition and its reliability.

Various statistical methods can be used to study patterns of relationships among specific variables or symptoms and syndrome (e.g., studies that use checklists or behavioral reports can use such techniques in an attempt to evaluate clinical groupings). These methods are most useful for the more common disorders. Such approaches can be used to evaluate the stability of specific dimensions or profiles, and use of dimensional techniques of assessment can be helpful in this regard.

Multiaxial Classification and Comorbidity

In working with children, the ability to use a multiaxial approach is very helpful. This can help clinicians be aware of many areas relevant to diagnosis. Thus, putting developmental disorders on a separate axis is intended to remind clinicians to look for such disorders on a regular basis. On the other hand, the distinction of what disorders are "developmental" can be problematic. Enuresis, for example, has strong developmental correlates but is generally included as a psychiatric rather than a developmental disorder.

One of the major benefits of a multiaxial system is that certain conditions are particularly likely to be overlooked (e.g., the child with a conduct disorder who also has learning problems). The presence of multiple disorders does, however, raise another problem—that of comorbidity. Having one problem may increase the risk for other difficulties. Particularly in the area of intellectual disability, there has often been a tendency to *underestimate* the presence of other problems. This difficulty, known as diagnostic overshadowing, can be very problematic because rates of psychiatric problems of specific types in individuals with mild mental retardation may be four- to fivefold increased! There are significant differences in ways in which diagnostic systems such as the DSM and ICD deal with comorbidity; on balance, the DSM tends to encourage multiple diagnoses, but the ICD system provides a single category for a child with what DSM might refer to as two conditions. The issue of comorbidity is a particularly complicated one for childhood-onset disorders given the importance of developmental factors and the potential for one condition or problem to contribute to others in complex ways. Potentially, an understanding of comorbidity might truly enrich our understanding of psychopathology; on the other hand, it can sometimes be trivial. For example, a child with autism should not receive an additional diagnosis of stereotypy-habit disorder because stereotyped movements are a diagnostic feature of autism. On the other hand, conduct disorder with depression does appear to be a more frequent and relevant combination with its own specific ICD code.

In summary, classification in child and adolescent psychiatry has multiple meanings and functions. Complications for classification of child and adolescent disorders are myriad: The child is often not the person complaining, different kinds of data may be used in making a diagnosis, developmental factors may have a major impact on the expression of disorders, and certain features (e.g., beliefs in fantasy figures) are normative at certain ages but not at others. Additional complications are posed by the unintended, but no less real, uses to which diagnostic concepts are put, such as their inclusion in legislation and their use as mandates for services in educational programs or for purposes of insurance reimbursement for services. Different kinds and levels of classification are needed for different purposes. Advances in diagnosis and classification since 1980 have significantly advanced the field, but important work remains to be done. The ability, over the next decade, to identify more clearly endophenotypes or intermediate endophenotypes may advance the already impressive potential for relating genetic and neurobiological features to disorders.

ASSESSMENT

The child or adolescent should be evaluated in the context of her or his functioning within the family, school, peer, cultural, and community settings with a goal of identifying specific forms or psychopathology and developing an appropriate treatment plan if one is needed. Depending on the clinical situation, the examiner may need to prioritize areas for assessment and intervention (e.g., the presence of suicidal thoughts or psychotic symptoms suggests immediate intervention needs).

Occasionally, an assessment is needed for a very specific purpose (e.g., custody assessments or evaluation of psychiatric problems of a child hospitalized on a pediatric ward). More typically, the assessment process is much broader and less focused, which requires the examiner to take a broad view, taking into account presenting complaints (of child, parents, teachers, and others), the child's history and level of development, and family and cultural factors.

There are several major ways in which the assessment of a child or adolescent differs from the psychiatric assessment of an adult. Typically, the child is not the person complaining of the problem; more typically, parents or sometimes schools have initiated a referral. The child may or may not be as troubled by the problem. Sometimes the problem arises more in the context of the family rather than in either child or parent. The assessment also depending on the child's chronological age and developmental level (e.g., the approach to a preschool child will often involve play or games; a school-age child may prefer some combination or discussion and activities; and an interview of adolescent may be more like that of the adult, although even in this situation, there will be some differences).

It is important that the child understand, at whatever level he or she can, the purpose of the assessment and that, as appropriate, the clinician conduct interviews in a way designed to facilitate discussion. Unlike adults, children can function very differently depending on the setting. A child who is having real trouble sitting still in school may be well behaved and popular on the playground. As a result, it is typical that multiple sources provide information (e.g., child, parent(s), school, and others); consequently, a major task for the clinician becomes the reconciliation of views when they diverge. Also, as a result of this process, the clinician needs to form a working relationship with multiple parties while maintaining, as appropriate, the child and family's confidentiality. This process, just by itself, can be quite revealing about the nature and extent of the difficulties and development of a treatment plan. In contrast to interviews with adults, developmental issues can loom large either as presenting complaints (e.g., continued bedwetting, delayed speech) or as important considerations in the assessment itself (e.g., a child with autism who is not verbal). For younger, typically developing children, it is important that the clinician have an awareness of normative cognitive processes and common childhood fears, beliefs, and fantasies. In some instances, skills can be lost (e.g., a child who is hospitalized and begins to wet the bed again or an adolescent who becomes psychotic and whose self-care skills diminish).

A final set of problems arises from the limitations of current diagnostic approaches. The categories included with DSM or ICD were usually developed from work with adults. Developmental considerations have not always been given central importance. For some conditions, this makes little difference, but for others, it can be a major complication (e.g., there may be differences in how major depression is experienced in children, with more somatic complaints and less overt self-deprecation) As discussed earlier in this chapter, there are important and legitimate tensions around issues of syndrome boundaries, problems of comorbidity, and diagnostic overshadowing.

The assessment should, of course, be tailored to the circumstances of the individual case, but several key components should be considered (Table 3.2) with the aim of identifying the variables relevant to the child's presentation.

Typically, the assessment begins with a review of the reasons for referral. This helps clarify the nature of the presenting problem(s), the "pool" of individuals relevant to contributing to the assessment process, and expectations (overt or covert) for what the assessment will provide. The history can be obtained from relevant persons and perspectives (e.g., child, parents, siblings, other family members, school personnel). The examiner should be alert to the context or circumstance in which problem behavior emerges. In some fundamental way, the examiner tries to assemble, and constantly revise, a narrative with first attention paid to the "facts" as they present themselves (the who, what, where, and when of the narrative) with an eventual formulation (the why). The clinician should be alert to important clues about what sets off or maintains problem behaviors. Problems can arise for many reasons, including psychiatric difficulties in the child but also because of some environmental circumstance. A history of previous treatment should be included if relevant. At some time, the examiner will also wish to obtain a developmental history to help clarify any potential developmental difficulties contributing to current problems and any long-standing issues that may shed light on current problems (e.g., the child's temperament; see Chapter 2).

A review of the past history should put current problems in an historical context (e.g., is this a new problem, an exacerbation of an old one, or some new problem that arises in the context of some other difficulty?). As noted earlier in this chapter, this last issue, of comorbidity, presents particular challenges for diagnostic systems and clinicians alike. Children (and parents) typically have not studied the DSM-IV, and clinical presentations usually include a range of difficulties. Accordingly, an important part of the assessment reflects the clinician's judgment, based on history and presentation, of how the presenting symptoms can be placed in a broader context. For example, although attentional problems are a hallmark of attention-deficit disorder (Chapter 8), they can also be seen in children with anxiety, autism spectrum disorders, stress, depression, or bipolar disorder or may arise because of some environmental factor (e.g., a child placed in an inappropriate classroom setting).

The medical history should include attention to the pregnancy, labor, and delivery. Sometimes parental expectations of the child even before birth may be relevant. Complications during delivery or the neonatal period should be noted as should any relevant medical conditions, hospitalizations, surgeries, and so forth. Response to medications and allergies to medications should be elicited. The clinician should be alert to any factors in the history that might contribute to current difficulties (e.g., a mother who drank during the pregnancy, putting the child at risk for fetal alcohol syndrome or a child with a history of significant prematurity who might be at risk for learning difficulties). Any sensory vulnerabilities should be noted (e.g., a child

TABLE 3.2

CONTENT COMPONENTS OF THE PSYCHIATRIC ASSESSMENT OF CHILDREN AND ADOLESCENTS

Content Component	Primary Informant	Additional Resources
Reason for referral	Usually parent or guardian; sometimes school or legal agency	Letter from school or other agency seeking evaluation
History of problem(s)	Child and parent	Referral source; contact from primary care provider
Past problems	Child and parent	Structured interviews; screening scales
Comorbid symptoms	Child and parent	Structured interviews; screening scales
Substance use	Child, parent	Laboratory screening (as relevant)
Previous assessment or treatment(s)	Child, parent, clinicians	Mental health records
Child's development, including psychomotor, cognitive, interpersonal, emotional, moral, trauma, harm (to self and others)	Parents, school staff	School records, including special education evaluations; home video (as relevant)
Family history	Parent	Genogram
Medical history	Parent, health care provider(s)	Review of symptoms checklist; laboratory tests (as relevant)
Child's strengths	Parent, child, teachers, coaches, peers	Activity video (e.g., sports, music); cognitive, school, neuropsychological testing
Child's media diet	Parent, child, caregivers, siblings	Media diary; "Tivo" records; DVD or CD collections; magazine subscriptions
Environmental supports	Parent, child, adults familiar to child	Activity schedules (scouting, teams); after-school or summer programs; mentorships such as Big Brother or Big Sister relationships
Mental status exam	Child	Mini-Mental Status Examination

Reprinted with permission from Bostic, J., & King, R. A. (2007). Clinical assessment of children and adolescents: Content and structure. In A. Martin & F. Volkmar (Eds.), *Lewis's Child and Adolescent Psychiatry: A Comprehensive Textbook*, 4th edition, pp. 324. Philadelphia: Lippincott Williams & Wilkins.

with recurrent ear infections who might present with language delay). The medical history should include a review of any significant accidents or injuries and any potential sequelae.

Family history should include a review of the parents' own histories of developmental or psychiatric problems, parenting styles, marital style, and methods for conflict resolution. Relevant cultural, ethnic, religious, or other information should be noted. Recent, or enduring, stresses and, for that matter, supports should be noted. Family moves can be disruptive of peer relationships and stressful for parents and children alike. Sometimes the death of a familiar figure (e.g., a grandparent) significantly changes child care patterns. If parents are divorced or if there has been chronic or sporadic marital conflict, it is important that the examiner attend to parental perceptions of how these have impacted the child. If a child is adopted, the history, to the extent available, of the child before the adoption is relevant. The child's understanding of the adoption should also be obtained. The clinician should be clear about the family constellation and inquire about other individuals present. A genogram can be helpful in this process.

Depending on the child's age and level of maturity, other issues may merit review. If the child is approaching adolescence or if adolescence is already well established, it is important to inquire about pubertal development. In some situations (e.g., feeding or eating problems), measures of height and weight can be very relevant. The child's use or exposure to alcohol, cigarettes, or illegal substances should also be reviewed. Media-related issues (broadly defined) may also be worth exploration (e.g., how does the child spend his or her time? What is the level of supervision?). The identification of favorite activities can also help inform the clinical interview with the child (e.g., by giving the examiner some obvious places to begin a discussion).

It is helpful for clinicians to have a general conceptual model to follow during the assessment. This aids both the assessment process itself and the written summary that should follow. It is important that the child or adolescent (and family members) understand exactly what is involved in a psychiatric assessment. Unlike a usual office visit to the pediatrician, a visit to a psychiatrist or other mental health professional is fraught with psychological "baggage" that may interfere with the assessment process. Accordingly, clarity and transparency on the part of the interviewer can be extremely helpful.

Often, parents may come for an initial interview without the child. This allows for both a review of the presenting problem and child's history and a chance for parents to convey their own concerns, expectations, and misconceptions. It can also provide an opportunity for talking with the parents about exactly what they will tell their child before she or he comes to the assessment.

The child may have major misconceptions about what is involved in speaking with a psychiatrist. She may worry that the parents are going to hospitalize her or send her away or that the assessment is a form of punishment. The child may be burdened with some secret—or not so secret—fear. It is helpful if parents can openly discuss their hopes for the meeting and indicate, if it is appropriate, what they know about what will happen and who the child will see. Depending on the context, other family members (siblings, parents) or child care workers (day care providers) or teachers and school personnel may be involved and may have their own, sometimes major, misconceptions about what will take place and what can be accomplished.

For younger children, information from the parents (e.g., about the child's favorite activities, TV shows, or games) may serve as an "ice breaker" for the clinician. Any special needs of the child should be discussed along with confidentiality issues.

Often, the initial parent interview focuses both on the question of how (did we get here?) but also of "Why now?" Parents should be helped to elaborate, in their own words, their understanding of how the child's difficulties have evolved over time. If there are major differences in perception (e.g., between the mother and father or between a parent and teacher), it is important that everyone have a chance to voice their own perspectives.

In addition to areas of weakness or vulnerability, the clinician should be alert to areas of strength and potential resources for the child. The latter may take the form of people who have special relationships with the child. Similarly, cultural or social resources should be noted (e.g., the presence of a supportive religious or ethnic community can be very relevant).

A host of factors can complicate the valuation process. These can include problems in the parents (e.g., highly divergent expectations or perspectives on the problem). Sometimes, sadly, often in custody situations, the child can become a "target" of parental struggle. As with the child, the specific developmental and personality issues of the parents may color the assessment process.

The clinician should be very sensitive to the potential for parents to feel embarrassed or ashamed (i.e., that they have failed in some way because their child has some problem or need). The clinician should be actively listening to parental concerns and to how these concerns are colored by the parents' own history. Some important aspects of the topics for parent and child interviewing are summarized in Appendix 1.

The Mental Status Examination

The mental status examination (MSE) is a key component of the assessment. It gives a perspective based on direct interaction as to how the child presents him- or herself. The MSE should be informative and descriptive. The MSE should include a description of how the child presents him- or herself (well organized, tidy, or studiously the reverse). How easy is it to engage the child? How cooperative is she or he? How does she act and interact with the clinician? What is her or his speech like? Are there concerns about mood or thought process disturbance? Although usually written up as a separate section from this history, the MSE is usually highly dependent on observations made throughout the assessment. Some aspects of the MSE require specific inquiry (orientation, memory, fund of knowledge, and so forth), but others can be collected continuously throughout the assessment. Table 3.3 provides an overview of components of the MSE. Depending on the results of initial examination, other assessments (e.g., of cognition, speech-communication functioning, academic skills, or learning problems) may require specific investigation.

The interview of the child is an important aspect of the assessment. It provides the child's view of the presenting problem or issues, provides an opportunity for additional history, and gives the clinician the child's perspective on the problem. Information derived from the child interview can be extremely helpful in developing an appropriate intervention program. The child may also reveal particular features or symptoms not necessarily either noted or commented on by the parents (e.g., movement problems and tics, thoughts of suicide, ruminations, hallucinations). In some situations (e.g., sexual abuse), the child can be the major informant on an event. It is important to realize, particularly with younger children, that idiosyncratic or developmentally appropriate views may color the child's reporting.

It is essential that the interview be tailored to the child's language and cognitive level. In some instances (e.g., with adolescents), a lack of trust or profound desire to avoid discussion of a painfully recalled traumatic event may complicate the interview process. In instances of abuse or neglect, the knowledgeable child may rightly understand the risk of removal to an out-of-home placement. It is important that the clinician rightly position him- or herself as on the one side the child's advocate while maintaining an ongoing dialog with the family. Typically, the child and parents are seen together before the interview of the child alone can proceed.

Once comfortable, the child can often readily have his or her parents leave (sometimes this is more of an issue for parents than children). The use of games or play materials or other objects or materials may facilitate the transition. After the parents have left, it is usually appropriate to begin with asking the child what she or he understand about the purpose of the interview. This also provides a chance for the clinician to ask why the child believes parents or other adults want this process. Adolescents present some important challenges for interviewing. Often, an adolescent feels that the various adults have, in some way, colluded against him or her. Accordingly, it may be more helpful with adolescents to have a short phone interview with the parents before the first visit of the adolescent with the clinician, who can then truthfully say that he or she has not met the parents but has heard from them at least a bit about what the concerns are. Both parents and adolescents may have information to share only with the clinician (e.g., relative to marital issues; concerns about substance abuse; or from the child's point of view, concerns they do not wish to share with the parents). It is important to maintain boundaries and appropriate confidentiality, always keeping in mind the importance of sharing certain kinds of information (e.g., relative to suicidality or dangerousness to others). Adolescents usually respond to a reasonably straightforward approach. Sometimes clinicians can "overdo" their ability to relate at the same level to the adolescent patient; in reality, there are often important generational differences not always easily bridged even by well-meaning adults. Typically with an adolescent, it is better to first discuss areas of strength before moving to problems. The clinician should maintain sensitivity to the child's developmental level at all times. This is partly, but not totally, a function of chronological age. Some younger children can be rather mature. Conversely, some adolescents can act much more like younger children. If the content of the interview becomes distressing using of other methods (play, puppets,

TABLE 3.3

THE MENTAL STATUS EXAMINATION IN CHILDREN

Category	Components	What to Assess
Appearance	Physical appearance	Gender; ethnicity; age (actual and apparent); cleanliness and grooming, hair and clothing style, presence of physical anomalies, indicators of self-care and parental attentiveness; jewelry, cosmetics, adornments
	Manner of relating to clinician and parents	Ease of separation from each parent, guardedness or warming up to clinician, eagerness to please, defiance, flirtatiousness, reactions to meeting the clinician
	Activity level	Psychomotor retarded to hyperactive, sustained or episodic, goal oriented or erratic; coordination, unusual postures or motor patterns (e.g., tics, stereotypies, compulsions, catatonia, akathisia, dystonia, tremors)
	Speech	Fluency (including stuttering, cluttering, speech impediments), rate, volume, prosody
Mood	Current affect	Predominant emotion and range (constricted to labile) during the interview and appropriateness to content (e.g., giggles while talks about sibling's illness); intensity; lability
	Persisting mood	Predominant emotion over days or weeks; whether current affect is unusual or consistent with mood; whether mood is reactive to situations or the same across a range of situations
	Coping mechanisms and regulation of affect	How child manages conflict or distress, age appropriateness of responses to and dependency on parents; sexual interests, impulses, aggression; control or modulation of urges (finding alternative or socially appropriate means of satisfying urges); how deals with frustration or when anxious
Sensorium	Orientation	Self (name), place (town, state), time (awareness of morning, day of week, month, year varies by age), situation (why at this appointment)
Intellect	Attention	Eye contact, need for redirection or repeating, how long sustained on activity, degree to which child shifts from activity to activity, distractibility (e.g., to outside noises)
	Memory	Immediate (repeat numbers, names back), short term (recall three objects at 2 and 5 minutes), long term (recall events of past week)
	Intelligence; fund of knowledge	Age-appropriate recognition of letters, vocabulary, reading, counting, computational skills; age-appropriate knowledge of geography, history, culture (e.g., celebrities, sports, movies); concrete to abstract thinking, ability to classify and categorize
	Judgment	Especially concerning the current problems (best assessed after rapport established because initial responses may be minimization or denial); what do if found stamped envelope next to mailbox or a fire started in a theater; what the child would say if he or she saw a man with big feet
	Insight	Ability to see alternative explanations, others' points of view; locus of control (internal vs. external); defense mechanisms
Thought	Form: *coherence*	Logical, goal directed, circumstantial or tangential (consider age appropriateness), looseness of associations, word salad (incoherent, clanging, neologisms)
	Form: *speed*	Mutism, poverty of thought (long latency, thought blocking), poverty of content (perseveration), racing thoughts, flight of ideas
	Perceptions	Altered bodily experiences (depersonalization, derealization), misperception of stimulus (illusion), no stimulus (hallucination: auditory [psychosis > PTSD > organic causes], visual [dementia > delirium], olfactory (neurologic, seizure disorder] gustatory [from medicine side effects])
	Content	Obsessions (ego dystonic), delusions (ego syntonic), thoughts of harm to self or others (magical thinking and fears at night are often age appropriate)

PTSD, posttraumatic stress disorder.
Adapted from Bostic, J., & King, R. A. (2007). Clinical assessment of children and adolescents: Content and structure. In A. Martin & F. Volkmar (Eds.). *Lewis's Child and Adolescent Psychiatry: A Comprehensive Textbook*, 4th edition, p. 329. Philadelphia: Lippincott Williams & Wilkins.

drawing) may be helpful. When carefully used, honest humor *and* empathy can help with the adolescent (sarcasm and the appearance of sarcasm should, in particular, be avoided). The goal is for the child to feel able to talk about her or his concerns in a straightforward way. The clinician must constantly be able to shift technique depending on the child's response.

Several different techniques are generally used in facilitating the clinical interview.

- *Engagement methods* help put the child at ease and elicit accurate and meaningful clinical information.
- *Projective* techniques help the child reveal underlying issues, particularly ones difficult for the child to verbalize.
- *Direct questioning* can be used for clarification and specific information.
- *Interactive techniques* are used to elucidate how the child relates to others.

It is important to attain a balance between, on the one hand, the child's needs and, on the other, the specific information required for the clinician to formulate a diagnosis and intervention program.

Child engagement can be a challenge. It is useful for the examiner to realize that the child is typically being seen in a strange place by strange people. Helping the child feel more comfortable will facilitate the interview. This can be done both in the office itself and the waiting room (e.g., with provision of a range of materials, including toys, magazines, and activities). The office should be "child friendly." Less experienced clinicians are often surprised to discover that generic, rather than highly specific, toys and play materials are helpful. Particularly, cartoon figures may, for example, initially elicit repletion of familiar scripts, video games, and TV programs, but less recognizable materials may stimulate greater imagination and conversation. Drawing materials and games such as board games, card games, or even chess can be used to provide an "overt" activity during which clinical interaction can be ongoing. In such activities, the clinician must always maintain appropriate awareness of the goals of the setting (i.e., the investment should be in the child rather than in winning the game!). As much as possible, the child should be allowed to set the tone and direct the content of the play and interview. This can provide helpful information about the child's ability to self-organize, relate to others, and develop a narrative. Observation of the child during this time will reveal much about gross and fine motor skills, speech-communication abilities, cognitive level, affect, attention span, and so forth. In some situations (e.g., children with autism), play may present major challenges, and the child may engage in solitary, repetitive activities.

For some children, more projective techniques may help supplement imaginative play. These methods allow the child to express concerns indirectly so that anxiety associated with important issues can be minimized. Drawing is probably the most frequently used projective technique. The child can be asked to draw a picture of him- or herself or family. The content of the picture can be revealing as is the process (e.g., if in family drawing, who is placed where can be important).

Play materials can also facilitate verbal projection (e.g., asking what a puppet or doll is thinking in play or asking the child about his or her favorite television character or superhero). Another approach is to ask the child what she or he would do if granted three magic wishes. Sometimes responses become rather generic (e.g., wishes for world peace), but these can be followed up with more specific discussion. Donald Winnicott invited the squiggle game in which the clinician begins a drawing (with a squiggle on a page), which the child can then add to. Over several rounds of back-and-forth addition, the picture may turn into something with relevance to the child.

Even with adolescents, discussion of favorite movies, musicians, or sports figures can allow an elaboration of the adolescent's desires and concerns. Discussion of what attracts the interest or admiration of the adolescents in an admired person can also speak to some of the adolescent's own hopes and concerns. Given the central importance of the peer group for adolescents, discussion of friends is important. The adolescent can be asked about the different cliques or groups at school and how she or he fits in with them. Adolescence is also a time when thinking abilities have undergone a significant shift and there is more potential for the adolescent to see things not only how they are but as how they should be (e.g., issues of judgment and justice may be prominent). For some adolescents, giving the potential for some displacement (e.g., by centering the discussion around a friend who had similar problems or what an admired adult might do in a situation) can sometimes be helpful.

Any child or adolescent can be asked about favorite activities, games, movies, books, and so forth. This discussion, particularly early on in the interview, can help "break the ice" and also may reveal common areas that the clinician can use to facilitate engagement. This discussion can also be continued over several interviews if, as is often the case, an evaluation extends over several sessions.

Direct questioning is the usual method used in interviews with adults and has an important role in interviewing children and adolescents as well. Good judgment is required on the part of the clinician (e.g., relative to inquiries about information that the child may be sensitive about or reluctant to disclose). In some situations, such as in the emergency department, a more leisurely approach to information gather may not be possible, but even in these cases, tact and sensitivity to the child's feelings and developmental level are important. Except in emergency or urgent situations, it is preferable to allow the child to initially control the level of detail in response to direct questions. Similarly, questions posed to the child may, at times, have to be very specific, but often more open-ended questions provide information.

Occasionally, particularly for younger children, helping the child establish a time frame may be useful (e.g., did this happen before you were out of school this summer?). With adolescents, issues of tact and timing are particularly important. As a general rule, the clinician should start off discussions with less threatening topics and areas of the adolescent's strength rather than immediately moving to areas of difficulty. Some sensitive issues (e.g., substance abuse, sexuality, risk-taking behaviors) are intrinsically the focus of direct question. Giving the child a more general question to respond to is often a good way to begin a line of inquiry. It is important in discussions of sexuality that the clinician be sensitive to the possibility of both homosexual and heterosexual relationships and experiences (e.g., questions should be phrased in a way to be gender neutral as much as possible). Risk taking can be approached by asking about things that were potentially dangerous or might have gotten the child or adolescent into trouble with parents or teachers.

The clinical interview gives the clinician a unique opportunity to observe how the child relates to a new person. Even responses to the usual social conventions provide information. The child's response to transitions can be assessed along with capacities for developing narratives, following rules (e.g., in play games), and dealing with a new adult. Adolescents may provide important information at the outset of the interview (e.g., with his or her style of dress). The clinician should not simply assume the meaning of particular styles but rather should take the opportunity to inquire about its meaning to the particular adolescent. With adolescents, it is also appropriate to ask about future plans and hopes.

Ending the interview in a mutually satisfactory and collaborative way can help the child have a positive feeling on leaving and may facilitate subsequent clinical encounters. Often, it is helpful to signal the approach end of an interview and ask the child or adolescent if there are any things she or he would like to talk about that have not been touched on. It also is very reasonable to ask the child or adolescent if he or she has any questions for the examiner. Occasionally, the child will ask about the clinician's recommendations or thoughts. Usually, it is best not to be overly specific until there has been a chance to talk with the child's parents; in addition, there may be additional studies (e.g., laboratory or psychological tests) that the examiner wishes to obtain.

The issue of confidentiality remains one of the most complicated ones for clinicians to address, particularly relative to adolescents. On the one hand, it is important that the clinician not be a "parental spy," but on the other hand, there may be some reporting requirements (e.g., in some cases relative to protection or child or for insurance reimbursement purposes; Bostic & King, 2007). Usually, an explanation to the adolescent or child of exactly what will be disclosed will be sufficient (e.g., recommendations for classroom modifications). On the other hand some information (e.g., relative to sexuality) may need to be confidential. Both the child and parents should understand that in some situations, usual confidentiality rules do not apply.

TABLE 3.4

LABORATORY TESTS TO CONSIDER IN CHILDHOOD PSYCHIATRIC DISORDERS

Lab Test	Disorder					
	MR or PDD	Mood	Psychosis	OCD Tics	Substance Abuse	Eating Disorders
Chromosomal testing	X		X			
Wood's (UV) lamp	X					
Monospot		X				
Thyroid		X	X			X
Lyme titer		X				
CBC	X	X	X		X	X
Serum chemistry	X	X	X		X	X
Lead level	X					
Throat culture ASO, antideoxyribonuclease B titers				X		
Urine drug screen		X	X		X	
CSF analysis		X	X			
Neuroimaging			X			
EEG	X					

ASO, antistreptolysin O antibody; CBC, completed blood count; CSF, cerebrospinal fluid; EEG, electroencephalography; MR, mental retardation; OCD, obsessive-compulsive disorder; PDD, pervasive development disorder; UV, ultraviolet.
Adapted from Bostic, J., & King, R. A. (2007). Clinical assessment of children and adolescents: Content and structure. In A. Martin & F. Volkmar (Eds.). *Lewis's Child and Adolescent Psychiatry: A Comprehensive Textbook*, 4th edition, p. 342. Philadelphia: Lippincott Williams & Wilkins.

Laboratory Studies and Collaborations with Primary Care Providers

Occasionally, results of laboratory studies may be helpful. Table 3.4 summarizes some of the situations in which laboratory studies might be obtained. Sometimes history or examination will suggest the potential presence of a medical condition (e.g., hypo- or hyperthyroidism). In actual practice, the "yield" of routine laboratory tests is relatively small, perhaps 1% of cases.

It is important that the evaluator maintain contact with the child's pediatrician or primary care provider, who will usually have had the longest history of professional contact with the child and family. Often, a pediatric physical examination will complement the results of the psychiatric assessment. Sometimes information in the pediatric medical record will be highly relevant to the psychiatrist (e.g., growth charts for a child with an eating disorder or documentation of a hearing loss or other sensory problem). It is also important for the pediatrician to know any medical interventions (e.g., in monitoring for side effects). The primary care provider can also consult regarding recommendations for additional tests or laboratory studies.

FORMULATION AND INTEGRATION: THE TREATMENT PLAN

The formulation of the case provides a context for understanding the child's symptoms and life circumstances, providing a set of hypotheses to be adapted and changed based on subsequent clinical encounters and additional information. A range of treatment options, including no treatment, is available. The formulation of the case should effectively communicate relevant information about the child and a rationale for treatment recommendations made. Core components of the formulation include the chief complaint, historical information, results of present evaluation, and so forth (see Table 3.5). The formulation can vary in length, breadth,

TABLE 3.5

CORE COMPONENTS TOWARD A FORMULATION OF A TREATMENT PLAN

Component	Details
Source	Patient, collaterals
Chief complaint	What brought the patient in
History of present illness	Symptoms, course, severity, pertinent negatives
Past psychiatric history	Previous evaluations, therapies, hospitalizations, medications and treatments; substance abuse history.
Past medical history	Treatments, illnesses, hospitalizations, surgeries, medications (including home remedies, homeopathy, and so on)
Family history	Pertinent positives and negatives in the family's psychiatric and medical history
Social history	Family constellation, peer relations, interactions with the law and social services
Education history	Schools, grades, report cards, special or regular education
Developmental history	Mother's pregnancy and labor, delivery, milestones during infancy; stages of motor, cognitive, social, and behavioral development
Psychological testing	IQ, tests of adaptive functioning, speech and language evaluation
Mental status exam	
Assessment	Diagnoses, hypotheses of causality
Plan	Treatment goals and options, collaterals to contact

Adapted from Bostic, J., & King, R. A. (2007). Clinical assessment of children and adolescents: Content and structure. In A. Martin & F. Volkmar (Eds.). *Lewis's Child and Adolescent Psychiatry: A Comprehensive Textbook*, 4th edition, p. 342. Philadelphia: Lippincott Williams & Wilkins.

and level of detail, depending on clinical circumstance. We have seen everything from two sentences ("child seen, diagnosis is autism") to a 30–page, single-spaced narrative of which 15 pages were detailed recommendations. The typical formulation usually occupies a middle ground between these two extremes. The formulation can follow any of several different models. Regardless of the model chosen, the formulation should endeavor to help parents, teachers, and other professionals (and the child or adolescent him- or herself) understand the patient's difficulties and explain them; these are two rather divergent goals. For example, at times, we may have a very good understanding of the child' experience but much less understanding of the cause of a particular symptom or syndrome.

The biopsychosocial approach is likely the most common formulation used in all of psychiatry. Developed originally by Engel, this model attempts a synthesis of biologic, psychological, and social factors in understanding the child's experience, symptoms, and life circumstances. Although this model emphasizes the importance of all three domains, in fact, the social domain is usually the one that received the least attention.

The four Ps model organizes the patient's condition into *predisposing, precipitating, perpetuating*, and *protective* factors. This model includes attention to vulnerability in the child; the factors that appear to precipitate current symptoms or difficulties; the factors that help the condition persist; and the areas of patient strength, resilience, and support. Provides a sample formulation based on the four Ps approach.

This approach has the advantage of allowing the biological, psychological, and social elements within each category. It has the disadvantages of a nonstandard format and less of an overall synthesis of understanding how all the various factors converge to explain the symptoms.

Both approaches are rather "agnostic" relative to diagnosis. In particular, the four Ps approach is less concerned with how and rather more concerned with why. Another approach focuses of four perspectives of psychiatry: *disease* (which entails knowledge about the specific clinical entity and its etiology, treatment, and prognosis), *dimensions* (based on vulnerabilities such as intellectual deficiency or personality style), *behaviors* that are either maladaptive or undesirable, and the *life story* or a reconstruction of narratives through talk therapy.

Sample Formulation Using the *Four* Ps approach

A 14-year-old boy presents to an emergency department (ED) from school, having been referred by his teacher first to a counselor and then to the ED after writing an essay in which he expressed suicidal ideation. Predisposing factors include a mother with a long history of depression treated with psychotherapy, a paternal uncle who committed suicide, and his parent's divorce with lengthy and often bitter custodial disputes. Precipitating factors include 3 weeks of poor sleep, decreased appetite, rumination about his guilt and helplessness in the context of his parent's divorce, as well as several recent stressors, including a test in school, which he is scared he might fail. Perpetuating factors include a desire not to engage in any sort of treatment because of stigma, his parents' denial that their conflicts affect their son, and a depression that has reached such depths that the patient is considering suicide. In his case, though, several protective factors can be identified, including the boy's popularity at school as a secretary of the student assembly and as catcher on the baseball team; his willingness to talk with a therapist after he comes in; his parents' care for his well-being despite their conflict; and the family's willingness to work together to help the boy through depression.

Reprinted with slight modification from Henderson, S. W., & Martin, A. (2007). Formulation and integration. In A. Martin and F. Volkmar (Eds.), *Lewis's Child and Adolescent Psychiatry: A Comprehensive Textbook*, 4th edition, p. 379. Philadelphia: Lippincott Williams & Wilkins.

A formulation based on the four perspectives would start with the clinical presentation and end with formulation of specific interventions.

In reality, of course, no single approach is entirely satisfactory. A disease model approach might work well for patients with schizophrenia or Rett syndrome but would work much less well in dealing with normative grief. Similarly, a behavioral approach can be used to target maladaptive behaviors, but the life story model would be more adaptable in dealing with stresses such as bereavement or dissatisfaction with one's life course. At present, a pluralistic approach acknowledges the multiple levels of explanation and need for more truly integrative scientific paradigms.

Regardless of which approach is adopted, the formulation should lead to specific, defendable treatment plan. The process of formulation should depending on an integrative process with an opportunity for the clinical to consolidate in understanding of the child and formulate a treatment plan. It should give the clinician an opportunity to understand and explain, to the extent possible, the presenting concerns. *Understanding* requires an intersubjective appreciation of the patient's experiences, hopes, and concerns while building an empathic relationship. *Explaining* has two dimensions, interpretation and explanation. The formulation can and should draw on various points of view in the attempt to understand the child and his or her difficulties. Finally, it should be emphasized that the format should take cultural context into account. This typically includes several components such as cultural identity, explanations of illness, adaptations to the environment, and any stresses. It is important for the clinician to be aware of areas of convergence and the cultures children participate in; few are more important than the culture of childhood itself. A good formulation will include the child's relationship to this rich culture, including the child's interactions with peers and participation in childhood rituals and his or her engagement with television, video games, sports, movies, and books.

For child psychiatry, in particular, a consideration of developmental factors is critical. The meaning of fantasy figures will, for example, differ markedly depending on the age of the child. It is one thing for a 3-year-old child to believe in Santa Claus or the Tooth Fairy and quite another for a 15-year-old adolescent to be receiving messages from the Mars Lander telling him how to behave. The formulation should attempt to place all major symptoms and problems within a broader context. The formulation of the case presents opportunities for synthesis of diverse observations and theoretical approaches and perspectives in an attempt to understand how a child or adolescent experiences the world and his or her own problems. In the best of circumstances, the formulation will be grounded in hard fact and observation and move to a level of hypothesis generation with the potential for modification based on experience and additional information. Particularly for children and adolescents, the question of the "right" diagnosis may be clarified only over time, but diagnosis aside, the formulation's aim should be providing a thoughtful, sympathetic portrait of the child.

APPENDIX 1

SAMPLE CLINICIAN QUESTIONS

Component	Example Parent Questions To Elicit ("Yes" responses warrant follow-up questions to clarify acts, context, intentions, and consequences.)	Example Child Questions ("Yes" responses warrant follow-up questions to clarify acts, context, intentions, consequences, and learning from these events.)
Reason for referral	Whose idea was it that [child] might need this evaluation? Who is most concerned about [child's] behavior? Has anyone else, such as other family members, school staff, or other agencies, encouraged this evaluation? What do you/they hope this evaluation will accomplish?	What did your parent(s) tell you about coming here today? Who wanted you to meet with me today? What did they say to you about us meeting? How do you feel about being here?
History of problem(s)	When did you first notice [child's] problem? How did the problem develop over time? How did you understand [child's] behavior?	What do you wish would be different? What is not going well for you? What do you think is making this such a hard time?
Functional assessment of problem behaviors	Where does the problem behavior occur most often? How does the problem impact [child] at home? At school? With peers? Is the problem behavior worse in one of these places? What usually occurs before right before the problem behavior? What happens after [child] does [problem behavior]? How do [parent, teacher, peers, friends] respond? Has anything changed to make the behavior worse or better?	When and where does the problem occur? What happens when you [exhibit symptoms]? What usually happens right before you [exhibit symptom]? How does your [parent, teacher, friends] respond when you [exhibit symptom]? How do you feel after you [exhibit symptom]?
Past problems	Did [child] have any problems this severe at an earlier point? What other significant difficulties has [child] had in the past?	Have there ever been any times when things were difficult? Have you had any times before where things were difficult? Has anyone ever been worried about you?

(continued)

APPENDIX 1
(CONTINUED)

Component	Example Parent Questions To Elicit ("Yes" responses warrant follow-up questions to clarify acts, context, intentions, and consequences.)	Example Child Questions ("Yes" responses warrant follow-up questions to clarify acts, context, intentions, consequences, and learning from these events.)
Comorbid symptoms	Does [child] have any other symptoms that trouble you? Does [child] have any other symptoms that interfere at home, school, or with friends? Have others identified any other problems they've noticed with [child]?	Is there anything else going on that you wish were different? Do you feel bad in any other ways? Do you have any difficulty sleeping, eating, or going to the bathroom? Is there anything you worry about? How often do you feel sad? Do you wish anything were different with your peers, family members, or teachers?
Substance use history	Has your child done anything to suggest use of substances? Have you detected your child to be drunk, high, or stoned/on drugs? Have you seen or found any drug paraphernalia that might be your child's? Has your child spoken about drinking, smoking, or substance use?	Have you ever been around any substances (alcohol, tobacco, marijuana, and so on)? Have you ever tried tobacco? Alcohol? Any other drugs? Do they help in any way? Have you ever been high, stoned, or intoxicated? Has that ever led to any problems for you? Have you ever tried to stop? How did that go?
Previous treatment(s)	What all has been attempted to address this in the past? Has [child] received any treatment(s) in the past for emotional or behavioral concerns?	Has anyone tried to help you with ___? Have you talked with anyone about these difficulties before? Have you ever taken any medicines for these difficulties?
Developmental history		
Basic functions	How did [child] progress with sleep? Did [child] always sleep through the night? How has [child's] appetite been? Has [child] ever been overweight? How do you feel about [child's] size or weight? What do you tell [child] about his or hr weight or appearance? How did toilet training progress with [child]? Has [child] had periods of wetting or soiling?	Do you have any trouble falling asleep? Staying asleep? How do you sleep through the night? Do you need or use a nightlight? Do you like it better when someone sleeps with you? How is your appetite? How do you feel about the way you look? What do others (peers, parents) say about your appearance? Do you have any difficulties going to the bathroom?
Psychomotor development	When did [child] start walking? What sports or activities has [child] participated in? Which ones have gone well? Not so well?	How do you do in sports? How do you do when you play with friends your age? Do you have any problems playing games, sports, music, or dancing?
Cognitive development	Did [child] show interest in things you pointed to? Did [child] point things out to you? When did [child] begin preschool or school? How did that go? How did [child] do with reading? With math? With writing? In which subjects did [child] do particularly well? Which subjects were more difficult?	Which subjects do you like best at school? Which subjects do you do best in at school? How do you like reading? Math? Writing? Is anything at school really hard for you to do? Is there anything you have trouble understanding? How do you get along with the other kids in your class? With your teacher?

APPENDIX 1
(CONTINUED)

Component	Example Parent Questions To Elicit ("Yes" responses warrant follow-up questions to clarify acts, context, intentions, and consequences.)	Example Child Questions ("Yes" responses warrant follow-up questions to clarify acts, context, intentions, consequences, and learning from these events.)
	How did [child] do each year in school? Did [child] ever receive any special educational services? Has [child] ever been suspended, expelled, or asked to leave as school? Did [child] ever have any periods of excessive absences? Did [child] ever fail in subjects or grades? Has [child] even had any summer school or after-school tutoring? Is there anything [child] particularly enjoys or does well at in school?	Has anyone ever helped you with school work? What do they do? Have you ever had to take any classes over? Have you ever done any grades over? Have you ever gone to school during the summer?
Interpersonal development	How did [child] relate to you as a child? How did [child] respond to your requests or directions? When did [child] start interacting with other children? How did that go? Did [child] have any significant attachments or relationships to others that ended? What kind of friends does [child] have at this point? How does [child] get along with these children? Does [child] get invited to play dates, birthday parties, or sleep-overs?	Who are some of your good friends now (when and where met, what do together, how often, and so on)? How often do you and [friend] play together? How long do you stay at [friend's house]? Do you spend the night at [friend's house]? How does that go (What do you do?)? Any rough spots between you and other kids? How come? Have you lost any good friends (because of moves, misunderstandings, and so on)?
Emotional development	Does [child] recognize when he or she is sad, really happy, etc.? How does [child] soothe him/herself when unhappy or in a bad mood? What is the child's prevailing or most common mood? How does the child respond to unexpected changes? Disappointments? Frustrations? Anxieties or depressed moods?	How often do you feel sad? Mad? Worried? Does anything in particular make you sad, mad, or worried? What do you do when you are feeling that way? Can you do anything to stop yourself from getting sad, mad, or worried? How do you calm yourself down?
Moral development	Does [child] recognize right from wrong? Does [child] describe any "principles" that guide his or her actions? How does [child] contend with mistakes or when confronted about doing something wrong? Has [child] ever deliberately hurt any animals or other kids? Bullied or been bullied by other kids? Does [child] show remorse after hurting someone? Does [child] anticipate consequences of his or her decisions? Does [child] consider consequences of decisions on others? Is [child] ever too perfectionistic or morally rigid?	Do you ever do things that you wish you hadn't? Do you ever hurt others even if it's not on purpose? What do you wish will happen when you [hit other, say something really mean, break or steal someone's toy]? What does happen when you do something that hurts or upsets [someone else]? Can you keep yourself from hitting or getting back at someone if you want to?

(continued)

APPENDIX 1
(CONTINUED)

Component	Example Parent Questions To Elicit ("Yes" responses warrant follow-up questions to clarify acts, context, intentions, and consequences.)	Example Child Questions ("Yes" responses warrant follow-up questions to clarify acts, context, intentions, consequences, and learning from these events.)
Trauma history	Has [child] ever been hurt or injured? Has [child] ever witnessed anything really bad or frightening? Has [child] described frightening dreams/nightmares? Has [child] ever made unusual comments about sex? Have you [parent] had any traumatic experiences that remind you of what [child] is going through?	Have you ever been hurt? Injured? Have you ever seen anything really bad? Frightening? Have you ever seen anyone get hurt badly? Do you ever have scary dreams or nightmares? Do you ever see or hear something that reminds you of something really scary? Has anyone ever tried to hurt you? Who did or would you tell if someone tried to hurt you?
Harm to self or others history	Has [child] ever talked about hurting himself? Others? Has [child] ever done things to inflict pain on himself? To hurt others? Has [child] ever hurt any animals? What happened? Has [child] ever been involved with school officials or police because of threats or harm toward others?	Have you ever thought about hurting yourself? Others? Have you every deliberately hurt yourself? How did you feel after you did ___? Have you ever hurt anyone else on purpose? How did you feel about that? How do you feel about that now? Have you ever hurt a pet or an animal? How did that feel? Has you ever gotten into trouble with anyone for talking about hurting yourself or someone else?
Family history	What were the circumstances surrounding the conception and pregnancy with [child]? Do [parents] agree on how to respond to [child]? Do you treat him or her differently than you were treated by your parents? Did [parents] grow up in similar type families? Is there anything [one parent] does quite differently from [other parent] or from your own parents? Has anyone on father's [mother's] side of the family had depression, anxiety, problems with attention or learning, tics, substance abuse problems, or any other mental illness? Has anyone in the family had serious medical problems? Has anyone in the family ever been psychiatrically or medically hospitalized? Incarcerated? [If relevant] What was that like for [the child]? What do you think [child] has inherited from [all parents, biological, and adoptive]?	Are you like anyone else in your family? Do you know if anyone in your family has ever felt like you do? How do your parents understand you?

APPENDIX 1
(CONTINUED)

Component	Example Parent Questions To Elicit ("Yes" responses warrant follow-up questions to clarify acts, context, intentions, and consequences.)	Example Child Questions ("Yes" responses warrant follow-up questions to clarify acts, context, intentions, consequences, and learning from these events.)
Family constellation history	Have there been any times when [child's parents] were separated or together? Have any changes in the family [loss or addition of parent, loss or addition of sibling or other in the home] contributed to [child's] symptoms? What kind of contact does [child] have with [parents, grandparents, primary caregiving relatives]? What does [child] say about [other parent, caregivers]?	Have either of your parents ever been away very long? Do you miss anyone from your family? Who do you get along best with in your home? Who do you have the hardest time with? Why?
Medical history	Has [child] ever had any medical illnesses or serious injuries? Been hospitalized? Had any operations? Was [child] physically ill before these symptoms started? Has [child] had any physical symptoms that occur with or since the emotional symptoms? Has [child] ever been allergic to anything?	Have you ever been really sick? Have you ever had to go to the hospital (what happened?) Have you ever had any surgeries (what was that like?)? Have you been physically sick since you have had problems with____?
Child's strengths	What is [child] good at? What does [child] do for fun? What does [child] do during the day? What does [child] want to do or wish he or she could do?	What do you most like to do? What are you really good at? What do your friends or other students think you are really good at? What would you like to be better at? Do you feel special in any way? What do you want to do when you grow up?
Child's media diet	What does [child] watch, read, or listen to? How much time does [child] spend watching television or movies? Listening to music? Reading magazines? How does television influence [child]? What effects do you think [child's] musical choices have on him or her? What impacts do you think those magazines have on [child]?	How much do you watch TV every day? Listen to music? Read for fun? What about [TV show, music, magazines] most appeals to you? How do you feel after watching, listening, or reading ____? Do you ever get into trouble after watching, listening, or reading ____?
Community and environmental supports	What is your neighborhood like? Do kids play outside much in your neighborhood? Are there any neighborhood problems or tensions? Is a language other than English spoken at home? If so, by whom, and does [child] also speak or understand that language? [If family is of recent immigrant origins], does [the child] still have close relatives there? Does he or she visit there often?	Outside of your home, where are you most happy? Are there any other adults who are special to you or work with you? Can you tell me about your best friends? Are there any kids that bother you or make you uncomfortable? Is there a group you feel a part of? Who do you "hang out" with? Is there a group you would rather be a part of? Are there particular others you'd like to hang out with?

(continued)

APPENDIX 1
(CONTINUED)

Component	Example Parent Questions To Elicit ("Yes" responses warrant follow-up questions to clarify acts, context, intentions, and consequences.)	Example Child Questions ("Yes" responses warrant follow-up questions to clarify acts, context, intentions, consequences, and learning from these events.)
	What is the family's religious tradition? Does [the child] attend services regularly or have strong religious identifications? What activities does [child] participate in? Are there others who work with [child]? Do you have any help or support managing these problems with [child]? How do your family members view [child's problems]? Does [child] benefit from interactions or participation with neighbors, scouting, hobbies, or shared interests with others?	Is there any place you really like to go to feel better? How have your symptoms affected your family?

Adapted from Bostic, J., & King, R. A. (2007). Clinical assessment of children and adolescents: Content and structure. In A. Martin & F. Volkmar (Eds.). *Lewis's Child and Adolescent Psychiatry: A Comprehensive Textbook*, 4th edition, pp. 333–326. Philadelphia: Lippincott Williams & Wilkins.

Selected Readings

Achenbach, T. (1991). *Manual for the Child Behavior Checklist/4-18 and 1991 Profile.* Burlington, VT: University of Vermont Department of Psychiatry.

American Psychiatric Association. (1994). *Diagnostic and Statistical Manual of Mental Disorders*, 4th edition. Washington, DC: Author.

Angold, A., Costello, E. J., & Egger, H. (2007). Diagnostic assessment: Structured interviewing. In A. Martin and F. Volkmar (Eds.). *Lewis's Child and Adolescent Psychiatry: A Comprehensive Textbook*, 4th edition, pp. 344–356. Philadelphia: Lippincott Williams & Wilkins.

Bell, R. Q., & Harper, L. V. (1977). *Child Effects on Adults.* Hillsdale, NJ: Erlbaum.

Bostic, J., & King, R. A. (2007). Clinical assessment of children and adolescents: Content and structure. In A. Martin & F. Volkmar (Eds.). *Lewis's Child and Adolescent Psychiatry: A Comprehensive Textbook*, 4th edition, p 324. Philadelphia: Lippincott Williams & Wilkins.

Bostic, J. Q., & Rho, Y. (2006). Target-symptom psychopharmacology: Between the forest and the trees. *Child and Adolescent Psychiatry Clinics of North America, 15*(1), 289–302.

Bostic, J. Q., Schlozman, S., Pataki, C., Ristuccia, C., Beresin, E. V., & Martin, A. (2003). From Alice Cooper to Marilyn Manson: The significance of adolescent antiheroes. *Academic Psychiatry, 27*(1), 54–62.

First, M. B., & Pincus, H. A. (2002). The DSM-IV Text Revision: Rationale and potential impact on clinical practice. *Psychiatric Services, 53*(3), 288–292.

Henderson, S. W., & Martin, A. (2007). Formulation and integration. In A. Martin and F. Volkmar (Eds.). *Lewis's Child and Adolescent Psychiatry: A Comprehensive Textbook*, 4th edition, pp. 377–382. Philadelphia: Lippincott Williams & Wilkins.

Hobbs, N. (Ed.). (1975). *Issues in the Classification of Children.* San Francisco: Jossey-Bass.

Indredavik, M. S., Vik, T., Heyerdahl, S., Kulseng, S., Fayers, P., & Brubakk, A. M. (2004). Psychiatric symptoms and disorders in adolescents with low birth weight. *Archives of Disease in Childhood Fetal Neonatal Edition, 89*(5), F445–F450.

King, R. A. (1997). Practice parameters for the psychiatric assessment of children and adolescents. *Journal of the American Academy of Child and Adolescent Psychiatry, 36*(10 suppl), 4S–20S.

King, R. A., & Schowalter, J. E. (2004). The clinical interview of the adolescent. In J. A. Wiener & M. K. Dulcan (Eds.). *Textbook of Child and Adolescent Psychiatry*, 3rd edition, pp. 113–116. Washington, DC: American Psychiatric Publishing.

Kupfer, D. A., First, M. B., & Regier, D. A. (2002). *A Research Agenda for DSM-V*. Washington, DC: American Psychiatric Publishing.

Pataki, C., Bostic, J. Q., & Schlozman, S. (2005). The functional assessment of media in child and adolescent psychiatric treatment. *Child and Adolescent Psychiatry Clinics of North America, 14*(3), 555–570, x.

Rutter, M. (1989). Annotation: Child psychiatric disorders in ICD-10. *Journal of Child Psychology and Psychiatry, 30,* 499–513.

Shemesh, E., Newcorn, J. H., Rockmore, L., et al. (2005). Comparison of parent and child reports of emotional trauma symptoms in pediatric outpatient settings. *Pediatrics, 115*(5), e582–e589.

Volkmar, F. R., Schwab-Stone, M., & First, M. (2007). Classification. In A. Martin & F. Volkmar, (Eds.). *Lewis's Child and Adolescent Psychiatry: A Comprehensive Textbook*, 4th edition, pp. 302–309. Philadelphia: Lippincott Williams & Wilkins.

Wallerstein, J. S., & Blakeslee, S. (2000). *The Unexpected Legacy of Divorce: A 25 Year Landmark Study*. New York: Hyperion.

Winnicott, D. W. (1971). *Therapeutic Consultations in Child Psychiatry*. London: Hogarth Press.

World Health Organization. (1992). Mental and behavioral disorders, clinical descriptions and diagnostic guidelines. In *International Classification of Diseases*, 10th edition. Geneva: World Health Organization.

CHAPTER 4 ■ AUTISM AND RELATED DISORDERS

BACKGROUND

Autism and the related disorders, also referred to as pervasive developmental disorders (PDDs) or autism spectrum disorders (ASDs), are a group of conditions characterized by significant social difficulties associated to varying degrees with communicative and behavioral problems. These conditions and their similarities and differences are listed in Table 4.1. Of these conditions, childhood autism (autistic disorder) has been the most extensively studied.

AUTISTIC DISORDER

Definition and Clinical Features

For a diagnosis of autism, characteristic problems in social interaction (autism) are required along with problems in communication and play as well as unusual restricted and repetitive interests. By definition, autism has its onset before age 3 years. Social problems are the central defining feature of autism and are weighted more heavily than other factors. International Classification of Diseases (ICD-10) criteria for the disorder are listed in Table 4.2. The condition was first described by Leo Kanner in 1943. Kanner noted that the children exhibited an apparently congenital inability to relate to others (autism) and were overly concerned with changes in the nonsocial environment. Hand flapping and other purposeless repetitive movements were common as were unusual aspects of language (when language developed at all). For example, Kanner mentioned that children with autism often repeated words or phrases, had trouble in pronoun use (referring to themselves in the third person), or had highly idiosyncratic language. For some years after his description, there was confusion about whether autism might represent the earliest form of childhood schizophrenia, but by the 1970s, it was clear that autism was a distinct condition. Similarly, there was speculation, particularly in the 1950s that parents might "cause" autism, such as through deviant parenting, but longitudinal data made it clear that autism was a strongly genetic, brain-based disorder.

Autism is an early-onset disorder. Most parents report concerns in the first year of the child's life, and about 90% are worried by age 2 years. Common concerns include language delay, social deviance, or odd interests in the nonsocial environment (Table 4.3). Although

TABLE 4.1

DIFFERENTIAL DIAGNOSTIC FEATURES OF AUTISM AND NONAUTISTIC PERVASIVE DEVELOPMENTAL DISORDERS

Feature	Autistic Disorder	Asperger Disorder	Rett's Disorder	Childhood Disintegrative Disorder	Pervasive Developmental Disorder Not Otherwise Specified
Age at recognition (months)	0–36	Usually >36	5–30	>24	Variable
Sex ratio	M > F	M > F	F (?M)	M > F	M > F
Loss of skills	Variable	Usually not	Marked	Marked	Usually not
Social skills	Very poor	Poor	Varies with age	Very poor	Variable
Communication skills	Usually poor	Fair	Very poor	Very poor	Fair to good
Circumscribed Interests	Variable (Mechanical)	Marked (facts)	NA	NA	Variable
Family history of similar problems	Sometimes	Frequent	Not usually	No	Sometimes
Seizure disorder	Common	Uncommon	Frequent	Common	Uncommon
Head growth decelerates	No	No	Yes	No	No
IQ range	Severe MR to normal	Mild MR to normal	Severe MR	Severe MR	Severe MR to normal
Outcome	Poor to good	Fair to good	Very poor	Very poor	Fair to good

MR, mental retardation.
Adapted with permission from Volkmar, F. R., & Cohen, D. Nonautistic pervasive developmental disorders. In R. Michaels & J. Cavenar (Eds.), *Psychiatry*, p. 4. Lippincott-Raven Publishers.

Kanner originally believed autism to be congenital but in a minority of cases (~20%), it appears that the child develops normally or near normally for some months before development slows or actually regresses. This phenomenon has been difficult to study given the reliance on retrospective report, but prospective studies of at-risk populations (e.g., siblings) should help to clarify aspects of this issue.

The social disturbance in autism is very distinctive and is an essential diagnostic feature. It cannot be accounted for simply by associated cognitive problems or intellectual deficiency (see Chapter 5). Normally developing infants are profoundly social from the first months of life, but those with autism appear to have little interest in the human face or social interaction. Early social problems can include lack of engagement as expressed in a failure to respond to name, failure to engage in joint attention, and reduced babble or vocal play; these problems are the basis for many early screening procedures (Coonrod & Stone, 2005; Volkmar & Wiesner, 2009).

Delays in speech are a common presenting problem, and communication problems are a major defining feature of the condition. In the past, about half of individuals with autism had little or no expressive speech; with earlier diagnosis and treatment, that number has decreased. Children who do talk have speech remarkable for echolalia (immediate or delayed repetition of words or phrases), problems with a monotonic voice, idiosyncratic language, pronoun reversal, and major difficulties with the social use of language (pragmatics). These problems are very specific to autism (i.e., they are not like those of children with other kinds of language delay).

Behavioral problems are often striking with a marked contrast between the child's lack of engagement with the social work (autism) and an overfocusing on aspects of the nonsocial environment (problems with change or preoccupations with sensory experiences). Often, the

TABLE 4.2

INTERNATIONAL CLASSIFICATION OF DISEASES (ICD-10) CRITERIA FOR CHILDHOOD AUTISM (F84.0)

A. Abnormal or impaired development is evident before the age of 3 years in at least one of the following areas:
   (1) Receptive or expressive language as used in social communication
   (2) The development of selective social attachments or of reciprocal social interaction; functional or symbolic play
B. A total of at least six symptoms from (1), (2), and (3) must be present, with at least two from (1) and at least one from each of (2) and (3).
   (1) Qualitative impairments in social interaction are manifest in at least two of the following areas:
       (a) Failure adequately to use eye-to-eye gaze, facial expression, body postures, and gestures to regulate social interaction
       (b) Failure to develop (in a manner appropriate to mental age and despite ample opportunities) peer relationships that involve a mutual sharing of interests, activities, and emotions
       (c) Lack of socioemotional reciprocity as shown by an impaired or deviant response to other people's emotions; lack of modulation of behavior according to social context; or a weak integration of social, emotional, and communicative behaviors
       (d) Lack of spontaneous seeking to share enjoyment, interests, or achievements with other people (e.g., a lack of showing, bringing, or pointing out to other people objects of interest to the individual)
   (2) Qualitative abnormalities communication as manifest in at least one of the following areas
       (a) Delay in, or total lack of, development of spoken language that is not accompanied by an attempt to compensate through the use of gestures or mime as an alternative mode of communication (often preceded by a lack of communicative babbling)
       (b) Relative failure to initiate or sustain conversational interchange (at whatever level of language skill is present) in which there is reciprocal responsiveness to the communications of the other person
       (c) Stereotyped and repetitive use of language or idiosyncratic use of words or phrases
       (d) Lack of varied spontaneous make-believe play or (when young) social imitative play
   (3) Restricted, repetitive, and stereotyped patterns of behavior, interests, and activities are manifested in at least one of the following:
       (a) An encompassing preoccupation with one or more stereotyped and restricted patterns of interest that are abnormal in content or focus or one or more interests that are abnormal in their intensity and circumscribed nature, although not in their content or focus
       (b) Apparently compulsive adherence to specific, nonfunctional routines or rituals
       (c) Stereotyped and repetitive motor mannerisms that involve either hand or finger tapping or twisting or complex whole-body movements
       (d) Preoccupations with part objects or nonfunctional elements of play materials (e.g., their odor, the feel of their surface, or the noise or vibration they generate)
C. The clinical picture is not attributable to the other varieties of pervasive developmental disorders; specific development disorder of receptive language (F80.2) with secondary socioemotional problems, reactive attachment disorder (F94.1), or disinhibited attachment disorder (F94.2); mental retardation (F70–F72) with some associated emotional or behavioral disorders; schizophrenia (F20) of unusually early onset; and Rett's syndrome (F84.12)

Reprinted with permission from: World Health Organization. (1993). *Mental and Behavioural Disorders (including disorders of psychological development): Diagnostic Criteria for Research.* ICD-10, pp. 147–149 (F84.0-F84.1). Geneva: WHO.

Key Concepts and Terms

Autism: being socially isolated; living in one's own world

Stereotyped movements: repetitive, apparently purposeless movements, particularly of the fingers or hands or whole body

Echolalia: repetition of words or phrases (as if echoed)

Idiosyncratic language: use of words or phrases in ways not generally understood by others

Resistance to change or **insistence on sameness:** lack of tolerance for changes in the physical environment; avoidance of novelty

child is very sensitive to nonspeech sounds but much less responsive to speech. Stereotyped (purposeless and repetitive) movements are common and include hand flapping, toe walking, and so forth, and they may consume much of the child's time. Unusual affective responses are also common, and play skills are often delayed.

Kanner initially believed children with autism probably had normal cognitive potential because the children often did well with nonverbal tasks (puzzles). The trouble they had with verbal activities was initially "written off" to negativism, but over time, it became clear that children with autism often have areas of cognitive strength and areas of great weakness and that poor performance should not simply be ascribed to lack of motivation. By around age 5 years, IQ scores (even when scattered) become more stable and begin to predict outcome. As with language development, earlier detection and intervention may well be leading to improved cognitive outcomes, presumably by way of minimizing the negative effects of autism on learning. Occasionally, unusual islets of marked ability (e.g., rote memory or block design) may be present. A few persons with "autistic savant skills" exhibit remarkable abilities in drawing, musical ability, or calendar calculation, but these abilities are usually accompanied by major deficits in other areas (see Hermelin, 2001). Typically, nonverbal skills are stronger than verbal skills. It is fairly common for autism to be associated with overall cognitive skills in the intellectual deficient range, although it appears that with early intervention, this number is decreasing.

Epidemiology and Demography

Many different studies of epidemiology have been conducted. The median rate of autism (strictly defined) is about one per 800 to 1000 people. Rates of autism appear to have increased in recent years, although this change also parallels greater recognition of cases, particularly in more able children as well as changes in diagnostic criteria; the latter were, in part, intended to improve detection in more cognitively able individuals.

There is a male predominance (three to five times more common), although in lower IQ groups, this is much less pronounced, and in high IQ cases much more pronounced. Among individuals with normal cognitive levels, the male predominance may be 25 or more to 1. Although cultural and ethnic issues may impact treatment and, to some extent, case detection, autism generally is remarkably similar around the world. The early impression that autism was more likely in children of parents with more education and higher occupational status proved to be incorrect and probably reflected bias in referral source.

Etiology

A host of findings support the importance of neurobiology in autism (Table 4.4 and Figure 4.1). Individuals with autism exhibit an increased frequency of physical anomalies, persistent primitive reflexes, and various neurologic soft signs, as well as increased abnormalities on electroencephalograms (EEGs). Neurobiological theories have focused on different brain regions related to social information processing. Given that some aspects of functioning are spared, it does it seems likely that some areas must be less affected (e.g., occasionally, a person

TABLE 4.3
SIGNS OF AUTISM IN THE FIRST THREE YEARS OF LIFE

	Age 0–12 Months	Age 12–36 Months
Social	Limited ability to anticipate being picked up Low frequency of looking at people Limited interest in interactional games Limited affection toward familiar people Content to be left alone	Abnormal eye contact Limited social referencing Limited interest in other children Limited social smile Low frequency of looking at people Limited range of facial expression Limited sharing of affect or enjoyment
Play	Little interest in interactive games	Limited functional play No pretend play Limited motor imitation
Communication	Poor response to name (does not respond when called) Does not frequently look at objects held by others	Low frequency of verbal or nonverbal communication Failure to share interests (e.g., through pointing, sharing, giving, or showing) Poor response to name Failure to respond to communicative gestures (pointing, giving, showing) Use of other's body as a tool (pulls hand to desired object without making eye contact, as if *hand* rather than person obtains object)
Restricted interests or behaviors	Mouths objects excessively Does not like to be touched	Unusual sensory behaviors Hyper- or hyposensitivity to sounds, texture, tastes, visual stimuli Inappropriate use of objects Repetitive interest or play

TABLE 4.4
NEUROBIOLOGICAL FINDINGS IN AUTISM

Increased (peripheral) serotonin levels
Persistent "primitive" reflexes
Increased head size (macrocephaly) in younger children
Changes in brain morphology or cytoarchitecture
Failure to activate fusiform face region
High rates of EEG abnormality or seizure disorder

EEG, electroencephalogram.
Reprinted from Volkmar, F. R., Lord, C., Klin, A., et al. (2007). Autism and the pervasive developmental disorders. In A. Martin & F. Volkmar (Eds.), *Lewis's Child and Adolescent Psychiatry: A Comprehensive Textbook*, p. 386. Philadelphia: Lippincott, Williams & Wilkins.

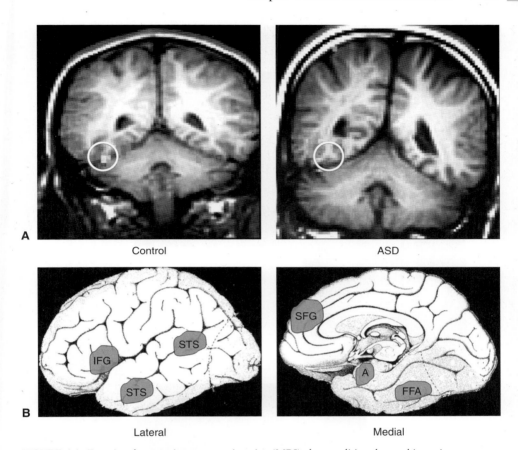

FIGURE 4.1. Functional magnetic resonance imaging (MRI) abnormalities observed in autism spectrum disorder (ASD). **A.** These coronal MRI images show the cerebral hemispheres above, the cerebellum below, and a *circle* over the fusiform gyrus of the temporal lobe. The examples illustrate the frequent finding of hypoactivation of the fusiform gyrus to faces in an adolescent boy with ASD (*right*) compared with an age- and IQ-matched healthy control subject (*left*). Note the lack of face activation in the boy with ASD but average levels of nonface object activation. **B.** Schematic diagrams of the brain from lateral and medial orientations illustrating the broader array of brain areas found to be hypoactive in ASD during a variety of cognitive and perceptual tasks that are explicitly social in nature. Some evidence suggests that these areas are linked to form a "social brain" network. A = amygdale (hypoactive during a variety of social tasks); FG = fusiform gyrus, also known as the fusiform face area (hypoactive during perception of personal identity); IFG = inferior frontal gyrus (hypoactive during facial expression imitation); pSTS = posterior superior temporal sulcus (hypoactive during perception of facial expressions and eye gaze tasks); SFG = superior frontal gyrus (hypoactive during theory of mind tasks, i.e., when taking another person's perspective). Reprinted from Volkmar, F., Lord, C., Klin, A., Schultz, R., Cook E. (2007). Autism and the Pervasive Developmental Disorders. In A. Martin & F. Volkmar (Eds.), *Lewis' Child and Adolescent Psychiatry*, p. 387. Philadelphia: Lippincott Williams & Wilkins.

severely impaired with autism may have unusual musical or drawing ability or remarkable memory skills). Increasingly, sophisticated neuroimaging methods have suggested a possible role for the amygdala (e.g., in social perception and social thinking) as well as in portions of the frontal lobe and areas of the brain involved in social information processing. Overall brain size in autism becomes increased in those with autism in the first years of life, possibly suggesting

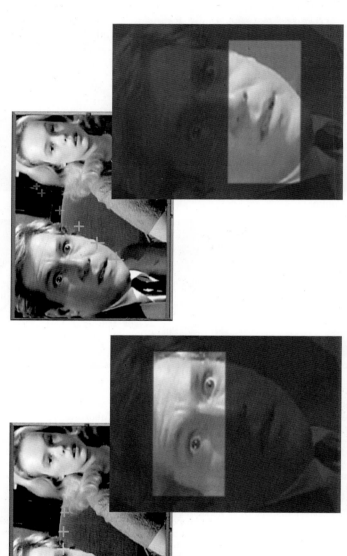

FIGURE 4.2. Successive visual focus of a typically developing individual (*top left*) and a person with autism (*top right*) shown a film clip of a young couple observing a frightening event. Whereas the individual who is typically developing focuses on the upper half of the face while the individual with autism is drawn to the mouth region. (Adapted and reprinted with permission from Klin, A., Jones, W., Schultz, R., Volkmar, F., & Cohen, D. (2002). Defining and quantifying the social phenotype in autism. *American Journal of Psychiatry*, 159:895–908.)

abnormalities in neural connectivity. Studies using functional magnetic resonance imaging (fMRI) have shown underactivation of the fusiform gyrus during facial recognition tasks, an observation consistent with a large literature suggesting important differences in processing of faces and face-like stimuli (Figure 4.2). Difficulties with social information processing are also suggested by studies of eye tracking in individuals with autism showing that individuals with autism are more preoccupied with less socially salient aspects of scenes and may overfixate on less relevant details. Available postmortem studies have revealed some abnormalities in the limbic system and other areas involved in social cognition. Some animal models (e.g., based on lesion work) have been proposed.

A strong role of genetic factors is suggested the greatly increased risk for autism in siblings. Similarly, risk is increased for monozygotic over same-sex dizygotic twins. It appears likely that multiple genes are involved. Considerable interest in the lay press has centered on the potential role of immunization, mercury exposure, or other environmental factors and autism, but supporting data are generally quite weak (see Offit, 2008 and Wing & Potter, 2008, for reviews).

Differential Diagnosis and Assessment

Autism must be differentiated from other PDD as well as other developmental disorders such as language disorders, severe deprivation, and sensory impairment (particularly deafness). Key diagnostic differences among the various PDDs are summarized in Table 4.1. In mental retardation without autism, social skills are usually on a par with cognitive development, and in language disorders, social skills may be well preserved even in the face of major language vulnerabilities.

Individuals with autism have problems in multiple areas of functioning. Cognitive assessment typically reveals significant scatter with social and language skills lower than would be expected given the child's nonverbal abilities. Efforts of a range of specialists are often needed to assess aspects of the child's development with the goal of developing a comprehensive intervention program. Various tests can be used to evaluate intelligence, communication, and motor skills; children with autism can be challenging to test, and experienced examiners are often needed. The assessment should address the issue of adaptive skills (i.e., the child's capacity to generalize skills to "real-world" settings). Observation of the child in more and less structured settings is helpful. Various rating skills and checklists can assist diagnosis but do not replace thoughtful assessment. Several excellent resources are available for parents, teachers, and professionals that summarize diagnostic assessments (Goldstein, Naglieri, & Ozonoff, 2009). Table 4.5 summarizes evaluation procedures.

The strongest associations of autism are with a handful of medical conditions. Probably the strongest connection is with epilepsy, which develops in about 20% of individuals with strictly diagnosed autism. Autism is also observed at higher than expected rates in connection with two strongly genetic conditions, fragile X syndrome and tuberous sclerosis. Brain size appears to be increased in toddlers with autism, although this difference becomes less pronounced over time. Medical assessment should include a careful medical and family history. Testing for fragile X syndrome and of hearing is typically indicated. More extensive genetic testing is indicated by physical examination or family history and has been increasingly productive as technology has advanced. Signs of possible seizures should prompt EEG and neurological examination. Neuroimaging studies may be indicated by examination or history.

Treatment

A growing body of work has supported the importance of behavioral and educational interventions in autism (Volkmar & Wiesner, 2009). Effective programs typically involve behavior modification and special education procedures designed to facilitate engagement and learning. Psychotherapy is not usually helpful except in carefully selected cases. Drug treatments may help with agitation and behavioral difficulties. For example, the drug risperidone has now been approved for use in autism after double-blind, placebo-controlled studies of the use of

TABLE 4.5

EVALUATION PROCEDURES: AUTISM AND PERVASIVE DEVELOPMENTAL DISORDERS

1. Historical information
   Early development and characteristics of development
   Age and nature of onset
   Medical and family history
2. Developmental and psychological assessment
   Intellectual level and profile of learning
   Communicative assessment (receptive and expressive language skills, use of nonverbal communication, pragmatic use of language)
   Adaptive behavior (ability to generalize skills to real-world settings)
   Occupational and physical therapy assessments as appropriate
3. Psychiatric examination
   Nature of social relatedness (eye contact, attachment behaviors, reciprocity, insight)
   Behavioral features (stereotypy or self-stimulation, resistance to change, unusual sensitivities to the environment)
   Language or communication difficulties (echolalia, presence of communicative speech, and so on)
   Play skills (nonfunctional use of play materials, symbolic play, and imagination)
4. Medical evaluations
   Search for associated medical conditions, genetic abnormalities, presence of seizures (with additional tests as needed)
   Hearing test (if indicated)
   Additional consultation (neurologic, pediatric, genetic) as indicated by history and current Examination (e.g., EEG, CT or MRI scan, chromosome analysis)

CT, computed tomography; EEG, electroencephalography; MRI, magnetic resonance imaging.
Reprinted with permission from Volkmar, F. R., Lord, C., Klin, A., et al. (2007). Autism and the pervasive developmental disorders. In A. Martin & F. Volkmar (Eds.), *Lewis's Child and Adolescent Psychiatry: A Comprehensive Textbook*, p. 391. Philadelphia: Lippincott, Williams & Wilkins.

this agent to deal with agitation and problem behaviors. Other drug treatments can also be helpful. Many alternative treatments (for which substantitive data are lacking) are available and frequently used by parents; it is important that parents understand that it is important not to pursue unproven treatments if this is done at the expense of interventions with proven effectiveness.

Course and Prognosis

The diagnosis of infants with autism is increasingly common but can be a challenge until ages 3 to 4 years (sometimes it is only by this age that all required features develop). Delays in case detection remain common, but increased public awareness and professional education have helped to address this problem. Often by school age, children with autism become more socially interested, although behavioral problems may also be more common. These can include agitation and sometimes self-injurious behaviors that may prompt drug treatments. Some adolescents make major gains in functioning, but others lose skills. As noted earlier, intervention and more intensive intervention do appear to be improving long-term outcome with more individuals, as adults, able to achieve personal independence and self-sufficiency.

Case Report: Autistic Disorder

John was the second of two children born to middle-class parents after a normal pregnancy, labor, and delivery. As an infant, John appeared undemanding and relatively placid; his motor development proceeded appropriately, but his language development was delayed. Although his parents indicated that they were first concerned about his development when he was 18 months of age and still not speaking, in retrospect they noted that compared with their previous child, he had seemed relatively uninterested in social interaction and the social games of infancy. Stranger anxiety had never really developed, and John did not exhibit differential attachment behaviors toward his parents. Their pediatrician initially reassured John's parents that John was a "late talker," but they continued to be concerned. Although John seemed to respond to some unusual sounds, the pediatrician obtained a hearing test when John was 24 months old, and levels of hearing appeared adequate for development of speech. John was referred for developmental evaluation. At age 24 months, John's motor skills were age appropriate, and he exhibited some nonverbal problem-solving skills close to age level. His language and social development, however, were severely delayed, and he was noted to be resistant to changes in routine and unusually sensitive to aspects of the inanimate environment. His play skills were quite limited, and he used play materials in unusual and idiosyncratic ways. His older sister had a history of some learning difficulties, but the family history was otherwise negative. A comprehensive medical evaluation revealed a normal electroencephalogram and computed tomography scan; genetic screening and chromosome analysis results were normal as well.

John was enrolled in a special education program, where he gradually began to speak. His speech was characterized by echolalia, extreme literalness, a monotonic voice quality, and pronoun reversal. He rarely used language in interaction and remained quite isolated. By school age, John had developed some evidence of differential attachments to family members; he also had developed a number of self-stimulatory behaviors and engaged in occasional periods of head banging. Extreme sensitivity to change continued. Intelligence testing revealed marked scatter, with a full-scale IQ in the moderately retarded range. As an adolescent, John's behavioral functioning deteriorated, and he developed a seizure disorder. Now an adult, he lives in a group home and attends a sheltered workshop. He has a rather passive interactional style but exhibits occasional outbursts of aggression and self-abuse.

Comment: With earlier intervention, more children with autism are doing better. Unfortunately, in this case, although the child developed speech, his overall outcome has not been as good as might have been hoped.

Adapted from Volkmar, F. R., Lord, C., Klin, A., & Cook, E. (2002). Autism and the pervasive developmental disorders. In M. Lewis (Ed.), *Child and Adolescent Psychiatry: A Comprehensive Textbook*, p. 595. Philadelphia: Lippincott Williams & Wilkins.

RETT'S DISORDER

Definition and Clinical Features

In Rett's disorder, early development is normal as is head circumference, but then in the first years of life (usually before age 12 months), head growth slows, and development deteriorates. Unusual and characteristic hand washing stereotyped mannerisms develop as purposeful hand

TABLE 4.6

INTERNATIONAL CLASSIFICATION OF DISEASES (ICD-10) CRITIERA FOR RETT'S DISORDER

A. Apparently normal prenatal and perinatal period and apparently normal psychomotor development through the first 6 months and normal head circumference at birth

B. Deceleration of head growth between 5 months and 4 years and loss of acquired purposeful hand skills between 6 and 30 months of age that is associated with concurrent communication dysfunction and impaired social interactions and appearance of poorly coordinated or unstable gait or trunk movements

C. Development of severely impaired expressive and receptive language together with severe psychomotor retardation

D. Stereotyped midline hand movements (e.g., hand wringing or washing) with an onset at or after the time that purposeful hand movements are lost

Reprinted with permission from (2003). *International Classification of Diseases, 10th edition.* Geneva: World Health Organization.

movements are lost. The child develops significant developmental delays, including language delays. The condition was first reported Rett in 1966, who initially believed that it might represent a form of autism; over time, it became clear that the more "autistic like" phase was generally confined to the preschool years. The clinical picture then varies over time, but generally, individuals have more noteworthy cognitive and motor problems, and social delays are much less striking. Diagnostic criteria for Rett's disorder are provided in Table 4.6.

Epidemiology and Demography

The disorder is relatively uncommon, with a prevalence of between one in 15,000 and one in 22,000 females. Although males can exhibit Rett's disorder, it probably often proves lethal in utero. Recognition of the gene causing Rett's disorder has led to an awareness of a greater range of clinical presentation.

Etiology

Since the disorder was included in *Diagnostic and Statistical Manual* (DSM-IV), it has been found to be associated with a specific genetic defect in the MECP2 gene on the X chromosome; this gene is present in most cases.

Differential Diagnosis and Assessment

The history and clinical presentation in more "classic" cases of Rett's disorder are highly distinctive. Other neurologic conditions that can lead to regression should be considered in the differential diagnosis. EEG abnormalities and seizure disorder are common. Other medical difficulties include problems with respiration, scoliosis, movement, eating, and growth.

Course and Prognosis

There is some potential for confusion with autism in the preschool years, although much less so by the time the child achieves school age. The clinical stages are summarized in Table 4.7.

Case Report: Rett's Disorder

Darla was born at term after an uncomplicated pregnancy. An amniocentesis had been obtained because of maternal age, and results were normal. At birth, Darla was in good condition; her weight, height, and head circumference were all near the 50th percentile. Her development during the first months of life was within normal limits. At around 8 months of age, her development seemed to stagnate, and her interest in the environment, including the social environment, waned. Her developmental milestones then became markedly delayed; she was just starting to walk at her second birthday and had no spoken language. Evaluation at that time revealed that her head growth had decelerated. Some self-stimulatory behaviors were present. Marked cognitive and communicative delays were noted on formal testing. Darla began to lose purposeful hand movements and developed unusual "hand washing" stereotyped behaviors. By age 6 year, her electroencephalogram was abnormal, and her purposeful hand movements were markedly impaired. Subsequently, she developed truncal ataxia and breath-holding spells, and her motor skills deteriorated further.

Comment: The discovery of the genetic basis of Rett's disorder has opened new possibilities both for diagnostic confirmation and research on the condition.

Adapted from Volkmar, F. R., Lord, C., Klin, A., & Cook, E. (2002). Autism and the pervasive developmental disorders. In M. Lewis (Ed.), *Child and Adolescent Psychiatry: A Comprehensive Textbook*, p. 595. Philadelphia: Lippincott Williams & Wilkins.

Treatment

No specific treatments are available, but supportive treatments can include special education and occupational, physical, and respiratory therapies. Care should be used regarding medications that might lower the seizure threshold. It is hoped that the discovery of the Rett's disorder gene may lead to new treatments.

TABLE 4.7

CLINICAL STAGES OF RETT'S DISORDER

Stage	Approximate Age	Clinical Profile
1. Onset	6–18 months	Motor growth slows, onset of hypotonia
2. Rapid destructive	1–4 years	Loss of acquired abilities, loss of purposeful hand movements, decline in social communication skills, ataxia or apraxia, breathing difficulties
3. Plateau	2–10 years	Autistic-like features diminish, seizure onset, communication skills may improve, scoliosis and truncal ataxia and apraxia
4. Late motor deterioration	10+ years	Progressive muscle wasting, scoliosis, decreased mobility, cognitive functioning stable, seizures may decrease

Adapted from Van Acker, R., Loncola, J., & Van Acker, E. (2005). Rett syndrome: A pervasive developmental disorder. In F. R. Volkmar, R. Paul, A. Klin, & D. Cohen (Eds.), *Handbook of Autism and Pervasive Developmental Disorders,* vol. 1, p. 133. Hoboken, NJ: Wiley.

ASPERGER DISORDER

Definition and Clinical Features

In 1944, Asperger described a group of boys who were verbally precocious but socially quite impaired. Unaware of Kanner's work, he referred to the condition as "autistic psychopathy" or "autistic personality disorder." The boys were socially isolated, tended to intellectualize their feelings, and engaged in long-winded conversations about topics of special interest to them. Asperger noted that the special interests interfered with learning and intruded on family life. These boys were motorically clumsy, and Asperger noted similar problems in fathers of his patients. Asperger's report was largely recognized until 1981, when Lorna Wing published an influential review. Although officially recognized, aspects of the definition of the disorder and its validity apart from autism (and other) conditions remain controversial. Criteria for Asperger disorder are provided in Table 4.8.

In Asperger disorder, there are severe impairments in social interaction and restricted interests, but there is no clinically significant delay in spoken or receptive language, cognitive development, self-help skills, or curiosity about the environment. All-absorbing and intense circumscribed interests as well motor clumsiness are typical of the condition but are not required for diagnosis. The criteria are the topic of much debate, and it is likely that changes will be made in future versions of the DSM. The diagnostic concept is, however, of much interest because, for research purposes, the constellation of marked social vulnerability in the face of good language (but not communication) skills may represent a different pathway into social vulnerabilities. It may have important treatment implications as well.

Asperger disorder requires significant impairments in social interaction of the type seen in autism associated with restricted patterns of interest and activities (often taking the form of highly circumscribed interests). However, in contrast to autism, there should be no clinically significant delay in language acquisition or in cognitive and self-help skills. Individuals with Asperger disorder are often socially isolated; they are often interested in social interaction but are unable to engage appropriately with others because of their eccentric social style. For older individuals, lack of social sensitivity may lead to innumerable social gaffes

TABLE 4.8

INTERNATIONAL CLASSIFICATION OF DISEASES (ICD-10) CRITERIA FOR ASPERGER SYNDROME

A. A lack of any clinically significant general delay in spoken or receptive language or cognitive development. Diagnosis requires that single words should have developed by 2 years of age or earlier and that communicative phrases be used by 3 years of age or earlier. Self-help skills, adaptive behavior, and curiosity about the environment during the first 3 years should be at a level consistent with normal intellectual development. However, motor milestones may be somewhat delayed, and motor clumsiness is usual (although not a necessary diagnostic feature). Isolated special skills, often related to abnormal preoccupations, are common, but are not required for diagnosis.
B. Qualitative abnormalities in reciprocal social interaction (criteria as for autism).
C. An unusually intense circumscribed interest or restricted, repetitive, and stereotyped patterns of behavior, interests, and activities (criteria as for autism; however, it would be less usual for these to include either motor mannerisms or preoccupations with part objects or nonfunctional elements of play materials).
D. The disorder is not attributable to the other varieties of pervasive developmental disorder, schizotypal disorder, or simple schizophrenia.

Reprinted, with permission, from WHO (1993). *International Classification of Diseases, 10th edition: Diagnostic Criteria for Research*. Geneva: WHO.

Case Report: Asperger Disorder

Tom was an only child. Birth, medical, and family histories were unremarkable. His motor development was somewhat delayed, but his communicative milestones were advanced; he talked before he walked. His parents became concerned about him at age 4 years when he was enrolled in a nursery school and was noted to have marked difficulties in peer interaction that were so pronounced that he could not continue in the program. In grade school, he was enrolled in special education classes and was noted to have some learning problems. His greatest difficulties arose in peer interaction; he was viewed as markedly eccentric and had no friends. His preferred activity, watching the weather channel on television, was pursued with great interest and intensity; this had been an interest since preschool. On examination at age 13 years, he had markedly circumscribed interests and exhibited pedantic and odd patterns of communication with a monotonic voice quality. Psychological testing revealed an IQ within the normal range with marked scatter evident and significantly higher verbal than nonverbal skills. Formal communication examination revealed age-appropriate skills in receptive and expressive language but marked impairment in pragmatic language skills. Tom has now gone on to college where he has, with considerable support, done well.

Comment: Preservation of language (if not always communication) skills in people with Asperger disorder presents some important strengths for treatment.

(e.g., as the individual makes true, but highly inappropriate, comments to a conversational partner).

In his original description, Asperger emphasized that often children with the condition talked before they walked or that words were the child's lifeline. Major difficulties in *communication* are typical as are differences in prosody (the musical aspects of speech) with a restricted intonation pattern. The usual form of restricted interest in Asperger disorder centers around collecting information about a specific, sometimes very esoteric, topic (e.g., weather, the stock market, the operas of Wagner, telegraph line pole insulators, deep fat fryers). Although the topic may change over time, it tends to dominate the individual's life and conversation and that of the family as well.

Epidemiology and Demography

If relatively stringently defined, the disorder is less common than autism (e.g., about four cases per 10,000). Boys are clearly more commonly affected than girls. Individuals with Asperger disorder appear to be at increased risk for depression in adolescence.

Etiology

The cause of Asperger disorder remains unknown, although Asperger highlighted the familiality of the condition. The highest rates of family comorbidity are reported if more stringent definitions of Asperger are used. There is some likelihood that autism and Asperger disorder are etiologically related, with case studies reporting both conditions in different family members. There appears to be a strong association of Asperger disorder with the nonverbal learning disability (NVLD) profile (see Chapter 6). Overlap with the concept of right hemisphere syndrome or developmental disabilities or semantic-pragmatic disorder have also been suggested.

Differential Diagnosis and Assessment

Several features help distinguish between autism and Asperger disorder. Both conditions share marked social vulnerabilities, but vocabulary and early language tend to be preserved in Asperger disorder (see Table 4.1). Similarly, parental concern develops later, and motor delays and clumsiness are often present in individuals with Asperger disorder. Psychological testing often reveals verbal skills that are much stronger than nonverbal, and the NLVD profile is more frequent; this profile can have important implications for intervention (e.g., favor verbally mediated strategies different than those more typically used in autism; Klin et al., 2005). As already noted, the greater cognitive ability and genetic and family history factors may increase the risk for depression in adolescents and young adults. Case reports have appeared in which Asperger disorder has been associated with specific abnormalities in the right hemisphere.

Course and Prognosis

Given the relative recency with which this condition has been officially recognized, it is not surprising that follow-up and longitudinal data are limited. Individuals can attend regular school and profit from supports around social and communication skills. Compared with individuals with autism, outcome in those with Asperger disorder is significantly better. Asperger disorder is frequently associated with other problems in childhood such as attentional problems, and overactivity may be present. In adolescents and adults, there has been a suggestion, based on case reports, of an increased risk of psychosis, but there is also a clear potential for misdiagnosis. There is also the potential for troubles with the legal system, although much of this stems from poor social judgment, inflexible styles, and, paradoxically, overly moralistic (rule governed) behavior.

Treatment

Treatment shares many similarities with that used for individuals with autism with the major exception related to preservation of verbal abilities in Asperger disorder (Klin, et al., 2005). Thus, verbal mediation can be extremely helpful through specific teaching and counseling. Academic strengths can be capitalized on, and areas of weakness (e.g., social skills, fine motor and gross motor problems) should be addressed. This pattern of strengths and weaknesses should inform the intervention program. Thus, the use of verbal scripts and routines may be helpful, and the tendency to rely rigidly on rules and routines can be used to teach. Roleplaying, homework, and supportive psychotherapy can be extremely helpful. Despite what appear to be good verbal abilities, the support of a speech-communication specialist can be extremely helpful. Use of laptops and organization aids can help individuals focus on communication and social skills.

CHILDHOOD DISINTEGRATIVE DISORDER

Definition and Clinical Description

In this rare condition an "autistic like" syndrome is preceded by years of normal development. The condition was first described by Heller in 1908. The term has also been described as disintegrative psychosis or Heller's syndrome. The condition was not included in either DSM-III or DSM-III-R, on the assumption that the condition was almost always the function of some identifiable medical condition, but review of cases has not supported this. Furthermore, in general, the child loses skills and then development stabilizes, and the outcome appears to be significantly worse than for individuals with autism. Early development is normal up to at least age 2 years. The condition's onset can be gradual or more acute, typically between ages 3 and 4 years. Skills must be lost in at least two areas, including communication, social interaction,

TABLE 4.9

INTERNATIONAL CLASSIFICATION OF DISEASES (ICD-10) CRITERIA FOR OTHER CHILDHOOD DISINTEGRATIVE DISORDER

A. An apparently normal development up to the age of at least 2 years. The presence of normal age-appropriate skills in communication, social relationships, play, and adaptive behavior at age 2 years or later is required for the diagnosis.

B. A definite loss of previously acquired skills at about the time of onset of the disorder. The diagnosis requires a clinical significant loss of skills (and not just a failure to use them in certain situations) in at least two of the following areas:
  (1) Expressive or receptive language
  (2) Play
  (3) Social skills or receptive language
  (4) Bowel or bladder control
  (5) Motor skills

C. Qualitatively abnormal social functioning manifest in at least two of the following areas:
  (1) Qualitative abnormalities in reciprocal social interaction (of the type defined for autism)
  (2) Qualitative abnormalities in communication (of the type defined for autism)
  (3) Restricted repetitive and stereotyped patterns of behavior, interests, and activities, including motor stereotypies and mannerisms

D. The disorder is not attributable to other varies of pervasive developmental disorder, acquired aphasia with epilepsy, elective mutism, schizophrenia, or Rett's disorder.

Reprinted with permission from WHO (2003). *International Classification of Diseases, 10th edition.* Geneva: World Health Organization.

toileting, or motor abilities. There may be a period of anxiety or agitation before onset. When it is established, it closely resembles autism. Social and communication problems of the type seen in autism are observed, as are stereotyped movements (Table 4.9).

Epidemiology and Demography

The condition is clearly rare, in the range of approximately one per 100,000 children. Boys are more likely to be affected.

Etiology

The cause is unknown, but neurobiological factors are likely. There are high rates of EEG abnormalities and seizure disorders. The condition has been associated with various general medical conditions, although usually despite an intensive search for such conditions, they are not typically found. Given the highly distinctive pattern of onset, a role for genetic factors seems likely.

Differential Diagnosis and Evaluation

Assessment and the differential diagnosis are similar to those for autistic disorder. However, a search for associated medical conditions is indicated but typically is negative. Many different medical conditions are potentially associated with regression (see Volkmar, Koenig, and State, 2005).

Case Report: Childhood Disintegrative Disorder

Bob's early history was within normal limits. By age 2 years, he was speaking in sentences, and his development appeared to be proceeding appropriately. At age 40 months, he was noted to exhibit, abruptly, a period of marked behavioral regression shortly after the birth of a sibling. He lost previously acquired skills in communication and was no longer toilet trained. He became uninterested in social interaction, and various unusual self-stimulatory behaviors became evident. Comprehensive medical examination failed to reveal any conditions that might account for this developmental regression. Behaviorally, he exhibited features of autism. At follow-up at age 12 years, he still was not speaking, apart from an occasional single word, and was severely retarded.

Comment: Despite the prolonged period of normal development and previously normal language, the outcome in this case is, unfortunately, rather typical for children who develop this "late onset" form of autism.

Adapted from Volkmar, F. R., Lord, C., Klin, A., & Cook, E. (2002). Autism and the pervasive developmental disorders. In M. Lewis (Ed.), *Child and Adolescent Psychiatry: A Comprehensive Textbook*, p. 595. Philadelphia: Lippincott Williams & Wilkins.

About 20% of children with autism exhibit some reported regression after some words develop. For childhood disintegrative disorder (CDD), early development should be clearly normal through at least 2 years of age. In Rett's disorder, head growth does slow, and the unusual hand washing or wringing movements are present. There may be some potential for confusion with very early onset childhood schizophrenia, although in this condition, the more autistic features do not usually develop.

Course and Prognosis

In about 75% of cases, the child's behavior deteriorates and then stabilizes with minimal recovery. Occasionally, significant recovery occurs but in instances associated with a progressive neuropathological process and then deterioration continues. Unless associated with such a condition, life expectancy is presumed normal. The outcome appears to be generally poor.

Treatment

Behavioral and educational interventions as used in autism are indicated. The focus is on helping the child relearn basic skills. Pharmacologic treatments may help with specific symptoms.

PERVASIVE DEVELOPMENTAL DISORDER NOT OTHERWISE SPECIFIED

The term *pervasive developmental disorder not otherwise specified* (PDD-NOS) and the equivalent term *atypical autism* refer to a residual category for individuals with difficulties suggestive of autism or autism spectrum diagnosis but who do not meet specific criteria for autism or another explicitly defined condition in this group. Historically, the concept has some overlap with Rank's term *atypical personality development*. Practically, the term refers to a relatively large group (probably about one in 150 children) of children with problems in social interaction and either communication or restricted interests and behaviors.

Case Report: Pervasive Developmental Disorder Not Otherwise Specified

Leslie was the oldest of two children. She was noted to be a difficult baby who was not easy to console but whose motor and communicative development seemed appropriate. She was socially related and sometimes enjoyed social interaction but was easily overstimulated. She was noted to exhibit some unusual sensitivities to aspects of the environment and, at times of excitement, exhibited some hand flapping. Her parents sought evaluation when she was 4 years of age because of difficulties in nursery school. Leslie was noted to have problems with peer interaction. She was often preoccupied with possible adverse events. At evaluation, she was noted to have both communicative and cognitive functions within the normal range. Although differential social relatedness was present, Leslie had difficulty using her parents as sources of support and comfort. Behavioral rigidity was noted, as was a tendency to impose routines on social interaction. Leslie was enrolled in a therapeutic nursery school where she made significant gains in social skills. Subsequently, she was placed in a transitional kindergarten and did well academically, although problems in peer interaction and unusual affective responses persisted. As an adolescent, she describes herself as a "loner" who has difficulties with social interaction and who tends to enjoy solitary activities.

Comment: Often the outcome of children with pervasive developmental disorder not otherwise specified is better than those with more classical autism. Comorbid attentional or affective problems can arise in adolescence.

Adapted from Volkmar, F. R., Lord, C., Klin, A., & Cook, E. (2002). Autism and the pervasive developmental disorders. In M. Lewis (Ed.), *Child and Adolescent Psychiatry: A Comprehensive Textbook*, p. 595. Philadelphia: Lippincott Williams & Wilkins.

There is considerable heterogeneity within this condition. Attempts have been made to define specific subgroups or subtypes (e.g., individuals with greater attentional difficulties). The disorder presumably reflects to some degree the manifestation of the "broader phenotype" of autism and may be important to study for genetic mechanisms.

Children with PDD-NOS often exhibit unusual sensitivities and atypical affective responses but with better cognitive and language abilities than in those with autism. Although some clinicians tend to equate the concept of Asperger disorder and PDD-NOS data from the DSM-IV field trial suggested, there are important areas of difference (e.g., with more severe social difficulties in individuals with Asperger disorder). As a practical matter, many of the interventions appropriate to individuals with autism can be readily applied. Although it can be a source of frustration from parents to learn that their child has PDD-NOS (e.g., rather than autism), the outcome is almost certainly better.

Differential Diagnosis

Autism and related conditions are differentiated from each other and other disorders on the basis of both history and current examination. The diagnosis of autism is most complicated in very low or high intellectually functioning individuals and in infants (who may not yet exhibit all required diagnostic features). In Asperger disorder, the diagnosis may be delayed because of the preservation of language skills, which may overshadow social deficits. The course and presentation of Rett's and CDD are usually very striking; evaluation of other potential causes of developmental deterioration is indicated.

SUMMARY

Considerable progress in understanding the biological bases of autism has occurred over the past decade. As a result of increased interest, research funding and productivity have significantly increased. As a result of early diagnosis and treatment, the outcome for individuals with autism is improving. Although research on autism is well established, knowledge regarding the other PDDs remains more limited.

Longitudinal studies have made it clear that the term *infantile autism* was, in many ways, a misnomer because infants grow up to be adults. Studies of adults with all the PDDs remain relatively uncommon; an entire generation or two of individuals with Asperger disorder were, essentially, missed. Studies of special groups are needed (e.g., children with regression and those who fail treatment). Newer diagnostic techniques, such as positron emission tomography and fMRI scanning, may help to elucidate underlying pathophysiologic mechanisms. The study of specific subgroups (e.g., CDD) may be particularly appropriate to for such research. Genetic studies remain an area of very high priority. It is quite possible that the final behavioral syndrome known as autism may well represent the effects of multiple insults on the developing central nervous system (CNS) acting through different pathways, and it will be critical to consider genetic work on specific endophenotypes in this regard. The explication of underlying CNS substrates for social behavior is a very active area of current work. The development of testable hypothesized mechanisms of CNS dysfunction will significantly advance our understanding of these complex disorders; the discovery of specific genes holds the promise for developing better animal models and increasing our understanding of how genetic risk is expressed in the developing brain and in behavior.

Selected Readings

Abrahams, B. S., & Geschwind, D. H. (2008). Advances in autism genetics: On the threshold of a new neurobiology [erratum appears in *Nature Reviews Genetics, 9*(6), 493]. *Nature Reviews Genetics, 9*(5), 341–355.

Amir, R. E., Van den Veyver, I. B., Wan, M., et al. (1990). Rett syndrome is caused by mutations in X-linked MeCP2, encoding methyl-CpG-binding protein 2. *Nature Genetics, 23,* 185–188.

Asperger, H. (1944). Die autistichen psychopathen im kindersalter. *Archive fur psychiatrie und Nervenkrankheiten, 117,* 76–136.

Autism Genome Project, Szatmari, C. P., Paterson, A. D., Zwaigenbaum, L., et al. (2007). Mapping autism risk loci using genetic linkage and chromosomal rearrangements. *Nature Genetics, 39*(3), 319–328.

Chawarska, K., Klin, A., & Volkmar, F. R. (Eds.). (2008). *Autism Spectrum Disorders in Infants and Toddlers: Diagnosis, Assessment, and Treatment.* New York: Guilford Press.

Coonrod, E. E., & Stone, W. L. (2005). Screening for autism in your children. In F. R. Volkmar, R. Paul, A. Klin, & D. Cohen (Eds.), *Handbook of Autism and Pervasive Developmental Disorders, vol. 2. Assessment, Interventions and Policy,* third edition, pp. 707–729. Hoboken, NJ: Wiley.

Fombonne, E. (2005). Epidemiological studies of pervasive developmental disorders. *Handbook of Autism and Pervasive Developmental Disorders,* vol. 1, pp. 42–69. Hoboken, NJ: Wiley.

Goldstein, S., Naglieri, J. A., & Ozonoff, S. (Eds.). (2009). *Assessment of Autism Spectrum Disorders.* New York: Guilford Press.

Grinker, R. R. (2007). *Unstrange Minds.* New York: Basic.

Gupta, A. R., & State, M. W. (2007). Recent advances in the genetics of autism. *Biological Psychiatry, 61*(4), 429–437.

Heller, T. (1908). Dementia infantilis. *Zeitschrift fur die Erforschung und Behandlung des Jugenlichen Schwachsinns, 2,* 141–165.

Hermelin, B. (2001). *Bright Splinters of the Mind: A Personal Story of Research with Autistic Savants.* London: Jessica Kingsley.

Kanner, L. (1943). Autistic disturbances of affective contact. *Nervous Child, 2,* 217–250.

King, B. H., Hollander, E., Sikich, L., et al. (2009). Lack of efficacy of citalopram in children with autism spectrum disorders and high levels of repetitive behavior: Citalopram ineffective in children with autism. *Archives of General Psychiatry, 66*(6), 583–590.

Klin, A., Jones, W., Schultz, R., et al. (2002). Defining and quantifying the social phenotype in autism. *American Journal of Psychiatry, 159*(6), 895–908.

Klin, A., Pauls, D., Schultz, R., & Volkmar, F. (2005). Three diagnostic approaches to Asperger syndrome: Implications for research. *Journal of Autism & Developmental Disorders, 35*(2), 221–234.

Lord, C., & Corsello, C. (2005). Diagnostic instruments in autism spectrum disorders. In F. Volkmar, A. Klin, R. Paul, & D. J. Cohen (Eds.), *Handbook of Autism and Pervasive Developmental Disorders,* pp. 730–771. Hoboken, NJ: Wiley.

McCracken, J. T., McGough, J., Shah, B., et al. (2002). Risperidone in children with autism and serious behavioral problems. *New England Journal of Medicine, 347*(5), 314–321.

Moy, S. S., & Nadler, J. J. (2008). Advances in behavioral genetics: Mouse models of autism. *Molecular Psychiatry, 13*(1), 4–26.

National Research Council. (2001). *Educating Young Children with Autism*. Washington, DC: National Academy Press.

Offit, P. (2008). *Autism's False Prophets*. New York: Columbia University Press.

Pinkham, A. E., Hopfinger, J. B., Pelphrey, K. A., et al. (2008). Neural bases for impaired social cognition in schizophrenia and autism spectrum disorders. *Schizophrenia Research, 99*(1–3), 164–175.

Schultz, R. T., Gauthier, I., Klin, A., et al. (2000). Abnormal ventral temporal cortical activity during face discrimination among individuals with autism and Asperger syndrome. *Archives of General Psychiatry, 57*(4), 331–340.

Volkmar, F. R., Klin, A., Siegel B, et al. (1994). Field trial for autistic disorder in DSM-IV. *American Journal of Psychiatry, 151*(9), 1361–1367.

Volkmar, F. R., Koenig, K., & State, M. (2005). Childhood disintegrative disorder. In F. Volkmar, A. Klin, R. Paul, & D. J. Cohen (Eds.), *Handbook of Autism and Pervasive Developmental disorders*. Hoboken, NJ: Wiley, 1, 70–78.

Volkmar, F. R., Lord, C., Klin, A., et al. (2007). Autism and the pervasive developmental disorders. In A. Martin & F. Volkmar (Eds.), *Lewis's Child and Adolescent Psychiatry: A Comprehensive Textbook*. Philadelphia: Lippincott, Williams & Wilkins, 384–400.

Volkmar, F., & Wiesner, L. (2009). *A Practical Guide to Autism*. Hoboken, NJ: Wiley.

Wing, L. (1981). Asperger's syndrome: A clinical account. *Psychological Medicine, 11*(1), 115–129.

Wing, L., & Potter, D. (2008). In S. Goldstein, J. A. Naglieri, & S. Ozonoff (Eds.), *Epidemiology of Autism: Assessment of Autism Spectrum Disorders*, pp. 18–54. New York: Guilford.

World Health Organization. (1993). *Mental and Behavioural Disorders (including disorders of psychological development): Diagnostic Criteria for Research*. ICD-10, pp. 147–149 (F84.0-F84.1). Geneva: WHO.

CHAPTER 5 ■ INTELLECTUAL DISABILITY (MENTAL RETARDATION)

BACKGROUND

Awareness of children with significant problems in learning and development can be traced to antiquity, although modern interest in what is now termed *intellectual disability* (ID) began at the time of the Enlightenment and increased greatly during the 19th century. This was a time of great social upheaval. This was also a time during which infant and child mortality began to decline and there was increased interest in children and in their education. Interest in children's development led to debates about the role of experience (nurture) versus endowment (nature). The interest was exemplified in the report of the French physician Itard who reported on Victor, child thought to be wild or "feral" (but who probably had autism). Specific methods for stimulating children's development were used, and facilities for caring for children with intellectual deficiency became available. Although initially the impetus was to provide rehabilitation, such facilities often became places for custodial care, a program that has now led to the emphasis on providing services within homes and communities.

The development of the first adequate test of intelligence early in the 20th century also stimulated interest in children with delayed development as it became possible to more precisely characterize levels of disability. In France, Alfred Binet developed the idea of the "mental age" by looking at knowledge that was normatively expectable for children at certain ages. Subsequently, the concept of Intelligence Quotient (IQ, originally produced by dividing mental age by chronological age and multiplying by 100) made it much easier to compare children of different ages and levels of ability. There was considerable faith in the IQ as a valid predictor of subsequent development (i.e., as a fixed measure), and this led to a number of problems and problems. Over time, it became clear that IQ scores did not become particularly stable, in large groups of children, until around the time the child entered school (this is not surprising because IQ tests were originally designed to predict success in school). Studies conducted in the 1930s and 1940s, often on children in orphanages or other institutions, began to show significant effects of experience. In the 1940s and 1950s, there was increased awareness that the IQ score was indeed the product of both experience and endowment, and therapeutic optimism again increased for improving the functioning of children with mental retardation (MR).

It also became apparent that IQ alone was not an adequate predictor of adult self-sufficiency. The focus on appropriate self-care or "adaptive" skills led the psychologist Edgar Doll to develop the Vineland Social Maturity Scale. The current version of this scale continues to

Howard Skeels and the Iowa Study

In a classic study, Skeels and Dye demonstrated this practically by transferring infants and young children from an orphanage to a home for the "feeble minded" to make the children "normal." This fantastic plan had been prompted by clinical observation that children in the home for the feeble minded received considerably more stimulation than those in the orphanage. Skeels later reported major differences in outcomes for these better-cared-for children, both in childhood and in later adult life.

serve as an important tool in the assessment of children with ID. Importantly, in contrast to IQ, adaptive skills can be readily taught.

Another body of work centered on the delineation of specific syndromes of ID. For example, Dr. Langdon Down reported on a syndrome (which now bears his name) that we now recognized as being the result of a trisomy of chromosome 21. At the time of his report, Dr. Down, of course, had no notion of chromosomes. Indeed, although his theoretical understanding was fundamentally flawed, Down's clinical observation has been remarkably robust. As time went on, more syndromes of ID were identified. It became clear that ID could result from a range of risk factors, including problems related to the developing fetus, and ranging from genetic factors (Down syndrome) to exposure to toxins in utero (fetal alcoholism) to maternal infections (congenital rubella). This is an area of active work, and advances in genetics and neurobiology have led to an increasingly detailed understanding of pathophysiological mechanisms.

A series of court cases and legal and social initiatives began to significantly change the care of individuals with ID. Over the past 50 years, there has been an emphasis on caring for children in their homes and communities and avoiding institutionalization. This movement has been further stimulated by the mandate of the U.S. federal government that schools provide appropriate education for all children with disabilities within integrated settings when possible. In the United States, many students with ID are largely or entirely integrated into classrooms with typically developing age mates, although there are marked state-to-state variations, and the benefits of mainstreaming remain debated as students with more severe disabilities may continue to have more restricted experiences. As noted subsequently, the study of mental health aspects of ID has increased substantially during this time, although adequate mental health services often remain difficult to obtain.

DEFINITION AND CLINICAL FEATURES

Intellectual deficiency (ID) (previously referred to as mental retardation) is defined on the basis of (1) subnormal intellectual functioning, (2) commensurate deficits in adaptive functioning, and (3) onset before 18 years. Subnormal intellectual functioning is defined by an IQ lower than 70, usually determined on an appropriate standardized test of intelligence. Deficits in adaptive skills (social and personal sufficiency and independence) are generally measured using instruments such as the recently re-revised Vineland Adaptive Behavior Scales. Specific tests of intelligence and adaptive behavior are discussed subsequently. Guidelines for diagnosis are summarized in Table 5.1.

Various levels of ID have been specified: mild (IQ, 50–70), moderate (IQ, 35–49), severe (IQ, 20–34), and profound (IQ <20) (Figure 5.1). Unspecified ID can also be noted if, as sometimes happens in very disabled individuals, it is not possible to administer usual tests of intelligence. Borderline ID can be noted as a V code in DSM-IV. Some flexibility is allowed for clinical judgment. Most persons with ID in childhood are those with mild ID (~85% of

TABLE 5.1

DIAGNOSTIC FEATURES OF INTELLECTUAL
DISABILITY AND MENTAL RETARDATION

Onset: in childhood or adolescence
Delayed or deviant cognitive functioning: IQ of 70 or below
  based on appropriate intellectual testing
Delayed or impaired adaptive functioning: inability to meet
  age-expected social, communication, academic,
  occupational, or other activities of daily living

cases); the remainder of cases include those with moderate (~10%), severe (about 4%), and profound (1%–2%) ID.

In the past, the distinction was made between educable (IQ, 50–70) and trainable (IQ <50). Although no longer commonly used, this distinction continues to be relevant. For example, persons with mild ID often have psychiatric difficulties that are fundamentally similar (if generally more frequent) to those seen in the general population; this is not true for more severely impaired persons. Similarly, whereas specific medical conditions associated with ID are more likely in the group with an IQ lower than 50, lower socioeconomic status is more frequent in the group with mild ID. The proportion of persons with severe and profound ID is higher than would be expected given the normal curve, reflecting the impact of genetic disorders and severe medical problems on development. By definition, the disorder has its onset in childhood or adolescence (e.g., a young adult who sustained a brain injury and subsequent IQ deficits would *not* receive a diagnosis of MR).

The clinical presentation varies depending on a host of factors, particularly the level of ID. Thus, children with severe and profound ID come to diagnosis earlier, are more likely to exhibit dysmorphic features and associated medical conditions, and have higher rates of behavioral and psychiatric disturbances. The latter can be quite different from those seen in the general population (e.g., self-injurious behaviors, unusual mood problems). Although individuals with mild ID have increased rates of psychopathology (compared with the general population), the nature of problems seen is fundamentally similar to those in normative samples. Persons with moderate levels of ID are intermediate between these two extremes.

Somewhat paradoxically, for many years, the diagnosis of ID tended to cause clinicians and researchers to overlook the presence of associated psychiatric and behavioral problems, a phenomenon known as "diagnostic overshadowing." As researchers began to look, it became clear

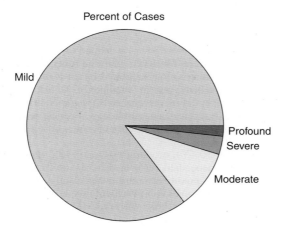

FIGURE 5.1. Proportional representation of levels of intellectual disability.

Case Report: Mild Intellectual Deficiency

Jimmy was born at term after an uncomplicated pregnancy, labor, and delivery. His early developmental milestones were slightly delayed. Jimmy did not walk until 15 months and did not use words until he was nearly 2 years of age. His parents expressed concern to their pediatrician, and Jimmy was seen for assessment when he was 3.5 years old. At that time, developmental testing suggested borderline cognitive ability with a fairly even profile. His strengths included his social engagement and motivation to please. Various medical evaluations were undertaken, and results were uniformly negative. There was no family history of ID nor did Jimmy exhibit any unusual physical findings or features. Genetic consultation was noncontributory. He was enrolled in a program in which he had special supports as well as opportunities for interaction with typically developing peers. By age 8 years, repeat psychological testing revealed a full-scale IQ of 68 with some areas of weakness and strength becoming more pronounced. Jimmy continued to receive some special help with classes and had a modified curriculum. Starting in adolescence, he began a part-time job working in a local restaurant, where he was well liked and popular. More and more of his work in school focused on vocational issues. He had some difficulties with depression and anxiety as a young adult but now lives largely independently from his parents, who see him on a regular basis. He has an active social life and continues to enjoy his job.

Comment: Often, the diagnosis of mild ID is not made until the child is nearing entry to school or preschool. Individuals with mild ID often are able to achieve considerable independence and personal self-sufficiency, particularly when, as in this case, efforts are made to encourage community and vocational skills.

that individuals with mild ID exhibited a four- to fivefold increase in mental health problems. In general, at least 25% of persons with ID may have significant psychiatric problems; these rates are much higher if persons with salient behavior problems are included. Although issues of diagnosis and assessment can be complex, it appears that rate of schizophrenia, depression, and attention-deficit/hyperactivity disorder are all increased relative to the general population. Various rating scales and checklists specific to psychiatric problems in this population have been developed (see Bouras and Holt, 2007, for a detailed discussion). Modifications of *Diagnostic and Statistical Manual* (DSM-IV) criteria for persons with ID have also been developed (Fletcher, Loschen, Stavrakaki, & First, 2007).

EPIDEMIOLOGY AND DEMOGRAPHICS

The use of both subnormal intellectual functioning and deficits in adaptive behavior in the definition of ID has important implications for epidemiology. If only the IQ criterion is used, the expectation, based on the normal curve, would be that 2.3% of the population should exhibit ID. However, this number is significantly decreased, particularly in adulthood, if the adaptive criterion is included. Figure 5.2 summarizes these differences in approach as exemplified in two different studies.

The prevalence ranges from three or four cases per 1000 for severe MR with rates from five to 10 children per 1000 for mild MR. The frequency is increased in boys over girls. Not surprisingly, times of case detection vary depending on several factors, including level of disability. Thus, profound or severe MR is likely to be recognized early in life, but mild ID is frequently not recognized until the school years. Rates of mild ID are increased in individuals at great environmental risk (e.g., because of poverty or lower socioeconomic status). Identifiable

Case Report: Severe Intellectual Deficiency

Jeff was born after a term pregnancy and uncomplicated labor and delivery. He had nursing problems. His early milestones were delayed, and he had recurrent ear infections. Referral for genetics consultation was made at age 2 years because of delays and the pediatrician's concern about his unusual appearance. Jeff had a short and wide head (bradycephaly), a flattened midface, and low-set ears. He also had short but broad hands. On developmental testing, he was significantly delayed in all areas. A diagnosis of Smith-Magenis syndrome (a deletion at 17p11.2) was made by testing and was consistent with the clinical picture. Jeff enjoyed being around adults and exhibited considerable attention-seeking behavior. When frustrated, he began to engage in head banging, although this decreased as he became older. Jeff had limited communication skills, and his frustration around communication issues seemed to exacerbate his behavioral problems. Jeff also had significant sleep problems.

When he was 6 years of age, IQ testing yielded a full-scale score of 32. At that time, he had a hoarse, deep voice and still exhibited some self-injurious behaviors. He was also noted by the psychologist to exhibit an unusual "self-hug" (often seen in children with this condition). As a school-age child, his sleep problems caused the family considerable difficulties; typically, he would be up and wander the house at night but then try to sleep during the day. Fortunately, he was somewhat gregarious and outgoing, although this sometimes caused issues with strangers.

Jeff has received considerable special help in school. He had difficulties with sequencing and change but did well with structure. His family plans are to try to help him transition to a nearby group home and sheltered workshop program when he is older.

Comment: In this deletion syndrome, there are several characteristic features, including the facial appearance, self-injury, sleep problems, and attention seeking. As adults, individuals with severe ID typically reside in group homes or other supervised care facilities.

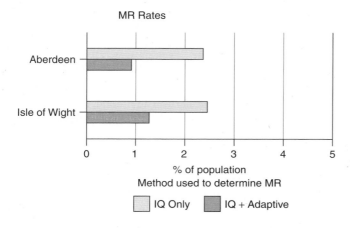

FIGURE 5.2. Comparison of studies using IQ alone or IQ and adaptive behavior for rates of intellectual disability in two different epidemiological studies in different locations in the United Kingdom.

medical syndromes become more frequently observed below an IQ of 50. As noted, the age of diagnosis often varies depending on the severity of the disability, so persons with more severe ID present for clinical assessment earlier than those with mild, or borderline, intellectual deficiency. The advent of more precise methods for genetic testing has shown, in some cases, that some individuals with specific genetic syndromes function in the mild or even borderline range.

ETIOLOGY

Much of the work on etiology has, in essence, continued to emphasize the nature versus nurture debate (i.e., with relative emphasis either on biological or experiential factors). So, for example, one focus has been on the cases of ID associated with known prenatal, perinatal, and postnatal insults. Indeed, in about half of cases, some medical factor can be implicated, particularly in individuals with more significant cognitive deficit. On the other hand, in cases with less severe ID, it often appears that social-cultural or experiential factors may predominate. In reality, of course, these issues are difficult to disentangle. Clearly, some cases of mild ID undoubtedly represent the tail end of the normal, Gaussian distribution of intelligence. In many respects, work on the cause of ID seems poised to enter a new era, with advances in genetics and neuroscience offering the potential for new models and theories. More than 1000 genetic causes have now been identified, and this number will undoubtedly increase. Table 5.2 summarizes some of the specific forms of ID, their causes, and relevant clinical features.

Advances have also occurred in the approach to behavioral characterization, and these features may in turn contribute to our understanding of gene or brain function. As noted in Table 5.2, some syndromes feature unique psychiatric vulnerabilities and thus hold promise for helping identify pathways to these psychiatric endpoints.

There has been increased interest in relating psychiatric and behavioral difficulties to specific genetic or other etiologies. Examples include hyperphagia and compulsivity in Prader-Willi syndrome, attentional and social problems in fragile X syndrome, inappropriate laughter in Angelman's syndrome, the unusual cry in 5p- syndrome, and the self-hug in Smith-Magenis syndrome. Sometimes aspects of syndrome expression can be been related to the genetic vulnerability underlying the disorder features of the syndrome, such as the severity of ID in fragile X syndrome and the type and severity of maladaptive behaviors in Prader-Willi syndrome. Furthermore, some of these connections between genetic disorder and behavioral outcome appear unique to a single syndrome, but others are "shared" between two or more syndromes. Thus, in some instances, features are relatively syndrome specific, such as the unusual handwashing stereotypies of Rett's syndrome or the extreme hyperplasia in Prader-Willi syndrome. More often, however, features are shared in two or more conditions. Thus, attentional problems are frequent in fragile X and Williams syndrome. Understanding the nature of "dual diagnosis" if of great interest given its potential for shedding light on fundamental mechanisms of psychopathology. These issues are, however, complex because the causal direction of most risk factors is unclear. Poor peer or social relations, for example, may be a precursor of psychopathology or a consequence of disruptive behavior.

Biological factors increasing risk include increased rates of seizure disorders, abnormal neurologic functioning that in most cases is undetected, high rates of sensory or motor impairments among persons with MR, biochemical or neurologic anomalies associated with unusual behaviors such as severe self-injury, and genetic causes that carry higher than usual risks of certain maladaptive or psychiatric vulnerabilities. Demonstrable brain abnormalities (e.g., as with neuroimaging) become more frequent as the degree of cognitive impairment increases. Some conditions are associated with gross brain atrophy, although more subtle difficulties may also be detected, particularly with the technical advances of recent years. Exposure to certain environmental toxins, obstetrical risk, poverty, and severe deprivation are other risk factors.

Psychosocial risk factors for development of additional behavior and mental health problems include unusual personality styles, unusual motivational styles, low expectancies for success, learned helplessness, negative self-concept, and long-standing reinforcement of maladaptive behaviors. Mental health problems also are compounded by difficulties in communication, peer difficulties, poor social judgment, isolation, and poor self-advocacy skills.

TABLE 5.2

AN OVERVIEW OF SELECTED CONDITIONS ASSOCIATED WITH INTELLECTUAL DEFICIENCY

Syndrome	Etiology	Physical and Clinical Examination Findings	Psychological Features
Down syndrome	Trisomy 21 (usually caused by nondisjunction)	Characteristic face with wide nasal bridge, upward slanting eyebrows, simian crease, short stature, low muscle tone, cardiac and other problems	Usually relatively sociable with better verbal skills that might otherwise be expected, increased risk dementia in adulthood
Fetal alcohol syndrome	Exposure to alcohol during pregnancy	Hypoplasia of the midface, microcephaly, short stature, long and smooth philtrum	Typically, mild to moderate ID with increased problems in attention
Fragile X syndrome	FMR-1 gene inactivation due to CCG repeats	Long face and large ears with high arched palate, large testes in boys	Difficulties with attention and social anxiety, mild to moderate ID
Williams syndrome	Deletion of part of long arm of chromosome 7 (~25 genes, including elastin gene)	Elfin-like face, short stature, stellate iris; renal, cardiac, and other abnormalities	Hyperacusis, anxiety, often sociable with better verbal skills
Prader-Willi syndrome	Deletion in 15q 11 (paternal origin in most cases)	Low tone; infants may have failure to thrive, but obesity develops; small hands and feet, small testes	Compulsive eating and other behaviors (hoarding), moderate to borderline IQ range, affective lability and agitation
Angelman's syndrome	Deletion in 15q13 (maternal original in most case)	Wide-set mouth, thin lips, and other characteristic faces; microcephaly; seizures frequent	Sleep problems, stereotyped movements (hand flapping), typically profound ID
Smith-Magenis syndrome	Deletion in chromosome 17	Broad face, but midface is flattened; characteristic deep voice	Severe self-injury and hyperactivity, severe IQ range, self-hugging
Lesch-Nyhan syndrome	Defect in gene for HGPRT, X linked	Gene defect; increased uric acid leading to gout, kidney problems; movement problems	Severe self-injury, aggression, anxiety with mild to moderate IQ delays
Phenylketonuria	Recessive defect in phenylalanine hydroxylase	High levels of phenylalanine; seizures; symptoms may not appear early in infancy	Language delay, agitation, aggression; can be prevented with diet

HGPRT, hypoxanthine-guanine phosphoribosyltransferase; ID, intellectual disability.

Considerable research has focused on different profiles of strength or weakness in relation to specific syndromes. For example, individuals with Williams syndrome show relative strengths in specific aspects of expressive language along with pronounced deficits in visual-spatial functioning but despite these problems have remarkably good facial recognition and memory skills. Similarly, individuals with Prader-Willi syndrome show remarkable skills solving jigsaw puzzles that may exceed the skills of typically developing peers. In many instances, of course, behaviors are not syndrome specific or are only partially so (e.g., people both fragile X and Prader-Willi syndromes appear to have relative weaknesses in certain short-term memory and sequential processing tasks, and inattention and hyperactivity are seen in those with Williams and fragile X syndromes). Individuals with ID are, of course, also individuals, and within-syndrome studies are of interest in illustrating the range of individual variation. Research is needed to identify the genetic, environmental, developmental, and psychosocial factors that help to explain individual behavioral differences in people with the same vulnerability.

A large body of work has focused on aspects of preventing ID. Recurrence risk in families varies depending on the situation. For example, in some situations, a clear genetic origin can be identified (e.g., fragile X syndrome), but in other cases, the cause may be nongenetic in origin (fetal alcohol syndrome or congenital rubella). When no specific cause is identified, there is still some increased risk. For some disorders, such as autism, there has been a growing appreciation of genetic factors, and it now appears that for parents who have one child with autism, the risk of having a second child with autism is between 2% and 10%. Siblings of children with ID who are not themselves affected may be at increased risk of other difficulties caused by increased family and personal stress. Support for siblings and for their parents is an important element of long-term treatment planning.

Differential Diagnosis and Assessment

The diagnosis of ID is based on the appropriate assessment of cognitive abilities and adaptive skills; clinical assessment also includes a careful developmental and family history, physical examination, and laboratory studies as appropriate. The clinician should be alert to any medical or environmental conditions that may be associated with developmental disability. For example, a strong family history or certain dysmorphic features in a child should raise the possibility of an inherited condition; a history of significant birth trauma, exposure to environmental toxins, or exposure to marked psychosocial adversity are some of the factors that should be considered. Metabolic and genetic testing may be obtained guided on history and results of physical examination (e.g., abnormal facial features or other physical anomalies should alert the clinician to the need for more extensive assessment).

Psychological assessment usually includes administration of a formal IQ test and measure of adaptive skills as well as less formal observation. Several excellent introductions to psychological testing are available for nonpsychologists as are some useful critiques of the limitations of IQ testing (see Selected Readings). For younger children, tests of cognitive ability are often used as developmental tests; by the time a child reaches 5 years or so, the more traditional tests of intelligence can be used. Also, the emphasis in many states for very young children is on providing services for children at risk rather than, for example, assigning a precise diagnostic label. Some examples of these tests are listed in Table 5.3. A distinction between developmental and intelligence tests is made for several reasons, including a recognition that tests are able to sample more skills and more school-related skills as children become older. Tests of intelligence usually provide an overall or "full-scale" IQ score, as well as additional scores (e.g., for verbal or nonverbal abilities). Many different intelligence tests are available, and the choice of the specific test can reflect many different factors. Psychologists are trained to administer tests in a standardized way so that results can be compared with normative samples. Clearly, the tests chosen for assessment of intellectual functioning should be appropriate, have clear reliability and validity, and be administered by appropriately trained examiners.

TABLE 5.3

SELECTED TESTS OF INTELLIGENCE AND DEVELOPMENT*

Name of Test	Comments
Wechsler Intelligence Scales: Wechsler Preschool and Primary Scale of Intelligence, 3rd edition (WPPSI-III, 2002); Wechsler Intelligence Scale for Children, 4th edition (WISC-IV, 2003), Wechsler Adult Intelligence Scale, 3rd edition, (WAIS-III, 1997)	Excellent series of tests covering preschool (around age 4 years) to adulthood; provide separate verbal and other scores; some tasks (both on the verbal and nonverbal sections) are timed, which is a challenge for many children with autism and related conditions (this actually may help document the need for untimed tests).
Stanford Binet Intelligence Scale, 4th edition (SBS-V) (Roid, 2003)	Excellent test that can be used with somewhat younger children; wide age range; nonverbal scale may underestimate abilities in ASDs
Kaufmann Assessment Battery for Children, 2nd edition (KABC-II) (Kaufman and Kaufman, 2004)	Excellent test that can be used from 3 to 18 years of age; some language is needed (but not much); somewhat more flexible administration; many of the materials interest children; language demands are minimized, and good sensitivity to possible cultural bias
Leiter International Performance Scale—Revised (Leiter-R) (Roid & Miller, 1997)	A test originally developed for deaf children that was recently redone; provides assessment of nonverbal cognitive ability (can be used for children with no expressive speech); some teaching is allowed Limitations: no verbal IQ, and the new materials are less interesting for children
Mullen Scales of Early Learning	Can be used with very young children; provide scores in nonverbal problem solving, receptive and expressive language, and gross and fine motor skills; scores from developmental tests such as this one are usually less predictive of later abilities
Differential Ability Scales, 2nd edition (DAS-II) (Elliott, 2007)	Well-done test that covers wide range of ages and taps a number of different skills.

ASD, autism spectrum disorder.
*Many other tests are available, and tests are constantly being revised and reissued.
Reprinted with permission from Volkmar, F., & Wiesner, L. (2009). *A Practical Guide to Autism*. Hoboken, NJ: Wiley.

   Measures of adaptive skills are generally based on parent or caregiver report, although in some cases, the person may be interviewed directly. In essence, the conceptual notion is that the term *adaptive skills* refers to the performance of day-to-day activities required for personal or social self-sufficiency. The inclusion of adaptive skills in the definition of ID rests on the observation that many persons with IQ scores below 70 may, as adolescents or adults, have learned sufficient adaptive skills that they are able to function totally or largely independently. Technically, then, such individuals would not meet criteria for ID. This situation is more typical of persons who, as children, score in the mildly range. The Revised Vineland Adaptive Behavior Scales is the most widely used of these instruments and assesses abilities in several areas, including communication (receptive, expressive, and written language), daily living skills (personal, domestic, and community), and social skills (interpersonal, play and leisure time, and coping) as well as optional gross and fine motor domains (for younger children) and an optional maladaptive behavior domain. Cultural and other factors may be important considerations both in terms of selecting specific assessment instruments and making a diagnosis of ID.

Treatment

As noted previously, treatment approaches have shifted dramatically over the past decade with more individuals living with their families, attending public schools, and staying within their communities. Placement in the community does not, of course, mean that special supports are not needed. Treatment should begin with a consideration of the underlying cause or associated medical condition(s) if it is known. For example, knowing that a child has trisomy 21 has immediate implications for medical care. For example, 50% of newborns will have congenital heard problems, and there is an increased risk for both leukemia and Alzheimer's disease. Similarly, persons with Prader-Willi syndrome also show particularly high rates of etiology-related health problems. Overall, in individuals with ID, there is increased risk for development of epilepsy.

Educational planning should be based on thoughtful assessment and ongoing monitoring. Children with ID are included in mainstream settings as much as possible. This can become more problematic for lower cognitively functioning individuals as they become older, particularly if behavior problems interfere. It is important that an explicit attention be paid to generalization and development of skills relevant to community life and adult self-sufficiency. Transition planning should formally start in adolescence.

Persons with ID are at increased risk of psychiatric problems, and these can be a major source of distress to the individual and family and may also limit opportunities for self-sufficiency. Up to 75% of persons with ID who are referred for psychiatric assessment also have undiagnosed or undertreated medical conditions and, conversely, about half take nonpsychotropic medications that could have behavioral side effects. As noted previously, the problem of diagnostic overshadowing is common and results in significant psychiatric problems being overlooked. The use of specific rating scales and assessment instruments can help focus attention on these problems. The psychiatric interview of persons with ID may need to be modified, particularly for those with more severe MR, but still needs to be comprehensive and multifocal. Associated medical problems or other difficulties may further complicate accurate psychiatric diagnosis. Particularly in individuals with more severe ID, the diagnostic picture can be complex because other psychiatric problems or vulnerabilities complicate the diagnostic picture. It is important that the clinician not overlook other difficulties that may be present and keep in mind that for individuals with ID, what appears to be a small problem may, in fact, have a major impact on the person's functioning.

Persons with ID benefit from employment or from structured programs that emphasize vocational, adaptive, or socialization skills, long after formal schooling. The transition from school to work is a vulnerable point for many persons and their families. Unlike the school years, when special education and related services (e.g., occupational, physical, and speech and language therapies) are typically provided at school under one roof, the services for adults risk being more fragmented. These young adults may particularly benefit from case coordination to avoid becoming isolated or lost between various cracks in services. A particularly troublesome outgrowth of adult service concerns residential placements. By 2030, about 1.5 million individuals will need residential placement as they age.

COURSE AND PROGNOSIS

The outcomes of people with ID vary considerably, depending on the level of severity of the MR; associated biological or other vulnerabilities; and aspects of the individual's psychological functioning, family support, and other factors. Levels of ability to cope with the tasks of daily life are important in determining independence and self-sufficiency. Social and community supports are important. For persons with mild ID, the diagnosis is often first made on school entry but then "lost" as adaptive gains are made in adolescence. Such persons may be self-supporting, may marry, and may raise families but may be at increased risk for educational and behavioral problems in adult life. As adults, persons with moderate levels of ID (IQ, 40–55) typically have more serious impairment. It is common for such persons to need services as adults. Moderate ID is more frequently identified in the preschool years, and medical causes are more frequently identified. Adult self-sufficiency is less likely than in mild ID, although it is possible, and many persons can live semi-independently or with partial support. In individuals with severe or profound ID, case identification often occurs in infancy or early childhood. Goals for these patients include facilitating self-care and other independent living skills as far as possible. Associated medical problems and behavioral difficulties are frequent; unfortunately, problems in communication are more common and further compound the problem of assessment and intervention.

SUMMARY

Considerable progress has been made in the identification and treatment of children with ID. In some ways this field of research has become much more active over the past decade. Areas of active investigation include the study of the interplay between genetic and environmental (including psychosocial) risk factors in the origin of ID as well as the study of basic neural mechanisms in ID. An understanding of basic processes that underlie phenotypic expression, including various forms of psychopathology, offers the opportunity to advance knowledge more generally about mechanisms of disorder. Although many advances in the care and treatment of persons with MR have been made, studies of treatment methods remain an important priority.

Selected Readings

Bouras, N., & Holt, G. (2007). *Psychiatric Behavioural Disorders in Intellectual and Developmental Disabilities*, 2nd edition. New York: Cambridge University Press.

Braaten, E., & Felopulos, G. (2004). *Straight Talk about Psychological Testing for Kids*. New York: Guilford Press.

Elliott, S. D. (2007). *Differential Ability Scales*, 2nd edition. San Antonio, TX: Harcourt Assessment.

Fletcher, R., Loschen, E., Stavrakaki, C. & First, M. (2007). *Diagnostic Manual-Intellectual Disability (DM-ID): A Clinical Guide for Diagnosis of Mental Disorders in Persons with Intellectual Disability*. Kingston, NY: NADD Press.

Gould, S. J. (1996). *The Mismeasure of Man*. New York: W.W. Norton & Company.

Hogan, T. P. (2003). *Psychological Testing: A Practical Introduction*. Hoboken, NJ: Wiley.

Kaufman, A. S., & Kaufman, N. L. (2004*). Kaufman Assessment Battery for Children*, 2nd edition. Circle Pines, MN: American Guidance Service.

Mullen, E. M. (1995). *The Mullen Scales of Early Learning*. Circle Pines, MN: American Guidance Service.

Roid, G. H. (2003). *Stanford Binet Intelligence Scales*, 5th edition. Itasca, IL: Riverside.

Roid, G. H., & Miller, L. J. (1997). *Leiter International Performance Scale–Revised*. Wood Dale, IL: Stoelting.

Skeels, H. M. & Dye, H. B. (1939). A study of the effects of differential stimulation on mentally retarded children. *Proceedings and Addresses of the American Association on Mental Deficiency* 44(1), 114–136.

Sparrow, S. S., Cicchetti, D. V., & Bella, D. A. (2005). *Vineland Adaptive Behavior Scales: Second Edition (Vineland II), Survey Interview Form/Caregiver Rating Form*. Livonia, MN: Pearson Assessments.

Sparrow, S. S, Cicchetti, D. V., & Bella, D. A. (2008). *Vineland Adaptive Behavior Scales: Second Edition (Vineland II), The Expanded Interview Form*. Livonia, MN: Pearson Assessments.

Wechsler, D. (1997). *Wechsler Adult Intelligence Scale*, 3rd edition. San Antonio, TX: Psychological Corporation.

Wechsler, D. (2002). *Wechsler Preschool and Primary Scale of Intelligence*, 3rd edition. San Antonio, TX: Psychological Corporation.

Wechsler, D. (2003). *Wechsler Intelligence Scale for Children*, 4th edition. San Antonio, TX: Psychological Corporation.

Wodrich, D. L. (1997). *Children's Psychological Testing*. Baltimore, MD: Brookes.

CHAPTER 6 ■ LEARNING DISABILITIES AND DEVELOPMENTAL COORDINATION DISORDER

LEARNING DISABILITIES

Interest in what now are termed the learning disabilities began in the 19th century with the increased emphasis on universal public education and with an awareness of adults with major problems in reading. The term *dyslexia* was used to describe the problem, and many different terms have subsequently been used. A strong link to language difficulties (aphasia) was assumed, and this was further emphasized in the 1920s by the neurologist Orton, who speculated that left hemisphere damage (to the language centers) was involved. The topic of definition and issues of broader conceptualization of learning problems remains an area of active debate and discussion. Samuel Kirk proposed the term *learning disabled* in 1963, and the concept promptly gained acceptance from parents who established the Association for Children with Learning Disabilities. As a practical matter, changes in U.S. federal law, in the late 1960s, began to use the term for children whose ability in some specific area, often reading or math, falls below that which might be expected given their skills in other areas.

Public Law 94-142 (the Education for All Handicapped Children Act) became law in 1975 and established the right of children to a free and appropriate education. This law, now amended several times, has been critical in helping children with disabilities obtain educational services. Before its passage, perhaps only 20% of children with disabilities received educational services in public school. At that time, schools provided education to only one in five children with disabilities, but by 2003 to 2004, more than 6.5 million children were serviced under this program. Children with specific learning disabilities make up 50% of all special education students served under this program.

Given the strong relationship to school and academic performance, these problems are, essentially, confined to school-aged children and adolescents but can persist into adulthood.

Additional difficulties arise because in addition to legal definitions (which themselves change over time), somewhat different approaches have been taken by the many different specialties dealing with these problems. Under current law, a child who exhibits a learning disability can qualify for special help and services in school, and an entire system for developing an Individualized Education Program (IEP) is implemented when it is clear after an assessment that the child qualifies for services.

Definition and Clinical Features

In 1980, the *Diagnostic and Statistical Manual* III (DSM-III) included a concept termed *academic skills disorder* Over time, this concept has evolved in both the DSM and International Classification of Diseases (ICD-10) to encompass several different disorders. Both the DSM-IV-TR and ICD-10 use an approach, now seen as somewhat outdated, in the learning disabilities field of basing diagnosis on a *discrepancy* model (i.e., in which the child's performance on an achievement test is significantly lower than IQ). In the DSM-IV-TR, a learning disorder is diagnosed ". . . when the individual's achievement on individually administered, standardized tests in reading, mathematics, or written expression is substantially below that expected for age, schooling, and level of intelligence." As a practical matter, this method is overly stringent and excludes many children who might profit from intervention. The current DSM-IV-TR approach recognizes three explicitly defined categories: Reading Disorder, Mathematics Disorders, and Disorder of Written Expression. A residual category (learning disorder not otherwise specified [NOS]) is also provided. These terms are generally equivalent, overall, to the term for learning disability (LD) recognized in federal regulations.

The DSM-IV-TR approach, now more than 15 years old, was based on then (1994) current methods that relied on discrepancy scores (e.g., of reading difficulties significantly below the level expected by overall cognitive ability). The ICD-10 approach to definition of these conditions is rather similar but includes an explicit requirement that the school environment is one that is appropriate to the child's ability to learn the skill. As defined in DSM-IV-TR, each of the conditions is characterized by achievement that is "substantially below" expectable levels given age, IQ, and educational level. By definition, the problem must be interfering in some way. Sensory deficits can be present, although the additional learning difficulty is diagnosed only when the achievement delays are even greater than would be expected.

Changes in definition in terms of eligibility for services have come from several sources. In the 2004 amendment to the Individuals with Disabilities Education Act (IDEA), a series of 13 categories were recognized, including specific learning disability. The notion of "specific" learning disabilities is used to emphasize the difference between these conditions and more general learning problems (e.g., intellectual deficiency). A specific learning difficulty should not be diagnosed if other factors (e.g. lack of exposure, language, or cultural issues) better account for the problem. An awareness of the potential problems led to then introduction of a new concept, Response to Intervention (RTI),in the 2004 amendment of IDEA

Other learning disorders of potential interest such as the nonverbal learning disabilities profile (Rourke et al., 2002), are not officially recognized. This diagnostic concept is of some interest given its rather different pattern of presentation and unique constellation of neuropsychological findings (strengths in verbal areas and weaknesses in nonverbal areas but with significant developmental shifts over time as children learn to use their strengths to compensate for their weaknesses). It is likely that substantial revisions in the learning disabilities category will occur in DSM-V.

Typically, children present with learning disabilities as they enter school environments and their progress in some specific area lags behind that in other areas. Recognition of learning difficulties and differences can be delayed in some circumstances (e.g., children who have higher cognitive abilities may present with problems sooner than those with lower abilities). Similarly, children whose problems are mild and associated with other conditions (see below) may have learning difficulties that are recognized only over time.

Epidemiology and Demographics

Reading problems are very common in childhood and account for the majority (75%–80%) of learning disorders. Mathematics learning difficulties and disorder of written expression are much less frequent. In math disorder, girls predominate, but in the other two conditions, boys are more likely to have the condition. Disorder of written expression is frequently associated with reading problems and, to some extent, math problems. As noted subsequently, the

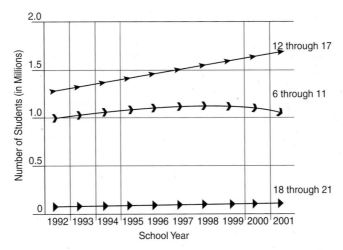

FIGURE 6.1. Recent dynamics of estimates for prevalence rates of learning disabilities in different age groups. (U.S. Department of Education, 25th Annual Report to Congress, 2003. Reprinted from Grigorenko, E. L. (2007). Learning disabilities, p. 412. In A. Martin & F. Volkmar (Eds.). *Lewis's Child and Adolescent Psychiatry: A Comprehensive Textbook*. Philadelphia: Lippincott Williams & Wilkins.)

developmental learning disorders are also strongly related to other conditions, notably attentional difficulties.

Figure 6.1 provides data on the prevalence of learning disabilities data by age group based on data provided to the U.S. Department of Education and then reported to congress. On balance, about 5% to 6% of the total school-age population has a learning disability of some kind. It is the case, however, that rates can vary dramatically from state to state and school district to school district. These differences reflect many different factors ranging from factors that increase the risk of learning disability in the first place (e.g., poverty, lack of exposure to written materials, poor educational programs) to more methodologic issues (failure to detect milder cases given a lack of resources). This diversity in rates also reflects the substantial differences in how local educational programs diagnose learning problems. The discrepancy approach, currently used in DSM-IV-TR, may lead to overdiagnosis of learning problems.

Etiology

Genetic and neurobiologic factors as well as experience play a role in the pathogenesis of learning difficulties. A large body of work has now underscored the importance of genetic factors in these conditions. These factors are presumed to act through one or more brain mechanisms to impact the neuropsychological processes that underlie reading, writing, and mathematics learning (Shaywitz & Shaywitz, 2005). Similarly, experience factors in terms of deprivation and lack of exposure to materials and opportunities to develop basic skills also contribute. Other factors may lead to learning disabilities (e.g., head trauma; treatment of childhood cancers, including central nervous system radiation). Most of the work on etiology has centered on specific reading disability. Various methods have been used to study the neurobiological correlates of reading problems (see Grigorenko, 2007, and Shaywitz & Shaywitz, 2005 for reviews).

Reading skills appear to involve a large network of brain areas, predominately in the left hemisphere of the brain (Figure 6.2), and involve brain regions involved in visual and auditory skills as well as more basic conceptual processing. The four areas that appear to be of greatest relevance to reading include the fusiform gyrus (Broadman area [BA] 37), a portion of the middle temporal gyrus (including part of BA 21 and portions of areas 21 and 37 along with

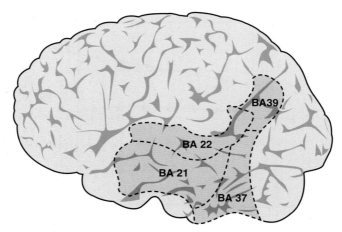

FIGURE 6.2. Areas of the brain that reportedly form the brain circuitry for reading. (Reprinted from Grigorenko, E. L. (2007). Learning disabilities, p. 413. In A. Martin & F. Volkmar (Eds.). *Lewis's Child and Adolescent Psychiatry: A Comprehensive Textbook.* Philadelphia: Lippincott Williams & Wilkins.)

the angular gyrus [BA 39] and the posterior aspect of the superior temporal gyrus [BA 22]). Differences in brain activation have strong developmental correlates, and more able readers seem to shift to frontal regions, but those with difficulty tend to use most posterior ones (in the parietal and occipital regions) (see Gabrieli, 2009).

Beginning in the 19th century, there was an awareness that specific reading difficulties did, at times, strongly run in families. Subsequent work in the area has confirmed this observation and used different approaches to search for specific mechanisms and patterns of inheritance. It seems likely that various genes contribute to the overall risk with a focus on specific areas on chromosomes 15q, 6p, 2p, 6q, 3cen, 18p, 11p, 1p, and Xq. Several genes have now been identified, all of which seem to be involved in neuronal migration and axon crossing.

Differential Diagnosis and Assessment

Intrinsic to the diagnosis of a learning disability is the need to establish that skills in reading or math or writing are discrepant in some way from overall cognitive ability. This simple concept is not always easy to operationalize in practice. Usually, tests of achievement (e.g., of reading or math skills) are examined in the context of overall IQ or cognitive ability. However, numerous problems immediately present themselves, such as how great does the discrepancy have to be? How reliable and appropriate are the instruments chosen to assess either cognitive abilities or achievement? Given the problems with the discrepancy approach, a number of alternatives have been proposed.

These have tended to center on finding the best approaches to teaching and remedial intervention rather than focusing solely on some specific cognitive defect. As a practical matter, schools have some freedom in selecting which approach to use. RTI has emerged as a leading alternative (Vaughn and Fuchs, 2003); it combines aspects of assessment with intervention. In this approach, the child's performance is compared with that of peers on academic tasks, and then students who differ from their peers in either their rate of skills gain or absolute level of skill are identified. The students so identified are then given individualized interventions and appropriate accommodations to help address their specific learning needs. Several types of interventions are used, ranging from less to more intensive. The learning disability diagnosis is made only if these various attempts to modify the child's regular classroom and program have not been successful or if the child's absolute performance or rate of skill gains remains problematic. Alternatives to the RtI approach use annual testing to identify students

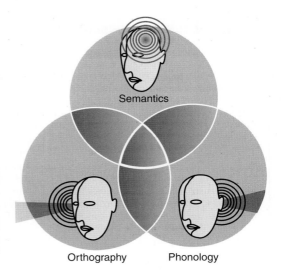

Semantics

Orthography   Phonology

FIGURE 6.3. Theoretical model grouping psychological processing and types of representations studied in Specific Reading Disability (SRD). (Reprinted from Grigorenko, E. L. (2007). Learning disabilities, p. 415. In A. Martin & F. Volkmar (Eds.). *Lewis's Child and Adolescent Psychiatry: A Comprehensive Textbook*. Philadelphia: Lippincott Williams & Wilkins.)

whose skills have not progressed as rapidly as would be expected and thus might need extra intervention. Another approach uses norm-references tests to establish which children score below a certain pre-established "threshold" and thus might merit more intensive evaluation or treatment. These issues continue to be widely debated in the field.

Theoretical models for understanding specific reading disability have been elaborated within psychology and special education. Clearly, reading involves several different processes, including orthography (translating the alphabetic, visual symbols code), phonology (translating these symbols into speech), and semantics (translating these in turn into meaning) (Figure 6.3).

Various research strategies and methods have been used to explore the various aspects of this model. Diagnosis of specific learning difficulties using the DSM-IV-TR focuses on highly specific and circumscribed learning problems. In contrast, the RtI approach (see below) focuses more on response to intervention—or the lack thereof—in identifying children with learning problems. The older approach—the discrepancy approach—tended to use an assumption that processes in learning in the specific learning disabilities were in some ways atypical or deficient representing a specific problem in understanding word meaning, or semantics, that needed intervention. In contrast, the RtI approach is less concerned with differentiation of specific processes. As already noted, school districts vary considerably in their approach to these issues. The services of psychologists and special educators in evaluating learning challenges is particularly helpful.

Learning disabilities are frequently associated with some other disorders and it is important the clinician keep this in mind in evaluating the child or adolescent with a learning problem. These conditions include attention-deficit/hyperactivity disorder (ADHD) as well as disruptive behavior disorders. Children who have experienced repeated school failures are also at increased risk for mood and anxiety problems. The presence of one or more of these disorders may have important treatment implications.

Treatment

There has been, particularly in recent years, an important emphasis on prevention as well as the provision of additional supports and special educational services. Psychopharmacologic treatments may be helpful in dealing with associated comorbid conditions (e.g., ADHD, depression) but do not address the underlying learning challenge. The RtI approach has some

Case Report: Learning Disability

Alex, a 9-year-old boy, was referred for evaluation because of persistent and worsening problems in school. For the past 2 years, he had been noted by his classroom teacher to have problems in reading and, to a lesser extent, in organization and attentional skills. He had an overall IQ in the low-average range, and achievement testing revealed somewhat lower than expected reading skills, although not at the level that would have, for his school, prompted eligibility for special services.

An interview with his parents revealed a normal pregnancy, labor, and delivery. Language and motor milestones had all been achieved within the normal range but slightly on the late side. In preschool, he seemed, at least compared with his sister, much less interested in reading and books and much more interested in rough-and-tumble play and various construction "projects." He particularly enjoyed helping his father around the house in carpentry and similar activities. Both of his parents noted that he had some mild motor coordination problems, and they were most noticeable when he was trying to play sports such as softball. His father had a history of significant reading problems.

On psychological testing, Alex's verbal IQ was in the low-average range with nonverbal skills being somewhat higher. Achieve testing revealed significant difficulties with word identification and pronunciation, and his comprehension of spoken language was poor. The psychologist also noted issues with low self-esteem and with self-organization and executive functions.

His school district had recently changed its approach to the diagnosis of students with reading disability and judged Alex to be qualified for special services. Several different interventions were put in place, including procedures to help him learn to sound out words more effectively. A summer program was provided as was a special reading tutor and the provision of some special education services.

At the conclusion of the academic year, Alex had made important gains in reading, and his self-esteem had also improved. A specific teaching strategy had been used to help him learn to sound out words, and for the first time, he was interested in reading on his own.

advantages in helping clarifying which approaches do and do not work for a certain child with a learning disorder. As a practical matter, a range of services can be provided in school from a very intensive level (e.g., special educational classes) to less intensive supported (e.g., additional help in the mainstream classroom, additional help with tutoring or homework). Other treatment approaches have been concerned with addressing what are presumed to be underlying problems in information processing, attention, and so forth. Learning differences often present children with challenges in various areas, including peer interaction, and support for learning in these areas, as well as the more specifically academic challenges, can be helpful.

Course and Prognosis

Given the various federal mandates for services, most children with significant learning challenges now receive special help. Accordingly, data on natural history and course of these conditions become somewhat more difficult to interpret and, as in other areas, the largest body of research work has centered on reading disability. There is some suggestion that early intervention can make a difference, although some vulnerability often persists, to at least some degree. Many different intervention strategies and accommodations are now available and can help children, adolescents, and adults with learning disabilities. These include various forms of assistance ranging from very low to very high technology (e.g., text-to-speech computers, organization software, visual aids, and schedules).

Unfortunately, many children with significant learning disabilities do not graduate from high school, and they have greater challenges entering the workforce.

DEVELOPMENTAL COORDINATION DISORDER

Definition and Clinical Features

Children with severe, isolated motor delays have been known since antiquity. The term *cerebral palsy* has been used frequently to refer to these conditions, which are typically associated with birth trauma or some other specific process. Other children have motor difficulties that are severe and less obviously associated with some specific medical cause. Various terms have been used to describe children with motor and coordination problems; these have included terms such as *dyspraxia* and *specific motor developmental disorder*. The concept of developmental coordination disorder, including dyspraxia, is defined on the basis of motor deficits greater than expected given a child's age or intellectual level and not attributable to some other condition such as an autism spectrum disorder. As with the learning disorders, performance must be below expected levels for age and IQ and may occur in gross or fine motor activities (or both).

The condition may be noted as an isolated phenomenon or in association with other conditions (often language-communication or learning disorders). The condition may be associated with attentional problems, and one autism spectrum variant with a significant motor component has been described as well.

Epidemiology and Demographics

The DSM-IV-TR suggests that the disorder may be as high as 6% of school-aged children. Boys are more frequently diagnosed than girls, although this may reflect societal emphasis on motor skills (sports skills) in boys. Boys may also be more likely to be evaluated for other problems and to have motor delays than noted as well.

Etiology

Motor skills problems can arise for many different reasons, ranging from birth difficulties to prematurity, and may be associated with speech-language difficulties (speech itself, of course, having a significant oral-motor component). Associations with specific learning disorders are also frequent. Some combination of developmental immaturity and specific motor skills vulnerabilities is often involved.

Diagnosis and Assessment

If motor skill deficits are severe, referral for neurologic evaluation may be warranted; this is indicated if there are unusual movements, if overall tone is high or low, or if there are specific neurologic signs or symptoms.

Several instruments for assessing motor skills are available. These include tests of both gross and fine motor skills as well as tests focused on visual-motor integration and dexterity. Documentation of deficits in these areas with standardized instrument can be helpful in establishing eligibility for services or obtaining specific remedial devices or programs. For example, rather than struggle with teaching cursive handwriting to a child with major fine motor or visual-motor vulnerabilities, it may be much more helpful, having documented the problem, to teach keyboarding skills.

Treatment

Occupational and physical therapy approaches can address the fine and gross motor needs of individuals with motor problems. Adaptive physical education can also be used in schools.

Course and Outcome

Several different factors and their interaction can impact outcome. Prognosis is best when motor difficulties are mild and when motor difficulties are an isolated finding (i.e., when comorbid conditions are not present). Unfortunately, secondary problems, such as peer problems and difficulties in sports, can lead to anxiety and mood difficulties.

SUMMARY

About half of all children identified as having disabilities under current federal guidelines exhibit a specific learning disability, usually a reading disability. Greater awareness and increased vigilance on the part of parents and schools have led to earlier identification and potentially more effective earlier intervention. The current DSM-IV-TR approach to diagnosis is based on a discrepancy model that has now, in some respects, been supplanted by changes in federal law. New approaches based on RtI hold promise, but studies of these methods remain in their early stages.

A continuing tension exists around, on the one hand, the desire to identify children with vulnerabilities and, on the other, an awareness of the degree to which the "pool" of resources is somewhat limited. The newer RtI may offer some advantages over current approaches in addressing this dilemma.

Selected Readings

American Psychiatric Association. (2000). *Diagnostic and Statistical Manual of Mental Disorders*, 4th edition, text revision. Washington, DC: American Psychiatric Association.

Deshler, D. D., Mellard, D. F., Tollefson, J. M., & Byrd, S. E. (2005). Research topics in responsiveness to intervention: Introduction to the special series. *Journal of Learning Disabilities, 38*, 483–484.

Ehlers, S., A. Nydén, A., Gillberg, C., et al. (1997). Asperger syndrome, autism and attention disorders: A comparative study of the cognitive profiles of 120 children. *Journal of Child Psychology & Psychiatry & Allied Disciplines 38*(2), 207–217.

Fletcher, J. M., Lyon, G. R., Barnes, M., et al. (2002). Classification of learning disabilities: An evidence-based evaluation. In R. Bradley, L. Danielson, & D. P. Hallahan (Eds.). *Identification of Learning Disabilities: Research to Practice*, pp. 185–250. Mahwah NJ: Erlbaum.

Franklin, B. M. (1987). The first crusade for learning disabilities: The movement for the education of backward children. In T. Popkewitz (Ed.). *The Foundation of the School Subjects*, pp. 190–209. London: Falmer.

Gabrieli, J. D. E. (2009). Dyslexia: A new synergy between education and cognitive neuroscience. *Science, 325*(5938), 280–283.

Gresham, F. M., Reschly, D. J., Tilly, D. W., Fletcher, J. et al. (2004). Comprehensive evaluation of learning disabilities: A response to intervention perspective. *The School Psychologist, 59*, 26–29.

Grigorenko, E. L. (2005). A conservative meta-analysis of linkage and linkage-association studies of developmental dyslexia. *Scientific Studies of Reading, 9*, 285–316.

Grigorenko, E. L. (2007). Triangulating developmental dyslexia: Behavior, brain, and genes. In D. Coch, G. Dawson, & K. Fischer (Eds.) *Human Behavior and the Developing Brain*, pp. 117–144. New York: Guilford.

Grigorenko, E. L., Wood, F. B., Meyer, M. S., et al. (1997). Susceptibility loci for distinct components of developmental dyslexia on chromosomes 6 and 15. *American Journal of Human Genetics, 60*, 27–39.

Grigorenko, E. L. (2009). Dynamic assessment and response to intervention: Two sides of one coin. *Journal of Learning Disabilities, 42*(2), 111–132.

Gurney, J. G., Krull, K. R., Kadan-Lottick, N., et al. (2009). Social outcomes in the Childhood Cancer Survivor Study cohort. *Journal of Clinical Oncology, 27*(14), 2390–2395.

Haight, S. L., Patriarca, L. A., & Burns M. K. (2002). A statewide analysis of eligibility criteria and procedures for determining learning disabilities. *Learning Disabilities: A Multidisciplinary Journal, 11*, 39–46.

Hallahan, D. P., & Mercer, C. R. (2002). Learning disabilities: Historical perspectives in Identification of learning disabilities. In R. Bradley, L. Danielson, & D.P. Hallahan, (Eds.) *Research to Practice*, pp. 1–67. Mahwah, NJ: Lawrence Erlbaum.

Jordan, N. C., & Levine, S. C. (2009). Socioeconomic variation, number competence, and mathematics learning difficulties in young children. *Developmental Disabilities Research Reviews*, 15(1), 60–68.

Lagae, L. (2008). Learning disabilities: Definitions, epidemiology, diagnosis, and intervention strategies. *Pediatric Clinics of North America*, 55(6), 1259–1268.

Mandlawitz, M. (2006). *What Every Teacher Should Know About IDEA 2004*. Boston: Allyn & Bacon.

Mercer, C. D., Jordan, K., Allsph, D. H., et al. (1996). Learning disabilities definitions and criteria used by state education departments. *Learning Disability Quarterly*, 19, 217–232.

Pennington, B. F. (2009). How neuropsychology informs our understanding of developmental disorders. *Journal of Child Psychology & Psychiatry & Allied Disciplines*, 50(1-2), 72–78.

Price, C. J., & Mechelli, A. (2005). Reading and reading disturbance. *Current Opinion in Neurobiology*, 15, 231–238.

Rourke, B. P., Ahmad, S. A., Collins, D. W., et al. (2002). Child clinical/pediatric neuropsychology: Some recent advances. *Annual Review of Psychology*, 53, 309–339.

Semrud-Clikeman, M. (2005). Neuropsychological aspects for evaluating learning disabilities. *Journal of Learning Disabilities*, 38, 563–568.

Shaywitz, S. (2003). *Overcoming Dyslexia: A New and Complete Science-Based Program for Reading Problems at Any Level*. New York: Random House.

Shaywitz, S. E., Morris, R., & Shaywitz, B. A. (2008). The education of dyslexic children from childhood to young adulthood. *Annual Review of Psychology*, 59, 451–475.

Shaywitz, S. E., & Shaywitz, B. A. (2005). Dyslexia (specific reading disability). *Biological Psychiatry*, 57, 1301–1309.

Shaywitz, S. E., & Shaywitz, B. A. (2008). Paying attention to reading: the neurobiology of reading and dyslexia. *Development & Psychopathology*, 20(4), 1329–1349.

Sternberg, R. J., & Grigorenko, E. L. (2002). Difference scores in the identification of children with learning disabilities: It's time to use a different method. *Journal of School Psychology*, 40, 65–83.

U.S. Office of Education. (1977). Assistance to states for education for handicapped children: Procedures for evaluating specific learning disabilities. *Federal Register*, 42, 65.

U.S. Office of Special Education Programs. (2000). *History: Twenty-five Years of Progress in Educating Children with Disabilities Through IDEA*. Washington, DC: U.S. Department of Education.

CHAPTER 7 ■ DISORDERS OF COMMUNICATION

Language is a uniquely human ability and one that is easily disrupted. As a result, disorders of language development are frequently associated with various other conditions, although they can occur in isolation as well. The concept of *communication* refers to language as well as gestures and body language; speech is an important part of the more general communication domain (Figure 7.1). Although animals can communicate (e.g., with calls signaling danger or warning), only humans truly use language to express ideas, thoughts and feelings. These utterances are often totally new, that is, they are created without being previously heard. Speech is one mode of language; writing provides another form of expression. For individuals who have already learned to communicate and write but then experience impediments to speech (e.g., after a stroke), written communication can be a substitute. The situation is more complicated when difficulties occur in the developmental period before these various forms of communication are established.

BACKGROUND

In the early 19th century, Gall differentiated children experiencing problems with language from those with cognitive-intellectual disability. The investigations of Broca and Wernicke led to important discoveries about the brain localization of language functions as they studied aphasia in adults. Indeed, in the first century of study of language difficulties, neurologists dominated the field, and the focus tended to be adults. This changed as Samuel Orton, a neurologist, began the scientific study of child language disorders. He noted the relevance of these problems to behavior and problems in learning, particularly reading and writing. In the mid 20th century, psychiatrists, psychologists, and pediatricians such as Arnold Gessel began to study what was termed "infantile aphasia." Benton developed the notion of a specific disorder of language learning in children similar to adult aphasia. In a parallel body of work, educators were struggling with the problem of best teaching methods for children who were deaf or who exhibited severe language problems. Attempts were made to start differentiating various types of children with language-speech problems. Around the same time, interest in child language began to increase, with Chomsky's work on transformational grammar.

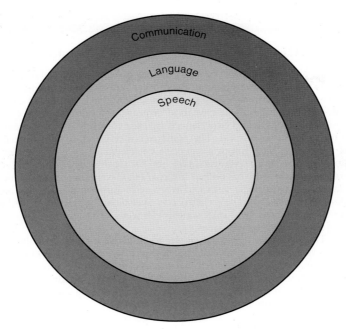

FIGURE 7.1. Domains of communication. Reprinted from Paul, R. (2007). Disorders of communication. In A. Martin and F. Volkmar (Eds), *Lewis's Child and Adolescent Psychiatry: A Comprehensive Textbook*, p. 418. Philadelphia: Lippincott Williams & Wilkins.

DEFINITIONS AND CLINICAL FEATURES

Communication disorders are broadly defined and impair the individual's ability to engage in interaction socially. The current *Diagnostic and Statistical Manual* (DSM-IV) approach recognizes several different disorders depending on the pattern and nature of the communication problem. It also emphasizes both functional impairment and a judgment of impairment relative to other developmental abilities and certain other conditions.

In *expressive language disorder*, scores on measures of expressive language must be "substantially" below those for nonverbal cognitive and receptive language ability. These problems must interfere and not be attributable to a mixed receptive–expressive language disorder or an autism spectrum condition. Care should be used in making this diagnosis in the face of intellectual disability, gross deprivation, or sensory-motor deficits. Individuals with this condition usually have limited expressive language with a limited vocabulary.

Key Concepts and Terms

Pragmatics: the social use of language
Syntax: the way words are put together
Semantics: the meaning of language
Phonology: the sounds of language
Morphology: word formation; system of word formation

Case Report: Expressive Language Disorder

Jimmy was an active, sociable 2.5-year-old child whose parents complained to his pediatrician about his language development. His mother had a normal pregnancy, labor, and delivery. His early developmental milestones were within normal limits except that his speech was delayed. He said his first word at around 15 months, but his understanding of language seemed fine. He had experienced two ear infections, but his hearing had recently been tested and was normal. The pediatrician referred him to a speech-language pathologist, who tested him. Jimmy's receptive vocabulary was above age level. He was able to follow age-appropriate commands, but his expressive vocabulary was significantly delayed and his expressive output limited. His parents were both concerned, and the speech-language pathologist began to work with Jimmy on a regular basis and included his parents in sessions to help them carry over techniques to home. By age 4 years, Jimmy's expressive language was only slightly delayed, although he had some difficulty in formulating more complex sentences.

Comment: The issue of when to intervene in children with more isolated expressive language delays is somewhat controversial. Many children who are late talkers go on to do well. In this case, the significance of the expressive delay prompted the parents and therapist to begin treatment, with a good result. Some children with this pattern of difficulties may go on to have other problems in school (e.g., with writing). Jimmy's excellent response to treatment is a good prognostic sign.

In *mixed receptive–expressive language disorder*, the requirements are the same as for expressive language disorder, but in the mixed type, receptive skills are also substantially below what would be expected given the individual's nonverbal cognitive abilities.

Thus, in expressive language disorder, the individual's expressive abilities are below what is expected given the child's nonverbal cognitive abilities. In contrast, language understanding is relatively preserved. Language may be slower to develop, and articulation problems may be noted as the child learns to speak. In mixed receptive–expressive language disorder, both receptive and expressive skills are below expected levels.

Phonological disorder (also referred to as *developmental articulation disorder* in the past) is characterized by a failure to produce and use "developmentally expected" speech sounds. These problems, which can include sound substitution, sound omission, and other errors in making sounds, must interfere with communication and academic or occupational achievement. As with expressive and mixed receptive–expressive language disorder, the diagnosis can be made in the presence of intellectual disability, neglect or deprivation, or sensory-motor problems only when they are greater than would otherwise be expected. Children with phonological disorders have delays or an inability to produce certain speech sounds. As a result, they often substitute sounds (W for R) or leave off the final consonant at the end of words. Sound distortions may also be present (i.e., an approximation of the sound is used). Less frequently, additions of sounds may be noted (e.g., "uh uh, give me that"). Some children have other sound production difficulties. Although many children improve with age (with or without treatment), the condition may be a source of distress and, in severe cases, may result in speech that is not intelligible.

Stuttering (previously referred to as stammering) is a condition characterized by disturbance in the flow of language (e.g., repetition of sounds or whole words, word substitutions). This problem must be a source of academic or occupational interference. It is often associated with behavioral difficulties and affective problems. Various speech dysfluencies may be involved, including blocking of sounds, hesitations, and tense pauses. Although many children exhibit

Case Report: Mixed Receptive–Expressive Language Disorder

Vinny had been noted to have delays in both his receptive and expressive language as a toddler. His family and primary care doctor adopted a "wait and see" attitude, partly because his father also had delays in language and then developed normally. By the time he was 4 years old and entering preschool, Vinny's difficulties with language remained striking. An evaluation was obtained. Although his problem-solving abilities were at the average level and he was noted to have strengths in the area of visual learning and problem solving, auditory processing was an area of weakness, and both receptive and expressive language were significantly delayed. A diagnosis of receptive–expressive language disorder was made, and speech therapy was begun. By 6 years of age, Vinny was exhibiting attentional difficulties in first grade, and his continued language difficulties posed further obstacles for his learning. Fortunately, his reading skills turned out to be a relative area of strength for him, and he used this, in part, to compensate for his language problems.

Comment: It is not unusual for children with mixed receptive–language disorder to have other problems, commonly other learning difficulties and attentional problems. Fortunately for this child, reading was an area of relative strength and provided some opportunities for compensatory learning.

dysfluencies early in life, these usually tend to involve larger linguistic units (words, phrases, and sentences). In contrast, for a child with persistent stuttering, these dysfluencies usually involve repetitions of sounds or syllables ("s-s-s-struck' or "vi-vi-vi-vi-video"). In other cases, sounds may be prolonged ("WWWWWait!"). There can also be blocks when the child is struggling to attempt to make a sound; often this is associated with observable signs such as blinks or grimaces. The prognosis is better if the dysfluencies are relatively effortless and if

Phonological Disorder

Larry was a pleasant but somewhat shy 4.5-year-old child seen for a kindergarten screening. His birth and early development were unremarkable. He had a few ear infections, but his hearing had recently been tested and found to be within normal limits. During the screening, he had shown some articulation errors and was referred to a speech pathologist, who noted difficulties with some of the later-developing consonant sounds (e.g., z, sh, th, r). Sometimes Larry would simply omit these sounds from words or put in other sounds in their place (e.g., w for r). His difficulties became more notable when he had to string together multiple words. His speech was best articulated when he was calm and spoke in a slow, deliberate fashion. Although his parents could understand almost all of his speech, the speech pathologist suggested that likely a classroom teacher and peers might only be able to understand 80% of it. Because of this and what appeared to be his own awareness of the difficulty, speech therapy was begun with a good result. Two years later, he was having only occasional difficulties.

Comment: Often the prognosis is good so that by age 6 years, many children with mild to moderate problems are doing well. Sometimes problems can persist, particularly if speech becomes more complex or rapid.

Case Study: Stuttering

Johnny, a 6-year-old boy, started to stutter around 3 years of age. Both his speech and motor milestones had been slightly delayed. As his language developed, he began to have difficulties with fluency, pausing at certain words. This problem was initially only occasional, but over time, it became frequent, and he began to repeat some sounds and got stuck on the initial sound in the word (e.g., "h–h–h–h-help me out"). There was a strong family history of stuttering. Eventually, intervention was obtained and focused on helping Johnny have better control over the rate of his speech.

Comment: It is common to observe a strong family history of stuttering. Prognostic factors, in addition to family history, include persistence of the difficulty over time, its association with other language problems, and the individual's or family's anxiety about the problem.

---

the child begins to improve within the first year. The International Classification of Diseases (ICD-10) diagnostic guidelines make a distinction between stuttering (where there are frequent repetitions or sound prolongation) and cluttering (where there are fluency breakdowns without repetitions or hesitations). There are some other differences as well. These differences between the DSM and ICD approaches reflects a continuing controversy about the nature of stuttering and its relationship (or lack thereof) to other speech disorders.

Although not recognized as an official diagnosis, the term *childhood apraxia of speech* is sometimes used to describe a subset of cases in which speech difficulties are severe and persistent. In these cases, the range of speech sounds is limited, there are difficulties in sound imitation, the rate of speech is slow, and there are many sound omission errors. This concept was originally thought of as an analogue of adult acquired neurologic disorders of speech. The validity of the concept has been controversial and newer techniques, including neuroimaging, have not supported the comparison to adult disorders. Similarly, in the past, terms such as *childhood aphasia* and *congenital aphasia* were used to describe language disorders with a straightforward connection to the acquired aphasias of adulthood.

Several features of the DSM-IV-TR approach to diagnosis should be noted. Interference is emphasized as is the role of formal language *and* psychological testing. Some degree of clinical judgement is also allowed. Given that communication difficulties are part of the definition of autism and related conditions, certain communication disorders cannot be diagnosed in the presence of autism or pervasive development disorder (PDD). In contrast, the American Speech-Language-Hearing Association defines *language disorder* somewhat differently as impairment in "comprehension and/or use of a spoken, written, and/or other symbol system." In this view, the problem could be in language form, content, or function—or combinations of these. Speech disorders refer to problems with sound production and thus are intrinsically more limited. Comprehension can often be intact, but speech fluency can be affected (stuttering) or pronunciation of specific sounds may be affected (phonological disorders).

EPIDEMIOLOGY AND DEMOGRAPHICS

Given differences in definition and method, it is not surprising that estimates of the prevalence of specific language disorders vary widely given different approach to definition. Clearly, language delays are the most common presenting complaint of parents of preschool children; estimates vary, but overall, the median prevalence rate is about 6%, with boys more likely than girls to be impaired. By school age, the prevalence of primary language disorders is about 4% to 7%. One complexity is that there can be overlap with other disorders (e.g., learning disabilities and dyslexia). Specific language disorders combined with learning disabilities are some of the most prevalent disorders of school-age children. Disorders of language expression are probably more common than those involving comprehension, although even when the problem seems to be primarily expressive, and there are often subtle difficulties in reception as well. The most frequent speech-communication disorders are the phonological disorders, which represent about 80% of referrals to speech clinics. About 5% to 6% of school-age children have articulation problems; in preschool, this number is at least double. The incidence of stuttering is highest between ages 2 and 4 years, affecting as much as 5% of the population.

Language difficulties can predispose to or be comorbid with a veritable host of other conditions. In one meta-analysis, Benner, Nelson, and Epstein (2002) reported that nearly 75% of children with emotional-behavioral disorders had clinically significant language problems. Similarly, more than 50% of children diagnosed with language deficits also have additional psychiatric problems. Explanations for these associations vary. The arrow of causality could point in either direction (e.g., language problems lead to emotional or behavioral ones or vice versa). Or some third factor could potentially underlie both conditions.

The psychiatric difficulties that most commonly coexist with language disorders include attention-deficit/hyperactivity disorder (ADHD), conduct and oppositional disorders, and anxiety disorders. Of the anxiety disorders, *selective mutism* has major communicative aspects. This condition is defined on the basis of persistent refusal to talk in one or more major situations despite the ability to speak and understand language (see Chapter 12). The condition is twice as common in girls. Interesting high rates of speech and language difficulties have been reported in this population with high rates of articulation and expressive language problems. These cases present special challenges in school, and mental health workers and speech pathologists often work together to provide effective interventions.

It is important to take relevant cultural, ethnic, and family situations into account. For example, children exposed to two languages (bilingual households) usually learn both languages without difficulty but may be somewhat delayed in becoming fluent in them. Standard measures of language-communication or intelligence should take such issues into account.

ETIOLOGY

Language disorders can exist in isolation but are frequently associated with other developmental disorders. If the focus is on specific language impairments (SLIs), there is strong evidence for neurobiological factors in syndrome pathogenesis. For example, the concordance rate of such disorders is higher in monozygotic than dizygotic twins; similarly, the risk for family members is increased. Although much speculation has centered on the role of environmental factors, the strongest associations are with lower socioeconomic status, larger family size, later birth order, and recurrent otitis media—all factors that deprive the child of language input at a critical stage in learning.

If the focus is broadened beyond isolated language problems, high rates of activity and attentional problems are observed. The nature of the role of cognitive factors has been debated. Some investigators suggest that the language difficulties reflect a more a general deficit in symbolic representation; the speed of responding also may contribute to problems in information processing. Leonard (1997) has argued that the difficulties may reflect abilities at the lower end of the normal range. Most investigators, however, would question this view given the frequent association of language impairment with problems in attention and activity and with "soft" neurologic signs. Another approach to understanding the etiology has focused on difficulties in auditory information processing, particularly rapid processing of the kind needed for speech processing.

Imaging work has been used to document differences in brain processing among children with and without specific language disorders. For typically developing persons, the brain is asymmetrical, with language structures (e.g., the planum temporale) tending to be larger in the left hemisphere; in contrast, children with SLIs typically have more symmetrical hemispheres. Adults with language difficulties are more likely to have an extra sulcus in Broca's area in either brain hemisphere, although it must be emphasized that no one pattern of brain architecture has been consistently demonstrated.

Stuttering clearly has a strong biological component with involvement of aspects of both the central and peripheral nervous system. There is also a genetic component with increased risk in first-degree relatives.

Language disorders can also have their onset during children, often as a result of focal brain lesions (e.g., caused by damage at birth or, much less commonly, postnatal brain insult). Delays are most common when damage is sustained in the left cortex. Usually, significant recovery or development of language can occur but with some mild residual deficits.

Some children who have had normal language suddenly or gradually lose language skills in association with seizure disorder. Testing usually shows normal hearing, but the child seems to attend less to speech. The child may regress in language ability or stop talking altogether, although nonverbal cognitive abilities are preserved. This syndrome of acquired aphasias with epilepsy (also known as Landau-Kleffner syndrome) typically onsets between 3 and 6 years of age. The outcome is usually better with later onset. Even if clinical seizures are not observed, abnormal electroencephalographic activity is evident. The child may slowly regain functional communication abilities, but with delays in some areas.

Prenatal exposure to toxins can result in communication disorders. For example, in fetal alcohol syndrome, communication difficulties are extremely common as are cognitive difficulties. Speech is often delayed, and the child has problems with vocabulary development, comprehension, and social language use. In children exposed to drugs prenatally, there is an increased risk for prematurity, low birth weight, intrauterine growth retardation, and a small head circumference. Children with a history of cocaine exposure may show delayed language acquisition, although this effect can be modified by a stimulating environment. Children with communication problems may be at increased risk for maltreatment. It is possible that the child's difficulties predispose the child to abuse presumably through their impact on the parent–child attachment. Maltreatment also constitutes a risk for language disorder. A history of maltreatment (see Chapter 21) is often associated with significantly lower language scores both in terms of vocabulary and sentence production.

DIFFERENTIAL DIAGNOSIS AND ASSESSMENT

As noted, language difficulties can be observed in relative isolation or in the context of other developmental problems. For example, delays and limitations in language may be an initial sign of intellectual disability (mental retardation). In general, children with intellectual disability seem to progress through normal sequences of language acquisition, although at a slower pace. Although many children with intellectual disability show language skills similar to their cognitive abilities, a fairly large group exhibits problems in language, particularly in language production or in both reception and expression of language. Phonological errors are more common in this group, but pragmatic (social language) skills are usually consistent with overall developmental level (in contrast to children with autism). Two of the most well-recognized syndromes of intellectual deficiency, Down syndrome and fragile X syndrome, are associated with language problems. In other conditions, such as Williams syndrome, language skills are relatively preserved compared with developmental level. Autism and related conditions are frequently associated with communication deficits (see Chapter 4). Indeed, the exclusionary rule of autism or PDD for a diagnosis of expressive language disorder or mixed receptive-expressive language disorder reflects the fact that communication difficulties are a core aspect of the definition of autism (see Chapter 4 for a discussion of language-communication problems in individuals with autism and related conditions). Essentially all children with autism have some form of communication problem. In the case of autism and related conditions, the motivation to communicate is affected, but signs and other alternative forms of communication can be used if the lack of motivation presents a major problem for intervention. Diagnostic controversies surround precise delineation of syndrome groups, and borders among language disorder, learning difficulties, and autism spectrum disorder can become blurred.

Given their lack of access to linguistic information, children with hearing impairments are understandably at risk for language disorders. A wide variation is observed in the oral ability of children with hearing impairments. Clearly, with appropriate supports (e.g., amplification through hearing aids), it may be possible to substantially improve the auditory signal. Cochlear implants and other aids can also be used to help individuals who would otherwise be deaf. Indeed, the earlier use of cochlear implants facilitates language development in children born with severe hearing losses. For children with hearing impairment, language development follows the usual sequence, although it is usually greatly delayed. This delay is observed in all areas, including articulation and spoken and written language. In contrast to children with autism spectrum disorders, children with hearing impairment usually do not have major problems in social communication. Given the language difficulties, reading and writing are often adversely affected, and the typical reading level of adolescents with uncorrected hearing impairments is usually at the third or fourth grade level; use of cochlear implants results in higher levels of achievement.

Many different tests of speech-language-communication abilities are available for individuals of different ages. It is important to understand the aims and intended uses of the specific instrument (e.g., the results of widely used tests of vocabulary, either receptive or expressive, may not convey the severity of actual communication levels). Newer tests assess even more complex aspects of language (e.g., the child's social language use or understanding of higher order language features such as figurative or ambiguous language). Typically, the tests are administered by a speech-language pathologist or psychologist. Similarly, nonverbal intelligence can be estimated from traditional tests of intelligence or tests specifically designed to assess nonverbal abilities (Table 7.1).

The clinician should be aware of other conditions frequently associated with speech and language problems. As noted previously, these include hearing loss, mental retardation, autism or a related condition, and other psychiatric problems such as ADHD. Some physical difficulties can contribute to communication problems (e.g., cleft palate, apraxia, cerebral palsy). And as already noted, maternal substance abuse can be a risk factor as is child maltreatment. Audiometric testing by a certified audiologist should be used to verify that hearing is intact. Chronic ear infections can be associated with speech-language problems, but it is important not to attribute this as the sole cause of difficulty because it appears that by itself, recurrent otitis media does not significantly increase the risk of language disorder in otherwise typically developing children.

A speech-language pathologist conducts an assessment of factors that can impact the speech mechanism and typically assesses the morphology, symmetry, and alignment of the facial features as well as structures involved in speech. Phonological disorders can be diagnosed through formal testing in which the speech-language pathologist will assess the child's ability to produce target words by naming objects or pictures. Phonological problems frequently coexist with other language disorders. For a diagnosis of expressive language disorder or mixed receptive expressive language disorder, individually administered, standardized tests should be used. In stuttering, phonological, receptive, and expressive language skills are age appropriate. If stuttering coexists with other speech and language problems, it may be appropriate to see if the dysfluency persists after other problems are resolved. Because preschool children commonly have dysfluency, it is often sensible to follow the child before recommending speech therapy; if, however, the child appears to show signs of struggling or self-consciousness, then referral is indicated.

TREATMENT

Treatment should follow a careful assessment with the goal of clarifying and the presence of any additional conditions (e.g., hearing impairment, mental retardation, autism). Apart from selective mutism, the treatment of children with speech-communication disorders typically involves individual or small group therapy provided by a certified speech-language pathologist. Given the frequency of comorbid conditions and difficulties, it is common for educational

TABLE 7.1

COMMONLY USED TESTS OF SPEECH-LANGUAGE-COMMUNICATION*

Name of Test	Comment
Peabody Picture Vocabulary Test, 4th edition (PPVT-4) (Dunn & Dunn, 2007)	Measures receptive vocabulary (what the child understands); age range, 2.5–90 years; this score may overestimate child's actual language ability.
Expressive One Word Picture Vocabulary Test (EOWPVT) (Brownell, 2000)	Measures naming ability (what the child can label); age range, 2–18 years; again, may overestimate child's actual language ability
Reynell Developmental Language Scales, U.S. edition (Reynell & Gruber, 1990)	Useful from 12 months through age 6 years; provides measures of actual language use; scores are often lower than when single-word vocabulary is assessed; provides scores for verbal comprehension and expressive language; materials are attractive to children
Preschool Language Scale–4 (PLS-4) (Zimmerman, Steiner, & Pond, 2002)	Used to assess receptive and expressive language; frequently used in schools; this is a direct assessment that is a good instrument for younger children; age range, 2 weeks–<7 years
Comprehensive Assessment of Spoken Language (CASL) (Carrow-Woolfolk, 1999)	Used from ages 3 to 21 years; only a verbal or nonverbal (pointing) response required (no reading or writing ability expected) with test of various language abilities, including pragmatic ability (social language use) and figurative language
Clinical Evaluation of Language Fundamentals, 4th edition (CELF-4) (Semel, Wiig, & Secord, 2003)	Used for children from 3 to 21 years (two versions); assesses various language skills related to school requirements; useful for older and higher functioning children
Test of Language Competence (TLC) (Wiig & Secord, 1989)	Focuses on more complex aspects of language (e.g., ambiguity, figurative language, abstract language); for ages 5–18 years
Goldman-Fristoe Test of Articulation-2 (Goldman and Fristoe, 2000)	Test of articulation; for ages 2–21 years

*Many other tests are available.
Reprinted with permission from Volkmar, F., & Wiesner, L. (2009). *A Practical Guide to Autism*, p. 66. Hoboken, NJ: Wiley.

tutoring, social skills training, or psychiatric intervention to be used as well. Intervention methods include both behavioral and educational approaches. Some clinicians may be more likely to use a strictly behavioral approach, but others use a more child-centered model with many opportunities for incidental learning. Most of the time, a mix of these two approaches is used. Effectiveness has been demonstrated in several small studies, but more work is needed on treatment efficacy, particularly relative to the choice of treatment methods for the individual child. For many children with milder difficulties (e.g., immature articulation), significant improvement can occur with the passage of time.

For persons who have chronic stuttering, the severity fluctuates, with stuttering becoming more severe when the person is pressed to communicate, is stressed, or is anxious. Although general anxiety reduction techniques are not particularly effective, reducing stress while speaking may be helpful. Speech therapy can be helpful. As a single treatment modality, psychotherapy is not effective, although it may help with the secondary effects of stuttering. For selective mutism, behavioral modification procedures have been used as are medications to target anxiety.

Manual sign can be used, particularly when a parent is deaf. This method provides an ability to communicate that is not otherwise available, often with considerable complexity and eloquence. Within the community of hearing impaired individuals, there is considerable debate regarding the role of sign language versus oral language instruction. In general, deaf children without cochlear implants who are taught sign will develop higher level language skills than those who were taught speech. Cochlear implant use has had a major impact because many such children can learn adequately through the auditory channel.

Various complementary and alternative approaches to treatment are available, and some make extravagant claims of dramatic improvement; data for such interventions are generally sparse or, in some cases, convincingly negative. Clinicians should help parents make informed treatment decisions and encourage healthy skepticism.

COURSE AND PROGNOSIS

Language is often delayed in children who go on to exhibit speech-language difficulties. Words may not appear until well into the second year of life, and the rate of new word acquisition is slower than usual. Language may be more like that of a younger child. Whereas a typical 2-year-old child has a vocabulary of about 200 words, a child with speech-language impairment may only have 20. Although vocabulary gradually increases, it frequently lags behind that of peers in school, and reading difficulties may be observed. Social language skills (pragmatics) are usually relatively preserved.

Phonological disorders are the most common speech-communication problems, and they involve difficulties with speech articulation and impaired production of developmentally expected speech sounds. This difficulty should not be solely attributable to cognitive disability, hearing problem, or problems with the oral-motor structures. In phonological disorder, speech is marked by distortions of sounds (e.g., the s sound is produced but with a lisp) or omissions of sounds (e.g., "play" is pronounced "pay") and incorrect sound substitutions (e.g., "cat" is pronounced "dat"). Many of these misarticulations are typical of normal young children as they are learning speech, but in children with phonological disorders, they persist longer than normal and are more common. In addition, the child may try to avoid producing some sounds or may rearrange and misorder the sounds in words or try to simplify words. More severe disorders are recognized earlier than mild ones; it is common for parents to be concerned when the child is about 4 years of age, but younger children are seen as well. Milder cases may not be picked up until the child attends school. Phonological disorders co-occur with many conditions or may exist in isolation. About half of children with phonological disorders have delays in expressive language, and a smaller number exhibit delayed language comprehension as well. Most children with phonological disorders "outgrow" their speech difficulties, but some continue to require services.

By school age, in children with a mild to moderately severe language disorder, the disorders are often centered in subtle difficulties of language organization and efficiency with problems in word retrieval, narrative and conversation, and written language observed. The range of communicative functions may be limited. The language difficulties may contribute to an impression that the child is rude or not polite given the child's difficulty in making use of nuances of social language. Academic difficulties often center on reading and writing, although many children cope, and most go on to high school or beyond and lead independent, productive lives. That being said, severe speech disorders have a much less favorable prognosis.

In stuttering, recovery usually occurs by adolescence so that although perhaps one in 30 children stutter, the rate in adolescence is 1%. Girls are more likely to recover without treatment than boys. Over time, boys are more likely to persist in stuttering. When children recover from stuttering, they typically do so in between 6 months and 3 years of age; in most cases, recovery occurs in 1 to 2 years. Boys are more likely to have stuttering associated with other communication problems such as problems in articulation and phonology.

SUMMARY

Clinicians should be alert to the presence of speech-language difficulties in young children. Many of these difficulties are developmental in nature, but some persist, and early intervention can facilitate the child's language development and help prevent other problems. Because of the central nature of speech-language-communication in organizing experience and learning from the world, disorders of communication can have a significant impact on children's development and increase risk for other disorders. Research on specific genetic and neural mechanisms of these disorders is likely to yield important new insights in the years ahead.

Selected Readings

Bartlett, C. W., Flax, J. F., Logue, M. W., et al. (2002, July). A major susceptibility locus for special language impairment is located on 13q21. *American Journal of Human Genetics, 71*(1), 45–55.

Benner, G., Nelson, J., & Epstein, M. (2002). Language skills of children with EBD: A literature review. *Journal of Emotional & Behavioral Disorders, 10,* 43–57.

Bishop, D. (1997). *Uncommon Understanding: Development and Disorders of Language Comprehension in Children.* East Sussex, UK: Psychology Press.

Bishop, D. V. (2009, March). Genes, cognition, and communication: Insights from neurodevelopmental disorders. *Annals of the New York Academy of Sciences, 1156,* 1–18.

Brownell, R. (2000). *Expressive One Word Picture Vocabulary Test (EOWPVT).* Los Angeles: Western Psychological Services.

Carrow-Woolfolk, E. (1999). *Comprehensive Assessment of Spoken Language* (CASL). Circle Pines, MN: American Guidance Service.

Clark, M. M., & Plante, E. (1998). Morphology of the inferior frontal gyrus in developmentally language-disordered adults. *Brain and Language, 61,* 288–303.

Dunn, L. M., & Dunn, L. M. (2007). *The Peabody Picture Vocabulary Test,* 3rd edition. Circle Pines, MN: American Guidance Service.

Fisher, S.E., & Scharff, C., (2009 April). FOXP2 as a molecular window into speech and language. *Trends in Genetics, 25*(4), 166–177.

Gardner, H. (1983). *Frames of Mind: The Theory of Multiple Intelligences.* New York: Basic Books.

Goldman, S., & Fristoe, M., (2000). *Goldman-Fristoe Test of Articulation 2.* Circle Pines, MN, American Guidance.

Laing, G., Law, W., Levin, A., et al. (2002). Evaluation of a structured test and a parent led method for screening for speech and language problems: Prospective population based study. *British Medical Journal, 325,* 1152–1156.

Leonard, L. (1997). *Children with Specific Language Impairment.* Cambridge, MA: MIT Press.

Newbury, D., & Monaco, A., (2002). Molecular genetics of speech and language disorders. *Current Opinion in Pediatrics, 14,* 696–701.

Peng, S., Spencer, L., & Tomblin, J. B. (2004). Speech intelligibility of pediatric cochlear implant recipients with 7 years of device experience. *Journal of Speech, Language, and Hearing Research, 47*(6), 1227–1236.

Paul, R. (1996). Clinical implications of slow expressive language development. *American Journal of Speech-Language Pathology, 5,* 5–21.

Paul, R., & Lewis, M. (2007). Assessing communication. In A. Martin & F. Volkmar (Eds.) *Lewis's Child and Adolescent Psychiatry: A Comprehensive Textbook,* 4th edition, pp. 371–376. Philadelphia: Lippincott, Williams & Wilkins.

Pennington, B. F., & Bishop, D. V., (2009). Relations among speech, language, and reading disorders. *Annual Review of Psychology, 60,* 283–306.

Presse, J. E., & Kikano, G. E., (2008, May 1). Stuttering: An overview. *American Family Physician, 77*(9), 1271–1276.

Reynell, J., & Gruber, C. (1990). *Reynell Developmental Language Scales,* U.S. edition. Los Angeles: Western Psychological Services

Rice, M., Warren, S., & Betz, S. (2005). Language symptoms of developmental language disorders: An overview of autism, Down syndrome, fragile X, specific language impairment, & Williams syndrome. *Applied Psycholinguistics, 26,* 7–27.

Semel, E., Wiig, E. H., & Secord, W. (2004). *Clinical Evaluation of Language Fundamentals,* 4th edition. San Antonio, TX: Pearson.

Sharp, H. M., & Hillenbrand, K., (2008, October). Speech and language development and disorders in children. *Pediatric Clinics of North America, 55*(5), 1159–1173, vii.

Van Dyke, D. C., & Holte, L. (2003, July). Communication disorders in children. *Pediatric Annals, 32*(7), 436.

Wiig, E. H., & Secord, W. (1989). *Test of Language Competence.* New York: Psychological Corporation.

Zebrowski, P. M. (2003, July). Developmental stuttering. *Pediatric Annals, 32*(7), 453–458.

Zimmerman, I. L., Steiner V. G., & Pond, R. E. (2002). *Preschool Language Scale-4.* San Antonio, TX: Psychological Corporation.

CHAPTER 8 ■ ATTENTION-DEFICIT/ HYPERACTIVITY DISORDER

Children with difficulties in attention and impulsivity have been recognized since the mid-1800s (i.e., as compulsory school attendance became the rule). The 19th century book *Struwwelpeter*, a "morality" book for children by Heinrich Hoffmann, included the tales of Fidgety Philip, who could not sit still, and Johnny Look-in-the-Air, who could not pay attention. The observation of difficulties after viral encephalitis in the early 20th century led to a presumption that these problems arose as a result of some subtle or "minimal" brain damage; Bradley's observation in the 1930s that such children could improve their attention after administration of amphetamine led to one of the first pharmacologic treatments for childhood mental disorders. This led to use of terms like *minimal brain dysfunction* to describe the condition even though evidence of gross brain damage was not demonstrable. Beginning in the 1970s, other terms, such as *hyperkinetic child syndrome*, began to be used. By 1980, the term *attention-deficit disorder* began to be used as was, subsequently, the term *attention-deficit hyperactivity disorder* (ADHD), although the current International Classification of Diseases (ICD-10) term, *hyperkinetic disorder*, emphasizes activity more than attention, reflecting continued controversies over how best to conceptualize this condition.

DEFINITION AND CLINICAL FEATURES

The syndrome of ADHD is characterized by problems with inattention, overactivity, and impulsivity along with other deficits in the set of skills usually termed *executive functioning*. The latter are a range of abilities involved in forward planning. Although similar in some ways, there are differences in approach between the *Diagnostic and Statistical Manual* (DSM-IV-TR) and ICD-10. Both approaches provide a list of 18 symptoms that can involve both attentional problems and hyperactivity (the combined type) or only inattention *or* impulsivity. In DSM-IV TR, the hyperactive type requires at least six of nine symptoms of overactivity, and the inattentive requires at least six of nine listed symptoms of inattention. In the combined type, six of each are required. The ICD-10 approach emphasizes the overactivity aspect. It is also, on balance, more stringent in making the diagnosis. The ICD-10 also adopts a different approach to the issue of frequent comorbidity associated with ADHD, including a special code for co-association with conduct problems (hyperkinetic conduct disorder). These approaches to diagnosis are summarized in Table 8.1. Within the DSM-IV-TR, the distinctions between the subtypes can be subtle, and debate continues about the best approach to conceptualizing

"Fidgety Phil"

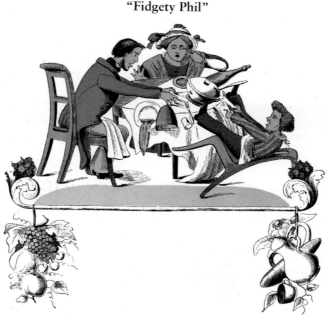

But fidgety Phil,
He won't sit still;
He wriggles and giggles,
And then, I declare
Swings backwards and forwards
And tilts up his chair.

Reproduced from Hoffmann, H. (1845). Der Struwwelpter. Frankfurt, Germany: Routledge & Kegan Paul Ltd. Courtesy of the Cushing/Whitney Medical Library, Yale University School of Medicine.

the condition(s). For example, some children with predominately inattentive symptoms may be less active. It is the case that children whose difficulties relate to overactivity are likely to be more disruptive and thus may be more frequently referred for treatment and earlier diagnosis. For a diagnosis of ADHD to be made, the symptoms must be present in more than one setting, must have started before age 7 years, must cause significant impairment, and cannot be exclusively attributable to another disorder or be better accounted for by it. As a practical matter, multiple sources of information are, accordingly, needed.

The degree to which any one (or none) of the three major areas of difficulty—overactivity, inattention, and impulsivity—will color the diagnostic presentation. Similarly, the child's age and levels of functioning are very important; for some children, difficulties only become apparent because of the age-expected demands placed by school for concentration and attention. A lack of precision regarding how "often" a behavior or feature must be present and how "persistent" it is means that there is considerable clinical judgment involved in making the diagnosis. Finally, the frequent presence of comorbid conditions, such as learning difficulties, conduct problems, language problems, and so forth, frequently complicates the clinical picture and can have important implications for treatment. For some children, the burden of

TABLE 8.1

APPROACHES TO DIAGNOSIS OF ATTENTION-DEFICIT/HYPERACTIVITY DISORDER IN THE *DIAGNOSTIC AND STATISTICAL MANUAL* (DSM-IV) AND INTERNATIONAL CLASSIFICATION OF DISEASES (ICD-10)

DSM-IV-TR
Onset and duration: Before age 7 years; symptoms must be present for at least 6 months
Symptom presentation and impairment: Symptoms must be present in more than on setting and result in significant impairment; symptoms must be persistent and not attributable to developmental level and not occurring exclusively during psychosis or better explained by another disorder)
Subtypes: Three possible subtypes (and a "not otherwise specified") category are identified: inattentive, hyperactive, or combined
For the **inattentive** type, at least 6 symptoms of inattention (e.g., in school work, social interaction, following through on activities, troubles in organization and activities that require forward planning, readily disorganized, by extraneous environmental events)
For the **hyperactivity** type, at least six symptoms such as inability to sit still, high activity level inappropriate to situation, trouble playing quietly, excessively verbal, trouble waiting turns, interrupts frequently, and so on.
In the **combined** type, both hyperactive and inattentive symptoms are present.
Exclusionary rules: Features not attributable solely to (or occur during) schizophrenia or psychotic disorder or autism or related condition or better viewed as part of some other condition such as anxiety or mood disorder

ICD-10
Onset and duration: Before age 7 years; symptoms last at least 6 months
Symptom presentation and impairment. Same symptoms list as DSM-IV, but symptoms must be present in *three* areas: inattention (six of nine), hyperactivity (three of five), impulsivity (at least one of four). The clinician must either observe problems in attention or activity directly or by report in setting outside home or school (or via documented deficits in attention on psychological testing).
Subtypes: No subtypes (although a special code is used for children with both overactivity *and* conduct problems)
Exclusionary rules: Anxiety or mood disorders, mania, pervasive development disorder not present

significant attentional and activity problems takes a toll on affective regulation as well as on peer relationships and social development. There has been growing awareness that, for many children, symptoms of overactivity may lessen with time, but attentional problems may persist. As a result, in adulthood, many individuals may continue to experience difficulties, although their impairment may be less immediately obvious.

In the office setting, the difficulties with attention and impulsivity may not seem markedly different than those in other children, although when a child's difficulties are severe, they are often noted even in office settings. For school-age children, problems with overactivity may be most dramatic in less structured settings (e.g., gym or recess), and problems with attention are reflected in academic areas. Rating scales, checklists, and some psychological tests (discussed subsequently) may be useful in helping to clarify the diagnosis. More complex academic tasks, which require organizational skills and forward planning, are particularly impacted by problems in attention and impulsivity. This is often reflected in forgotten homework or many different projects started but never finished and can be demonstrated on psychological testing. As a practical matter, the clinician should keep in mind the core features of the condition—hyperactivity, inattention, and impulsivity—and have a reasonable sense of what is and is not within the normal range for a child of a given age.

Case Report: Attention-Deficit/Hyperactivity Disorder

Jasper, a 6-year-old boy, was referred at the request of his teacher because of disruptive behavior in the classroom. Jasper was the third child and only boy in the family. Although not particularly worried about his behavior until he entered school, his parents did report that "his engine was running all the time." As a toddler and preschool child, he had had several accidents. He had been enrolled in a relatively unstructured nursery school program, where some concern had been expressed about his ability to "stick with" activities, although the teachers and his parents viewed him as bright.

On entering first grade in a public school setting, Jasper had significant difficulty sitting still. He often did not seem to be listening to the teacher and had difficulty waiting his turn (e.g., in line). His teacher was concerned that he was behind other students in this class in emerging reading abilities. His parents initially provided him with a tutor after school, but after two sessions, the tutor suggested that the parents seek an evaluation. Psychological testing was performed in school and revealed an IQ in the high-average range but with lower than expected achievement scores. He had difficulty with tasks on the IQ test that required sustained attention. The examiner noted in her classroom observation that because of his behavioral difficulties, he tended to be a "loner" in the class, even at recess on the playground.

Apart from several ear infections, his birth, developmental, and medical history were unremarkable. His hearing had been tested and found to be within the normal range. Jasper's father reported that Jasper had attentional difficulties in school and had been treated for many years with methylphenidate.

On examination, Jasper's behavior became more disorganized after he became more comfortable with the examiner and the setting. With support, he was able to attend to tasks, but without this support, his attention was fleeting. He complained that other children in school made fun of him and said he had "ants in his pants."

Stimulant medications were begun along with family counseling. Because of his concern about being called out of class to the nurse's office to take medication, a long-acting stimulant was eventually prescribed and was well tolerated. Additional psychological testing was requested and resulted in several steps to improve his organization and attention in the classroom setting. Peer relationships and Jasper's self-image improved.

As an adolescent, Jasper's difficulties with overactivity improved, even during summers when he did not usually take medication. On the other hand, his problems with sustained attention and organization were more persistent. In college, Jasper was able to obtain additional supports, including a tutor, untimed tests, and some other modifications.

Comment: Although the presenting complaint was related to classroom difficulties, the history revealed previous problems, probably dating back to the toddler years (numerous accidents). Many features of the condition responded to stimulant medication, but even though some aspects of overactivity seemed to improve with time, other problems persisted into adolescence or adulthood. Treatment included medication, parent guidance, educational support, and other measures. The family history of the disorder is relatively common.

By definition in the DSM-IV-TR, the disorder must have its onset before age 7 years. Determination of the actual age of onset is difficult because these data are invariably retrospective in nature. Most of the time, parents will have noted some difficulties in the preschool period, when the child may have had a "driven" quality as she or he rapidly explored the room. Often, parents provide detailed reports of outings and parties during which the child's difficulties have led to major disruptions. In situations in which the major difficulties relate to sustained attention and organization, it may be only as the child enters school when difficulties pose a serious obstacle for learning and lead to diagnosis. Some children have difficulty remaining seated during class. Even in situations such as recess and sports, the child's difficulties with attention and impulsivity may take a toll on social relationships. Difficulties may continue into adulthood.

EPIDEMIOLOGY AND DEMOGRAPHICS

ADHD is one of the more common psychiatric disorders in childhood, affecting 5% to 12% of children. Various issues complicate the interpretation of epidemiologic studies, including significant differences in diagnostic approach in the ICD-10 (which is more stringent, resulting in reduced rates). Boys are more likely be affected than girls (2:1 or 3:1 ratio) and are more likely than girls to present with disruptive behaviors. ADHD is also found more frequently in younger children and in children from families with a lower socioeconomic status. Symptoms of hyperactivity decrease with age. As adults, many, perhaps more than 50% of individuals, continue to have symptoms. Younger individuals are more likely to show features of the hyperactive subtypes; attentional problems become more marked over time so that the combined type becomes predominant. By the junior high and high school years, the inattentive type is most common. Compared with many other disorders, ADHD is often a diagnosis made by history from parents and teachers or, with adolescents and adults, by self-report. A child with ADHD can appear calm and well organized in a novel setting, so reports of parents and teachers are often used in making the diagnosis.

As noted previously, ADHD is frequently associated with other conditions including oppositional defiant or conduct disorder (~50% of cases), anxiety disorder (25%–30%), and learning disabilities (20%–25%). The risk for developing Tourette's disorder is also increased. Clearly, conduct and oppositional defiant disorder are the most frequent associations and can present major obstacles to treatment. Some children may also exhibit specific learning difficulties (see Chapter 6). It is important that these be documented when they are present, because they may require additional interventions apart from those for ADHD. As children become older, they are at increased risk for mood disorder. Comorbidity can present some practical challenges for both diagnosis and treatment. Comorbidity can arise from various sources (e.g., from genetic or environmental factors that contribute to both disorders or because ADHD increases risk for other problems). For example, ADHD can negatively impact peer relationships, leading to social isolation and mood problems.

ETIOLOGY

Both genetic and environmental factors have been implicated in the etiology of ADHD. Early studies of genetics were limited, but more recent research shows a strong genetic component. The importance of genetic factors has been demonstrated using various strategies, including adoption studies. Children of adults with ADHD have a higher risk for the disorder. Recent research has been more sophisticated in its examination of potential genetic mechanisms and neuropsychological profiles presumed to underlie syndrome expression. Various regions on the human chromosome have been implicated in available linkage studies. One line of work has focused on dopaminergic brain mechanisms. The association of ADHD with pre- and perinatal complications and with neurologic soft signs and, of course, its early history of association with the after effects of brain infection or trauma suggest an important role for neural mechanisms. Table 8.2 summarizes some of the soft neurologic signs observed in ADHD.

One body of work has focused on structural brain abnormalities (e.g., after damage to the prefrontal cortex given the important role of this area in executive function abilities). Findings have included reduced volumes in dorsolateral prefrontal cortex, caudate, pallidum, corpus callosum, and cerebellum (see Spetie & Arnold, 2007 for a detailed review). Other neuroimaging approaches have included single-photon emission computed tomography (SPECT), positron emission tomography (PET), functional MRI (FMRI), and proton

TABLE 8.2

SOFT NEUROLOGIC SIGNS IN ATTENTION-DEFICIT/HYPERACTIVITY DISORDER*

Clinical Finding	Putative Explanation
Difficulties performing repetitive motor tasks (e.g., hand flipping, foot rocking, serial thumb to finger opposition)	Impaired ability to use cognitive control to alternately inhibit and excite motor activity to maintain a regular cadence
Difficulties performing sequential timed tasks (e.g., foot rocking, hand flipping, serial finger)	Impaired ability to use cognitive control to adjust motor performance flexibly in a multistep task
Difficulties maintaining gait and balance (sustained motor stance, tandem balance)	Difficulties maintaining balance, integrating proprioceptor input or body position sense, abnormal vestibular function

Reprinted from L. Spetie and E. J. Arnold (2005). Attention-deficit/hyperactivity disorder. In A. Martin & F. Volkmar (Eds). *Lewis's Child and Adolescent Psychiatry*, 4th Ed. Philadelphia: Lippincott Williams & Wilkins, p. 439.

magnetic resonance spectroscopy (PMRS) to focus on brain metabolism during cognitive activities. Most studies have suggested hypoperfusion of the frontal and possibly striatal areas as well as deficits in activation of the brain inhibitory control areas. Because dopamine has had such an important apparent role in the treatment of the condition, another line of work has focused on dopamine and the dopamine transporter and has found increased binding of the transporter in the striatum of individuals with ADHD.

Changes in electroencephalograms (EEG) and event-related potentials have also been reported. The most consistent finding has been higher levels of slow-wave activity relative to normal children with reduced alpha- and beta-wave activity. Some studies have explored the possibility of use of the EEG diagnostically to examine, for example, ratios of theta to beta activity. Related work has focused on evoked potentials, although this line of work is less advanced. There does appear to be a strong hereditary component to EEG measures. It is possible that in the future, endophenotypes might be defined using such approaches.

Psychosocial adversity and other environmental factors have also been associated with ADHD. It is possible that various environmental factors interact with biological ones to increase risk for the disorder. Lead toxicity can, for example, lead to attentional difficulties. Similarly, maternal smoking during pregnancy increases the risk for ADHD in the child.

Neuropsychological theories of ADHD have focused on deficits in inhibitory control (a general pattern of difficulties in inhibition) or in delay aversion (an inability to tolerate delay). Another approach focuses on the interaction of information processing and processes such as effort, arousal, and activation (the cognitive energetic model). Another approach differentiates ADHD with and without hyperactivity and focuses on delays in information process and information retrieval (the sluggish cognitive tempo theory).

DIFFERENTIAL DIAGNOSIS AND ASSESSMENT

The differential diagnosis of ADHD can be complex. Difficulties include varied symptom presentation, age-related changes, and associations with other conditions (e.g., mood problems; anxiety disorder, particularly posttraumatic stress disorder; conduct problems; and developmental difficulties of various kinds). Accordingly, careful history and examination are important.

Various parent and teacher rating instruments have been developed and other procedures are used to document various features of ADHD. For example, activity monitors have been used to document high activity levels which do then diminish with drug treatment Instruments like the Continuous Performance Test (Cornblatt et al., 1988) can be used to measure

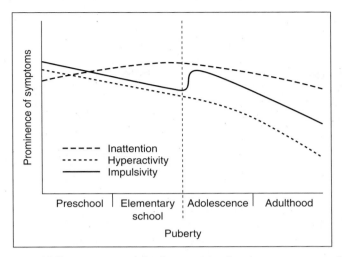

FIGURE 8.1. Course of different attention-deficit hyperactivity disorder symptoms over the life span. Hyperactivity tends to wane with maturity, being replaced by a feeling of restlessness. Impulsivity also tends to wane except for a possible blip in adolescence under the influence of "raging hormones." The most persistent cluster of symptoms is inattentiveness, with the main adult manifestations being disorganization and difficulty managing money, keeping schedules, and sticking with a relationship or job. (Reproduced from Arnold, L. E. (2004). *Contemporary Diagnosis and Management of ADHD*. Newtown, PA: Handbooks in Health Care, with permission.)

inattention, although correlation with classroom performance is not as robust as might be hoped. Instruments such Connor's (2008), which now exists in a third edition for use in children from 6 to 18 years of age, can be completed by parents, teachers, and the child him- or herself. Neuropsychological testing reveals a number of areas of vulnerability in individuals with ADHD. These include difficulties with tasks that require response inhibition and execution, shifting of set and task, interference control, planning and organization, and working memory.

COURSE AND PROGNOSIS

In more than half of cases, symptoms persist into adulthood, although there may be changes in syndrome expression. In the adult population, the male–female discrepancy is much less marked than in childhood. As adults, hyperactivity symptoms often diminish substantially, persisting only as an internal experience of restlessness. However, the problems of inattention, disorganization, and distractibility are more likely to persist. An area of controversy has been the need for different diagnostic approaches or criteria in the adult population. Figure 8.1 summarizes the course of different ADHD symptoms over the lifespan.

Development of comorbid conditions is a risk for adults with ADHD. There is an increased risk, especially for boys and men, to develop substance abuse problems or antisocial behaviors. Difficulties with attention and impulsivity may lead to job difficulties, problems in daily living, and accidents. In women, impulsive behavior can lead to increased risk for unplanned pregnancy. Adults with ADHD may also have higher rates of mood disorders.

TREATMENT

Given the chronic nature of the disorder, treatment must be flexible and comprehensive. The child and family should be involved in treatment planning. Both behavioral and pharmacologic treatments can be helpful. The American Academy of Pediatrics' flow chart for evaluation and treatment is reproduced in Figure 8.2. In short- and medium-term studies, medications

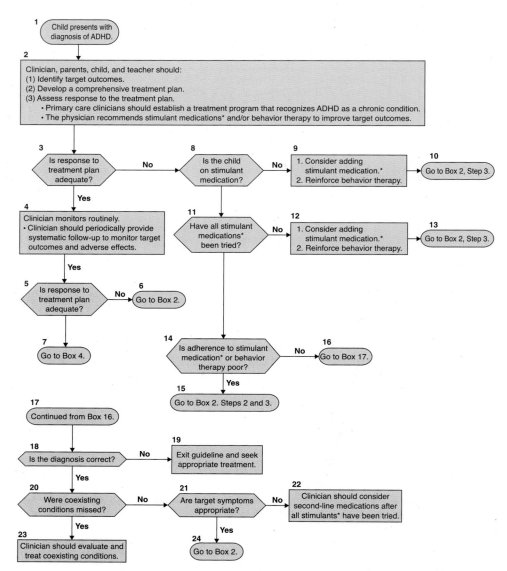

FIGURE 8.2. Clinical guidelines of the American Academy of Pediatrics, which were written before availability of atomoxetine, which, as a Food and Drug Administration–approved treatment for attention-deficit hyperactivity disorder, should be considered after a stimulant before resorting to off-label drugs. (From American Academy of Pediatrics. (2001). Clinical practice guideline for the school-age child with ADHD. *Pediatrics, 108,* 1033–1048, with permission.)

TABLE 8.3

DRUGS WITH FDA APPROVAL FOR ATTENTION-DEFICIT/HYPERACTIVITY DISORDER

Generic Name	Brand Name	Usual Daily Dose (mg) (mg/kg)
Stimulants		
Amphetamine (racemic), dextroamphetamine	Dexedrine Dextro Star	10–40 (0.2–0.7)
Levoamphetamine mixture	Adderall	5–40 (0.2–1)
	Adderall XR	5–40 (0.2–1)
Methamphetamine	Desoxyn	5–25 (0.2–0.7)
Methylphenidate, racemic	Ritalin	10–60 (0.3–1.5)
	Methylin	10–60 (0.3–1.5)
	Ritalin LA	20–60 (0.6–1.5)
	Metadate	10–60 (0.3–1.5)
	Metadate CD	20–60 0.6–1.5)
Methylphenidate, osmotic release	Concerta	18–72 (0.4–1.8)
Dextro-threomethylphenidate	Focalin	5–30 (0.2–0.7)
	Focalin XR	5–30 (0.2–0.7)
Pemoline	Cylert	37.5–112.3 (1–3)
Nonstimulant		
Atomoxetine	Strattera	18–100 (0.7–1.4)

Adapted from Spetie, L., & Arnold, E. L. (2007) Attention deficit/hyperactivity disorder. In A. Martin & F. Volkmar (Eds.). *Lewis's Child and Adolescent Psychiatry: A Comprehensive Textbook*, p. 443. Philadelphia: Lippincott Williams & Wilkins.

(stimulants and atomexetine) typically outperform behavioral treatments. However, 75% of children with ADHD can be managed with only behavioral interventions. The combination of behavioral and pharmacologic intervention also provides some advantages (see Chapter 21).

Behavioral interventions include a host of interventions designed to reinforce desired behaviors, assist the child with organization, and support the child's attempts to cope adaptively. These may include visual supports, charts, organizational aids, behavioral reward systems, and so forth. These can vary from simple to much more complex systems (e.g., token economies or a daily report card from school on the child's behavior). Parent management training offers many advantages (see Chapters 6 and 23).

Although a number of psychoactive medications have been used to treat individuals with ADHD, only a handful have received U.S. Food and Drug Administration (FDA) approval (Table 8.3). The psychostimulants and the one nonstimulant (atomoxetine) have been shown to be effective and are reasonably well tolerated.

For school-age children, it is common to start with a small dose of a stimulant medication and gradually increase the dose. The size of the child is only an approximate guide, and it is important to balance benefits and side effects for the individual child. For example, some children experience an "evening rebound" with stimulant medications that may be avoided by an extended-release preparation or the use of atomoxetine. These agents also have the advantage of minimizing the need for the child to take pills at school. Various side effects have been reported, including appetite suppression, troubles with sleep, irritability, and tics. Occasionally, children treated with high doses develop psychotic-like conditions, but this is uncommon. Although continuous use in nonschool settings is more frequent in recent years, the judicious use of drug holidays for stimulants (e.g., over school vacation and during the summer) provides an opportunity to provide observation in a drug-free state.

Various other agents are sometimes used in the management of individuals with ADHD. Occasionally, the antipsychotic medications have been used, but they have greater risk of side effects and usually are less beneficial. Other drugs not yet FDA approved but with some apparent efficacy include tricyclics, monoamine oxidase inhibitors (MAOIs), and bupropion; these may be particularly helpful when comorbid depression or anxiety is present. In general, the danger of significant adverse effects with foods does limit the use of MAOIs in children. α-Agonists, mainly clonidine and more recently guanfacine, have been used, particularly when agitation and aggression are present; of the two, guanfacine has a longer half-life and less sedation.

Learning difficulties and challenges should be addressed as part of the treatment program. This may include provision of special supports or an Individual Education Program (IEP). For children with clear learning disorders, provision of special supports is particularly important. Education of other family members as well as of the patient is also essential.

SUMMARY

ADHD is one of the most commonly encountered psychiatric disorders in children. Although significant advances in both research and treatment have been made over the past decades, in some respects the disorder appears poorly understood. It is likely that the various factors (environmental, genetic, neurobehavioral, and developmental) contribute, in varying degrees, to the expression of the condition in the individual case. Effective treatments are available. Clinicians should be alert to the possible presence of comorbid conditions and be aware that sometimes the problems of ADHD can mask or mimic or other conditions. Treatment planning should be comprehensive.

Selected Readings

Barkley, R. A. (1997). Behavioral inhibition, sustained attention, and executive function: Constructing a unified theory of ADHD. *Psychological Bulletin, 121,* 65–94.

Barkley, R., Smith, K., Fischer, M., & Navia, B. (2006). An examination of the behavioral and neuropsychological correlates of three ADHD candidate gene polymorphisms (DRD4 7+, DBH TaqI A2, and DAT1 bp VNTR) in hyperactive and normal children followed to adulthood. *American Journal of Medical Genetics Part B (Neuropsychiatric Genetics), 141B,* 487–498.

Barry, R., Johnstone, S. J., & Clarke, A. R. (2003). A review of electrophysiology in attention deficit hyperactivity disorder—event related potentials. *Clinical Neurophysiology, 114,* 184–198.

Cherkasova, M. V., & Hechtman, L. (2009). Neuroimaging in attention-deficit hyperactivity disorder: Beyond the frontostriatal circuitry. *Canadian Journal of Psychiatry, 54*(10), 651–664.

Cook, E. H., Stein, M. A., Krasowski, M. D., et al. (1995). Association of ADHD and the dopamine transporter gene. *American Journal of Human Genetics, 56,* 993–998.

Conners, C. K. (2008). Conners 3, *Conors,* 3rd edition. North Tonawanda, NY: MHS.

Conners, C. K., Epstein, J. N., March, J. S., et al. (2001). Multimodal treatment of ADHD in the MTA: An alternative outcome analysis. *Journal of the American Academy of Child & Adolescent Psychiatry, 40,* 159–167.

Connor, D. (2002). Preschool ADHD: A review of prevalence, diagnosis, neurobiology and stimulant treatment. *Developmental and Behavioral Pediatrics, 23,* 1S.

Cornblatt, B. A., Risch, N. J., Faris, G., Friedman, D., & Erlenmeyer-Kimling, L. (1988). The continuous performance test, identical pairs version (CPT-IP): I. New findings about sustained attention in normal families. *Psychiatric Research, 26*(2), 223–38.

DuPaul, G. J., Weyandt, L. L., O'Dell, S. M., & Varejao, M. (2009). College students with ADHD: Current status and future directions. *Journal of Attention Disorders, 13*(3), 234–250.

Faraone, S. V., Biederman, J., & Zimmerman, B. A. (2005). Correspondence of parent and teacher reports in medication trials. *European Journal of Child and Adolescent Psychiatry, 14,* 20–27.

Faraone, S. V., & Doyle, A. E. (2001). The nature and heritability of ADHD. *Child and Adolescent Psychiatry Clinics of North America, 10,* 299–316, viii–ix.

Faraone, S. V., & Mick, E. (2010). Molecular genetics of attention deficit hyperactivity disorder. *Psychiatric Clinics of North America, 33*(1), 159–180.

Floet, A. M., Scheiner, C., & Grossman, L. (2010). Attention-deficit/hyperactivity disorder. *Pediatrics in Review, 31*(2), 56–69.

Kieling, C., Kieling, R. R., Rohde, L. A., et al. (2010). The age at onset of attention deficit hyperactivity disorder. *American Journal of Psychiatry, 167*(1), 14–16.

Mostofsky, S., Cooper, K., Kates, W., et al. (2002). Smaller prefrontal and premotor volumes in boys with attention deficit hyperactivity disorder. *Biological Psychiatry, 52,* 785–794.

The MTA Cooperative Group. (1999). A 14-month randomized clinical trial of treatment strategies for attention-deficit/hyperactivity disorder. *Archives of General Psychiatry, 56,* 1073–1086.

Rojas, N. L., & Chan, E. (2005). Old and new controversies in the alternative treatment of attention-deficit/hyperactivity disorder. *Mental Retardation and Developmental Disabilities Research Reviews, 11,* 116–130.

Sharp, S. I., McQuillin, A., & Gurling, H. M. (2009). Genetics of attention-deficit hyperactivity disorder (ADHD). *Neuropharmacology, 57*(7-8), 590–600.

Sonuga-Barke, E. J. S. (1994). On dysfunction and function in psychological accounts of childhood disorder. *Journal of Child Psychology and Psychiatry and Allied Disciplines, 35,* 801–815.

Spetie, L., & Arnold, E. L. (2007) Attention deficit/hyperactivity disorder. In A. Martin & F. Volkmar (Eds.). *Lewis's Essential of Child and Adolescent Psychiatry: A Comprehensive Approach,* pp. 430–453. Philadelphia: Lippincott Williams & Wilkins.

CHAPTER 9 ■ OPPOSITIONAL DEFIANT AND CONDUCT DISORDERS

For developing children, the ability to learn to postpone gratification and to modulate aggressive impulses are important development tasks. This effort is fostered by the social context of the family; appropriate modeling by parents and others; and the child's own increased capacities for symbolic thinking, forward planning (appreciation of consequences), and moral development. For most children, this process goes forward relatively smoothly as the child learns to channel aggressive feelings in appropriate ways and learn the complex rules that govern aggressive behavior (e.g., on the sports field). For some children, this process does not go so smoothly, and aggressive behavior is a major clinical problem that may persist into adulthood (see Blader & Jensen, 2007, for a review).

BACKGROUND

Conduct disorder (CD) and oppositional defiant disorders (ODDs), sometimes termed the *disruptive behavior disorders*, represent a major challenge for society in general and the mental health system in particular. Historically referred to as *juvenile delinquency*, the study of criminal behavior and antisocial acts of children is more than a century old and yet remains an important area for both research and clinical work.

In many, but not all, cases, children with these problems go on to have similar problems in adulthood. Early attempts to understand such behavior led to early speculation that such behavior represented a failure in moral development and was potentially genetic. The term *psychopathy* was used by Cleckley to describe individuals without remorse, who did not have close relationships, and whose inner levels were impoverished. Interest in children with these difficulties increased in the early 1900s with the establishment of clinics to help juvenile courts rehabilitate children. Interest in early experience led John Bowlby and others to study early attachments of such children. In one critically important longitudinal study, Lee Robins (1966) was able to document the long-term stability of such behaviors from childhood to adulthood. Early distinctions within this category had to do with the nature of the conduct problems, such as aggressive (fighting) versus nonaggressive (property destruction) and group versus individual behavior.

The term *conduct disorder* was introduced in the *Diagnostic and Statistical Manual* (DSM-III) to describe a condition in which children persistently violated the rights of other or social rules and norms. The term *oppositional defiant disorder* has been used for children whose difficulties included problems with authority figures, provocative behavior, negativity, and so forth. In reality, ODD and CD share many features. Many children who go on to have CD "begin" with ODD, although other children will not do so.

DEFINITION AND CLINICAL DESCRIPTIONS

Guidelines for the diagnosis with a comparison of the somewhat different approaches in DSM-IV and International Classification of Diseases (ICD-10) are listed in Table 9.1. These systems have major similarities and some important differences. In both systems, a diagnosis of CD precludes a diagnosis of ODD. The ICD-10 approach is explicit in suggesting that ODD is a milder form of CD. Similarities in criteria are noteworthy, but differences arise because of requirements for symptom duration and exclusionary features. As a practical matter, the DSM-IV approach is more stringent, possibly too much so. In addition to categorical approaches, dimensional methods using rating scales and checklists have been extensively used in the study of children with conduct problems (see Chapter 3). Such methods have many advantages for research purposes. Attempts have also been made to identify specific subtypes of CD. Instead of the current approach (of less severe ODD and the more severe CD), the DSM-III subdivided CD into three subtypes depending on the presence or absence of socialization and aggressive behavior (e.g., one subtype was unsocialized aggressive). Another approach in DSM-III-R was to distinguish solitary versus group types. In DSM-IV, there is provision for differentiating childhood versus adolescent onset.

The problem of comorbidity (see Chapter 3) is particularly an issue for CD and ODD. It is clear that rates of several other disorders are markedly increased in association to these conditions, notably attention-deficit/hyperactivity disorder (ADHD (10-fold increase), major depression (sevenfold increase) and substance abuse (fourfold increase). It remains unclear which of the two (DSM-IV vs. ICD-10) competing approaches works best. Whereas the DSM-IV encourages multiple diagnoses, the ICD-10 discourages this practice. As a result, the ICD-10 provided codes for mixed categories. This is not a trivial issue because boys with both ADHD and CD have early onset of problem behaviors and worse outcome than those with CD alone.

Children with CDs exhibit a range of problem behaviors sometimes starting from an early age. In contrast to the normative "terrible twos" for whom negativism and defiance is a passing phase, young children with CD repeatedly lose their tempers, are angry, are readily annoyed by others, and are typically defiant. The signs of ODD usually appear relatively early with persistent stubbornness by age 3 years and temper tantrums by 5 years; the signs of CD appear somewhat later (e.g., lying may appear around age 8 years, bullying by age 9 years, and stealing by around 12 years of age). Although aggressive behaviors can be observed before puberty, the severity of such behaviors often markedly increases thereafter. Antisocial behaviors such as stealing and truancy also become more prevalent over time, particularly in adolescence. Some children exhibit decreases in problem behaviors over time, although in general, the symptoms of CD are relatively stable.

For some children, features of ODD symptoms begin when they are infants and then evolve into CD after puberty. For others, these symptoms do not progress to CD; this may be more likely in girls. For some children, the problem behaviors are restricted to one context (e.g., the home), but for others, the behavioral difficulties occur in multiple contests and situations.

EPIDEMIOLOGY

As expected, prevalence estimates of both ODD and CD vary considerably depending on various factors. Table 9.2 summarizes recent studies using the DSM-IV approach and reveal generally consistent results with about 5% of children (6–18 years old) meeting criteria for either one of these conditions in the previous 3 to 6 months. It is clear that ODD and CD are increased at least two- to threefold in boys. Epidemiologic studies also reveal that ODD is not necessarily more prevalent in children and CD in adolescence; in fact, the prevalences are rather similar in both groups.

TABLE 9.1

DIAGNOSTIC GUIDELINES FOR OPPOSITIONAL DEFIANT DISORDER (ODD) AND CONDUCT DISORDER (CD) ACCORDING TO THE *DIAGNOSTIC AND STATISTICAL MANUAL* (DSM-IV-TR) (21) AND INTERNATIONAL CLASSIFICATION OF DISEASES (ICD-10) (20)

Symptoms[1]

1. Often loses temper (ICD-10: "*unusually frequent or sever temper tantrums for developmental level*")
2. Often argues with adults
3. Often actively defies or refuses to comply with adults' requests or rules
4. Often deliberately annoys people
5. Often blames others for his or her mistakes or misbehavior
6. Is often touchy or easily annoyed by others
7. Is often angry and resentful
8. Is often spiteful and vindictive
9. Often bullies, threatens, or intimidates others
10. Often initiates physical fights (ICD-10: "this does not include fights with siblings")
11. Has used a weapon that can cause serious physical harm to others
12. Has been physically cruel to people
13. Has been physically cruel to animals
14. Has stolen while confronting a victim (including purse snatching, extortion, mugging)
15. Has forced someone into sexual activity
16. Has deliberately engaged in fire setting with the intention of causing serious damage
17. Has deliberately destroyed other's property (other than fire setting)
18. Has broken into someone's house, building, or car
19. Often lies to obtain goods or favors or to avoid obligations
20. Has stolen items of nontrivial value without confronting a victim (ICD-10: "within the home or outside")
21. Often stays out at night despite parental prohibitions, beginning before age 13 years
22. Has run away from home overnight at least twice while living in parental or parental surrogate home (or once without returning for a lengthy period) (ICD-10: "or has run away once for more than a single night [this does not include leaving to avoid physical or sexual abuse]")
23. Often truant from school, beginning before age 13 years
    - *DSM-IV ODD*: Four or more of symptoms from 1 to 8, lasting at least 6 months; symptoms do not occur exclusively during a psychotic or mood disorder episode.
    - *ICD-10 ODD*: Four or more symptoms must be present during 6 months, but no more than two must be from symptoms 9 to 23.
    - Symptoms must be developmentally inappropriate in both DSM-IV and ICD-10.
    - *DSM-IV CD*: Three or more of symptoms from 9 to 23 in the past 12 months (at least one present in past 6 months).
    - *ICD-10 CD*: Three or more symptoms must be present and at least three must be from 9 to 23. At least one symptom from 9 to 23 must be present for 6 months. Symptoms 11, 12, 14, 15, 16, 17, and 18 need only have occurred once for the criterion to be fulfilled.
    - *Impairment*: Symptoms must cause significant functional impairment in both taxonomies.

[1]Symptom descriptions are summarized slightly. When description is different between DSM-IV and ICD-10, relevant ICD-10 wording is added.
Shaded areas refer to ODD.
Reprinted from Rey, J. M., Walter, G., & Soutullo, C. (2007). Oppositional defiant and conduct disorders. In A. Martin & F. Volkmar (Eds.), *Lewis's Child and Adolescent Psychiatry: A Comprehensive Textbook*, 4th edition, p. 456. Philadelphia: Lippincott Williams & Wilkins.

Fire Setting

Fire setting is a particularly problematic behavior with potential danger both for the child and others placed at risk. Unfortunately, about half of individuals arrested for arson are younger than 18 years of age, with boys more likely than girls to set fires. Many children have an interest in fire and matches and benefit from education and modeling of safe behaviors and supervision. For other children, fire setting occurs in the context of psychiatric problems. Children with an early interest in fire setting can move along several different pathways, with factors in the school, family, and community all impacting fire setting activity (Barreto, et al., 2007). Treatment is typically multimodal, including aspects of education and attention to associated psychiatric and behavioral problems. It is important that professionals specifically inquire about fire-setting activities.

Case Report: Oppositional Defiant Disorder

Jason, age 7 years, was brought to the child guidance clinic by his mother with a chief complaint that he was "out of control." Jason was exhibiting frequent (usually daily) temper tantrums, which had been escalating in frequency and duration over the past year. The real precipitating event for the visit was that, for the first time, his mother was concerned that he might hit her during their most recent argument (although he did not actually do so).

Jason was living in a single-parent household. The youngest of two sons, he had no contact with his father, who was serving a 20-year sentence for armed robbery. Jason had some trouble in school as academic demands had increased. He has a few, but not many friends, because he has trouble tolerating the demands of others. His mother works two jobs, and he is left either with various babysitters or in the school's after-school program because his much older brother also is working, partly to save money for vocational school. His mother reports that developmental milestones were within normal limits, although he spoke "on the late side."

On examination, Jason tends to minimize his troubles and blames his mother and "deadbeat" father for his problems. He often interrupts his mother when present with her. When seen by himself, he is personable but irritable and angry. He complains that his older brother is the favorite one who can do nothing wrong. He denies feelings of depression or anxiety and appears to have adequate language and attentional skills. He and his mother confirm that it is at home where he has the most difficulty.

Comment: As in this case, children with ODD usually present clinically before about age 8 years. It is more typical for problems to be confined to one setting (often the home). Problems tend to be most noteworthy, and parents, other family members, and the child may appear well organized during the clinical interview. As symptoms become more severe, the likelihood of persistence into conduct disorder increases.

Case Report: Conduct Disorder

Timmy, age 13 years, was brought to the emergency department by the police. He had been truant from school for several days and then ran away from home. This has happened several times during the past year. When contacted by phone, his mother's first comment is, "He is in trouble again." She relates a history of long-standing problems in behavior going back to his first year in school, when he stole some money from a teacher's purse. He has been picked up by the police several times, including once, at age 11 years, for shoplifting in the local mall.

Timmy is an only child. His mother reports that his early developmental milestones were normal but that he was a fussy and demanding infant "just like his father," who she has not seen in 10 years. Timmy had special services in school, and the question of attention-deficit disorder was raised in the past, although his mother refused medications for it. His mother indicates that he is now failing school, which she says is not a surprise because "he never goes to class." She mentions that he hangs out with older kids on the street, and she suspects he is starting to "do drugs." His mother also notes that she was referred to child protective services when Timmy was 8 years old but that nothing came of this.

On examination, Timmy is an angry teenager who appears to just be going through puberty. He minimizes his troubles and explains that life is better on the street than at home. He reports that school is a "drag", and he does not want to have any part of it. Although angry and somewhat dismissive of the psychiatrist, his speech is logically organized. He denies substance abuse, but toxicology screen results are positive.

Comment: Timmy exhibits a history with multiple risk factors for conduct disorder. In addition, his problems with attention and now with substance abuse are fairly frequent in children with conduct problems. As noted by Robins (1966), these problems are, compared with many other psychiatric difficulties, some of the most difficult to treat and can be very persistent.

The issue of time-related (secular) changes is of interest for these disorders given the common perception that children, particularly girls, have more recently exhibited higher rates of OCD and CD. Epidemiologic studies suggest some ethnic or cultural differences (e.g., in the United States vs. the United Kingdom). The classic Isle of Wight study from the 1960s reported a rate of CD (4.2% in 10- to 11-year-old children) that was rather similar to those noted in Table 9.2.

ETIOLOGY

A host of factors have been implicated in the pathogenesis of ODD and CD (Table 9.3). In some ways, the rather daunting list of potential etiologic factors is similar to other aspects of medicine. For example, Dodge and Pettit (2003) have argued that in many respects problems are similar to those involved in study of heart disease with issues in definitions and heterogeneity of clinical phenomena but with a range of relatively easily identified outcomes.

There does appear to be a strong genetic component to ODD and CD, with heritability estimates of about 50%. Other risk factors are listed in Table 9.3. Important risk factors include poverty, attentional problems, intellectual or cognitive difficulties, and family factors. There are likely complex interaction among risk factors and among risk and protective factors. What might otherwise be relatively small risks in isolation may act together to multiply risk.

TABLE 9.2

POINT PREVALENCE (PERCENT) OF *DIAGNOSTIC AND STATISTICAL MANUAL (DSM-IV)* OPPOSITIONAL DEFIANT DISORDER (ODD) AND CONDUCT DISORDER (CD) IN RECENT EPIDEMIOLOGIC STUDIES USING DSM-IV CRITERIA

Sample	Oppositional Defiant Disorder					Conduct Disorder				
	Male	Female	Children	Adolescents	Total	Male	Female	Children	Adolescents	Total
3171 Australian children ages 6 to 17 years (55)						4.4	1.6	4.4[2]	2.4[2]	3.0
1420 children from North Carolina ages 9 to 13 years (51)	3.1	2.1	2.0[1]	3.0[2]	2.7	4.2	1.2	2.4[1]	2.7[2]	2.7
10438 British children ages 5 to 15 year old (56)	3.2	1.4	2.6[3]	1.4[4]	2.3	2.1	0.8	0.9[3]	3.3[4]	1.5
1886 children ages 4 to 17 years from Puerto Rico (57)					2.0					5.5
1251 children ages 7 to 14 years attending school in Southeastern Brazil (58)					3.2					2.2
Average across studies	3.2	1.8	2.3	2.2	2.6	3.4	1.2	2.6	2.8	3.0

[1]9 to 12 years of age.
[2]13 to 16 years of age.
[3]5 to 12 years of age.
[4]13 to 15 years of age.

Reprinted from Rey, J. M., Walter, G., & Soutullo, C. (2007). In A. Martin & F. Volkmar (Eds.), *Lewis's Child and Adolescent Psychiatry: A Comprehensive Textbook*, 4th edition, pp. 458. Philadelphia: Lippincott Williams & Wilkins.

TABLE 9.3

SUMMARY OF FACTORS ASSOCIATED WITH THE DEVELOPMENT OF DISRUPTIVE BEHAVIOR DISORDERS AND OPPORTUNITIES FOR PREVENTION

Risk Factor	Potential Prevention Interventions
Biological ■ Genetic ■ Low birth weight ■ Antenatal and perinatal complications ■ Brain injury, brain disease ■ Male sex	■ Improved antenatal, prenatal, and obstetric care ■ Quit cessation and drug treatment programs targeted to intending parents ■ Programs to reduce domestic violence
Individual ■ Below average IQ ■ Difficult temperament ■ Aggressiveness ■ Impulsivity and hyperactivity ■ Attentional problems ■ Language impairment ■ Reading problems	■ Early identification and adequate support and services for families and individuals with mental retardation ■ Quality home visiting programs that aim to facilitate attachment and enhance parenting skills ■ Parent management training programs ■ "Head Start" type programs ■ Early speech and reading remediation programs
Family ■ Parental antisocial behavior or substance use ■ Domestic violence ■ Single parent, divorce ■ Harsh discipline, maltreatment, or neglect ■ Parent–child conflict ■ Lack of parental supervision ■ Excessive parental control ■ Maternal depression and anxiety ■ Early motherhood	■ Quality home visitation programs ■ Parent management training programs ■ Programs to reduce domestic violence ■ Drug treatment programs ■ Child protection initiatives ■ Early identification and treatment of maternal depression ■ Prevention of teenage pregnancy ■ Support programs for teenage mothers
Social and school ■ Poverty ■ Association with deviant peers or siblings ■ Rejection by peers ■ History of victimization or of being bullied ■ Disorganized, disadvantaged, or high-crime neighborhoods ■ Dysfunctional or disorganized schools ■ Intense exposure to media violence	■ Measures to reduce poverty and provide a social "safety net" ■ Enhance the quality of schools ■ School programs to reduce bullying and prevent behavior problems ■ Initiatives to reduce access to firearms and gang activities ■ Programs to reduce school truancy ■ Initiatives to enhance neighborhood cohesion ■ Law enforcement initiatives to reduce crime targeted to high-crime areas ■ Public campaigns to reduce media violence and education about how to monitor and prevent children's exposure to it

Reprinted from Rey, J. M., Walter, G., & Soutullo, C. (2007). In A. Martin & F. Volkmar (Eds.), *Lewis's Child and Adolescent Psychiatry: A Comprehensive Textbook*, 4th edition, pp. 459. Philadelphia: Lippincott Williams & Wilkins.

Although genetic factors are also important, they can interact with environmental factors. Genetic factors may appear weaker in children coming from supportive environments. And to complicate things further, the genetic factors may themselves act to influence the environment. Disentangling these variables is complex (e.g., higher income levels may contribute to better parental supervision). Physiologically, one of the best replicated correlates of antisocial social behavior is low resting heart rate.

Neuroimaging research has focused on the frontal lobe; differences have been noted in the prefrontal cortex and orbital frontal lobe. The neurotransmitter serotonin has also been of interest given a potential link between higher levels of aggression and low central nervous system serotonin levels.

DIFFERENTIAL DIAGNOSIS AND ASSESSMENT

The clinician should be careful to use multiple sources of information and relevant questionnaires and other data in making the diagnosis of ODD or CD. Symptoms may be exhibited in only one context (e.g., the home). Requests for assessment may come from a wide range of persons, including parents, teachers, and juvenile justice or social service agencies. It is particularly important to clarify the purpose of the assessment and be sure that it is understood by the child or adolescent. As a group, these individuals can be difficult to interview given their anger at authority figures and minimization of their own difficulties. Often, referral comes only after years of difficulty. It is common to have conflicting reports from children, parents, and teachers.

A search for potential etiological risk factors (e.g., psychosocial adversity, parent-child problems, maternal depression, abuse) should be conducted. Information on the child's relationship with his or her parents and peers is important. Individuals with intellectual deficiency or subaverage cognitive ability present special problems for diagnosis. In contrast to boys, who are more likely to be aggressive, girls may be more inclined to use less overt methods involving social ostracism and so forth (a factor possibly accounting for lower observed rates in girls). Such behaviors can, however, be serious, with grave consequences for other children. Although it is possible to make a diagnosis of ODD or CD in preschoolers, these diagnoses are usually first made in school-age children or adolescents.

A diagnosis of CD is not made if the difficulties are simply an understandable reaction to a problematic situation (e.g., in some situations such as theaters of war or high-crime areas); these behaviors may be protective and not necessarily indicative of psychopathology. It is important that the clinician keep the possibility of comorbidity in mind in assessing children and adolescents with delinquent or disruptive behaviors. As noted previously, frequent disorders also observed include ADHD, depression, substance abuse, and anxiety and somatoform disorders. Some children on the autism spectrum, probably particularly those with Asperger disorder, may run into trouble with the law often because, paradoxically, they are too rigid and rule governed or because of some isolated special interest and poor social judgment. Occasionally, a child or adolescent with an acute psychotic episode may present with a major violation of social or societal norms or a crime of violence. Similarly, individuals with bipolar disorder have high rates of behavioral difficulties. The issue of comorbid CD or ODD and bipolar disorder in prepubertal children remains very controversial. Some children with major depression or anxiety may be irritable or noncompliant. A host of rating scales and questionnaires are available for use in evaluating children with ODD or CD (see Rey et al., 2007). The evaluation of the child or adolescent should include a careful medical history, review of educational records, and so forth. Apart from drug toxicology screens in adolescents, routine laboratory studies are not generally indicated. Occasionally, children with seizures may present with unusual behavior. Screening for sexually transmitted diseases is indicated if the child has been sexually active or sexually abused.

TREATMENT

Typically, many different approaches are used in the management of children with ODD or CD. These include psychological, behavioral, and pharmacologic approaches, sometimes alone but often in combination. Both the child and family may be involved in the treatment. Traditional psychotherapy appears to have relatively little utility. Research on effective interventions has been limited by problems in study design, difficulties with definitions, and so forth. As with other treatments, fidelity to the treatment model outside the academic center can also be problematic. Dependent variables for these studies have included symptoms ratings or, for adolescents, variables such as aggressive outbursts, arrest rates, and so forth.

ODD and CD tend to be chronic conditions. Typically, psychosocial interventions are used initially and then continued even if medications are added. Intervening early in the disorder may be more effective (i.e., before symptom patterns are well established). Treatment should also typically involve parents and thoughtful attention to any comorbid conditions (e.g., ADHD, depression). Goals of treatment should be realistic and progressive, e.g., preventing escalation or a move to another phase of difficulty, such as substance abuse, may be important as a first step in the treatment process. Attention should also be paid to school and peer groups; facilitating appropriate participation with typical peers is important.

Interestingly, children and adolescents with CD and ODD commonly present to emergency departments (EDs) after a legal, parental, school, or some other crisis. Often, this had led to aggressive behavior and problems with others or destruction of property. Children who present to the ED with such problem are more likely to have more severe difficulties or comorbid problems. The differentiation of ODD versus CD can be difficult but usually is less relevant in the emergency situation. Crisis intervention and psychosocial interventions should be attempted before use of medications. Restraint or seclusion should be used only as a last resort.

Table 9.4 summarizes evidence for treatment efficacy in children with ODD and CD.

Parent management training (PMT) uses positive reinforcement and aspects of social-learning theory and operant conditioning and is the most extensively researched treatment for these conditions. This method helps parents use positive reinforcement to effect more productive disciplinary strategies. It can produce significant improvement in both the home and school with indirect effects in other areas such as relationships with siblings and marital satisfaction.

Problems with the method include high drop-out rates and difficulties in use in the most complicated families. It has also been used more in younger children. Various PMT programs are available, with five to 15 sessions followed by phone follow-up; it can be used in group settings or individually (see Chapters 22 and 23).

Multimodal interventions may augment PMT for example by targeting peer relations or academic context. This approach has shown better results than PMT along. Sample programs include multisystemic therapy (MST) and Families and Schools Together (FAST Track). MST tends to target adolescents and more severe conduct problems, but the FAST program focuses on children with CD starting school; this program is designed to intervene to prevent worsened functioning. The MST approach is intensive with a home-based approach 7 days a week for about 4 months. This resource-intensive program appears to be cost effective.

Yet another approach is to place teens in special foster care programs. These relatively short (6-month) placements may reduce subsequent criminality. Various other programs including residential treatments and intensive wilderness or "boot camp" type programs have not been well evaluated. Individual approaches have focused on problem-solving skills training during which children are helped to use various techniques to derive more adaptive solutions to problems; these methods have at least a modest benefit.

Drug treatments are used only when other interventions fail and as part of an overall, comprehensive program (e.g., for children with other comorbid conditions such as ADHD or in emergency situations). Pharmacotherapy should be cautious with careful monitoring. The risk for substance abuse suggests considerable care in prescribing stimulants to adolescents with CD. It is important that trials of medication be adequate, and polypharmacy should be avoided. The strength of evidence for drug treatments in summarized in Table 9.4. Frequently

TABLE 9.4

SUMMARY OF TREATMENTS FOR OPPOSITIONAL DEFIANT AND CONDUCT DISORDERS

Treatment	Strength of Recommendation[1]	Quality of Evidence[2]	Comments
Psychosocial			
Parent management training	* * *	A	Limited empirical data for adolescents
Multisystemic therapy	**	A	Usually targets severely disordered or delinquent youth, resource intensive
FAST Track	*	B	Children starting school
Problem-solving skills training	*	B	
Therapeutic foster care	*	A	Usually targets severely disordered or delinquent youth,
Anger management programs	#	C	
Wilderness programs, boot camps, and similar programs	#	C	Usually target severely disordered or delinquent youth
Pharmacologic			
Antipsychotic drugs	*	B	Uncertain evidence; good short-term results with risperidone for individuals with mental retardation
Mood stabilizers and anticonvulsants	#	B	Heterogeneous participants (e.g., aggressive adolescents, CD with various comorbidities); inconsistent results; somewhat better data for lithium
Stimulants	#	B–	In children with comorbid ADHD
Atomoxetine	#	B–	In children with comorbid ADHD
Clonidine	#	B–	In children with comorbid ADHD
SSRIs	#	E	In children with comorbid major depression

[1] * * * (good supporting evidence) through # (uncertain evidence).
[2] A (supported by meta-analysis of several, sound, randomized controlled trials) through C (systematic open studies) to E (expert opinion).
ADHD, attention-deficit/hyperactivity disorder; CD, conduct disorder; FAST, Families and Schools Together; SSRI, selective serotonin reuptake inhibitor.
Reprinted from Rey, J. M., Walter, G., & Soutullo, C. (2007). In A. Martin & F. Volkmar (Eds.), *Lewis's Child and Adolescent Psychiatry: A Comprehensive Textbook*, 4th edition, p. 462. Philadelphia: Lippincott Williams & Wilkins.

used medications include atypical neuroleptics such as risperidone, which may have a short-term benefit, particularly for aggressive behavior. Mood-stabilizing medications have also been used, although results are less consistent.

COURSE

By definition in DSM-IV, adult antisocial personality disorder is preceded by CD. Although debated, the relationship of the two conditions has been well recognized for many years. In addition, childhood ODD and CD are associated with a range of other psychiatric difficulties in adulthood, including substance abuse, mood disorders, and psychosis. Other complications include suicide, educational problems, unemployment, and teen pregnancy. It appears that for many individuals, childhood difficulties become entrained in a cycle of difficulties, leading to progressively less favorable outcomes. In general, the more frequent and severe the behavioral difficulties in childhood, the worse the adult outcome. Fortunately, most adolescents with CD do not go on to develop adult antisocial personality disorders. For reasons that remain unclear, these behaviors often diminish in early adult life. The relationship of childhood ODD to adult difficulties is much less clear.

Given the societal and clinical significance of these conditions, considerable efforts have been made in the area of prevention. It is clear that such efforts must be comprehensive and multifaceted. There are many advantages to prevention, so one important role for mental health professionals is education of policy makers about the wisdom of investing in prevention efforts. The behavioral problems associated with ODD and CD cannot be viewed in isolation. Rather, they must be addressed systematically in the context of the families, schools, and communities where they occur. Schools have a particularly important role in prevention. As noted in Table 9.3, there are many areas of potential preventive efforts. More research on prevention is needed, but the available data suggest potential for improved child functioning. Many of the treatments already used can be adapted for preventive purposes.

SUMMARY

Conduct problems and oppositional behavior are important societal problems. CD, unfortunately, can be one of the most persistent childhood psychiatric diagnoses. A minority of individuals will go on to have overt antisocial personality disorder. Even for those who do not, there may be continuing difficulties both in social relationships and work settings. Although many treatments have been proposed, rigorous study of these treatments has been less common. Efforts at prevention, through many different modalities, remain important.

Selected Readings

Barreto, S. J., Zeff, K. R., Boekamp, J. R., & Paccione-Dyszlewski, M. (2007). Fire behavior in children and adolescents. In A. Martin & F. Volkmar (Eds.), *Lewis's Child and Adolescent Psychiatry: A Comprehensive Textbook*, 4th edition, pp. 483–493. Philadelphia: Lippincott Williams & Wilkins.

Barton, J. (2003). Conduct disorder: Intervention and prevention. *International Journal of Mental Health Promotion, 5*:32–41.

Blader, J. D., & Jensen, P. S. (2007). Aggression in children: An integrative approach. In A. Martin & F. Volkmar (Eds.), *Lewis's Child and Adolescent Psychiatry: A Comprehensive Textbook*, 4th edition, pp. 467–483. Philadelphia: Lippincott Williams & Wilkins.

Breslow, R. E., Klinger, B. I., & Erickson, B. J. (1999). The disruptive behavior disorders in the psychiatric emergency service. *General Hospital Psychiatry, 21*, 214–219.

Dodge, K. A., & Pettit, G. S. (2003). A biopsychosocial model of the development of chronic conduct problems in adolescence. *Developmental Psychology, 39*, 349–371.

Eyberg, S. M., Nelson, M. M., & Boggs, S. R., et al. (2008). Evidence-based psychosocial treatments for children and adolescents with disruptive behavior. *Journal of Clinical Child & Adolescent Psychology, 37*(1), 215–237.

Fazel, S., Doll, H., Langstrom, N., et al. (2008). Mental disorders among adolescents in juvenile detention and correctional facilities: A systematic review and metaregression analysis of 25 surveys. *Journal of the American Academy of Child & Adolescent Psychiatry, 47*(9), 1010–1019.

Fergusson, D., Swain-Campbell, N., & Horwood, J. (2004). How does childhood economic disadvantage lead to crime? *Journal of Child Psychology and Psychiatry, 45,* 956–966.

Frick, P. J., Lahey, B. B., Loeber, R., et al. (1993). Oppositional defiant disorder and conduct disorder: A meta-analytic review of factor analyses and cross validation in a clinical sample. *Clinical Psychology Review, 13,* 319–340.

Kazdin, A. E. (1997). Parent management training: Evidence, outcomes and issues. *Journal of American Academy of Child and Adolescent Psychiatry, 36,* 1349–1356.

Moffitt, T. E. (1993). Adolescence-limited and life-course-persistent antisocial behavior: A developmental taxonomy. *Psychological Review, 100,* 674–701.

Moffitt, T. E., Arseneault, L., Jaffee, S. R., et al. (2008). DSM-V conduct disorder: Research needs for an evidence base. *Journal of Child Psychology & Psychiatry & Allied Disciplines, 49*(1), 3–33.

Rey, J. M., Walter, G., & Soutullo, C. (2007). Oppositional defiant and conduct disorders. In A. Martin & F. Volkmar (Eds.), *Lewis's Child and Adolescent Psychiatry: A Comprehensive Textbook*, 4th edition, p. 462. Philadelphia: Lippincott Williams & Wilkins.

Robins, L. N. (1966). *Deviant Children Grown Up*. Baltimore: Williams & Wilkins.

Rutter, M., Tizard, J., & Whitmore, K. (1970). *Education, Health and Behavior*. London: Longman.

CHAPTER 10 ■ CHILDHOOD SCHIZOPHRENIA AND CHILDHOOD PSYCHOSIS

Interest in psychotic disorders in childhood is a relatively recent historical phenomenon. As commonly used, the term *psychotic* can itself be problematic given the changing nature of children's conceptions of reality. At one time, the term *childhood psychosis* was used quite broadly, but more recently the term and related diagnostic concepts have been more narrowly defined. The prototypic disorder is childhood-onset schizophrenia, but in other psychotic conditions, much less well defined and transient psychotic phenomena are common. When present in children, schizophrenia and related psychotic conditions have the potential for serious disruption of development and hence may be more severe than in adulthood. This chapter focuses on schizophrenia of onset in childhood and adolescence and, more briefly, of children with psychosis resembling schizophrenia but not meeting current *Diagnostic and Statistical Manual* (DSM-IV-TR) criteria for the disorder. Psychosis related to mood disorder is discussed in Chapter 11.

Before age 5 years, psychotic phenomena are uncommon and often stress related. Hallucinations may be seen as isolated phenomena and generally are relatively much more prognostically benign. By school age, the presence of psychotic phenomena is more concerning because such symptoms may persist. In this age group, potential factors such as drug exposure or other mental disorders should be considered (e.g., hallucinations and psychotic phenomena may also be observed in mood disorders). By the end of middle childhood, the presence of psychotic phenomena becomes much more predictive of subsequent schizophrenia

DIAGNOSIS AND CLINICAL FEATURES

Kraeplin's (1899) description of "dementia praecox" (what today is termed *schizophrenia*) was a watershed in psychiatric taxonomy. He explicitly noted that in some cases, onset was in childhood, and a downward extrapolation of the concept to children ("dementia praecossisma") quickly followed. Severe psychiatric disturbance in childhood became equated with schizophrenia. Kanner's description of the syndrome of infantile autism was taken by some as a description of the first manifestations of schizophrenia in infants and young children. However, with the pioneering work of Kolvin (1971), Rutter (1972), and others, it became clear that autism (see Chapter 4) is quite different from schizophrenia of childhood onset and was, if anything, much less common than autism. As a result, a category for childhood schizophrenia (which before the DSM-III in 1980 included what would now be termed autistic disorder) was dropped, and infantile autism was officially recognized.

The DSM-IV-TR defines schizophrenia in basically the same way for children as for adolescents and adults. The DSM-IV-TR definition includes the various signs and symptoms traditionally associated with schizophrenia. These include both positive and negative symptoms (i.e., hallucinations as well as flattening of affect). By definition, the condition must be present for at least 6 months (it is noted that treatment may shorten the active psychotic phase) and must cause dysfunction in expected levels of functioning. For children, this can take the form of failure to achieve expected academic or social skills (i.e., rather than being restricted to a loss of skill). By definition, the disorder is not better accounted for by a mood disorder or schizoaffective disorder or by a general medical condition or substance abuse. A diagnosis of autism or pervasive development disorder can only be made if hallucinations and delusions are prominent for at least 1 month (or less if successfully treated). It is possible to specify various subtypes of the disorder (e.g., paranoid, disorganized, catatonic, undifferentiated) as well as the potential for some additional diagnostic codes (e.g., specifying course after 1 year). Other conditions included in this section of DSM-IV-TR include schizophreniform disorder (which is similar to schizophrenia except a decline in function is not required, and symptoms last from one to 6 months). Apart from psychotic disorder not otherwise specified (NOS), the other disorders in this group are rarely diagnosed in children. The DSM-IV-TR notes that late adolescent onset is frequent but that onset before adolescence is rare, particularly before puberty. It also notes that although the essential features are similar in children, adolescents, and adults with the condition, children may have less elaborated hallucination and delusions and that difficulties with language or attention or other developmental problems can complicate the diagnosis. Younger children may also be less likely to exhibit some of the "negative" symptoms. Incoherence and poverty of thinking are also somewhat less common than in adults.

Several different patterns of onset have been identified. These include a pattern of acute onset, another with gradual onset, and finally a pattern that includes a gradual onset followed by acute exacerbation of symptoms. The insidious onset pattern is more common. Sometimes symptoms emerge in a child who has previously had other developmental or behavioral problems. These can take the forms of developmental disorders (e.g., of learning or language or of the disruptive behavior disorders). Sometimes autistic-like symptoms are reported retrospectively (e.g., echolalia or hand flapping), but these tend to be of brief duration. Social oddity is also sometimes noted. Several groups have now confirmed these various premorbid features in many cases.

Auditory hallucinations are reported most frequently (~80% of cases). As with adults, the content might include voices, often with persecutory content, commenting about the child. Somatic and visual hallucinations are less frequent. The content of the hallucinations is usually less elaborate in children and often reflects age-appropriate concerns (e.g., monsters or toys rather than more sexual themes). In childhood schizophrenia, auditory hallucinations are most consistently reported.

Delusions in children with schizophrenia are often less bizarre and systematic than those observed in adults. There may be concerns with thought broadcasting, thought insertion, and thought withdrawal.

EPIDEMIOLOGY AND DEMOGRAPHICS

Among school-age children, schizophrenia is relatively rare. Although solid epidemiologic data are critically needed, the childhood form of the disorder is probably 50 times less frequent than adult-onset schizophrenia. Clearly, the rate increases with age with onset frequent in adolescence. The condition appears to be somewhat more common in boys, particularly with younger children. As with adult schizophrenia, boys also appear to have an earlier onset than girls. Also, as with adults, there is probably some bias for increased rates in families with lower socioeconomic status.

ETIOLOGY

As might be expected, it appears that the familial risk for schizophrenia and schizophrenic-like illness is greater in childhood onset cases, with higher rates of cytogenetic abnormalities than seen in adults. Many potential candidate genes have been identified in adults and may be operative in childhood schizophrenia as well, although small sample sizes can complicate genetic studies. Associations have been reported with various conditions, including Smith-Magenis syndrome (17p11.2del), and 15q11-q13 deletions or duplications as well as with the 22q11 deletion syndrome (22q11DS) the velocardiofacial syndrome, which is associated with a high risk for schizophrenia. Mosaic Turner's syndrome has also been noted at a higher than expected rate in the National Institute of Mental Health (NIMH) series of cases (see Gogray and Rapoport, 2007).

Various studies have examined the neuropsychological correlates of childhood-onset schizophrenia. Children with schizophrenia have more difficulty with tasks that involve greater attention, fine motor coordination, and working memory. Attentional difficulties have been explored using Event Related Potentials, showing decreased early receptor potential amplitude when children are engaged in these tasks; these results are similar to those seen in adults.

The NIMH group has looked for various risk factors associated with schizophrenia in adults within their childhood-onset sample. Interestingly, they failed to find increased obstetric risk (relative to healthy sibling control subjects), although there was a suggestion of differences in smooth pursuit eye movements. As with adult-onset schizophrenia, there appeared to be a significant genetic component, with higher than expected rates of schizophrenia spectrum disorders in family members. In their samples, the NIMH group assessed neurocognitive functioning and found that siblings of individuals with childhood-onset schizophrenia had poorer performance on a battery of neuropsychological assessments than community control subject. However, the rates of neuropsychological abnormalities did not differ between childhood- and adult-onset schizophrenia.

Neuroimaging studies have been conducted in individuals with childhood-onset schizophrenia and fairly consistently reveal increased volume of the lateral ventricles along with reduced gray matter but with increased volume of the basal ganglia. Some of the observed changes may, however, relate to medication effects). The longitudinal studies of the NIMH cohort of cases have been particularly helpful in document progressive changes over a period of several years.

DIFFERENTIAL DIAGNOSIS AND ASSESSMENT

Although rare, schizophrenia of childhood onset should be considered if a child or adolescent manifests obvious psychotic symptoms. Sometimes, particularly early on in the course, the psychotic symptoms may not be dramatic, but there may be a noteworthy loss or deterioration of functioning. As already noted, various modifications of the DSM-IV criteria can be made for children. Despite these modifications, the diagnosis can, at times, be difficult. Several other conditions should be considered as part of the differential diagnosis. Hallucinations can be observed both in children with bipolar disorder and major depression, but these hallucinations are usually mood congruent and less disorganized. The course of the disorders also provides clarification. Particularly among adolescents but even among younger children, substance abuse, various medical conditions, or even side effects of medications may lead to psychotic phenomena. Hallucinations can be seen as isolated phenomena in some conditions (e.g., conduct disorders), but other symptoms of schizophrenia should not then be present. Similarly, the thoughts and compulsions of obsessive-compulsive disorder may occasionally be taken to suggest schizophrenia, although careful inquiry should then fail to find the characteristic psychotic symptoms. Occasionally children with autism and autism spectrum disorders seem odd or eccentric, particularly more verbal children with Asperger disorder; usually in these cases, careful review of history and current examination will clarify the diagnosis. It is common for the clinician to arrive essentially at a diagnosis of psychosis NOS given some of these difficulties and the rarity and complexity of diagnosis of psychosis in childhood. Various terms have been used to refer to this group of cases; the NIMH group has used the term *multidimensionally impaired.*

As noted previously, developmental issues and comorbid disorders can pose complexities for diagnosis. Hallucinations may be seen in young children (e.g., associated with stress) and tend to be visual and tactile rather than auditory. It is also important for the evaluator to realize that younger children, particularly younger than age 6 years, may have not yet have full knowledge of discourse rules (sometimes leading to difficulties following the child's line of thinking); also, in this age group, beliefs in fantasy figures and what Piaget termed *magical thinking* are relatively common (see Chapter 1). Some of the characteristic features associated with schizophrenia, such as disorganized behavior or speech, can be observed in children for various reasons. This can lead to a potential for overdiagnosis in school-age children, but schizophrenia in adolescents can sometimes be missed because of substance abuse. Unfortunately, sometimes adolescents attempt to medicate emergent psychotic symptoms. Further complicating matters, many children who are psychotic clearly do not meet strict application of DSM-IV-TR criteria for schizophrenia. Diagnosis is more complicated in younger children. With the onset of adolescence, the diagnosis becomes easier to make. Specific assessment instruments (e.g., for assessment of thought disorder) have also been developed (Caplan and Guthrie, 2000).

In addition to being alert to signs of possible substance abuse, clinicians should also conduct a reasonable search for medical conditions that might be associated with psychosis or be mistaken for schizophrenia. Partial complex seizures, for example, may present with changes in sensorium and features suggestive of psychosis.

Evaluation of children with possible schizophrenia should include a careful history, including premorbid functioning, nature and type of onset, and family and medical history. Psychological testing may be used to document thought disorder (i.e., projective testing and IQ and achievement testing may help clarify issues relevant to intervention). The mental status examination and history should be done carefully to include inquiry relative to both positive and negative symptoms. Sometimes just giving the child a pencil and drawing materials is sufficient to elicit psychotic signs (Figure 10.1). Unusual features, such as prominent mood

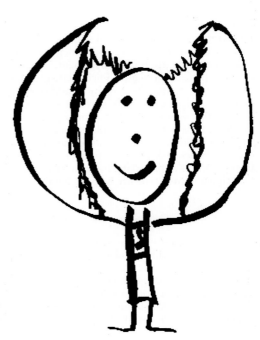

FIGURE 10.1. Drawing by a 9-year-boy with schizophrenia. He believed a radio transmitter had been implanted in his head (see antennae). He had persecutory delusions as well. (Reprinted from Lewis, M., & Volkmar, F. (1990). *Clinical Aspects of Child Development*, 3rd edition, p. 353. Philadelphia: Lea and Febiger.)

symptoms, should be noted. The physical examination should include consideration of conditions with a potential to cause psychosis. The child should be evaluated for possible substance abuse, and electroencephalography and neurologic consultation may be considered. It is important for clinicians to be aware of the potential for unusual presentations (e.g., delirium may be mistaken for psychosis and schizophrenia, and occasionally a child may present with catatonic symptoms; see Williams, 2007).

COURSE AND PROGNOSIS

The course of childhood-onset schizophrenia tends, unfortunately, to resemble that of adult cases with poor outcome (i.e., symptoms tend to be severe and persistent). Very early onset (before age 10 years) is associated with the worst prognosis. Although some variability in course is noted, the most typical pattern is one with periodic acute exacerbations occurring in the context of a steady deterioration in functioning. Sometimes stabilization occurs.

Several different factors may contribute to the worsened prognosis of schizophrenia with childhood onset. These include the possibility of increased genetic risk or the disruption that the disorder causes for subsequent learning and development. It appears the earlier onset, particularly when associated with preexisting difficulties, is a major sign of a bad prognosis. There is some suggestion that association with more affective symptoms, acute onset, later onset, and well-differentiated symptoms are associated with a better outcome.

TREATMENT

Research on treatment of childhood-onset schizophrenia is relatively limited. This reflects several factors, including the difficulty in obtaining adequate samples for well-controlled studies as well as other factors. The few studies available confirm that the first-generation antipsychotics are superior to placebo, and one small group of patients was noted to respond better to clozapine over haloperidol. The difficulties with clozapine in this population effectively severely restrict its use. Well-controlled studies with the newer atypical neuroleptics are needed.

As with adult-onset schizophrenia, comorbid conditions are frequent and can be an important consideration in management. Anxiety and mood disorders can significantly impact both the presentation and clinical management of cases; anxiety disorders, in particular, seem to persist over time. Treatment of additional conditions, when present, can be particularly helpful. Clinicians should be careful to titrate medication doses to achieve a balance of control of psychotic symptoms while avoiding sedation and other side effects. Clinicians should also be alert to the potential for side effects (e.g., neuroleptic malignant syndrome).

Many children with schizophrenia have significant issues in learning and development than can be addressed through a comprehensive educational plan. Special education services should be provided as appropriate. Integration of the treatment program and thoughtful involvement of a clinician over time are helpful. Family involvement is also important.

SUMMARY

The diagnosis of childhood schizophrenia in children with severe cognitive limitations or language disorder is particularly challenging. Other conditions can present with psychotic features (e.g., adolescents with borderline personality can exhibit psychotic phenomena, although these usually are less enduring and less frequently associated with thought disorder). Significant advances in our understanding of childhood schizophrenia have been made but much work remains. Prospective studies of at risk populations may be particularly helpful in this regard.

Case Report: Childhood-Onset Schizophrenia

Kristine was the second of two children born to upper middle class parents after a term pregnancy complicated by maternal viral illness and prolonged labor. At birth, she was noted to be in good condition. She was a somewhat fussy baby whose motor and communication development appeared to proceed appropriately. She appeared to be normally related socially and enjoyed social interaction games with her parents and older sister. She was enrolled in a nursery school program at age 4 years and subsequently in regular kindergarten and first grade classes; although she was noted to be somewhat shy, no other concerns were raised about her cognitive or emotional development. At age 6 years, 11 months, she exhibited an episode of acute delusions and hallucinations. This had been preceded by a period of several weeks during which she was noted to be somewhat withdrawn and occasionally talked to herself. The hallucinations were predominately auditory in nature but not very elaborate, consisting mostly of single words. Delusional beliefs centered around being kidnapped. She became progressively more anxious and developed some complicated rituals apparently revolving around her delusional fears. She was hospitalized for evaluation.

Extensive medical evaluations failed to reveal an explanation for her difficulties. Various studies, including electroencephalography, were normal. A positive family history of schizophrenia in a maternal aunt was noted. The clinician in charge of her care prescribed a low dose of an atypical neuroleptic with partial remission of the hallucinations and delusions. Kristine remained rather withdrawn. She was seen for ongoing supportive psychotherapy and medication management

At age 10 years, she was seen for comprehensive assessment. IQ testing revealed borderline intellectual functioning. She had some communication problems. Projective testing revealed some continued difficulties with reality testing. She had occasional hallucinations and a fairly complicated set of delusional beliefs. Her affect was relatively bland. She exhibited some unusual mannerisms.

As an adolescent, Kristine had an exacerbation of her difficulties. She became overtly suicidal and after hospitalization, a residential placement was arranged.

Comment: Early onset schizophrenia is, as this case illustrates, often associated with relatively poor outcome. In this case, the child had a relatively prolonged period of normal development before the onset of psychotic symptoms; this is a different pattern than that observed in autism.

Adapted from Volkmar, F., & Tsatsanis, K. (2002) Childhood schizophrenia, In M. Lewis (Ed.), *Child and Adolescent Psychiatry: A Comprehensive Textbook*, 3rd edition, pp. 745–754. Baltimore: Williams & Wilkins.

Selected Readings

Arango, C., Moreno, C., Martínez, S., et al. (2008). Longitudinal brain changes in early-onset psychosis. *Schizophrenia Bulletin, 34*(2), 341–353.

Asarnow, J. R., Tompson, M. C., & McGrath, E. P. (2004). Annotation: Childhood-onset schizophrenia: Clinical and treatment issues. *Journal of Child Psychology & Psychiatry & Allied Disciplines, 45*(2), 180–194.

Calderoni, D., Wudarsky, M., Bhangoo, R., et al. (2001). Differentiating childhood-onset schizophrenia from psychotic mood disorders. *Journal of the American Academy of Child & Adolescent Psychiatry, 40*(10), 1190–1196.

Campbell, M., Young, P. I., Bateman, D. N., et al. (1999). The use of atypical antipsychotics in the management of schizophrenia. *British Journal of Clinical Pharmacology, 47*(1), 13–22.

Caplan, R., Guthrie, D., Tang, B., et al. (2000). Thought disorder in childhood schizophrenia: replication and update of concept. *Journal of the American Academy of Child & Adolescent Psychiatry, 39*(6), 771–778.

Davis, J. M., Chen, N., & Glick, I. D. (2003). A meta-analysis of the efficacy of second-generation antipsychotics. *Archives of General Psychiatry, 60*(6), 553–564.

Egan, M. F., Goldberg, T. E., Gscheidle, T., et al. (2001). Relative risk for cognitive impairments in siblings of patients with schizophrenia. *Biological Psychiatry, 50*(2), 98–107.

Eggers, C., Bunk, D., & Kraus, D. (2000). Schizophrenia with onset before the age of eleven: Clinical characteristics of onset and course. *Journal of Autism and Developmental Disabilities, 30*, 29–38.

Gochman, P. A., Greenstein, D., Sporn, A., et al. (2004). Childhood onset schizophrenia: Familial neurocognitive measures. *Schizophrenia Research, 71*(1), 43–47.

Gogtay, N., & Rapoport, J. (2007) Childhood onset schizophrenia and other early onset disorders. In A. Martin & F. Volkmar (Eds.), *Lewis's Child and Adolescent Psychiatry: A Comprehensive Textbook*, 4th edition, pp. 493–502. Philadelphia: Wolters Kluwer.

Jacobsen, L. K., Giedd, J. N., Castellanos, F. X., et al. (1998). Progressive reduction of temporal lobe structures in childhood-onset schizophrenia. *American Journal of Psychiatry, 155*(5), 678–685.

Kolvin, I. (1971). Studies in the childhood psychoses. I. Diagnostic criteria and classification. *British Journal of Psychiatry, 118*(545), 381–384.

Kraeplin, E. (1899). *Psychiatrie: Ein Lehrbuch fur Studirende und Aerzte. Sechste, vollstandig umgearbeitete Auflage.* Leipzig: Verlag von Johann Ambrosius Barth.

Kumra, S., Oberstar, J. V., Sikich, L., et al. (2008). Efficacy and tolerability of second-generation antipsychotics in children and adolescents with schizophrenia [see comment]. *Schizophrenia Bulletin, 34*(1), 60–71.

Kumra, S., Wiggs, E., Bedwell, J., et al. (2000). Neuropsychological deficits in pediatric patients with childhood-onset schizophrenia and psychotic disorder not otherwise specified. *Schizophrenia Research, 42*(2), 135–144.

Murphy, K. C., Jones, L. A., & Owen, M. J. (1999). High rates of schizophrenia in adults with velo-cardio-facial syndrome. *Archives of General Psychiatry, 56*(10), 940–945.

Rapoport, J. C., Addington, A. M., & Frangou, S. (2005). The neurodevelopmental model of schizophrenia: Update 2005. *Molecular Psychiatry, 10*(6), 614.

Remschmidt, H. (2001) *Schizophrenia in Children and Adolescents.* Cambridge, U.K.: Cambridge University Press.

Ross, R. G., Heinlein, S., Tregellas, H. (2006). High rates of comorbidity are found in childhood-onset schizophrenia. *Schizophrenia Research, 88*(1-3), 90–95.

Ross, R. G., Novins, D., Farley, G. K., & Adler, L. E. (2003). A 1-year open-label trial of olanzapine in school-age children with schizophrenia. *Journal of Child & Adolescent Psychopharmacology, 13*(3), 301–309.

Rutter, M. (1972). Childhood schizophrenia reconsidered. *Journal of Autism & Childhood Schizophrenia, 2*(4), 315–337.

Schaeffer, J. L. & Ross, R. G. (2002). Childhood-onset schizophrenia: premorbid and prodromal diagnostic and treatment histories. *Journal of the American Academy of Child & Adolescent Psychiatry, 41*(5), 538–545.

Sowell, E. R., Toga, A. W., & Asarnow, R. (2000). Brain abnormalities observed in childhood-onset schizophrenia: A review of the structural magnetic resonance imaging literature. *Mental Retardation and Developmental Disabilities Research Review, 6*(3), 180–185.

Sporn, A., Greenstein, D., Gogtay, N., et al. (2005). Childhood-onset schizophrenia: smooth pursuit eye-tracking dysfunction in family members. *Schizophrenia Research, 73*(2-3), 243–252.

Sporn, A. L., Vermani, A., Greenstein, D. K., et al. (2007). Clozapine treatment of childhood-onset schizophrenia: Evaluation of effectiveness, adverse effects, and long-term outcome. *Journal of the American Academy of Child & Adolescent Psychiatry, 46*(10), 1349–1356.

Usiskin, S. I., Nicolson, R., Krasnewich, D. M., et al. (1999). Velocardiofacial syndrome in childhood-onset schizophrenia. *Journal of the American Academy of Child & Adolescent Psychiatry, 38*(12), 1536–1543.

Volkmar, F. R., & Tsatsanis, K. (2002). Psychosis and psychotic conditions in childhood and adolescence. In D. T. Marsh & M. A. Fristad (Eds.), *Handbook of Serious Emotional Disturbance in Children and Adolescents*, pp. 266–283. New York: John Wiley & Sons, Inc.

Williams, D. T. (2007) Delirium and catatonia. In A. Martin & F. Volkmar (Eds.), *Lewis's Child and Adolescent Psychiatry: A Comprehensive Textbook*, 4th edition, pp. 647–654. Philadelphia: Lippincott Williams & Wilkins.

CHAPTER 11 ■ MOOD DISORDERS

BACKGROUND INFORMATION

Childhood mood disorders have the potential for severely impacting development. Although described in adults (as melancholia and mania) since antiquity, the recognition of mood disorders in children is a much more recent historical phenomena and one that continues to be controversial in some ways.

Studies of childhood depression began to appear in the 1980s. Until that time, it was assumed, largely for theoretical reasons, that children either did not develop depressive disorders or that they presented in other ways (so-called "masked" depression). Although childhood depression can, at times, present in ways somewhat different than adults, it became clear that many of the symptoms are similar and that childhood depression is frequent, is a major source of suffering, and can be associated with suicide (see Chapter 24).

Similarly, although bipolar disorder in adults has been recognized since antiquity and was classically described by Kraepelin in the late 19th century, it was assumed for many years that children and adolescents did not experience it. However, work with adults suggested that, as with depression, symptoms often begin in childhood. Although bipolar disorder manifests itself somewhat differently in children, it clearly is observed. Differences from adults include manic periods that are shorter and more frequently interspersed with periods of subsyndromal mania, hypomania, or depression. As a result, case detection and treatment are frequently delayed as is diagnostic recognition of the condition.

DEPRESSIVE DISORDERS

Definition and Clinical Description

In children and adolescents, the hallmarks of depressive disorder include chronic, pervasive, and all-encompassing sadness; lack of pleasure in life and activities; and sometimes irritability. Depressive disorders differ from transient feelings of low mood based on their degree of pervasiveness, association with impairment, and lack of responsiveness to the usual activities that would make youth feel less depressed. The *Diagnostic and Statistical Manual* (DSM-IV-TR) recognizes several specifically defined depressive disorders as well as a not otherwise specified (NOS) category and mood associations with other conditions (e.g., medical conditions and substance abuse). Some of the relevant clinical features of these conditions are provided in Table 11.1.

TABLE 11.1

DEPRESSIVE DISORDERS IN CHILDHOOD AND ADOLESCENCE: AN OVERVIEW OF CLINICAL AND DIAGNOSTIC FEATURES[1]

Major Depressive Episode

Multiple persistent symptoms in four areas:
  Mood: depressed or irritable (loss of pleasure, suicidal thoughts, feelings of guilt)
  Activity: retarded or agitated
  Cognitive: difficulties in attention, decision making
Somatic: weight loss, lack of energy, fatigue
Duration: multiple symptoms over 2 weeks
Exclusionary features: not simply attributable to bereavement, substance abuse, or general medical condition
For children, irritable mood can be experienced, and failure to make appropriate weight gain (rather than weigh toss) may also be encountered
Various specifiers are available for coding: single vs. recurrent episode(s), presence of unusual features (e.g., catatonia), and severity (mild, moderate, severe)

Dysthymic Disorder
Major feature is chronic depressed mood (most of the day more often than not) associated with at least two features of depression (mood, concentration, somatic or vegetative symptoms) For children, irritable mood may count (rather than overt depressed mood) 1 year duration required (for children and adolescents; longer for adults) Diagnosis is not made if better accounted for by major depression or if manic or mixed mood episode has been present; diagnosis is also not made if features are better accounted for by substance use or abuse or a general medical condition; and it cannot occur exclusively in association with psychotic features Symptoms must be a source of distress or impairment Onset before or after age 21 years can be specified as can atypical features

[1] Depressive disorder not otherwise specified can be used in patients not corresponding to diagnostic criteria; in addition, depression can be associated with other conditions, including adjustment disorder, bereavement, substance-induced mood disorder, and so forth, can also sometimes be appropriately used in children and adolescents. Defined similarly in DSM-IV-TR and ICD-10.
DSM, *Diagnostic and Statistical Manual of Mental Disorders*; ICD, International Classification of Diseases.

By definition, history of a manic, mixed, or hypomanic episode is an exclusionary criterion (in these cases, a bipolar diagnosis, discussed subsequently, is appropriate). It is possible to use various specifiers for severity (mild, moderate, severe), for the presence or absence of psychotic features, and for remission status (partial or full) for the most recent episode. Various other specifiers less relevant to children can also be made. For major depressive disorder, a child or adolescent must exhibit at least one major depressive episode (a period of 2 weeks of depressed or irritable mood or loss of interest or pleasure in activities). By definition, several additional symptoms of depression (e.g., weight loss or gain, loss of appetite, sleep problems, feelings of guilt or worthless, suicidal ideas or attempts, loss of energy, agitation, difficulties concentrating) must be present. Some modification of these criteria is made for children (e.g., failure to gain anticipated weight or irritability rather than depression).

For dysthymic disorder, a depressed or irritable mood must be present for at least 1 year and be associated with at least two depressive symptoms, such as appetite (under- or overeating) or sleep (insomnia or hypersomnia) disturbances, lack of energy, low self-esteem, difficulties with concentration or decision making, or hopeless feelings. By definition, the child or adolescent cannot be free of these symptoms for more than 2 months at a time. For a diagnosis of depressive disorder NOS, there must be a period of at least 2 weeks of depressed or irritable mood with some symptoms of major depressive disorder also present. Thus, the "subthreshold" depression NOS is comparatively mild, but dysthymic disorder is somewhat more serious based on its chronicity and greater number of symptoms. In this group, the most severe condition is major depression in which multiple other symptoms are present; these may include withdrawal from social activities, suicidal thoughts, changes in need for sleep, feelings of guilt or worthlessness, lowered motivation or trouble concentrating, and decreased interest in food. Psychotic symptoms can be present in major depression, and the content of hallucinations or delusions usually has a marked depressive "flavor" (although sometimes paranoid thinking is observed); psychotic symptoms are less common in children. Major depression is often preceded by dysthymic disorder. The association with mania is another important consideration.

Other conditions with significant depressive aspects include adjustment disorders with depressed mood (e.g., after stress). Mood disorders can also be associated with general medical conditions (e.g., hypothyroidism). Various other conditions associated with depression can be diagnosed but are more common in adults.

There are some differences with the International Classification of Diseases (ICD-10)approach to the diagnosis of depressive disorders. The ICD 10 does not include criteria specific to children such as irritability and failure to make expected weight gain. Other differences include symptom thresholds and duration requirements. On balance, the DSM-IV-TR approach is somewhat more inclusive and likely more appropriate for children.

One of the great complications in understanding depression is the complex relationships depression has with other conditions. Anxiety disorders are very frequently observed in association with (often preceding) depression. Depression is also associated with attention-deficit/hyperactivity disorder (ADHD) and conduct disorder (CD) as well as with substance abuse problems and has a strong familial basis. The nature of this comorbidity remains somewhat poorly understood. It might, for example, relate to commonalities in the various conditions or might reflect the fact that our nosology is attempting overly fine-grained distinctions.

Epidemiology and Demographics

The prevalence of depressive disorders ranges from about 1% to 2% in childhood to somewhere between 4% and 8% of adolescents. By the end of adolescence, about 20% individuals will have been depressed. Starting in adolescence, female predominance emerges (female: male ratio, 3:1), possibly as a result of differential effects of hormones in the central nervous system (CNS), higher rates of anxiety disorder in girls, or an interaction of genetic and other risk factors.

Recent work has underscored the potential for depression to exist even in young children, although in this age group, either irritability or sadness may be prominent. Before puberty, depression is strongly associated with a range of other problems, including psychosocial adversity, chronic family fighting, parental substance abuse, or criminality. Prepubertal depression also increases the risk of adult antisocial disorder. In some cases, familial transmission is striking with associations to other disorders such as anxiety and bipolar disorders.

Etiology

Genetic factors are a major risk factor for depressive disorders. Studies in twins show a heritability of about 40% to 65% with higher concordance rates in identical twins. Early onset (before puberty) may be more mediated by environmental factors. Depressive disorders are also strongly related to anxiety symptoms, and there is some suggestion that anxiety symptoms might increase the risk by making individuals more susceptible perhaps via specific genetic factors.

Cognitive factors have also been implicated in the pathogenesis. In contrast to individuals without depression, those with depression tend to develop cognitive biases associated with depressive symptoms (e.g., in response to stressors). These distortions are seen in both children and adolescents, but they often persist in the adolescent group even after the depressive episode

Case Study: Depressive Disorder

Tommy was a 12-year-old boy who had exhibited difficulties in school over the past year. He was seen in the emergency department (ED) and complained of chronic depression, difficulties with sleeping and attention, lack of energy, and social isolation. He was overtly depressed with a sad mood. He cried easily and talked about his difficulties in school, which seemed related to his mood problems. He recently had been refusing to go to school. The visit to the ED was precipitated when his mother found Tommy's diary open on his computer and saw that he was having thoughts of suicide (planning to jump in front of a train on tracks near their house). There was a strong family history of depression and anxiety problems. His mother herself had been treated for many years with a selective serotonin reuptake inhibitor (SSRI), and as an adolescent, she had one episode of suicidal ideation that led to hospital admission.

After the initial assessment, Tommy agreed to a no suicide contract, and both his parents and evaluator were comfortable with the arrangements the family had made to ensure his safety. Rapid follow-up was arranged, and he was enrolled in a partial hospital program quickly. A combination of an SSRI and cognitive behavior therapy led to remission of his symptoms, and he began attending school more regularly and transitioned into a less intense outpatient treatment program. At the time of last follow-up (age 15 years), he remained on medications but was free of depression and had returned to his previous levels of social and academic achievement in school.

itself has passed. Neuropsychological differences have also been identified in relation to specific memory and affective tasks.

Studies of twins have also shown the importance of environmental factors. Indeed, shared environmental effects appear at least as strong as genetic ones. So, for example, having a depressed mother might provide not only a genetic risk but also a model for depression. Families in which depression exists without a strong family history are more likely to have had various forms of psychosocial adversity. Similarly, child neglect and abuse increase the risk for depression as does loss of a parent or significant other (particularly if a strong family history of mood disorder exists). On the other hand, protective factors include good connections to family, community, and school; engagement with supportive peers; and appropriate parental expectations and supervision. Studies of the noradrenergic and serotonergic neurotransmission systems have noted some differences in children with depression. Sleep complaints are very frequent in early-onset depression but somewhat surprisingly are not strongly correlated with sleep patterns observed in sleep laboratories. There is some suggestion of differences in cortisol secretion in adolescents.

Neuroimaging studies have noted several potential areas of difference. For example, depressed adolescents exhibit differences in several brain areas, including the prefrontal cortex, as well as changes in the pituitary and amygdale. In one study by Thomas and colleagues (2001), differences were found in amygdala activation for depressed and anxious children.

Differential Diagnosis and Evaluation

Assessment of childhood and adolescent depression begins with the comprehensive evaluation of the child and often separate interviews with the parents. The focus is on both the depression and other comorbid diagnoses. As noted previously, symptoms must meet certain requirements in terms of duration and number and must be a source of impairment (e.g., on school performance or peer relationships). The focus on impairment is essential in differentiating normative mood changes from a clinical disorder. As noted previously, the DSM-IV-TR allows irritable mood (rather than depression per se) to qualify for this diagnosis in children; when irritability is the presenting symptom, the clinician should be alert to the potential for depressive disorders to present in this fashion and alert to the possibility that the child or adolescent has relatively little awareness of the impact of his or her irritability on others. Similarly, the parents may not initially believe the child to be depressed and may view irritability as a sign of normal adolescent "storm and drung" (although the latter is not, in fact, necessarily normative; see Chapter 2). The adolescent may have somewhat greater insight given the increased cognitive capacities in this age group. Difficulties in school may result from chronic fatigue and difficulties with concentration and memory. Similarly, weight loss or failure to gain expected weight may be seen (excessive weight gain is more typical in adults). The individual may complain of feeling isolated or worthless. Adolescents are more likely than younger children to exhibit psychotic features or suicide attempts, but the latter is possible at any age (see Chapter 24). Given the complexities in how depression may present, it is common for the initial complaint to be one focused on school work or behavior change or substance abuse; sometimes a suicide attempt or expression of suicidal thoughts is what prompts parents or teachers to seek evaluation.

Comorbidity is frequent and is a complication for assessment. As many as half of depressed youth may have at least two comorbid conditions, and a single comorbid condition is even more frequent. For example, it is common for an anxiety disorder to precede depression and to be comorbid with it. Other frequent conditions include substance abuse, attentional disorders, and conduct problems. The presence of comorbid conditions can have important implications for treatment and thus their presence is an important aspect of the initial assessment. The clinician should also be alert to the possibility that children and adolescents with bipolar disorder may present with a depressive episode. Accordingly, careful inquire about manic or hypomanic symptomatology should be conducted, and the clinician following the child over time should be aware of the potential for bipolar disorder to develop after an initial period of depression. In taking a history, the clinician should be alert to the importance of potential stressors (e.g., for adjustment disorder with depressed mood), Similarly, bereavement can result in depressive symptoms. Substance use and withdrawal can also be associated with irritability or feelings of depression (substance-induced mood disorder can be diagnosed, but again the clinician should be alert to the possibility that the child has essentially been self-medicating depression). The role of routine laboratory tests is relatively limited with the exception of symptoms that suggest hypothyroidism, which should prompt testing. Features that suggest substance abuse or the presence of a general medical condition might prompt other laboratory studies. A host of other medical problems can include a significant component of depression (e.g., seizure disorders, infections, other endocrinologic conditions, and autoimmune disorders, among others). Children with infections such as mononucleosis may also complain of chronic fatigue, difficulties concentrating, and mood problems suggestive of depression. Finally, a variety of medications (including antibiotics, steroids, oral contraceptives, and others) can be associated with symptoms suggestive of depression. When depression can be reasonably attributed to any of these conditions, a diagnosis of mood disorder associated with a general medical condition is made.

The task of the clinician is complicated by the considerable symptom overlap between depressive disorders and a range of other conditions including eating problems associated with eating or feeding disorders (see Chapter 14); sleep problems associated with stress or other psychiatric conditions (see Chapter 20); and mood and self-esteem problems that are frequent in children with developmental, learning, or attention-deficits disorders.

Several rating scales and checklists are available. These include Children's Depression Rating Scale-Revised (CDRS-R), a clinician-administered assessment of various symptom areas; this scale can be used at baseline and then for monitoring treatment efficacy.

Treatment

Effective treatments are available, including both pharmacologic and psychotherapeutic methods. These are used alone and in combination. In addition to medications, cognitive behavior therapy (CBT) and interpersonal therapy (IPT) have been shown to be useful (see Chapters 22 and 23). Treatment studies in prepubertal children have been more limited than those in somewhat older children. Several studies have now questioned the effectiveness of the tricyclic antidepressants (TCAs) relative to placebo, although other studies using the selective serotonin reuptake inhibitor (SSRI) antidepressants have indicated benefit. Fluoxetine has been the most intensively studied agent in this class. There is some suggestion of age-related differences in response to the various available antidepressants in older individuals, and the differences in children and adolescents may be a manifestation of these developmental effects, with adolescents responding more favorably to these agents. In the Treatment of Adolescents with Depression Study (TADS), fluoxetine was more effective than either placebo or CBT. Interestingly, in that study, combined treatments were, overall, most effective. Although the SSRIs appear to be of greater benefit than placebo, the overall effect size is not high, reflecting a robust placebo response rate. Other SSRIs have been studied as well, although less extensively, and show benefit, although effect sizes are relatively small. Children appear to respond less well than adolescents. Side effects and adverse events are a source of concern. In a meta review conducted by the Food and Drug Administration, there were higher rates of suicide-related adverse events, mostly early on in treatment. Although the risk-to-benefit ratio appears to be acceptable, caution and careful monitoring, particularly early in treatment, are indicated. Other adverse effects include agitation and restlessness, sleep and gastrointestinal problems, and some risk for increased bruising. If combinations of serotonergic agents are used, there is an increased potential for serotonin syndrome, a potentially life-threatening toxic condition caused by excess CNS serotonin with autonomic, cognitive, and other effects. There is also some risk of eliciting mania. Some work in adults has suggested poorer response to the SSRIs if the short serotonin transporter variant is present. One of the potential advantages of agents such as fluoxetine is the potential for targeting anxiety, which may precede depression.

Two psychotherapeutic interventions have strong empirical support. CBT (see Chapter 22) uses a range of techniques to address maladaptive cognitions and long-standing behavior patterns that contribute to depression. The emphasis is on remediation of "distortions" and use of a range of strategies to cope more effectively with negative feelings and mood states. A number of different techniques can be used, and techniques and procedures are frequently modified for children. These treatments differ in some details, such as relative to length of treatment, format (individual or group), and so forth, and these differences complicate comparisons across studies. Work with adolescents has found these approaches superior to wait list control groups. For youth with depression and CD, several well-controlled studies have now appeared. In the TADS, CBT was compared with fluoxetine, a combination treatment (drug plus CBT), and placebo. In this study, CBT was not superior to placebo (35%), although both the combination treatment (most effective) and drug treatment alone (with fluoxetine) were. It is possible that the differences observed had to do with differential assignment of more severely impacted patients to the CBT or that the particular approach used for CBT was overly generic. Modifications of CBT have also been used in prevention interventions with some suggestive of benefit for youth at risk.

IPT for adolescents (IPT-A) is the other psychotherapeutic intervention with substantive empirical support. This approach (see Chapter 22) adapts IPT, a well-known treatment used in adult unipolar depression, for adolescents. This approach emphasizes the interpersonal context of depression and has some similarities with as well differences from CBT. The interpersonal focus of IPT-A has some unique advantages for teenagers for whom peer relationships are particularly important and peer conflicts are frequent. Several studies have now demonstrated the benefits of this approach, and the ability to move this treatment readily into school-based mental health clinics is an important advantage.

Data on other interventions are less substantive. Some work has been done using family-based intervention as well as on light therapy (for seasonal affective disorder). As with adults, there may be a role for electroconvulsive therapy (ECT) in refractory depression, particularly in adolescents.

Given the generally strongly response to placebo or supportive treatment, it appears that for mild depression, supportive counseling and education are indicated. As depressive disorders become more severe or last longer, several treatment options are available, including SSRIs, CBT, or IPT-A. Response should be assessed after a reasonable period so that a move to a different strategy can be considered if the response is not satisfactory. Unfortunately, the dearth of clinicians trained in CPT and IPT-A methods is a practical problem. Medications should be considered if depression is severe with problems in sleep, appetite, and concentration. The support for combined treatments in adolescents is less strong than for adults. Caution is indicated if a family history of mania or hypomania exists or when the adolescent or child exhibits hypomanic or psychotic symptoms. In such cases, use of a mood stabilizer before use of antidepressants might be considered.

Of the various pharmacologic agents, fluoxetine has been most intensively studied. It is usual to begin with a relatively smaller initial dose to be sure the agent is tolerated and then to gradually increase it. If the individual fails to respond, a trial of another SSRI is indicated (although in such a circumstance, the clinician should be alert to other factors, such as noncompliance, which is frequent in adolescents and might account for the lack of responses). Drug treatments are reviewed in detail in Chapter 21.

Course and Prognosis

In samples obtained in the community, the typical duration of depression episodes ranges between 3 and 6 months and is somewhat longer in clinically referred samples. Depressive episodes are long in the presence of some comorbid conditions, including anxiety and substance abuse disorders. Other factors associated with longer durations include family history (e.g., parental depression and family discord), initially greater severity, and the presence of suicidal ideation or behavior. In about one in five cases in adolescents, depression lasts for 2 years or more.

Unfortunately, recurrence risk is high in children and particularly in adolescents (up to 70% of cases over 1 to 2 years). Factors that increase the risk for recurrence include parental history of early-onset mood problems, lack of total remission of symptoms, social difficulties, sexual abuse history, and chronic family strife. Between one in 10 and one in five individuals with early-onset depression go on to exhibit bipolar disorder. The risk for this is increased if there is a family history of bipolar disorder or if the initial presentation includes some hypomanic or psychotic symptoms. Hypomania can develop after treatment with antidepressant medications. Other difficulties include increased risk for substance abuse, conduct disorders, personality disorders, suicidal behavior, as well as social, occupational, and academic difficulties.

BIPOLAR DISORDER

Definition and Clinical Description

Various issues make the definition of bipolar disorder in children and adolescents complex and controversial. These include the degree to which cardinal adult features (grandiose thinking and elated mood) must accompany irritability (the later feature being common in childhood and a shared feature with childhood depression). Similarly, the issues of how best to define manic episodes in terms of symptoms, duration, and relation to issues of cycling remain controversial. To some extent, these issues are unique to children, but other controversies are shared with the adult bipolar literature.

The applicability of the current DSM-IV-TR approach has been widely questioned. Despite these controversies, some children and adolescents clearly do meet current DSM-IV-TR criteria even though, when these criteria were published in 1994, there was relatively little work on manifestations of the condition in younger age groups. So, for example, many of the criteria for either a manic or hypomanic episode could be viewed as applying to children in general, at least to some extent. Accordingly, in considering the diagnosis in youth, it is important that developmental factors, context, and degree of mood abnormality relative to usual mood are taken into account Other symptoms must be viewed in a developmental context as well (e.g., prepubertal children are not going to be making unwise business decisions or driving recklessly). On the other hand, unusual behaviors, including sexual behaviors, may be noted, and high-risk behaviors, arising from feelings of grandiosity and a sense of invulnerability, may contribute to dangerous behavior. Table 11.2 summarizes current approaches to diagnosis. More so, in some ways, than in adults, the putative distinction between manic and hypomanic episode can be difficult. Again, a consideration of developmental issues can be helpful because the threshold for minimal duration and severity may otherwise be difficult to judge. Parents, teachers, and other caregivers have important roles to play in providing information. One meta-analytic review of symptoms for mania in youth revealed that excessive energy and distractibility were the most likely symptoms exhibited, and hypersexuality was the least. Issues of differences in method, sample, informants, and so forth contribute to variability across studies. Psychosis is observed in a minority of cases. The lack of specificity of common symptoms of mania in children is also suggested by studies comparing bipolar disorder and ADHD, with no significant differences in a number of areas, including irritability, accelerated speech, distractibility, and unusual energy levels. Accordingly, a simple frequency count of symptoms does not capture the complexity of the clinical phenomena and has some potential to mislead less experienced clinicians. As a result of these controversies, some have argued for an emphasis on the core features of elevated mood and grandiosity. Unfortunately, although these features are usually present, there is more variability in children. Clearly, longitudinal and follow-up studies are needed to address issues of best diagnostic practice.

Other complexities arise in relation to features such as irritability. Although almost always present, it is not, unfortunately very specific because irritability is common in children with depression, conduct problems, anxiety, and stress-related disorders. This is an area of considerable disagreement, with some advocating reliance on irritability alone (if severe) as a primary feature but others emphasizing the lack of specificity in pediatric populations. A final controversy arises relative to the degree to which features are chronic or episodic. Some investigators suggest that symptoms are long lasting, up to several years for manic or mixed episodes. Others have emphasized that the duration of strictly defined episodes is much shorter than this. The technical DSM-IV-TR requirement for manic, mixed, or hypomania episode requires some clear period of abnormal mood and associated symptoms; some include an episodic course as a cardinal feature. Unfortunately, high rates of comorbidity, rapid periods of fluctuation, and complicated symptoms presentations are often involved The issue of associated depressive symptoms is of great interest, particularly because most studies of adults with bipolar disorder suggest that they exhibited noteworthy depressive symptoms in their youth. Clearly, some youth with bipolar disorder have clear periods of depression sufficient to qualify for a major depressive episode and it is sometimes the case that bipolar disorder first presents with a depressive episode. Similarly, another source of controversy has been the approach to youth who present either with mixed features or complicated cycling patterns. Difficulties arise relative to differentiating mixed states from lability or transient dysphoria. Technically, in the DSM-IV-TR, a mixed episode diagnosis requires that the child or adolescent meet the criteria for manic episode as well as for a major depressive episode on an almost daily basis for a substantial (1-week) period. Issues of symptom (and criterion) overlap and comorbidity complicate the issue of deciding the best way to conceptualizing the symptoms. Yet other issues arise because at times youth have some manic symptoms, but either the symptoms do not last long enough or are not sufficiently distinctive or associated with other features; therefore, the question of whether full criteria are met is unclear. Often, a diagnosis of bipolar disorder NOS ends up being assigned, but clearly, more work is needed to more precisely delineate syndrome boundaries.

Epidemiology and Demographics

Given the controversies surrounding the diagnosis, it is not surprising that epidemiologic data are limited. Retrospectively, more than half of adults with the condition report symptom onset

TABLE 11.2

BIPOLAR DISORDERS IN CHILDHOOD AND ADOLESCENCE: AN OVERVIEW OF CLINICAL AND DIAGNOSTIC FEATURES

Manic Episode

Elevated, expansive, or irritable mood for 1 week (or less if individual needs hospitalization)

Symptoms must include multiple of the following: grandiosity, diminished need for sleep, pressure of speech, racing thoughts or flight of idea, decreases in attention, agitation (psychomotor or sexual, although the latter is less common in children), risk taking

Difficulties must cause impairment or cause hospitalization but must not be attributable to substance use or abuse or a general medical condition, and the individual cannot meet the criteria for mixed episode

Note: No special modifications are made for mania in children

Mixed Episode

Individual exhibits both manic and major depressive episode features for at least 1 week and almost every day

Difficulties cause impairment or require hospitalization and are not attributable to substance use or abuse or a general medical condition

Hypomanic Episode

A marked period of elated, expansive, or irritable mood (lasting at least 4 days) that represents a change from baseline functioning (must be a distinct change and noticed by others)

Features must include multiple of the following: grandiosity, diminished need for sleep, pressure of speech, racing thoughts or flight of idea, decreases in attention, agitation or increased activities, risk taking

Episode does *not* cause marked impairment or need for hospitalization and is not attributable to effects of substance use or abuse or a general medical condition

Hypomanic episodes associated with medication use (e.g., antidepressants, do *not* qualify for a diagnosis of bipolar II disorder)

Bipolar I Disorder

One or more manic or mixed episodes present

Frequently, a depressive or hypomanic disorder will have been present (but is not required for diagnosis)

Difficulties must cause impairment or distress

A number of coding modifiers can be used to specify the nature of the most recent episode, severity, features of onset, rapid cycling, and so forth

Bipolar II Disorder

Major depressive episode(s) associated with at least one hypomanic episode (*not* a manic episode)

Difficulties must cause impairment or distress

A number of coding modifiers can be used to specify the nature of the most recent episode, severity, features of onset, rapid cycling, and so forth

Cyclothymic Disorder

Symptoms of hypomania and depression are generally present for at least 1 year (in children and adolescents)

These must be the source of distress or impairment

The diagnosis is not made if the individual has met criteria for a major depressive episode, if better accounted for by a psychotic condition such as schizophrenia, or if it is attributable to substance use or abuse or a general medical condition

Bipolar Disorder Not Otherwise Specified

This residual category can be used for cases not meeting full criteria but when the difficulties cause impairment or distress

---

Case Study: Bipolar Disorder

Tim was a 15-year-old boy with a history of depressive episodes and one prior suicide attempt (overdose of his mother's medication). Over the past year, he had seemed to do well in an outpatient treatment program without medication, but over the past several weeks, he had been sleeping less and was more grandiose. He had attempted to board a train without a ticket because he decided he was ready to go to college. The police had become involved when he presented his father's credit card to pay for a ticket, and his degree of obvious disturbance led the police to transport him to the nearest emergency department (ED).

On meeting the clinician, Tim began to talk very rapidly about his interest in becoming a physician, a lawyer, and an MBA. He attempted to explain his desire to board the train to get to college, but his account was difficult to follow, and his speech was pressured. After his parents arrived, they reported that he had seemed to need less sleep over the past week and was up in the middle of the night engaged in various projects. They had been somewhat concerned about his mood because of a strong family history of bipolar disorder and had made an appointment for him that day for follow-up but had awoken to find that Tim had left the house and had left them a note saying he was going off to college.

Tim's father reported that in the past, Tim has been somewhat reserved with girls, but over the last several weeks, had been e-mailing various girls in his class nonstop asking them to date him. He had lost weight over the past several weeks as his need for food seemed to diminish.

Tim became more and more agitated in the ED, eventually threatening various staff. He and his parents denied substance use and a tox screen was negative. Tim was initially treated with an antipsychotic and begun on a mood stabilizer. He responded well to this regimen and was hospitalized for 10 days. Follow-up indicated that for a period of almost 2 years, he was symptom free, but an attempt on his part to stop his mood stabilizer at that time led to rehospitalization for a second manic episode.

---

before age 20 years. The age of first onset also appears to be decreasing over time. The available studies generally suggest rates of about 1% to 2% of the general population if a strict definition is used and up to 6% if a less stringent approach is adopted focusing on subsyndromal symptoms. These estimates must be regarded with caution, however. In clinical populations, there is considerable variation, presumably reflecting sundry factors related to ascertain and methodology.

Etiology

A strong role for genetic factors is suggested by the high rates of bipolar disorder in family members (eight to 10 times more common than in the general population). Similarly, both adoption and twin studies show strong genetic components with children of parents who have bipolar disorder having about a sevenfold increase in risk for bipolar as well as high risk of anxiety, mood, attentional, and other problems. Finally, relatives of youth with bipolar disorder have first-degree relatives with higher risk for the condition. The heritability of the condition has been estimated to be more than 80%. Several potential linkages on chromosomes 13, 9, 10, and 14 have been identified, although results are not always consistent. It appears likely that several loci interact in conferring risk.

Other work has focused on structural and functional neuroimaging to clarify potential brain mechanisms. There have been findings in several areas, including cortical and subcortical regions. Studies of neural circuiting using Proton magnetic resonance spectroscopy have noted possible changes in frontostriatal region, cingulate cortex, and other brain regions, and some of these markers have also been noted to be present in children of parents with the condition. Studies of neurocognitive functioning suggest a range of associated neuropsychological deficits in visual-spatial and verbal memory as well as executive functioning, although, as is true of the neuroimaging findings, small sample sizes and other factors may limit the generalizability of these results. The small literature on psychosocial risk does suggest associations with socioeconomic stress, negative life events, and high "expressed emotion" that are apparently associated with worse outcomes.

Differential Diagnosis and Evaluation

As with depressive disorder, pediatric bipolar disorder is very frequently associated with other conditions, including AHDD, CD, and anxiety disorders. In adolescents, rates of substance abuse also gradually increase. Treatment should carefully consider the implications for co-morbid conditions for planning care. The variability in clinical presentation and high rates of comorbidity raise major practical problems for differential diagnosis.

Various conditions that can lead to mood variability and behavioral challenges should be considered in the differential diagnosis (and sometimes are present in addition to the bipolar disorder). In addition to the conditions noted previously, these include depressive disorders; autism and related conditions; and other psychotic conditions, particularly schizophrenia. Substance abuse and borderline personality disorder can also sometimes be confused with pediatric bipolar disorder, although the history and presentation usually help to clarify the diagnosis. Various medical conditions can present with affective and behavioral change suggestive of mania (e.g., hyperthyroidism; CNS tumors and trauma; side effects of a number of medications, such as antidepressants, steroids and corticosteroids, and stimulant medications). ADHD can usually be differentiated based on the later onset of bipolar disorder (usually before age 10 years in those with ADHD), abrupt symptom onset, association with mood change and fluctuation in course, psychotic features, family history, and so forth. Similarly, in disruptive behavior disorder, unusual aspects of the presentation (fluctuating course), positive family history of bipolar disorder, and psychotic thinking are also suggestive of bipolar disorder (see Birmaher et al., 2007 for a discussion). Sometimes the presentation of more "classic" bipolar symptoms such as grandiosity, decreased need for sleep, and hypersexuality may help with the differential diagnosis, as, over time, does the course. At the time of initial presentation of depression, it is clear that some youth will go on to develop bipolar disorder, but as a practical matter, the issue of which ones are at risk for doing so is difficult to sort out. The clinician should be alert for the presence or history of symptoms suggestive of mania or hypomania. Positive family history and history of psychotic thinking or apparent manic symptoms in relation to drug treatments are further possible warning signs. In the presence of substance abuse, the clinician should be alert to the possibility that the child or adolescent is, essentially, self-medicating an underlying mood or other problem.

A number of approaches have been developed to systematize assessment. These include various structured and semi-structured interviews as well as checklists and other rating scales. The Kiddie Schedule for Affective Disorders and Schizophrenia for School Age Children—Present and Lifetime Version (K-SADS-PL) and the Washington University KSADS (WASH-U-KSADS) are widely used for research purposes but are lengthy to administer. Rating scales include the Young Mania Rating Scale (YMRS) and the KSADS Mania Rating Scale. Parent and teacher report scales have also been used (e.g., the Child Mania Rating Scale for Parents). Other approaches rely on diaries or "mood timelines" to chart the course of mood and its association with life events and stressors and in response to treatment. For some children and adolescents, hospitalization is indicated (e.g., if suicidal or homicidal symptoms, significant agitation, psychosis, substance dependence are present). In some instances (e.g., when families are unable to be supportive and stabilizing), hospitalization may be considered even if levels of symptomatology are somewhat lower than would usually prompt hospitalization.

Treatment

Treatment goals and priorities vary depending on the state of the illness. In the acute situation, the primary focus is on acute symptoms; in the subsequent phases, the goal shifts to avoiding relapses and maintaining gains made. Treatment is also guided by the severity, associated conditions, age of the child or adolescent, and family and individual factors. Particularly when response is poor, it is important to be aware of other factors that may be impacting treatment (e.g., lack of compliance, associated disorders, ongoing stress). At all times, it is important to provide education and support. Preparation for potential recurrence and mood fluctuations is a part of this process for the child and parents alike. This helps improve treatment compliance and helps parents gain some perspectives on the origins of frequent mood changes and steps that can be taken to help avoid recurrence. For example, parents and patients alike should be helped to understand the potential of sleep deprivation's exacerbating the difficulties. Several books written for patients and their families are now available and may be helpful for educators as well (see Selected Readings).

The literature on the acute treatment phase is, unfortunately, based on studies using varying methods and having important limitations. A few randomized, controlled trials (RCTs) are available, and as larger such studies become more available, recommendations may well change. In general, doses of mood stabilizers and the atypical antipsychotics are similar to those used in adults, although some youth may need slightly higher serum lithium concentrations for greatest efficacy. If possible, doses of medications are begun at a low level and gradually increased. The various mood stabilizers (see Chapter 21) are relatively similar in the treatment of mania or mixed nonpsychotic episodes with up to 50% of those treated responding. The atypical antipsychotics are also effective and may provide benefit more rapidly. For an acute manic or mixed episode, the combination of mood stabilizer with atypical antipsychotic ranges from 60% to 90% response. Often, lithium or valproate is used initially with nonresponders then switched to a different mood stabilizer or to a combination with an atypical antipsychotic. The combination of mood stabilizers or use of mood stabilizer and antipsychotic may be indicated if symptoms are severe or there has been only a partial response to the single mood stabilizer. The presence of psychosis also typically suggests the need for a mood stabilizer and antipsychotic. In some situations (e.g., with severe illness that is refractory to drug treatment), ECT can be considered. Studies of pharmacologic intervention for hypomania or depressive symptoms are limited.

There is some suggestion that, as with adults who have depression associated with bipolar disorder, mood stabilizers or atypical antipsychotics can be combined with the SSRIs, but data are limited. Unfortunately, there is also some suggestion that the SSRIs can elicit manic or hypomanic symptoms, especially if used in isolation. At present, use of a mood stabilizer or atypical antipsychotics is frequently the initial pharmacologic intervention in depression associated with bipolar disorder.

It should be noted that many of the psychosocial interventions effective for depression also can be used in this situation. Other psychosocial interventions have been developed for children and adolescents with bipolar disorder, including special family treatment programs and CBT approaches. Psychosocial treatments can be helpful for associated condition such as substance abuse, anxiety, and CDs.

Compared with the adult literature, RCTs of pharmacologic agents in the continuation and maintenance phases are uncommon. There are high relapse rates in adolescents who discontinue lithium compared with those who maintain it. A handful of studies have also addressed the issue of moving from multiple drugs to monotherapy. Most experts presently suggest considering a medication taper after 1 to 2 years of remission, although various factors such as severity might suggest reasonable modifications of this time frame in either direction. Chapter 21 reviews issues of psychopharmacology in greater detail. Lithium can be associated with toxicity if levels are elevated; this can be associated with brain and kidney damage and can be fatal. Signs and symptoms of toxicity are most frequently seen at 1.5 mEq/L and above but sometimes at even lower levels. Both the child and family should be aware of basic signs of toxicity, which often appear to mimic alcohol intoxication. If toxicity is suspected, a lithium level should be obtained, fluid encouraged, and the lithium dose held or reduced if there are problems in taking fluid or with fluid loss through vomiting. Education regarding adequate hydration and basic precautions relative to vigorous exercise should be emphasized. Prescription and some nonprescription drugs can increase lithium levels. Routine laboratory studies are needed to monitor possible renal, thyroid, and other potential side effects. The other mood stabilizers similarly have a range of side effects (see Chapter 21).

In contrast, the atypical neuroleptics have rather different side effect profiles but as a group share many side effects in common. These include both metabolic effects and extrapyramidal symptoms. There is also potential risk for tardive dyskinesia and neuroleptic malignant syndrome. Children taking these agents should be followed on a regular basis for the presence of abnormal movements as well as metabolic effects.

Complex issues for treatment can arise in the presence of associated comorbid disorders, and the literature on this topic is, unfortunately, quite limited. Sometimes attentional difficulties or other problems associated with bipolar disorder resolve or substantially diminish if the bipolar disorder is effectively treated. If this is done and attentional symptoms continue after the mood disorder is stabilized, consideration can be given to whether treatment of a comorbid condition is indicated. Both pharmacologic and nonpharmacologic treatment can be used, and it is important for clinicians to have a full sense of the entire clinical picture (e.g., sometimes clinicians use many different medications to treat symptoms that might, more parsimoniously, be thought of as manifestations of a single condition).

Course and Prognosis

Despite the various diagnostic complexities and controversies, it appears that between 70% to 100% of youth with bipolar disorder largely recover within about 2 months; unfortunately, as many as 75% or so will have a recurrence in the next several years. There are frequent problems with substance abuse, legal issues, school, and family relationships. Recent research has also noted that although cycles of recovery and recurrence are noted, some youth have fluctuating courses with subsyndromal symptoms, particularly with depressive and mixed symptoms. Rapid mood fluctuations appear more pronounced than in adults, presumably accounting for some of the complexities of diagnosis. Negative prognostic factors include early onset, comorbid conditions, the presence of familial psychopathology and low socioeconomic status, duration of symptoms, psychotic thinking, and mixed or rapid cycling.

SUMMARY

Mood disorders in children and adolescents represent a significant public health problem. These disorders often have a chronic course and can be the source of considerable morbidity and mortality. Advances have been made in a number of areas. Studies of the brain using neuroimaging have helped clarify brain regions and circuits involved in pathogenesis. Similarly, family and genetic studies have helped clarify important aspects of risk and offer important leads for future research. Although noteworthy progress has been made in treatment, much work remains to be done in the areas of clarifying mechanisms of action and the best ways that clinical intervention can be tailored to the needs of the individual child. Although many children respond positively to treatment, there remains a considerable risk of relapse or of only partial treatment response. This work also has important implications for prevention, early intervention, and public health practices given the severity of the disorder and its association with suicidality. These difficulties are particularly noteworthy in treatment approaches for youth with bipolar disorder, who can present with a wide range of symptoms and symptom severity and in whom important issues of clinical phenotype remain the topic of considerable debate. For mood disorders, the high rates of comorbidity are not surprising but do present important challenges for implementation of treatment programs.

Selected Readings

Angold, A., Costello, E. J., Erkanli, A., & Worthman, C. M. (1999). Pubertal changes in hormone levels and depression in girls. *Psychological Medicine, 29*, 1043–1053.

Baldessarini, R. J., Bolzani, L., Cruz, N., Jones, P. B., Lai, M., Lepri, B., Perez, J., Salvatore, P., Tohen, M., Tondo, L., & Vieta, E. (2010). Onset-age of bipolar disorders at six international sites. *Journal of Affective Disorders, 121*(1-2), 143–146.

Baroni, A., Lunsford, J. R., Luckenbaugh, D. A., Towbin, K. E., & Leibenluft, E. (2009). Practitioner review: The assessment of bipolar disorder in children and adolescents. *Journal of Child Psychology & Psychiatry & Allied Disciplines, 50*(3), 203–215.

Birmaher, B. (2007). Longitudinal course of pediatric bipolar disorder. *American Journal of Psychiatry, 164*(4), 537–539.

Birmaher, B., Axelson, D., & Pavuluri, M. (2007). Bipolar disorder. In A. Martin & F. Volkmar (Eds.), *Lewis's Child and Adolescent Psychiatry: A Comprehensive Textbook*, 4th edition, pp. 513–528. Philadelphia: Lippincott Williams & Wilkins.

Brent, D. A., & Birmaher, B. (2002). Adolescent depression. *New England Journal of Medicine, 347*, 667–671.

Brent, D. A., Poling, K., McKain, B., McKain, B., & Baugher, M. (1993). A psychoeducational program for families of affectively ill children and adolescents. *Journal of the American Academy of Child and Adolescent Psychiatry, 32*, 770–774.

Brent, D. A., & Weersing, V. R. (2007). Depression disorders. In A. Martin & F. Volkmar (Eds.), *Lewis's Child and Adolescent Psychiatry: A Comprehensive Textbook*, 4th edition, pp. 503–512. Philadelphia: Lippincott Williams & Wilkins.

Brown, G. W., & Harris, T. O. (2008). Depression and the serotonin transporter 5-HTTLPR polymorphism: A review and a hypothesis concerning gene-environment interaction. *Journal of Affective Disorders, 111*(1), 1–12.

Carlson, G. A., & Glovinsky, I. (2009). The concept of bipolar disorder in children: a history of the bipolar controversy. *Child & Adolescent Psychiatric Clinics of North America, 18*(2), 257–271.

Caspi, A., Sugden, K., Moffitt, T. E., Taylor, A., Craig, I. W., Harrington, H., McClay, J., Mill, J., Martin, J., Braithwaite, A., & Poulton, R. (2003). Influence of life stress on depression: Moderation by a polymorphism in the 5-HT gene. *Science, 301*, 386–389.

Costello, E. J., Mustillo, S., Erkanli, A., Keeler, G., & Angold, A. (2003). Prevalence and development of psychiatric disorders in childhood and adolescence. *Archives of General Psychiatry, 60*, 837–844.

Dietz, L. J., Birmaher, B., Williamson, D. E., Silk, J. S., Dahl, R. E., Axelson, D. A., Ehmann, M., & Ryan, N. D. (2008). Mother-child interactions in depressed children and children at high risk and low risk for future depression. *Journal of the American Academy of Child & Adolescent Psychiatry, 47*(5), 574–582.

Emslie, G., Heiligenstein, J. H., Wagner, K. D., Hoog, S. L., Ernest, D. E., Brown, E., Nilsson, M., & Jacobson, J. G. (2002). Fluoxetine for acute treatment of depression in children and adolescents: A placebo-controlled, randomized clinical trial. *Journal of the American Academy of Child and Adolescent Psychiatry, 41*, 1205–1215.

Evans-Lacko, S. E., Zeber, J. E., Gonzalez, J. M., & Olvera, R. L. (2009). Medical comorbidity among youth diagnosed with bipolar disorder in the United States. *Journal of Clinical Psychiatry, 70*(10), 1461–1466.

Fergusson, D. M., & Woodward, L. J. (2002). Mental health, educational, and social role outcomes of adolescents with depression. *Archive of General Psychiatry, 59*, 225–231.

Fristad, M. A., Gavazzi, S. M., & Mackinaw-Koons, B. (2003). Family psychoeducation: an adjunctive intervention for children with bipolar disorder. *Biological Psychiatry, 53*, 1000–1008.

Fristad, M. A., Weller, E. B., & Weller, R. A. (1992). The Mania Rating Scale: Can it be used in children? A preliminary report. *Journal of the American Academy of Child and Adolescent Psychiatry, 31*, 252–257.

Fristad, M. A., Goldberg-Arnold, J. S., & Gavazzi, S. M. (2003). Multi-family psychoeducation groups in the treatment of children with mood disorders. *Marital Family Therapy, 29*, 491–504.

Geller, B., Tillman, R., Craney, J. L., & Bolhofner, K. (2004). Four-year prospective outcome and natural history of mania in children with a prepubertal and early adolescent bipolar disorder phenotype. *Archives of General Psychiatry, 61*, 459–467.

Geller, B., Williams, M., Zimerman, B., Frazier, J., Beringer, L., & Warner, K. L. (1998). Prepubertal and early adolescent bipolarity differentiate from ADHD by manic symptoms: Grandiose delusions; ultra-rapid or ultradian cycling. *Journal of Affective Disorders, 51*, 81–91.

Geller, B., Warner, K., Williams, M., & Zimerman, B. (1998). Prepubertal and young adolescent bipolarity versus ADHD: Assessment and validity using the WASH-U-KSADS, CBCL, and TRF. *Journal of Affective Disorders, 51*, 93–100.

Geller, B., Zimerman, B., Williams, M., Bolhofner, K., & Craney J. L. (2001). Bipolar disorder at prospective follow-up of adults who had prepubertal major depressive disorder. *American Journal of Psychiatry, 158*, 125–127.

Glowinski, A. L., Madden, P. A. F., Bucholz, K. K., Lynskey, M. T., & Heath, A. C. (2003). Genetic epidemiology of self-reported lifetime DSM-IV major depressive disorder in a population-based twin sample of female adolescents. *Journal of Child Psychology, Psychiatry and Allied Disciplines, 44*, 988–996.

Harrington, R., Rutter, M., & Fombonne, E. (1996). Developmental pathways in depression: Multiple meanings, antecedents, and endpoints. *Development and Psychopathology, 8*, 601–616.

Harrington, R., Fudge, H., Rutter, M., Pickles, A., & Hill, J. (1990). Adult outcomes of childhood and adolescent depression I. Psychiatric status. *Archives of General Psychiatry, 47*, 465–473.

Harrington, R., Rutter, M., Weissman, M., Fudge, H., Groothues, C., Bredenkamp, D., Pickles, A., Rende, R., & Wickramaratne, P. (1997). Psychiatric disorders in the relatives of depressed probands I. comparison of prepubertal, adolescent and early adult onset cases. *Journal of Affective Disorder, 42*, 9–22.

Hollon, S. D., Garber, J., & Shelton, R. C. (2005). Treatment of depression in adolescents with cognitive behavior therapy and medications: A commentary on the TADS project. *Cognitive Behavioral Practice, 12,* 149–155.

Kaufman, J., Birmaher, B., Brent, D., Rao, U., Flynn, C., Moreci, P., Williamson, D., & Ryan, N. (1997). Schedule for Affective Disorders and Schizophrenia for School-Age Children—Present and Lifetime Version (K-SADS-PL): Initial reliability and validity data. *Journal of the American Academy of Child and Adolescent Psychiatry, 36,* 980–988.

Kovacs, M. (1996). Presentation and course of major depressive disorder during childhood and later years of the life span. *Journal of the American Academy of Child and Adolescent Psychiatry, 35,* 705–715.

March, J. S., Silva, S., Petrycki, S., Curry, J., Wells, K., Fairbank, J., Burns, B., Domino, M., McNulty, S., Vitiello, B., & Severe, J. (2004). Fluoxetine, cognitive-behavioral therapy, and their combination for adolescents with depression. Treatment for Adolescent Depression Study (TADS) randomized controlled trial. *Journal of the American Medical Association, 292,* 807–820.

Miklowitz, D. J., George, E. L., Axelson, D. A., Kim, E. Y., Birmaher, B., Schneck, C., Beresford, C., Craighead, W. E., & Brent, D. A. (2004). Family-focused treatment for adolescents with bipolar disorder. *Journal of Affective Disorders, 82,* 113–128.

Pavuluri, M. N., Graczyk, P. A., Henry, D. B., Carbray, J. A., Heidenreich, J., & Miklowitz, D. J. (2004). Child- and family-focused cognitive-behavioral therapy for pediatric bipolar disorder: Development and preliminary results. *Journal of the American Academy of Child and Adolescent Psychiatry, 43,* 528–537.

Prager, L. M. (2009). Depression and suicide in children and adolescents. *Pediatrics in Review, 30*(6), 199–205; quiz 206.

Rice, F. (2009). The genetics of depression in childhood and adolescence. *Current Psychiatry Reports, 11*(2), 167–173.

Thomas, K. M., Drevets, W. C., Dahl, R. E., Ryan, N. D., Birmaher, B., Eccard, C. H., Axelson, D., Whalen, P. J., & Casey, B. J. (2001). Amygdala response to fearful faces in anxious and depressed children. *Archives of General Psychiatry, 58,* 1057–1063.

Weissman, M. M., Wolk, S., Wickramaratne, P., Goldstein, R. B., Adams, P., Greenwald, S., Ryan, N. D., Dahl, R. E., & Steinberg, D. (1999). Children with prepubertal onset major depressive disorder and anxiety grown up. *Archives of General Psychiatry, 56,* 794–801.

Young, R. C., Biggs, J. T., Ziegler, V. E., & Meyer, D. (1978). A rating scale for mania: reliability, validity and sensitivity. *British Journal of Psychiatry, 133,* 429–435.

Zuckerbrot, R. A., Cheung, A. H., Jensen, P. S., Stein, R. E. K., Laraque, D., & GLAD-PC Steering Group (2007). Guidelines for Adolescent Depression in Primary Care (GLAD-PC): I. Identification, assessment, and initial management. *Pediatrics, 120*(5), e1299–e1312.

CHAPTER 12 ■ ANXIETY DISORDERS AND OBSESSIVE-COMPULSIVE DISORDER

The experience of anxiety is a universal experience and has both psychological and physiological components. Anxiety is characterized by a variety of terms that refer to dystonic mood (e.g., fear, worry, apprehension) and is generally experienced in reaction to a specific fearful stimulus. The term *fear* is usually used when a specific threat is present. Anxiety is normally associated with stress but also has important adaptive functions. When excessive or prolonged, the experience of anxiety can stop being adaptive and become a source of distress or impairment that qualifies as an anxiety disorder.

One of the challenges for clinical definitions of these conditions is the common experience of fear and anxiety as a normative phenomenon as opposed to a clinical condition. Normative anxiety has strong developmental correlates beginning with issues of separation and stranger anxiety in very young children and then the development of various fears and concerns as children age. This trend continues with changes in the character of worry and anxiety manifestations in adolescents as cognitive capacities and social and personal expectations increase.

Probably the major point of differentiation of normal anxiety and anxiety disorder is the issue of impairment, that is, the condition must be of sufficient severity or intensity that it causes the child or adolescent some difficulties in daily functioning. The issue of "distress" is also included as a diagnostic feature but is, in many ways, much more difficult to operationalize, particularly in children.

Although frequently viewed as one of the anxiety disorders, obsessive-compulsive disorder (OCD) actually occupies a position somewhere between this and various other conditions (particularly tic disorders). The grouping with anxiety disorders here reflects a primary clinical awareness of the degree to which anxiety is a major aspect of the condition.

DEFINITIONS AND CLINICAL DESCRIPTION

Various different anxiety disorders are presently recognized. With some important exceptions, the approaches to diagnosis are similar in children and adults. These exceptions include separation anxiety disorder (SAD), which is essentially confined to children. A modification of the guidelines for generalized anxiety disorder (GAD) makes it easier to diagnose the condition in children and adolescents. As Krain et al. (2007) point out, the *Diagnostic and Statistical*

TABLE 12.1
KEY CHARACTERISTICS OF ANXIETY DISORDERS

DSM-IV-TR Disorder	Key Characteristics[1]
Separation anxiety disorder	■ Excessive anxiety concerning separation from a loved one ■ Possible risk factor for development of panic disorder or agoraphobia in adulthood
Social phobia (social anxiety disorder)	■ Persistent fear of social or evaluative situations ■ Behavioral inhibition may be a temperamental predictor of social phobia in childhood or adulthood
Generalized anxiety disorder	■ Excessive and uncontrollable worry about multiple issues ■ At least one somatic complaint ■ Close genetic link with depression
Specific phobia	■ Extreme fear of a specific situation or object ■ Five types of phobias, some corresponding to evolutionary dangers (i.e., snakes, blood)
Panic disorder with or without agoraphobia	■ Unexpected panic attacks accompanied by worry about future attacks ■ Agoraphobia is diagnosed if individual avoids places in which escape would be difficult or embarrassing ■ Panic attacks can be caused by medical conditions (e.g., hyperthyroidism, cardiac abnormalities)

[1] All *Diagnostic and Statistical Manual* (DSM-IV-TR) anxiety disorder diagnoses require clinically significant distress or impairment in social, academic, or other areas of functioning.
Reprinted from Krain, A., Ghaffari, M., Freeman, J., Garcia, A., Leonard, H., & Pine, D. S. (2007). Anxiety disorders. In A. Martin & F. Volkmar (Eds.), *Lewis's Child and Adolescent Psychiatry: A Comprehensive Textbook*, 4th edition, p. 540. Philadelphia: Lippincott Williams & Wilkins.

Manual of Mental Disorders (DSM-IV-TR) approach may well underestimate the importance of developmental differences in the ways anxiety is manifest. The utility of the current distinctions has been widely debated, particularly in light of frequent associations with other problems (e.g., mood disorders). Table 12.1 provides an overview of diagnostic features for the anxiety disorders in children (OCD is discussed in the final section of this chapter).

Separation Anxiety Disorder

This condition is defined based on a judgment that separation anxiety (a normative developmental phenomenon manifest in stranger anxiety and attachment behaviors; see Chapter 2) has become excessive and "developmentally inappropriate." Typically, this takes the overt form of distress around separation and excessive worry about a major attachment figure, often the mother. Symptoms at separation include overt distress, repeated somatic complaints, nightmares, or sleep refusal. Referral is made when somatic complaints are prominent or when school refusal occurs. In the DSM-IV-TR, the condition must last at least 1 month and be a source of significant impairment. Onset typically is after age 6 years and before 18 years (i.e., in the developmental period but generally after the time when separation fears are normative). One argument for recognizing SAD as a category is the subsequent risk for panic disorder or agoraphobia later.

Social Anxiety Disorder (Social Phobia)

Social anxiety disorder is defined based on a persisting fear of exposure to unfamiliar persons in social situations. The term was added in DSM-IV-TR as an alternative to the term *social phobia*

Case Study: Separation Anxiety Disorder

Tommy, a 6½-year-old boy, was referred by his family physician because of a long-standing pattern of shyness and inhibition that had become dramatically worse on his entering school. He expressed fear that his mother would be harmed or become ill and had several times come home early from school or had tremendous difficulty separating from his mother at the start of school. His mother had a history of anxiety-related difficulties as a child and even at present described herself as rather like Tommy with many worries and concerns about the future.

When left at school, Tommy quickly would begin to complain of headaches or more frequently gastrointestinal upset. He often left the classroom to go to the nurse's office because he felt nauseous and was afraid he would vomit in the classroom. It was a struggle for his mother to drop him off at school in the morning; he would be reluctant to bring his backpack, would lose his lunch, and would become upset on leaving the car. He had never been willing to take the bus with other children on his street.

His teacher reported that when he was in school and working, his academic abilities appeared to be at age level. She was, however, concerned that his degree of difficulty with separation and his numerous physical complains were taking a toll on his peer relationships and would eventually also impact his academic progress.

His mother noted that Tommy had a long history of anxiety-related difficulties, only falling asleep when one of his parents (usually his mother) was in bed with him. He often woke during the night and would come into his parents' bed complaining of nightmares. Although his father had tried to interest him in soccer, Tommy was reluctant to have his father leave him.

Although he would play with children in the neighborhood, he wanted his mother around. His parents had difficulty leaving him with a babysitter.

Tommy and his parents engaged in a course of treatment focused both on his anxiety and, for his parents, ways to help him cope more effectively. Issues for the parents included a careful review of ways in which their behavior had frequently supported Tommy's anxiety and lack of independence. For Tommy, a course of cognitive behavior therapy was helpful combined with the work with his parents. Although Tommy remained a somewhat anxious child, he began to be able to attend school on a regular basis and became more independent at home as well. His sleeping difficulties decreased. After Tommy had completed his treatment, his mother chose to pursue treatment for her own long-standing anxiety difficulties, which had seemed to play some role in Tommy's problems.

---

to underscore the difference of this condition and the specific phobias. In social anxiety disorder, even the risk of exposure to a social situation can provoke severe anxiety or a panic attack. Commonly feared social situations include performance or public speaking as well as simply meeting new people or attending parties, meetings, and other social gatherings. The condition gives rise to significant problems because of attempts to avoid these situations and gives rise to preoccupations about rejection, negative judgments by others, and so on. Somatic symptoms can include heart palpitations, gastrointestinal complaints, and so forth; these can readily result in school refusal and other difficulties.

Toddlers who are behaviorally inhibited (withdrawing from novel or challenging situations) may be particularly likely to develop social anxiety disorder. As a result of failure to engage with others, individuals may develop noteworthy social deficits, and there is some suggestion (e.g., in family studies) of a connection to autism and related disorders that are characterized by marked problems in social interaction as well as anxiety.

Generalized Anxiety Disorder

In this condition, excessive and uncontrollable worry leads to impaired daily functioning. In addition to extreme worry, there must be one somatic symptom, and the extreme anxiety must last for a period of at least 6 months. The anxiety often centers on issues of approval, events in the future, worries about lack of competence, or worries about new or unfamiliar situations. Although reassurance may be sought and may briefly seem to help, relief is brief. The somatic complaints are variable and can include the usual array of anxiety-related symptoms. Children with this condition frequently initially present to their pediatrician.

Various studies have revealed a strong association with depression. This has been taken to suggest that what is inherited may be a more general predisposition because, for example, adolescents with GAD often later develop depression.

Specific Phobia

In this condition, a marked and persistent fear is excessive or unreasonable and results in interference. Various objects or situations may be the source of the fear (e.g., heights, specific

---

Case Study: Generalized Anxiety Disorder

Todd, an 11-year-old boy, was referred for assessment by his primary care provider because of symptoms she suggested might reflect an anxiety disorder. The third and final child and only boy of professional parents, his parents had become concerned about Todd in the fifth grade as his school work had seemed to deteriorate. A successful participant in the martial arts and music, Todd had always been popular at school, although this year, in his private school, the level of work dramatically increased, and the school shifted from what had been narrative reports to an actual report card on which he was getting Bs and Cs. His parents were puzzled because not only his previous narrative reports but periodic achievement testing suggested higher levels of academic ability. His parents initially presented their worry to the pediatrician that he had developed learning problems, but in her discussions with Todd, the pediatrician noted that he complained of many worries and concerns. Although he had a number of physical complaints, the physical examination, including electrocardiography, had been unremarkable.

During the psychiatric assessment and over several sessions, Todd acknowledged being much worried about school this year, partly because he also had begun to feel pressure from his parents about grades and college; in addition, they had suggested he take an additional language in school. Todd had a number of somatic complaints (headaches, recurrent aches and pains), and his parents reported that he was more irritable at home. He indicated that his worries had gradually increased but had been noteworthy over the past 6 months.

Review of the previous year's psychological testing revealed above-average intelligence and even somewhat higher achievement scores. Todd's mother, an attorney, reported a history of depression and anxiety and was currently taking a selective serotonin reuptake inhibitor with good effect.

Todd was referred for a course of group cognitive behavior therapy with good results. In addition, his parents and school were encouraged to review his academic load and discontinue the additional course work. There was also an opportunity to discuss with his parents the potential role that increased expectations and premature worries about college might serve as an additional source of anxiety to him. Follow-up in several months revealed that Todd was doing well in school and at home with no apparent recurrence of anxiety-related symptoms.

animals). Typically, features of anxiety, up to and including panic attack, are quickly pro-voked by exposure to the fear-producing stimulus. In children, the anxiety can lead to distress, tantrums, marked inhibition, or clinging to parents. Unlike adults with phobias, children do not always appreciate that the fear is abnormal or maladaptive. To make the diagnosis, the condition must be present for at least 6 months.

Various phobia types have been identified: one group centers on animals another on natural environmental phenomena, another on fears related to blood and injury, another on specific situations, and a final residual category includes the remainder. There has been speculation that these various types have evolutionary correlates.

Case Report: Phobia in a Boy with Asperger Disorder

Jimmy, age 9 years, was the oldest of three children. His parents had become worried about him in preschool when he had major difficulties in peer interaction despite being academically gifted. A diagnosis of Asperger disorder was eventually made. Jimmy had multiple and long-standing special interests, including cars, the stock market, and dogs. Interestingly, Jimmy had been bitten by a dog at age 3 years, having, according to his mother, lunged on top of the dog from behind in an attempt to ride it. Since that time, he had been acquiring considerable information on dogs and knew a tremendous amount about dog breeds. However, over time, he had become more and more anxious about seeing or being near actual dogs. At first, his parents noticed that he became anxious and fearful even if seeing a dog from some distance. Over time, he became so upset that his parents would have to cross the street with him if a person was walking a dog on the sidewalk. At other times, he might have a tantrum or cling to them for safely. The family could not visit friends with dogs, and even travel in the car with Jimmy had become a burden because he would become very agitated at even seeing a dog in a yard or behind a fence. Somewhat paradoxically, his long interest in dogs was not particularly helpful because his knowledge was highly academic rather than practical, and it had become a sore point in the family because both his younger siblings highly desired having a pet dog. Various attempts to "reason" with him had been unsuccessful because he was convinced that every dog would bite him.

Jimmy was referred for a course of cognitive behavior therapy (CBT), which included a focus on explicit teaching about ways to monitor his anxiety, a graduated desensitization program with eventual exposure to a large but profoundly placid dog, and training in ways to approach dogs successfully. The family was also put in touch with a special agency that provided dogs for children with autism and similar social disabilities, and although Jimmy remained wary of other dogs, he came to be very close to this one. His parents noted that his ability to ably verbalize specific rules from the CBT (e.g., "The first rule is to ask the owner if the dog is friendly. The second rule is to ask if I can pet the dog. The third rule is to . . . ") also encouraged them to seek additional treatment over time, which helped him cope with other problem situations.

Comment: At times, the special interests of children with Asperger disorder (see Chapter 4) revolve about something they were, or initially were, afraid of. This may partly be a coping mechanism but can have, as in this case, varying degrees of success because the knowledge acquired is of a very factual rather than social-interaction or practical nature. For a diagnosis of phobic disorder to be made in children, the *Diagnostic and Statistical Manual of Mental Disorders* (DSM-IV-TR) makes two modifications in its diagnostic guidelines: (1) children do *not* have to recognize that their fear is unreasonable, and (1) children may express anxiety through crying, freezing, and tantrums rather than through panic attacks.

Panic Disorder with or without Agoraphobia

Panic disorder is characterized by recurrent and unexpected panic attacks. Unlike panic attacks associated with phobias or other conditions, there is not a specific environmental event that triggers the attack. The period of intense fear and anxiety is associated with a minimum of four somatic or cognitive symptoms. For adolescents, the somatic symptoms might include palpitations, trembling, feeling faint or nauseous, or sweating or feeling short of breath; cognitive symptoms include fears of dying or losing one's mind. When the patient is avoiding places or situations where he or she might have difficulty escaping (usually involving larger groups of people), a diagnosis of panic disorder with agoraphobia is made. The issue of differentiating cues and noncues or unexpected panic attack is needed to differentiate this condition from other anxiety disorders; but as a practical matter, this is not so easily accomplished in children. Panic attacks can also be associated with various medical conditions, including endocrine disturbances, seizures, vestibular problems, and cardiac conditions; accordingly, physical examination and appropriate laboratory testing may be needed.

Case Study: Selective Mutism

In this condition, an individual, usually a child, is unable to speak in specific situations (e.g., in school). Although originally thought of as a communication disorder, the condition has been more recently viewed as an anxiety-related disorder given the frequency with which it is associated with anxiety. The original term for the condition, *elective mutism*, also implied that the problem was one of deliberate choice rather than reflecting significant emotional difficulties.

Typically, the child functions normally in many ways but because of his or her shyness and inhibition may be unable to participate with peers. The child may, for example, be highly verbal at home or when he or she is comfortable but is largely nonverbal in school. Girls are more likely to exhibit the condition. Various gradations are noted, with some children speaking to adults but not peers or vice versa. Although there is some potential for confusion with autism, children with this condition can and usually do speak in situations when they are comfortable. The unusual motor mannerisms seen in autism are not observed in selective mutism, and when the child does talk, his or her language is not unusual, as it is in autism. It is important to establish that the situation is not better explained by another condition (e.g., psychosis or concern over a speech impediment). Children with selective mutism often have a history of behavioral inhibition and anxiety difficulties. Potential risk factors include underlying speech or language problems. Unfortunately, the condition tends to be self-reinforcing and rather persistent. Early intervention is important and should include a speech-language assessment (to clarify any potential underlying vulnerabilities) as well as a psychiatric assessment with special attention to anxiety-related issues. Treatment approaches vary with the age of the child and other relevant features. Unfortunately, well-meaning but poorly informed treatments that attempt to "force" speech often only make the child more anxious. Behavioral approaches have been used to encourage the gradual generalization of speech to other settings; the child might, for example, be initially encouraged to whisper and then gradually speak more forcefully.

Family members often have a history of anxiety disorders, particularly social anxiety disorder. It is important to note that transiently, many children are rather quiet and shy on entering school, and selective mutism should not be diagnosed in this initial period because many children go on to communicate normally.

Epidemiology and Demographics

Along with the mood disorders, to which they are closely related, anxiety disorders are some of the most common mental health problems in children and adolescents, impacting as many as one in five in this age group. Data from various epidemiologic studies randomly suggest that between 3% and almost 30% of children in community samples have some anxiety disorder. Rates vary significantly, reflecting differences in method and other factors.

One of the more robust differences is the consistent gender difference, with higher rates reported in females. This preponderance is noted even before puberty, even earlier than depression with the possible exception of GAD, which, similar to depression, becomes more frequent in girls during adolescence. SAD has an earlier onset than other conditions in this group, and its frequency markedly decreases over time. On the other hand, social phobia becomes more frequent in adolescents.

Lower socioeconomic status (SES) has been associated with both more normative fears and specific phobia. In other anxiety disorders, SES and cultural differences are not consistent. In addition to their frequency, these conditions can have multiple negative effects and are associated with an increased risk of problems in adulthood.

Etiology

Etiologic models for anxiety disorders must encompass many different potential risk factors. These risks have complicated interrelationships with each other and may interact or predispose the developing child to increased vulnerability (or resilience). For purposes of discussion, these factors can be discussed separately, but as Figure 12.1 indicates, there are actually complex interactions among them.

Work on the genetics of these conditions indicates a strong role for genetic factors, with increased risk for children whose parents have anxiety disorders and high rates of concordance in twin studies. It seems likely that these risk factors act by impacting specific psychological and developmental processes, which then put the child at increased risk. Studies have focused on specific genes, including the serotonin transporter gene (5HTT). In addition to genetic factors, environmental or experiential ones also have a major role in pathogenesis. One of

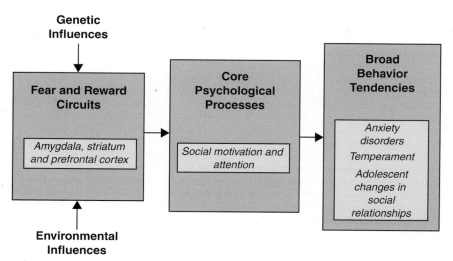

FIGURE 12.1. Etiologic model of pediatric anxiety disorders. (From Krain, A. L., Ghaffari, M., Freeman J., et al. (2007). Anxiety disorders. In A. Martin & F. Volkmar (Eds.), *Lewis's Child and Adolescent Psychiatry: A Comprehensive Textbook*, 4th edition, p. 324. Philadelphia: Lippincott Williams & Wilkins.)

the complexities here is that parents who are anxious may behave in ways that facilitate the development of anxiety in children (through parenting style, modeling, and so forth). As with genetic factors, there are many potential mediators of these effects. Much interest has centered on disentangling the complex relationships of environmental and genetic vulnerabilities and the mediating events in pathogenesis.

Psychological processes such as modeling and fear conditioning (i.e., learning) may also impact specific brain regions, including the limbic and paralimbic systems, striatum, amygdala, orbitofrontal cortex, and anterior cingulate cortex, areas that are highly interrelated and central in integration of emotional experiences. For example, the amygdala has been shown to be fundamentally involved in fear conditioning, and in neuroimaging studies, children with anxiety disorders exhibit greater activation of this structure in response to stimuli such as faces; the degree of signal change correlates positively with self-reported anxiety. Similarly, differences have been noted using structural imaging techniques relative to reduced amygdala volume in children with anxiety disorders. The orbitofrontal cortex has a role in mediating negative and as well as positive reinforcement, and several studies have shown increases in activation in this area as well as the prefrontal cortex. The anterior cingulate cortex plays a role in regulation of response to emotion and is thought to be involved in the experience of anxiety. It is presumed that changes in neural mechanisms impact information processing so that, for example, fearful and anxious responses are associated with a bias for attending to features in the environment associated with it. This might also be reflected in a tendency to misinterpret and become anxious in situations when it is not appropriate (e.g., in responding to ambiguous situations, children with anxiety disorders are more likely to become anxious). The basic psychological process interact with, and perhaps shape and are shaped by, basic temperamental factors (see Chapter 2) so that, for example, infants and toddlers who are unusually behaviorally inhibited are more likely to exhibit later anxiety disorders.

Differential Diagnosis and Evaluation

Differentiation of the various anxiety disorders can sometimes be difficult; challenges arise due to the frequency of anxiety in typically developing children, differentiation (largely based on impairment) of normative and clinically significant difficulties, the rapid pace of change in childhood, and the tendency of disorders to themselves become further risk factors for other problems. Anxiety as a result of realistic worries is not a disorder, and children's worries naturally change over the course of development, often being more concrete and tangible in younger children and more anticipatory and less tangible in older children and adolescents.

SAD can usually be differentiated given the onset, duration, severity, and the degree of impairment or distress. The nature of the anxiety may also be helpful in differentiation (e.g., in separation anxiety it often centers around parents and separation from parents). In contrast to OCD, the anxiety is not associated with compulsions. At times, severe distress or behavioral difficulties at times of separation can lead to some potential confusion with oppositional defiant disorder or even bipolar disorder, although in both cases, the marked concerns about separation are an important diagnostic indicator. In contrast to SAD, GAD involves a range of concerns and worries (i.e., rather than being confined to separation). In some ways, this category can be most difficult to distinguish from normative, if excessive, anxiety and worry. The impairment, difficulties in self-regulation, and degree of anxiety should be clearly more than what would be normally expected in GAD. Another clue is the usually wide ranging nature of the worries (i.e., of a range of topics rather than a single one as in phobia). School attendance issues can arise with both separation anxiety and GAD, in the first case because of issues relative to or about separation and in the second because of concerns about academic performance.

Issues of differentiation can be particularly complex in younger children who have separation issues and in older children who have social anxiety difficulties as well. Sometimes the worries about school or academic performance may initially be taken to suggest the perfectionism usually seen in OCD, but in OCD, the worry is usually not related to having good enough academic work but related to having error-free (i.e., perfect), work. But at times, a degree of perfectionism can be a source of confusion. The DSM-IV-TR has a somewhat lower "threshold" for the diagnosis of GAD in children than in adults along with a shorter duration requirement, although as in adults, some degree of interference must be present. Physical symptoms are particularly common in children with GAD. Several good rating scales and interviews for anxiety disorders are available and can aid in diagnosis and monitoring treatment (see Krain et al., 2007, for a review).

In some ways, phobias are simpler to diagnosis given the specificity of the fear. At times, however, the degree of anxiety and the efforts take to avoid exposure may be severe and complicate the diagnostic picture. Fears of some situations and objects are normative and may not be pathological but are not associated with high levels of impairment.

Social anxiety disorder and separation anxiety both involve anxiety centered in some ways about social situations. In SAD, anxiety focuses on caregiver separation; in social anxiety disorder, there is more generalized anxiety that involves concerns about being inadequate in some public situation. Although some degree of anxiety in school and other situations is normative (and can be adaptive) in social anxiety disorder, there is impairment or significant distress. Although children with GAD may worry about various social issues, peers, and how peers and teacher view them, they usually have a range of other concerns as well. Selective mutism has been increasingly viewed as a variant of social anxiety.

A further complication for the differential diagnosis come from the high rates of comorbidity reported within the various anxiety disorders, although high, the rate in youth is somewhat lower than in adulthood (partially reflecting continued development of anxiety disorders into adulthood). Rates of comorbidity are higher in clinical samples than in more normative samples. Panic attacks are frequently associated with various other anxiety disorders. Depression also frequently co-occurs with anxiety disorders. GAD and depression together frequently persist into adulthood. Interestingly, about 20% of children with anxiety disorders also exhibit attentional or conduct problems. Children with selective mutism also frequently exhibit social anxiety, and school refusal is frequent in cases of SAD. Children with autism and related conditions are frequently anxious, particularly in social situations, but an anxiety disorder should be diagnosed only if the degree of anxiety-related difficulties is greater than would be expected given the presence of the other condition.

Given the frequency with which somatic complaints are associated with anxiety problems in children, it is not unusual for the child or adolescent to have had laboratory and other studies (e.g., electrocardiography). The yield of these studies is usually minimal, but sometimes anxiety disorders can be substance induced or caused by a general medical condition, so a careful history and thoughtful assessment are needed. Depending on the context, urine for drug screening and thyroid function assessment may be indicated.

Treatment

Effective treatments, both behavioral (e.g., CBT) and pharmacologic, are available. Although some treatment studies focus on one particular condition, most include youth with a range of (and sometimes multiple) anxiety disorders. As described in Chapter 22, an impressive body of research now supports the effectiveness of CBT for childhood anxiety disorders. Often, the methods used have been extrapolated to children from original work in adults with modifications to encompass developmental issues. Approaches are used that help children understand and identify their feelings and responses to anxiety-provoking situations. Various behavior strategies are provided to help children learn to cope more adaptively (e.g., relaxation skills training). The use of practical homework and other procedures also helps children, and use of imagined or real-life exposure to anxiety-provoking situations helps the child use these skills outside the consulting room. Both individual and group treatment approaches have been used with success.

As drug treatments for adult anxiety disorders have advanced, efforts have been made to extend this work to children and adolescents. Several well-designed and adequately powered placebo-controlled studies have documented the effectives of drug treatments. Some of the drugs frequently used in adults, such as the benzodiazepines, have proven less useful in children, often because of potential adverse effects. Similarly, apart from some work using clomipramine for pediatric OCD (see below), work on the tricyclic antidepressants for pediatric anxiety disorders is rather limited, particularly given their potential side effects. Most of the available research has centered on the selective serotonin reuptake inhibitors (SSRIs) in the treatment of social phobia, SAD, and GAD (see also Chapter 21). Several different agents have now been systematically evaluated and found effective. Data on treatment of panic disorder in the pediatric population are, unfortunately, somewhat more limited, although some work suggests potential usefulness here as well.

Course and Prognosis

Longitudinal studies have repeatedly documented the risk that pediatric anxiety disorders represent for a range of adult anxiety, mood, and other disorders. The overall strength of this risk is, however, moderate, with some children going on *not* develop such problems, and adult risk is, for example, less than that posed by conduct disorder. Studies have often grouped pediatric anxiety disorders into a single overall category, so outcome data relative to specific pediatric anxiety disorders are more limited, but it does appear that GAD represents a significant risk for adult anxiety disorders; major depression data for other pediatric anxiety disorders is more limited.

OBSESSIVE-COMPULSIVE DISORDER

Obsessions and compulsions have been recognized since antiquity and were sometimes regarded as evidence of demonic possession. Early theorists, including Freud and Maudsley, were interested in this clinical problem, and Freud's attempt to derive a theory strongly emphasized developmental factors. Both the use of the SSRIs as effective pharmacologic treatment and advances in brain research have increased interest in this condition.

Diagnostic and Clinical Features

Obsessions are defined as undesired impulses, thoughts, worries, memories, words, or images that come to mind involuntarily and become the source of distress and impairment. Although the "flavor" of these mental contents may be highly unusual, the individual retains a strong awareness of reality while simultaneously seeing the obsession as some aspect of his or her own mind. Compulsions arise in response to what the individual views as a need to engage in certain activities or rituals, sometimes in connection to an obsession (i.e., in which some activity is meant to deal with or "ward off" the obsession); sometimes, particularly in children, a mental component is not identified. As with obsessions, *compulsions* are seen as involuntary and forced. Sometimes the individual develops a complicated set of rules and routines in response to these phenomena, which also become a source of functional impairment as well as of distress. Table 12.2 summarizes clinical and diagnostic features. Some modifications are made relative to children in the DSM-IV-TR definition (e.g., with regard to the awareness and insight into the meaningless nature of their behaviors).

The list of potential obsessions and compulsions is endless. Although occasionally an individual has only one or the other (usually obsessions), individuals often have both, usually multiple ones. Symptoms change over time and with development. For adolescents with OCD issues, dirt or germs, symmetry, and religion are common; in adulthood, aggressive and sexual topics become more common. Compulsive behaviors in adolescents include cleaning, repeating actions, and checking; in adulthood, checking, cleaning, counting, or a focus on numbers and repetitions become more common.

Studies using rating scales have explored the relationships of obsessions and compulsions and have often revealed four subtypes: (1) organized around issues of aggression, religion,

TABLE 12.2

OBSESSIVE-COMPULSIVE DISORDER: OVERVIEW OF DIAGNOSIS AND CLINICAL FEATURES IN CHILDREN AND ADOLESCENTS

Diagnostic Features

Obsessions (recurrent thoughts or impulses images experienced) are present; these are the source of distress and anxiety but are not usual realistic life concerns; the individual attempts to avoid these thoughts and sees them as coming from him- or herself (rather than as from outside as in psychosis).

Compulsions (recurrent and inappropriate behaviors performed in response to obsessional thinking) are present.

These features consume significant time (in DSM-IV-TR. it specified at least 1 hour a day) or interfere with some aspects of functioning or are a cause of distress.

The obsessions or compulsions are not simply caused by substance abuse or some medical condition, and if another mental disorder is present, the obsessions or compulsions are not simply a reflection of it.

In children, there is no requirement that the individual appreciates that the thoughts or behaviors are inappropriate.

Subtypes

There are probably at least four groups: (1) checking compulsions with obsessions around aggression, religion, sexuality, or somatic preoccupations; (2) symmetry obsessions and counting, ordering, and repetition compulsions; (3) cleanliness and washing preoccupations; and (4) hoarding

Onset

Usually in childhood, adolescence or young adulthood.

Neurobiology

Significant genetic component; connection to Tourette's syndrome may reflect a common underlying predisposition.

---

sexuality, and somatic obsessional behavior as well as associated checking; (2) another group in whom obsessions center on symmetry and compulsions take the form of counting, ordering, and repetition; (3) a group organized around cleanliness and washing; (4) and a final type including compulsions that involve hoarding. Most studies suggest that obsessions and compulsions should been seen as manifestations of the same problem (i.e., rather than as separate). The first and second groups have an earlier onset, but the hoarding subgroup seems rather distinctive from the rest and may eventually deserve its own diagnostic category. Although there is some suggestion that children can change types over time, the strong connections of the potential subtypes to other conditions remains an important topic for research because the types potentially relate to aspects of treatment, genetic vulnerability, and neuropsychological profiles. Longitudinal and follow-up studies may help clarify some of these issues. By adulthood, there is more stability of the specific clinical presentation.

Children with OCD often have some areas where life skills are relatively little impacted (e.g., academic and other school-related activities may not be impaired, although peer relations can be adversely impacted, particularly if symptoms are more severe). The apparent preservation of academic skills often masks the degree to which children with OCD suffer. For example, the child may be doing well in school but spending hours a day outside of school engaged in rituals and routines. Sleep may be impacted, and physical injury can result from repeated cleaning and other activities. Often, the apparently good academic skills combined with the child's tendency to hide the difficulties delays diagnostic assessment and treatment. Similarly, the fact that the

Case Report: Obsessive-Compulsive Disorder

Luke was a 13-year-old boy who lived with his parents and older sister. He was referred by his primary care provider for assessment in light of long-standing difficulties. His pediatrician reported that for as long as he had known him (since toddlerhood), Luke has been a worrier, but over the past several years, things had "taken a turn for the worse," and his parents were urged by the pediatrician to seek psychiatric assessment.

Luke's parents reported that he was a bright and academically successful boy who had always been "a bit of a worrier." He worried about various bad things that might happen early in life and was also very meticulous, wanting his projects and school work to be perfect. He constantly sought feedback on his performance and would repeatedly check his work, sometimes to the point that his teachers would tell him things became worse if he fussed over them too much. With the onset of adolescence, Luke had become more worried about his appearance and cleanliness. He wanted to have a girlfriend but was worried that his body odor (not notable to his parents or physician) would turn them off to him. At around this time, his entry into junior high school had also meant a somewhat more challenging academic load with more need for forward planning and less tolerance of his difficulties "getting stuck" on assignments (in contrast to the past, he now had to deal with many teachers as opposed to just one).

Even small mistakes in his work would result in his redoing his assignment. He became more meticulous about his clothing and seemed to his parents more withdrawn and preoccupied. He seemed to be taking longer and longer to get things done and seemed to lose many of his connections with peers as a result. He could spend several hours in the shower each day. Because he was unwilling to talk with his parent, they talked with his pediatrician, who made the referral for psychiatric assessment.

In talking with the parents, it emerged that the there was a family history of depression, and a paternal uncle had Tourette's syndrome, which was well controlled with medication. The parents ran a small business (in which Luke occasionally had worked). They were also devout members of a fundamentalist Christian church.

On examination, but only over several sessions, Luke began to talk more freely with the child psychiatrist. He had a number of obsessions and compulsions and was preoccupied with cleanliness because he felt dirty most of the time. It emerged that part of his feelings of dirtiness also were involved in sexual thoughts about girls. Part of his difficulty related to an inability to communicate with his parents because he thought that they would think he was a bad person and destined for Hell. He noted that he had become very stressed over the past months in his new school. Although always a perfectionist, he now realized that his previous perfectionism had begun to interfere with his school work. He was also aware of engaging in a number of rituals, including counting the number of drafts of each paper and showering a specific number of times each day. He was worried that if did not engage in these acts, his life would "fall apart." Although there was no indication of thought process disorder or of suicidal ideation, the psychiatrist was concerned that Luke's mood seemed to be increasingly depressed.

The parents initially expressed some shock at the diagnosis, but Luke indicated that he would prefer to keep working with the psychiatrist and was interested in trying medication. Fluoxetine was begun and gradually increased to a reasonable dose level with gradual improvement. In addition, a course of CBT was instituted, and within 2 months, Luke reported substantial improvement. He and his parents were pleased with his progress. He chose to remain in periodic, longer term treatment, partly to deal with a range of adolescent issues and continued to do well.

Comment: In adults, the *Diagnostic and Statistical Manual of Mental Disorders* (DSM-IV-TR) requires that adults with obsessive-compulsive disorder have some recognition that the obsessions or compulsions are unreasonable; this is not required for children. By definition, the difficulties must significantly interfere and take more than 1 hour a day.

child has insight into the lack of rationality of the symptoms may falsely reassure the parents. The lack of obvious difficulties in the pediatrician's office can similarly result in advice that minimizes or trivializes the problem. Parents may not initially see symptoms as severe but, over time, may become entrained in complicated ways in the child's preoccupations and rituals (see Towbin & Riddle, 2007, for a discussion).

Epidemiology and Demographics

As Freud and others observed, phenomena suggestive of OCD are common in younger children and indeed in the general population. In the normal population, this may take the form of getting things "just right" or being focused on rules, symmetry, and other phenomena suggestive of OCD. These phenomena do, however, decline as children move into the elementary school years. There is some possibility that this may not happen in children at risk for developing the disorder.

Issues in definition and method complicate interpretation of the available epidemiological data. Prevalence rates vary from 0.4% to 1%. In children, the prevalence rate is probably on the order of 0.6% to 1%. Although male and female rates are roughly equal, males seem to have an earlier onset. One of the complexities for research (and intervention) is that symptoms often exist for many years before clinical attention is sought.

Etiology

Several lines of evidence strongly implicate genetic factors in pathogenesis. The role of genetic factors was only appreciated over time as methodologic issues were addressed. More recent studies reveal higher rates in monozygotic as opposed to dizygotic twins and higher rates in family members. In addition, there are higher rates of "subthreshold" OCD phenomena in first-degree relates. In one well-done study that involved direct examination rather than self-report, Pauls and colleagues (1995) noted rates of 10% in relatives of OCD patients as opposed to 2% of the relatives in unaffected probands; these rates increased if "subthreshold" OCD was included. Greater genetic risk has also been associated with an earlier onset. A connection to Tourette's syndrome is also suggested by observation of high rates of OCD among relatives of patients with Tourette's syndrome.

Studies of neuropsychological functions in OCD have suggested problems in the functions usually associated with the prefrontal cortex. Difficulties include problems in executive functioning (forward planning and set shifting), visual-spatial and nonverbal memory, motor inhibition, and response suppression. Brain regions implicated include the dorsolateral prefrontal cortex, orbitofrontal cortex, cingulate, and parietal lobes. Neuropsychological and functional magnetic resonance imaging (fMRI) differences have also been reported in relation to the potential subtyping approach previously discussed. For example, basal ganglia functions were more involved in patients with aggressive and checking symptoms, but those with cleanliness preoccupations had the ventromedial prefrontal cortex, cingulated, and other areas involved. The anterior cingulate gyrus has been particularly well studied. Structural MRI studies have noted increased volume in this region. Although positron emission tomography and single photon emission computed tomography studies are not performed in children, some work has been done in adults. fMRI studies of children and adolescents have been generally consistent with observed neuropsychological deficits.

Another line of research has focused on the neurochemical correlates of OCD, reflecting an awareness that the SSRIs have proven to be effective pharmacologic interventions. This work has included studies of cerebrospinal fluid serotonin metabolites and use of medications, such as lithium and L-tryptophan, that augment serotonergic transmission. Studies of peripheral serotonin (e.g., through platelet levels) and studies of imipramine binding have not produced consistent results. Other work has focused on the potential contribution of dopamine given the apparent involvement of the basal ganglia and the frequent observation of OCD-type behaviors in patients with disorders that impact this brain region. The dopamine-blocking agents have also been used to successfully augment response in patients not responding to SSRIs; some evidence suggests that the SSRIs have both serotonergic and dopaminergic effects. The excitatory neurotransmitter glutamate has also been thought to be involved in pathogenesis.

A different line of research has focused on the pediatric autoimmune responses to streptococcal infection (PANDAS) because some children seem to develop OCD symptoms after these infections. These symptoms are usually associated with tics and have some similarities to the behaviors reported in Sydenham's chorea. It has been proposed that that this condition may arise as an autoimmune disorder. This observation is of interest for many reasons and has some support from scanning data. Some preliminary reports note a positive response to immunoglobulin or plasmapheresis treatment. This hypothesis has, however, been controversial because some findings have not proven easily to replicate. Current etiologic approaches attempt to integrate the various and diverse findings and posit connections among several brain regions potentially involved in OCD pathogenesis.

Differential Diagnosis and Evaluation

There is potential for OCD to be confused with (or overlap with) a number of conditions (Table 12.3). The DSM-IV-TR's approach to the problem of comorbidity and differential diagnosis is a requirement that the "obsessions" not be "restricted" to any other disorder that is present. Although this helps in some ways, it complicates the task of diagnosis in other ways because the issue of how restricted a problem is can be difficult to sort out. Given the heterogeneity with OCD and the association of similar symptoms with other disorders, a careful diagnostic assessment is needed. It is also important to realize that OCD phenomena that do not rise to the level of a disorder are very frequent, perhaps seen in more than 75% of the normal population.

TABLE 12.3
DISORDERS MANIFESTING OBSESSIONS OR COMPULSIONS

Anorexia nervosa
Body dysmorphic disorder
Delusional disorder (all types)
Depression
Hypochondriasis
Obsessive-compulsive personality disorder
Organic mental disorder[1]
Panic disorder
Pervasive developmental disorder
Phobias
Posttraumatic stress disorder
Schizophrenia
Schizotypal personality
Somatization disorder
Somatoform disorders
Trichotillomania
Tourette's syndrome

[1]Specifically arising from central nervous system trauma, tumors, or toxins.
Reprinted from Towbin, K., & Riddle, M. (2007). Obsessive compulsive disorder. In A. Martin & F. Volkmar (Eds.), *Lewis's Child and Adolescent Psychiatry: A Comprehensive Textbook*, 4th edition, p. 556. Philadelphia: Lippincott Williams & Wilkins.

Trichotillomania

Trichotillomania (TTM; "hair-pulling madness" in Greek) has many clinical similarities and possibly more basic relationships to obsessive-compulsive disorder (OCD). The suggestion of a relationship is also made by the observation that OCD is a risk factor for TTM. This diagnosis requires hair pulling that results in noteworthy and readily observable hair loss. There are feelings of increased tension before and gratification after the hair pulling. Interestingly, hair pulling without the psychological component is relatively prevalent (perhaps 4% of the population), although if strictly defined, as in the *Diagnostic and Statistical Manual of Mental Disorders* (DSM-IV-TR), the rate is between 0.6% and 1%. The condition is more common in females, and there are two apparent peaks of onset, early childhood and adolescence. The condition is often observed with OCD and with tic disorders. There is some suggestion of a genetic component and some suggestion of difficulties with cognitive flexibility on psychological testing. Some magnetic resonance imaging differences have been noted as well.

The relative infrequency of the condition and the difficulties of generalizing from clinical samples (presumably the most severe) limits what is known about the condition.

The condition is often chronic. Treatment approaches have used behavioral interventions (e.g., cognitive behavior therapy [CBT]) as well as drug treatment (e.g., with the selective serotonin reuptake inhibitors) but only with modest benefit. CBT has a relatively robust initial response rate, but over time, the condition tends to recur.

Similarly, there is potential for confusing obsessive-compulsive personality disorder (OCPD) with OCD; an essential difference is that in OCPD, the features do not generate distress, anxiety, or impairment as in strictly defined OCD. Impairment arises in OCPD more from the impact of the behavior on others. There is some suggestion that some children and adolescents with OCD may develop OCPD later in life.

Boundaries among an obsession or compulsion and psychotic thinking or behavior can be difficult to sort out at times. Patients with OCD usually have some degree of insight; DSM-IV-TR does allow the diagnosis of OCD when delusional disorder or schizophrenia is present. Some patients with OCD do not have high levels of self-awareness and insight.

As noted previously, it is common for children with OCD to be delayed in coming to assessment and treatment. The child's concerns about privacy, fears about disclosure, and feelings of shame or guilt may lead to minimization or underreporting. Giving the child or adolescent ample time and respecting his or her need for a thoughtful and methodical approach usually mean multiple evaluation sessions are needed. In addition to interviews with the child him- or herself, history from the parents, and potentially other family members, can be helpful. Teachers can provide information on peer interaction as well as academic performance (but may not be aware or only minimally aware of the child's distress and difficulties). Siblings can also be good sources of information. The clinician should take a careful history that examines all of the various contexts in which symptoms may be present and a source of difficulty. The impact of symptoms on school, peers, home life, and self-concept are all important areas for inquiry. It is important to keep in mind that the assessment process can be prolonged, and forming a working relationship with the patient is essential. Interviews with the family may clarify ways that symptoms emerge and are sometimes, unwittingly, encouraged or sustained. Sometimes family therapy is helpful. If a parent's own difficulties are severe enough to impact the child's treatment, the suggestion of parental referral might be considered. Meeting with the parents without the child also gives an opportunity to obtain important information (e.g., on family history of similar problems) and gives the clinician a chance to provide information and reassurance to the parents, who may be seriously concerned that their child is becoming psychotic.

Several assessment instruments specific to OCD have been developed. They augment but do not replace a thoughtful clinical assessment. The Leyton Obsessional Inventory—Children's Version (LOI-CV) and the Children's Yale-Brown Obsessive Compulsive Scale (CY-BOCS) have been most widely used. Personality tests and psychopathology rating scales and checklists, such as the Child Behavior Checklist (CBCL), may be useful in obtaining a broader view of potentially associated symptomatology.

There are no specific laboratory studies for OCD, although such tests and other studies may be obtained based on findings from the history and examination. Often, psychological testing can be used to document intellectual strengths and weakness.

Treatment

A range of treatment modalities can be used effectively. It is important to maintain a working treatment alliance with the child and family. At the time of diagnosis, the clinician can review the meaning and implications for treatment with special attention to associated features or conditions that might need to be addressed. The condition is typically chronic, and it is important that the patient and family be aware of this and be in agreement with clinicians about short-, medium-, and long-term objectives. At the same time, the clinician can describe the increasing number of treatment options available.

CBT is often the initial treatment for youth with mild to moderate OCD. A series of studies have now demonstrated the efficacy of this approach in children and adolescents. Various specific techniques can be used to achieve significant and sustained symptom reduction in the majority of cases. The available data suggest that CBT is about as effective as medication, but the need for an experienced therapist is essential.

Drug treatment has had a major role in treatment of patients with OCD, with about half of patients having a significant benefit. It is important for patients to understand that although many patients experience a marked reduction in symptoms, these are not totally eliminated. The issue of choice of medication is guided, in large part, by the specifics of the clinical situation (e.g., the presence of comorbid conditions or other factors that might suggest a particular agent over another). The presence of coexistent psychosis, tics, depression, or anxiety problems is highly relevant in evaluating the efficacy of a medication. It is important to educate patients about the need for an adequate drug trial (i.e., adequate both in terms of dose and length of trial). In some cases, patients should also be warned about the potential difficulties of stopping some agents abruptly (i.e., causing a withdrawal reaction); this is particularly true if the medication has a shorter half-life.

The serotonin reuptake inhibitors (SRIs) have been most intensively studied. Well-designed placebo-controlled trials have been conducted in children using a number of different agents. There is some suggestion of differential response based on clinical subtype (e.g. in one study patients, who engaged in hoarding were less likely to respond). The choice of agent may also be guided by side effect profiles. In adolescents, clomipramine has been well studied with a reasonably good symptom reduction in most patients, but anticholinergic side effects can be problematic. Fluoxetine also appears effective but with a few side effects; these most frequently included agitation, sleep issues, and other problems. Concern about the potential for suicidal ideation has also been raised. Typically, this agent is begun at with 5 mg/day and gradually increased to a maximal dosage (of about 60 mg/day). Various SRIs (and SSRIs; see Chapter 21) are now available. In general, differences between the agents appear relatively minimal within the SSRIs; clomipramine appears to have a somewhat more robust response rate but at the cost of significant side effects so that it is not typically a first choice drug in the pediatric age range.

A number of patients do not respond to adequate drug trials with SRIs. Unfortunately, there can be considerable variability in response so that individuals sometimes respond better to one agent than another; typically, at least two different agents should be given adequate trials. After two agents are used, many clinicians consider augmentation (i.e., use of a second agent to augment the response to the SRI). It is important that this be done carefully given the potential for drug interaction. Work by McDougle and colleagues (1994) demonstrated better response to combination of an SRI with a dopamine blocker in patients with tics or a family history of tics if the patient had not responded to the SRI alone. Fluoxetine should not be combined with L-tryptophan because serious toxicity has been reported.

In some cases, hospitalization may be indicated. This is particularly the case if the situation seems to be rapidly worsening and the ability of the child and family to cope seems seriously compromised. This step should not be taken lightly, but either partial or inpatient hospitalization may, at times, be helpful. The hospitalization has some potential for "detoxifying" the situation, giving parents and child some relief, providing a relatively rapid assessment and initial treatment plan, and providing an opportunity for all concerned to regroup before moving forward with treatment.

Course and Prognosis

A wide range of outcome is possible. The episode of OCD can go into total and permanent remission or can signal the beginning of an ongoing struggle. Many patterns between these two extremes are also observed, including partial remission, remission with occasional recurrent episodes, and so forth. Studies of the natural history of the condition are limited (e.g., often the most severe patients have been studied, so it is unclear how generalizable results are). In one longitudinal study of adults, about one-third of patients had an onset before age 20 years, although other studies suggest this rate may be much higher. The limited data available suggest that adolescents with "subclinical" OCD were usually stable, and those OCD often significantly improved. Other reports, particularly some of the earlier ones are, however, less optimistic. Negative prognostic factors include comorbid conditions, greater initial psychosocial difficulties, early onset, association with tics, and higher levels of parental psychopathology.

SUMMARY

The development of anxiety and its disorders is a complex process that likely involves biologic vulnerabilities as well as environmental influences. Significant advances in basic research have provided a neurobiological framework on which to base hypothesized etiologic models. Additionally, advanced research technologies in genetics and neuroimaging have allowed us to test these models with ever-increasing sophistication and detail.

Over the last several decades, significant advances have been made in understanding and treating anxiety disorders and OCDs in children and adolescents. Both behavioral and pharmacologic treatments have been shown to be helpful. An increasing focus of research has been the issue of which treatment approach (or combination of approaches) works best and for which children. Although understanding of basic mechanisms remains somewhat limited, there has been noteworthy progress in disentangling the rather complex interaction of neurobiologic and experiential factors. Advances in research should lead to further refinement of diagnostic categories or approaches and new strategies to prevent and treat children with these conditions.

Selected Readings

Achenbach, T. M. (1983). *Manual for the Child Behavior Checklist and Revised Behavior Profile.* Burlington, VT: Thomas Achenbach.
Benun, J., Lewis, C., Siegel, M., & Serwint, J. R. (2008). Fears and phobias. *Pediatrics in Review, 29*(7), 250–251.
Berg, C. J., Rapoport, J. L., & Flament, M. (1986). The Leyton Obsessional Inventory-Child Version. *Journal of the American Academy of Child Psychiatry, 25*(1):84–91.
Biederman, J., Rosenbaum, J. F., Chaloff, J., & Kagan, J. (1995). Behavioral inhibition as a risk factor for anxiety disorders. In J. March (Ed.), *Anxiety Disorders in Children and Adolescents,* pp. 61–81. New York: Guilford Press.
Bloch, M. H. (2009). Trichotillomania across the life span. *Journal of the American Academy of Child & Adolescent Psychiatry, 48*(9), 879–883.

Costello, E. J., Egger, H. L., & Angold, A. (2004). Developmental epidemiology of anxiety disorders. In T. H. Ollendick& J. S. March (Eds.), *Phobic and Anxiety Disorders in Children and Adolescents*, pp. 61–91. New York: Oxford University Press.

Costello, E. J., Egger, H. L., & Angold, A. (2005). The developmental epidemiology of anxiety disorders: Phenomenology, prevalence, and comorbidity. Child *and Adolescent Psychiatric Clinics of North America, 14*, 631–648, vii.

Crino, R., Slade, T., & Andrews, G. (2005). The changing prevalence and severity of obsessive-compulsive disorder criteria from DSM-III to DSM-IV. *American Journal of Psychiatry, 162*(5), 876–882.

Davis, M. (1997). Neurobiology of fear responses: The role of the amygdala. *Journal of Neuropsychiatry Clinics of Neuroscience, 9*, 382–402.

Farrell, L. J., Schlup, B., & Boschen, M. J. (2010). Cognitive-behavioral treatment of childhood obsessive-compulsive disorder in community-based clinical practice: clinical significance and benchmarking against efficacy. *Behaviour Research & Therapy, 48*(5), 409–417.

Gullone, E. (2000). The development of normal fear: A century of research. *Clinical Psychology Review, 20*, 429-451.

Klein, R. G. (2009). Anxiety disorders. *Journal of Child Psychology & Psychiatry & Allied Disciplines, 50*(1–2), 153–162.

Krain, A., Ghaffari, M., Freeman, J., Garcia, A., Leonard, H., & Pine, D. S. (2007). Anxiety disorders. In A. Martin & F. Volkmar (Eds.), *Lewis's Child and Adolescent Psychiatry: A Comprehensive Textbook*, 4th edition. Philadelphia: Lippincott Williams & Wilkins.

Leckman, J. F., Zhang, H., Alsobrook, J. P., & Pauls, D. L. (2001). Symptom dimensions in obsessive-compulsive disorder: Toward quantitative phenotypes. *American Journal of Medical Genetics, 105*(1), 28–30.

Lewinsohn, P. M., Gotlib, I. H., Lewinsohn, M., Seeley, J. R., & Allen, N. B. (1998). Gender differences in anxiety disorders and anxiety symptoms in adolescents. *Journal of Abnormal Psychology, 107*, 109–117.

Lin, H., Williams, K. A., Katsovich, L., Findley, D. B., Grantz, H., Lombroso, P. J., King, R. A., Bessen, D. E., Johnson, D., Kaplan, E. L., Landeros-Weisenberger, A., Zhang, H., & Leckman, J. F. (2010). Streptococcal upper respiratory tract infections and psychosocial stress predict future tic and obsessive-compulsive symptom severity in children and adolescents with Tourette syndrome and obsessive-compulsive disorder. *Biological Psychiatry, 67*(7), 684–691.

Lissek, S., Powers, A. S., McClure, E. B., Phelps, E. A., Woldehawariat, G., Grillon, C., & Pine, D. S. (2005). Classical fear conditioning in the anxiety disorders: A meta-analysis. *Behaviour Research and Therapy, 43*, 1391–1424.

March, J. S. (1995). Cognitive-behavioral psychotherapy for children and adolescents with OCD: A review and recommendations for treatment. *Journal of the American Academy of Child and Adolescent Psychiatry, 34*(1), 7–18.

March, J. S. (2004). Review: Clomipramine is more effective than SSRIs for paediatric obsessive compulsive disorder. *Evidence Based Mental Health, 7*(2), 50.

McDougle, C. J., Goodman, W. K., Leckman, J. F., Lee, N. C., Heninger, G. R., & Price, L. H. (1994). Haloperidol addition in fluvoxamine-refractory obsessive-compulsive disorder. A double-blind, placebo-controlled study in patients with and without tics. *Archives of General Psychiatry, 51*(4), 302–308.

Milham, M. P., Nugent, A. C., Drevets, W. C., Dickstein, D. P., Leibenluft, E., Ernst, M., Charney, D., & Pine, D. S. (2005). Selective reduction in amygdala volume in pediatric anxiety disorders: a voxel-based morphometry investigation. *Biological Psychiatry, 57*, 961–966.

Miller, M. C. (2009). Treatment that works for anxious children. *Harvard Mental Health Letter, 25*(7), 8.

Nestadt, G., Addington, A., Samuels, J., Liang, K. Y., Bienvenu, O. J., Riddle, M., Marco Grados, M., Hoehn-Saric, R., & Cullen, B. (2003). The identification of OCD-related subgroups based on comorbidity. *Biological Psychiatry, 53*(10), 914–920.

Pauls, D. L., Alsobrook, J. P., Goodman, W., Rasmussen, S., & Leckman, J. F. (1995). A family study of obsessive-compulsive disorder. *American Journal of Psychiatry, 152*(1), 76–84.

Pigott, T. A., Pato, M. T., Bernstein, S. E., Grover, G. N., Hill, J. L., Tolliver, T. J., & Murphy, D. L. (1990). Controlled comparisons of clomipramine and fluoxetine in the treatment of obsessive-compulsive disorder. Behavioral and biological results. *Archives of General Psychiatry, 47*(10), 926–932.

Pine, D. S. (2002). Treating children and adolescents with selective serotonin reuptake inhibitors: How long is appropriate? *Journal of Child and Adolescent Psychopharmacology, 12*, 189–203.

Rachman, S. L., & Hodgson, R. J. (1980). *Obsessions and Compulsions*. Englewood Cliffs, NJ: Prentice-Hall Inc.

Rosenthal, J., Jacobs, L., Marcus, M., & Katzman, M. A. (2007). Beyond shy: When to suspect social anxiety disorder. *Journal of Family Practice, 56*(5), 369–374.

Salkovskis, P. M., & Harrison, J. (1984). Abnormal and normal obsessions—A replication. *Behaviour Research and Therapy, 22*(5), 549–552.

Scahill, L., Riddle, M. A., McSwiggin-Hardin, M., Ort, S. I., King, R. A., Goodman, W. K., Cicchetti, D., & Leckman, J. F. (1997). Children's Yale-Brown Obsessive Compulsive Scale: Reliability and validity. *Journal of the American Academy of Child and Adolescent Psychiatry, 36*(6), 844–852.

Segool, N. K., & Carlson, J. S. (2008). Efficacy of cognitive-behavioral and pharmacological treatments for children with social anxiety. *Depression & Anxiety, 25*(7), 620–631.

Thomas, K. M., Drevets, W. C., Dahl, R. E., Ryan, N. D., Birmaher, B., Eccard, C. H., Axelson, D., Whalen, P. D., & Casey, B. J. (2001). Amygdala response to fearful faces in anxious and depressed children. *Archives of General Psychiatry, 58*, 1057–1063.

Towbin, K. (2007). Trichotillomania. In A. Martin & F. Volkmar (Eds.), *Lewis's Child and Adolescent Psychiatry: A Comprehensive Textbook*, 4th edition. Philadelphia: Lippincott Williams & Wilkins.

Towbin, K., & Riddle, M. (2007). Obsessive compulsive disorder. In A. Martin & F. Volkmar (Eds.), *Lewis's Child and Adolescent Psychiatry: A Comprehensive Textbook*, 4th edition. Philadelphia: Lippincott Williams & Wilkins.

Vasey, M. W., & MacLeod, C. (2001). Information-processing factors in childhood anxiety: A review and developmental perspective, pp. 253–277. In M. W. Vasey & M. R. Dadds (Eds.), *The Developmental Psychopathology of Anxiety*. London: Oxford University Press.

CHAPTER 13 ■ TIC DISORDERS

BACKGROUND

Tics are sudden, repetitive movements that typically are brief but occur in bouts. They may be quite mild or very severe. They can take the form of gestures or vocalizations. The can be very simple movements (e.g., eye blinking) or much more complex. They can include self-injurious behaviors or take the form of obscene movements (copropraxia). Vocal tics, when present, can range from barely audible throat clearing to the sometimes explosive expression of obscene words or phrases (coprolalia). Vocal tics can involve repetition of one's own words (palilalia) or the words of others (echolalia). The individual may be able to suppress the tics temporarily and may sense the tic before it happens—a "premonitory urge." The person may also have some sense of relief after the tic.

In addition to varying in severity, these disorders are often associated with other problems (e.g., in attention and overactivity). These conditions have traditionally been treated by both neurologists and psychiatrists; this reflects the somewhat unique way in which these conditions seem to be at the interface of "mind and body."

Tics have been observed for hundreds of years and were once viewed as examples of demonic possession. The modern study of tics began in France with the work of Itard and Gilles de la Tourette. It was Tourette who noted the co-occurrence of motor and vocal tics, the association with obsessive-compulsive features, and the strong genetic component to tics.

DEFINITIONS AND CLINICAL DESCRIPTIONS

Several types of tic disorder are presently recognized. The distinctions among these types have to do with the persistence of tics (chronic or transient) and whether vocal as well as motor tics are observed (both are seen in Tourette's disorder). A diagnosis of tic disorder is not made if the tics are caused by central nervous system disease (e.g., postviral encephalopathies) or psychoactive medication or substance use or abuse.

In transient tic disorder, one or more tics occur (off and on) for weeks to months. These tics are usually motor tics and typically are confined to the head, neck, and upper body. The onset typically is between ages 3 and 10 years, and the diagnosis is frequently missed or unrecognized. In some cases, tics go on to become chronic. Features of transient tic disorder are provided in Table 13.1.

In chronic vocal or motor tic disorder, the tics (either vocal or motor but not both) have lasted for at least 1 year without a long symptom-free period (arbitrarily set at 3 months).

Did Samuel Johnson Have Tourette's Disorder?

Dr. Samuel Johnson, the most famous writer in 18th century England and subject of one of the greatest biographies in the English language, may have had Tourette's disorder. His biographers have noted that throughout his life, Dr. Johnson exhibited various unusual movements and gestures as well as many verbal "eccentricities." Dr. Johnson had many different symptoms, including bouts of melancholy (depression) as well as some obsessions (e.g., with his feelings of guilt and lack of faithfulness). In his biography of Johnson Boswell noted his "convulsive cramps" and unusual gestures as well as his tendency to talk to himself. His contemporaries commented that his unusual gestures were so extraordinary that he attracted the attention of spectators who would come to watch him. Throughout his life, Dr. Johnson feared that he might become insane, but his contemporaries regarded his difficulties as reflecting some medical illness (e.g., such as a form of seizure disorder).

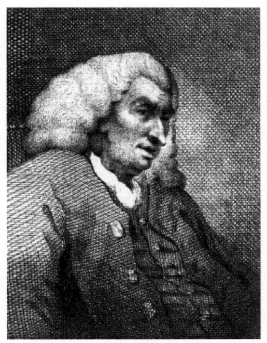

Samuel Johnson. (Courtesy of Yale British Art Center.)

The tics wax and wane over time and can be simple or more complex with a broad range of severity. Motor tics are more common than vocal tics and usually involve the head and upper body. As with other tic disorders, the tics can be voluntarily suppressed for period of time and are exacerbated by stress. The condition may persist into adulthood and become noticeable at times when the individual is fatigued or anxious. Table 13.1 reviews diagnostic features of chronic tic disorder.

TABLE 13.1

DIFFERENTIAL DIAGNOSTIC FEATURES: TIC DISORDERS[1]

	Transient Tic Disorder	Chronic Motor or Vocal Tic Disorder	Tourette's Disorder
Onset	<18 years	<18 years	<18 years
Tic frequency or duration	Many times a day >4 weeks <12 months	Many times a day >12 months not without tics >3 months	Many times a day >12 months not without tics >3 months
Tic forms	Motor, vocal, or both	Motor *or* vocal (not both)	Motor *and* vocal
Comorbid conditions			OCD and ADHD frequent

[1] By definition, the tics should not be caused by substance use or abuse (e.g., as a side effect of stimulants) or by a condition (e.g., Huntington's chorea or encephalitis).
ADHD, attention-deficit/hyperactivity disorder; OCD, obsessive-compulsive disorder.

If both motor and vocal tics are present, a diagnosis of Tourette's disorder is made. Tourette's disorder is the best known of the tic disorders. In Tourette's disorder, both vocal and motor tics must be present. Table 13.1 summaries distinctions among these various categories of tic disorders.

Of these conditions, Tourette's disorder is the best known and most frequently studied. It usually has its onset in childhood with simple motor tics, often involving the head or face (e.g., eye blinking or head jerks). Gradually, tics come to involve other regions of the body, often following a "rostral to caudal" progression (i.e., head to rest of body). As motor tics persist, they may have a negative impact on the child's functioning. Typically, vocal or phonic tics usually begin after the motor tics but then have a progression from more simple manifestations (throat clearing) to much more complex forms such as echolalia and coprolalia in a minority of cases. The severity of symptoms tends to a peak in middle childhood (Figure 13.1). As noted subsequently, various other disorders may coexist with Tourette's disorder and may, in some ways, pose even greater obstacles for treatment.

Transient tics are frequent in childhood but often are of brief duration. On the other hand, sometimes the onset of motor tics marks the onset of Tourette's disorder often between ages 5 and 7 years. In this condition, motor tics persist and generally progress down and away from the midline (e.g., head, neck, arms, and last and least frequently, the lower extremities). Phonic tics usually appear some time after motor tics (between ages 8 and 15 years) and are rare in isolation. Tic complexity changes with age, although most individuals with Tourette's disorder have a diagnosis in childhood. It is important to note that the severity of tics in Tourette's disorder waxes and wanes over time. Tics can be voluntarily suppressed for brief periods and are exacerbated by stress, fatigue, and lack of sleep. Tic episodes occur in bouts, which also often cluster. The pattern of tics is highly unique to the person. Most cases are diagnosed by 11 years of age. Often, as children with Tourette's disorder become older, they develop a sense that a tic is about to happen and may be able to exert some control over them, although this also serves as a source of anxiety and worry and can require much effort. The unusual behaviors are often very noticeable to others (as well as to the individual) and may pose significant problems. It is usual for attentional problems to be noted before the tics develop, but the obsessive-compulsive symptoms usually develop somewhat later, often around the same time the tics become most severe.

The severity of the tics waxes and wanes, and the tics themselves are highly variable. Tic episodes tend to happen in bouts, and these bouts themselves may cluster together. Individuals with tic disorders are very sensitive to stress, and a vicious cycle of tics leading to stress leading to more tics can be observed.

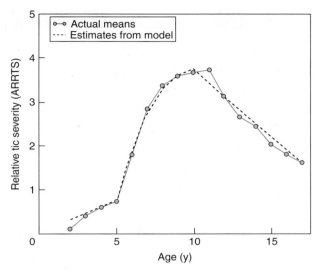

FIGURE 13.1. Plot of mean tic severity, ages 2 to 18 years. The *solid line* connecting the *small circles* plots the means of the annual rating of relative tic severity scores (ARRTS) recorded by the parents. The *dashed line* represents a mathematical model designed to best fit the clinical data. Two inflection points are evident that correspond to the age of tic onset and the age at worst-ever tic severity, respectively. (Adapted with permission from Leckman, J. F., Zhang, H., Vitale, A., et al. (1998) Course of tic severity in Tourette syndrome: the first two decades. *Pediatrics, 102*(1 Pt 1):14–19.)

EPIDEMIOLOGY AND DEMOGRAPHICS

Transient tic behaviors may be seen in 4% to 24% of school-age children. The prevalence of chronic motor tics is about 1%. Estimates of the frequency of Tourette's disorder (vocal and motor tics) vary considerably depending on the age group studied and definitions used; it appears that among older adolescents and adults, the rate is on the order of 4.5 per 10,000. This number is higher for younger children, many of whom improve over time or are not impaired by the condition. Boys are more commonly affected with tic behaviors than girls. Estimates of prevalence of Tourette's disorder vary dramatically between 10 to 100 per 10,000.

Case Report: Transient Tic Disorder

Marty was a 6½-year-old boy who had recently developed a facial tic. This occurred while he was away at summer camp, and several people and his camp counselor had commented on his unusual eye movements. His father and uncle had histories of tics. By the time Marty returned from camp, the movements had largely disappeared. His pediatrician sought consultation and was told that there was some chance the tics would return but also a good chance that these were transient in nature.

   Comment: Transient tics are very common in the population. In this case, the consultant is right to note, particularly given the history, that there is some chance that the tics would return.

Case Report: Chronic Motor Tic Disorder

Bob was a 15-year-old boy with a periodic tics since age 6 years. These included some unusual head movements and eye blinking and occasional upper body (shoulder) movements. He had recently started football, and his tics seemed to increase when he was anxious, although they were subtle at some points. He developed some compensatory strategies when they became more prominent but overall had made a good adjustment to them, although complaining, occasionally, when they were worse. He had never gone for more than 1 month without tics. He had never developed vocal tics.

Comment: The differentiation between chronic motor (or vocal) tic disorder and Tourette's disorder rests on the latter's including *both* vocal and motor tics. Some child begin with motor tics and then progress over time to have both vocal and motor tics. In such cases, a diagnosis of Tourette's disorder would be made. In this case, chronic motor tic disorder is the correct diagnosis, and a conservative approach (avoiding the potential side effects of medication) is warranted.

Tics may be only one part of a constellation of problems (e.g., obsessive-compulsive disorder [OCD] or attention-deficit/hyperactivity disorder [ADHD]). Indeed, 50% or more of referred children with Tourette's disorder are diagnosed with comorbid ADHD in clinical samples, although epidemiologic studies show a much lower rate (Fig. 13.2). At least more than 40% of individuals with Tourette's disorder experience recurrent symptoms of OCD. Patients with OCD and comorbid tics have higher rates of intrusive violent or aggressive thoughts and images, preoccupations, and compulsions. Tic disorders are several times more common in boys than in girls.

ETIOLOGY

Tic disorders have a strong genetic component. A child of a parent with Tourette's disorder has a 10% to 15% chance of having Tourette's disorder and a 20% to 30% chance of having tics. A higher risk has been shown in twin and family studies, similarly suggesting genetic factors. In monozygotic twin pairs, the concordance of Tourette's disorders is at least 50%; in dizygotic twin pairs, it is about 10%, If a broader definition of tic disorders is used, these values increase to 75% and 30%. Recently, a gene, *SLITRK1*, was identified as a candidate gene. Investigations into the effects of perinatal complications into the later development of

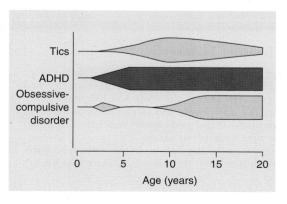

FIGURE 13.2. Age at which tics and coexisting disorders affect patients with Tourette's disorder. The width of the bars shows schematically the amount the disorder affects a patient at a particular age. (Adapted with permission from Leckman, J. F. (2002). Tourette's syndrome. *Lancet* 360(9345): 1577–1586.)

Tourette's disorder are complicated but suggest some potential role of such factors. Studies of the brain have focused on the basal ganglia and corticostriatal thalamocortical (CSTC) area. Tics are believed to arise from imbalances in focal populations of basal ganglia circuits such that microstimulation at numerous sites of the putamen produced ticlike stereotyped movements in awake monkeys.

Postmortem specimens in humans have also demonstrated abnormalities in basal ganglia development. Neuropharmacologic support for this idea comes from the effectiveness of dopamine-depleting agents and dopaminergic receptor antagonists in the suppression of tics and, on the other hand, by the exacerbation of tics caused by administration of dopamine agonists (L-DOPA) and stimulants. Neuroimaging studies also support the involvement of the basal ganglia (e.g., reductions in the size of the caudate nucleus are noted in affected vs. nonaffected twins, and caudate volume in childhood may be related to adult tic severity).

Group A β-hemolytic streptococci (GABHS) can trigger immune-mediated disease, and speculation concerning a postinfectious cause of tics dates from the late 1800s. One case-control study found an increased proportion of GABHS infections (odds ratio, 3.1) in children newly diagnosed with Tourette's disorder compared with control subjects. However, these cases likely represent at most a small subgroup of all pediatric Tourette's disorder and OCD cases.

DIFFERENTIAL DIAGNOSIS AND ASSESSMENT

In assessing a child with tics, it is important that the tics not overshadow other aspects of the child's life. The assessment should focus on strengths and weaknesses; the presence of comorbid medical conditions; and the impact of the condition on the family, academic performance, and peer relationships. For older individuals, there may be a long history of medication trials. Table 13.1 summarizes clinical features of patients with tics. Various rating scales are available and maybe useful in gaining a developmental perspective on the tics. Direct observation and videotape may be helpful in documenting tics. The medical history should pay careful attention to risk factors and movement disorders associated with other conditions.

Motor tics must be differentiated from a host of other movement difficulties, including tremor, chorea, athetosis, dystonias, and akathitic movements. Movement problems are observed in certain genetic disorders (e.g., Huntington's chorea) and after infection (e.g. Sydenham's chorea). Movement problems can arise as a result of drug side effects or may be noted in myoclonic seizures. Occasionally, stereotyped movements (e.g., as in individuals with autism or severe intellectual deficiency) may be confused with tics but usually are of earlier onset, are bilateral (not unilateral), and do not wax and wane; however, the diagnosis can sometimes be difficult. The presentation and history typically aid in the differential diagnosis. There are no specific laboratory tests. Several different rating scales useful in assessment are available (see Bloch & Leckman, 2007, for a review).

Various conditions may coexist with tic disorders (e.g., ADHD, OCD). Often, parents report attentional difficulties in the years before onset of tics. Diagnosis can be difficult given the difficulties in distinguishing the complex behaviors associated with Tourette's from other conditions. Around 40% of individuals with Tourette's disorder exhibit OCD symptoms. There is some suggestion of differences between OCD with and without a history of tics, with an earlier onset in Tourette's disorder–related OCD. Individuals with Tourette's disorder and OCD often have more has more violent or aggressive thoughts and images as well as concerns with symmetry and various rituals (counting) and touching or tapping compulsions. OCD observed in conjunction with tics appears less responsive to the selective serotonin reuptake inhibitor alone and may require augmentation with antipsychotic agents.

TREATMENT

The approach to treatment of patients with tic disorders should be comprehensive and flexible. The diagnosis may sometimes be clarified only over time (e.g., a child may initially present with simple motor tics and only some time later develop vocal tics of Tourette's disorder).

Initially, education and supportive treatment are used with drug treatments held in reserve because the severity of the condition varies among individuals and within the same individual over time. In some cases, tics are barely noticeable; in others, they are extremely disruptive. Tics may be transient, and even when chronic tics are present, they may not necessarily require specific intervention. On the other hand, as tics become more severe and disabling and when they are associated with other conditions, they may require more intensive treatment. Supportive treatment involves education of the individual and family as well as teachers. The child's self-esteem can be fostered by an understanding and supportive school environment with appropriate accommodations made for any needs for support (e.g., situations where the child is anxious will make tics more likely, and an alternative might be found for oral presentations). Helping the child and peers understand the problem is important. Many educational recommendations can be made that will be helpful.

Habit reversal training has been used to reduce tic severity with some success. This method involves helping the individual become more aware of the tics and then practicing competing responses.

Drug treatments are usually not the first line of intervention, and even when medications are used, the comorbid conditions (ADHD, OCD) may be the first targets of treatment. Various medications are now available, and the choice of medication should include consideration of the expected benefits and potential side effects. The most consistently effective medications include the dopamine D_2 receptor antagonists, which were first noted in the 1960s to suppress tics. Several drugs in this group have been evaluated in double-blind clinical trials, including haloperidol, pimozide, and tiapride, and the U.S. Food and Drug Administration has approved Tourette's disorder as an indication for the use of both haloperidol and pimozide. Typically, treatment is started at a low dose (0.25 mg of haloperidol or 1 mg of pimozide) at bedtime with gradual increases (0.5 mg of haloperidol or 1 mg of pimozide) every 1 to 2 weeks depending on clinical response. Potential side effects include dystonic reactions, sedation, depression, school and social phobia, and tardive dyskinesia. By starting with a low dose and gradually increasing it, the clinician may be able to minimize these problems. It is important to realize that the goal is not to totally eliminate the tics but to make them less troublesome to the individual. The atypical neuroleptics hold promise given their better side effect profile and a few double-blind clinical trials have now been conducted for several of these agents. Although avoiding some of the difficulties of the first-generation agents, these atypical neuroleptics may be associated with weight gain or sedation (e.g., with risperidone and olanzapine) or with QT prolongation (with ziprasidone).

Another pharmacologic approach has used the potent α_2-receptor agonists clonidine and guanfacine, which are presumed to decrease central noradrenergic activity. Initial, open-label studies were more favorable than subsequent double-blind studies. There can be a significant reduction in symptoms, particularly motor tics. This effect appears over some weeks. The usual starting dose is 0.05 mg in the morning followed by a gradual increase (in 0.05-mg increments) every 3 to 4 hours on a weekly basis up to a total dose of about 5 μg per kg or if the total dose for the day exceeds 0.25 mg. Although less effective than the neuroleptics, these agents are often better tolerated. The most frequent side effect, sedation, is observed in 10% to 20% of cases but often abates with continued use. Other potential side effects include hypotension. It is important for parents to realize that clonidine should be tapered rather than stopped abruptly because there may be a blood pressure rebound. Guanfacine has been used particularly in individuals with Tourette's disorder and comorbid ADHD and is generally less sedating than clonidine. As with clonidine, it is typical to begin guanfacine with a starting dose of 0.5 mg at night and then gradually increase it by 0.5 mg each week using thrice-daily dosing up to a daily maximum of about 4 mg.

Drug treatments for individuals with comorbid conditions present special consideration. The use of stimulants for attentional problems in children with tic disorders remains a source of controversy. Some children do well with stimulants, but other children with attentional problems appear to develop tics for the first time after stimulant administration or stimulants may exacerbate tics. As noted previously, the α_2-agonists may be used as can be the antidepressants nortriptyline and atomoxetine and bupropion. For individuals with tic disorders and OCD, cognitive behavioral therapies can be used alone or in combination with serotonin

Case Report: Tourette's Disorder

Jimmy, a 10-year-old boy, was referred for evaluation of multiple problems. Starting at age 6 years, he had attentional difficulties (noted in school) that seemed initially to respond well to stimulant medications. By the time he was in second grade, he had developed an unusual eye blinking movement and, over time, other motor tics as well. Starting a few months ago, he began to exhibit an odd "coughing" movement, which was eventually diagnosed as a tic. Both his motor and vocal tics varied over time. They disappeared while he was asleep and could be voluntarily suppressed for short periods. He became somewhat rigid and compulsive. His popularity at school suffered considerable with the onset of the vocal tics, and peers frequently made fun of him. A reward system was instituted at school to attempt to control the tics but did not meet with success. Jimmy was treated with a low dose of haloperidol, and the tics diminished markedly. He became somewhat sedated on the haloperidol, and several adjustments were made to balance the benefit of the medication on this tics and the sedative effect.

Comment: In Tourette's disorder, both vocal and motor tics must be present. It is common for attentional difficulties to precede the tics. Learning difficulties and obsessive-compulsive phenomena are also common. Waxing and waning of the tics is characteristic as is the ability to voluntary suppress the tics for short periods. Medications can be helpful in controlling the tics, but side effects can be problematic.

reuptake inhibitors (SRIs), although as a group, these individuals response less well than do patients with OCD without tics. Occasionally, small doses of haloperidol or risperidone may be added to augment the SRI's effect.

Other approaches to treatment include botulinum toxin injections to temporarily weaken muscle groups involved in tics; such injections may also reduce the individual's awareness ("premonitory urge") associated with the tic. Rarely, neurosurgical interventions are used when tics are severe or life threatening.

COURSE AND PROGNOSIS

The course of tic disorders is quite variable. Transient tics are, of course, by definition just that. As noted previously, the tics in Tourette's disorder follow a developmental progression. The intensity and frequency of tics in affected individuals parallels this progression. In general, it appears that the tics of Tourette's disorder reach their peak in early adolescence (ages 10 to 15 years) and tend to decrease after that time to a lower level where tics come and go over time. Some individuals—more than half—with Tourette's disorder become largely asymptomatic in adulthood with some becoming symptom free. In other cases, the tics typically persist but are reduced in both frequency and intensity. Occasionally, tics become much worse in adulthood.

The associated behavioral and emotional problems of these disorders are also important in determining outcome. By late adolescence, many individuals regard comorbid OCD, ADHD, and other behavioral or learning difficulties as more problematic than the tics. Probably 50% of children with Tourette's disorder also exhibit ADHD in clinical settings (the rate is lower in epidemiologically based samples). Having both conditions presents more of a challenge for the child, family, and clinicians. These children are particularly likely to have peer problems and social difficulties and are at increased risk for other disorders (e.g., mood and anxiety problems) later in life. There is also an increased risk for conduct problems. ADHD appears to be a powerful mediator because children with Tourette's disorder but without ADHD do substantially better even if their tics are more severe.

The symptoms of Tourette's disorder are sometimes difficult to distinguish from those of OCD and, as already noted, the two conditions may coexist. In many cases, adults with Tourette's disorder experience moderate levels of symptoms of OCD. If OCD symptoms are present in children with Tourette's disorder, they tend to persist into adulthood even more so than the tics themselves. The presence of associated attentional difficulties or learning problems may also impact outcome. Similarly, stressful and nonsupportive social environments and exposure to certain illicit drugs (e.g., cocaine) are associated with a worse prognosis.

SUMMARY

The recent identification of a gene associated with Tourette's disorder provides important opportunities for research. Similarly, the advent of nonpharmacologic treatment is an important area for future work. Studies using deep brain stimulation have been undertaken for the most refractory adult patients with Tourette's disorder. It is hoped that with the elaboration of genetic mechanisms and animal models, treatment will improve and we will gain an understanding of the neural basis of this and related disorders.

Selected Readings

Abelson, J. F., Kwan, K. Y., O'Roak, B. J., et al. (2005). Sequence variants in SLITRK1 are associated with Tourette's syndrome. *Science, 310*(5746), 317–320.

Ackermans, L., Temel, Y., Cath, D., et al. (2006). Deep brain stimulation in Tourette's syndrome: Two targets? *Movement Disorder, 21*(5),709–713.

Bawden, H. N., Stokes, A., Camfield, C. S., Camfield, P. R., & Salisbury, S. (1998). Peer relationship problems in children with Tourette's disorder or diabetes mellitus. *Journal of Child Psychology and Psychiatry, 39*(5), 663–668.

Bloch, M. H. (2008). Emerging treatments for Tourette's disorder. *Current Psychiatry Reports, 10*(4), 323–330.

Bloch, M. H., & Leckman, J. F. (2007). Tic disorders. In A. Martin & F. Volkmar (Eds.), *Lewis's Child and Adolescent Psychiatry: A Comprehensive Textbook*, 4th edition, pp. 569–583. Philadelphia: Lippincott Williams & Wilkins.

Bloch, M. H., Peterson, B. S., Scahill, L., et al. (2006). Adulthood outcome of tic and obsessive-compulsive symptom severity in children with Tourette syndrome. *Archives of Pediatrics & Adolescent Medicine, 160*(1), 65–69.

Leckman, J. F., King, R. A., Scahill, L., Findley, D., Ort, S., & Cohen, D. J. (1998). Yale approach to assessment and treatment. In J. F. Leckman & D. J. Cohen (Eds.), *Tourette's Syndrome Tics, Obsessions, Compulsions: Developmental Psychopathology and Clinical Care*, pp. 285–309. New York: John Wiley and Sons.

Mell, L. K., Davis, R. L., & Owens, D. (2005). Association between streptococcal infection and obsessive-compulsive disorder, Tourette's syndrome, and tic disorder. *Pediatrics, 116*(1), 56–60.

Pauls, D. L., & Leckman, J. F. (1986). The inheritance of Gilles de la Tourette's syndrome and associated behaviors: Evidence for autosomal dominant transmission. *New England Journal of Medicine, 315*(16), 993–997.

Piacentini, J. C., & Chang, S. W. (2006). Behavioral treatments for tic suppression: Habit reversal training. *Advanced Neurology, 99*, 227–233.

Sacks, O. (1995). A surgeon's life. In *An Anthropologist on Mars: Seven Paradoxical Tales*, pp. 77–107. New York: Random House.

Swain, J. E., Scahill, L., Lombroso, P., King, R., & Leckman, J. (2007). Tourette syndrome and tic disorders: A decade of progress. *Journal of American Academy of Child Adolescent Psychiatry, 46*(8), 947–968.

CHAPTER 14 ■ EATING AND FEEDING DISORDERS

Issues with eating and growth can arise throughout life, although given the rapid pace of development, they are often particularly important when they occur in children and adolescents. In many ways, these conditions are unique because they exist at the boundaries of psychiatry and general medicine. Anorexia nervosa and bulimia nervosa are probably the most well known of these disorders, but the *Diagnostic and Statistical Manual of Mental Disorders* (DSM-IV-TR) also includes three conditions that arise in early childhood: pica, rumination, and feeding disorder of infancy or early childhood. As Woolston and Hasbani (2007) have noted, this is an area of tremendous complexity. Other conditions such as obesity have very strong behavioral or psychiatric components but are recognized as medical rather than psychiatric conditions. Although the DSM-IV-TR strives for diagnostic purity in distinguishing among conditions related, or not, to general medical conditions, in reality, various medical conditions can present with difficulties in growth or eating (e.g., gastroesophageal reflux). Disentangling "medical" from "psychiatric" conditions in an arbitrary way can be problematic. Further issues arise given the highly social nature of early eating and feeding experiences as well as the potential for important cultural contributions to beliefs and practices. The tendency to use rigid dichotomies and overreductionism has resulted in simplistic formulations that underestimate the complexity of clinical situations (Woolston and Hasbani, 2007).

Advances in understanding mechanisms of hunger and satiety have furthered work in this area. The identification of the *ob* gene and leptin, its protein product, has helped clarify regulation of mechanisms that regulate both metabolic rate and food intake. An awareness of the entire range of eating issues, including problems with overeating and obesity, has also enriched work in the area.

PICA

Definition and Clinical Description

Pica is defined as the persistent eating of non-nutritive substances for at least 1 month. The word *pica* is derived from the Latin word for magpie, a bird once thought to eat anything.

TABLE 14.1

CLINICAL FEATURES OF PICA, RUMINATION, AND FEEDING DISORDER

	Pica	Rumination Disorder	Feeding Disorder
Essential clinical features	Persistent ingestion of substances without nutritive value (not culturally sanctioned)	Repeated regurgitation or rechewing of food (not because of reflux)	Failure to eat and significant weight loss or failure to gain (not caused by a general medical problem)
Frequency or duration	At least 1 month	At least 1 month (after some period of normal functioning)	At least 1 month
Developmental issues	Not developmentally appropriate	Not developmentally appropriate	Onset before 6 years of age
Risk factors	Poverty, psychosocial adversity, intellectual deficiency	Intellectual deficiency, lack of stimulation	Poverty, psychosocial adversity, oral-motor issues
Complications	Lead exposure, parasites, vitamin or mineral deficiency	Aspiration, nutritional issues, dental problems	Malnutrition (note importance of search for potential medical factors such as cystic fibrosis)

The behavior must be inappropriate to the child's developmental level (i.e., young infants tend to put almost anything into their mouths). In addition, the behavior must not be a part of a cultural practice (e.g., in some cultures, young women may eat clay or other non-nutritive substances). In reality, pica is a condition found in very different populations including toddlers ingesting lead in paint chips, developmentally disabled young adults who eat clothing, and even typically developing adults who eat unusual substances (tissues, pencil erasers).

In many respects, the most well-known example of pica is the eating of paint chips and lead poisoning. This behavior may be more common in less stimulating environments or with parental difficulties, both often co-occurring with poverty. In toddlers, it is typical for pica to begin from ages 1 to 3; the behavior may persist well into childhood, although it is frequently time limited. In persons with intellectual disability, the behavior may appear somewhat later but then may not diminish until middle age; in this population, a greater degree of cognitive impairment is more frequently associated with pica.

Substances ingested may include chalk, dirt, paper, soap, feces, and so forth. Some authorities also classify excessive eating of things that might, in small quantities, be thought of as food (e.g., starch, ice, flour, salt). Various terms for the different forms of pica exist, including *coprophagia* (consumption of feces) and *geophagy* (consumption of soil, clay, or chalk). Differential features of pica and other feeding disorders more frequent in young children are provided in Table 14.1.

Epidemiology and Demographics

Pica behavior is relatively common, occurring in as many as one-third of young children and from 10% to 25% of institutionalized adults with intellectual deficiency. The risk in intellectual deficiency increases in parallel with severity of the IQ deficit.

Etiology

Intellectual disability is a risk factor for pica. There has been some speculation that iron deficiency may be associated with it, although this has not been clearly established (this connection is more firmly established in animals). Pica can be increased by various factors, including stress and anxiety, mood problems, and lack of stimulation.

Differential Diagnosis and Assessment

Various medical problems can be associated with pica. As noted previously, lead exposure is a concern for infants and younger children. Other medical complications may include vitamin or mineral deficiency as well as ingestion of parasites. For some individuals, ingestion of nonfood substances can result in intestinal obstruction and require surgical correction. In some cases, cultural beliefs may be central. Thoughtful medical assessment is needed (e.g., to look for mineral deficiencies, anemia, and so forth).

Treatment

Infants and toddlers who are understimulated or poorly supervised may respond well to greater attention and careful monitoring. The environment should be carefully examined to address possible hazards. For individuals with intellectual disability, attention to the antecedents and contexts of the behavior may be helpful. Some intellectual disability syndromes (e.g., Prader-Wili Syndrome; see Chapter 5) can be associated with overeating. Most of the treatments used have been behavioral in nature, although some studies have used antidepressants in the treatment of patients with pica. Nutritional counseling can be helpful for older individuals and those with higher cognitive abilities.

Course and Prognosis

The course of the disorder depends on the context. For individuals with intellectual disability, the behavior may diminish over time, particularly if an appropriate behavioral program is put into place and an appropriately stimulating environment is provided. In infants and toddlers with pica, the disorder is often very time limited.

RUMINATION DISORDER

Definition and Clinical Description

Rumination disorder is defined in the DSM-IV-TR on the basis of repeated regurgitation and rechewing of food that occurs for a period of at least 1 month after some period of normal functioning. By definition, this cannot be attributable to an associated gastrointestinal (GI) or some other general medical condition. As with pica, rumination is seen in several rather different contexts. It can be observed in otherwise typically developing infants and very young children. It can also be observed in persons with intellectual deficiency, particularly more severe intellectual deficiency.

Epidemiology and Demographics

Information on clinical features is mostly derived from single case reports or small case series; thus, the available data are limited in important respects. The condition appears to be relatively rare. The issue of whether there is a gender predominance remains controversial. In infants

Case Report: Rumination Disorder

Steve was seen for evaluation at 7 months of age by his pediatrician because his grandmother was concerned that he was not eating well. Steven had been born to his 16-year-old mother after an unexpected pregnancy. Labor and delivery were unremarkable, and his maternal grandmother assumed care on a day-to-day basis but worked much of the time, and a series of relatives provided much of his care. One month previously, he had been regurgitating food after feeding. At first, this was occasional but now routine. He continued to gain weight, but his grandmother was concerned about the regurgitation. On examination, he was alert but somewhat apathetic and less interested in people and the environment than would be typical. Observation of him after a feeding did demonstrate regurgitation and rechewing of his food. Consultation with a behavioral psychologist recommended several steps to interrupt the regurgitation. In addition, arrangements were made for placement in a stable family day care setting. Both interventions resulted in relatively prompt resolution of the symptoms.

who are apparently typically developing, the onset is usually before age 1 year. In individuals with intellectual deficiency, the onset can be much later, including in adulthood. Rumination may be seen in association with other eating or feeding problems.

Etiology

Several different mechanisms appear to be involved in the process of rumination (Woolston, 2007). To further complicate issues of diagnosis the presumption, in DSM-IV-TR, is that there be no underlying GI disease, although the boundaries and potential connections of gastroesophageal reflux (GER), rumination and operant vomiting have yet to be clarified. Several models have emerged from behavioral psychology that might account for rumination. There is some suggestion that rumination is more common in infants who experience an environment that is not appropriately stimulating.

Differential Diagnosis and Assessment

As noted, the clinician should be alert to various factors (medical and psychosocial) that might contribute to rumination. The medical evaluation should include evaluation for possible GER and other gastroenterologic disorders.

Treatment

Various behavioral techniques have been used, with varying degrees of success, to treat rumination. These include both aversive and non-aversive techniques. High rates of success have been reported in at least some studies.

Course and Prognosis

The course of rumination disorder is highly variable. In some instances, the problem resolves fairly quickly. In other cases, medical complications (e.g., from aspiration or nutritional problems) may assume major significance. Dental problems are common in individuals with chronic rumination.

FEEDING DISORDER OF INFANCY OR EARLY CHILDHOOD

Definition and Clinical Description

As a diagnostic concept, feeding disorder of infancy has its origins in work on failure to thrive (FTT) in infancy, a condition marked by decreased rate of weight gain and associated developmental problems (decelerated weight gain rather than head or linear growth changes was traditionally the major defining feature). The DSM-IV-TR diagnostic concept has the advantages and disadvantages associated with any novel diagnosis. On the one hand, 5 decades of work on FTT had resulted in a large but confused literature. On the other hand, the applicability of some aspects of this literature is put into question. Over the decades, a number of different terms had been used to refer to this concept. In addition to *FTT*, similar terms included *psychosocial deprivation dwarfism*, *maternal deprivation syndrome*, *analytic depression*, *hospitalism*, and *organic* and *non-organic FTT*. The various terms were used, often interchangeably, even though they were not precisely synonymous. They variably emphasize one or more of the features associated with feeding difficulties in infants. Some have the advantage or disadvantage of essentially specifying an etiology. Differences in definition can, not surprisingly, have major implications for research, so, for example, if a diagnosis of FTT is made based solely on decelerated weight gain, it is rather less frequent to find associated developmental difficulties in the child. Similarly, the various terms used reflect a continued debate of the relative contribution of social-emotional factors (e.g., maternal deprivations) on the one hand and malnutrition on the other. There are several potential difficulties with the definition used in the DSM-IV-TR. Clinical judgment is used to decide if failure to gain weight is significant, exclusionary rules are simplistic, and there are probably at least two subtypes or disorders (an early onset and later onset form that appear to differ in important ways). Some authorities (e.g., Chatoor et al, 1998a, 1998b) have suggested that three distinctive feeding disorders may well exist.

Although the DSM-IV-TR specifies that the onset must be before 6 years of age, the condition usually has its onset in the first years of life. In early-onset cases, attention to problems in caloric intake (or medical conditions accounting for slower growth) may result in rapid weight gain. When psychosocial problems are major components of the clinical picture, relapse can occur if these problems are not addressed. Later onset is much more likely to be associated with more obvious interactional difficulties.

Epidemiology and Demographics

Pediatric hospital admissions for FTT have been noted to account for 1% to 3% percent of all admissions (Woolston, 2007). Although most studies report equal sex ratios, there may be male predominance in later-onset cases. Risk factors include psychosocial adversity, parental psychopathology, and social isolation of the family. Some feeding problems clearly occur in the context of supportive families without obvious risk. In these cases, problems in the child or in the "fit" of the child and parents likely contribute.

Etiology

Feeding disorder of infancy and early childhood clearly has both physical and behavioral and developmental components. Although inadequate caloric intake is a primary cause of slower than expected growth, other factors (e.g., poverty) may also be associated with developmental delays, and difficulties in the child can contribute to feeding problems in the parent–child dyad.

Differential Diagnosis and Assessment

Medical evaluations should be guided by the clinical examination and history, although the yield from extensive laboratory and clinical studies is relatively low. Although the current DSM-IV-TR criteria "rule out" medical causes of feeding disorder, the reality is complex because various medical issues can contribute to feeding problems and malnutrition. In the past, efforts were made to distinguish between "organic" and "non-organic" FTT, but this distinction proved somewhat arbitrary and cumbersome. Initial laboratory studies usually include a complete blood count and urinalysis as well as lead level and testing for cystic fibrosis. Premature infants may appear to have poor growth if gestational age is not considered; correction should be made for weight until 2 years of age. Children who are premature or small for gestational age can develop feeding problems, and such infants often already have significant clinical risk factors (e.g., maternal substance abuse, psychosocial adversity) and may have difficulties nursing. Observation of the infant in the act of nursing may help demonstrate difficulties with sucking (see Woolston and Hasbani, 2007).

Treatment

Intervention should begin with being sure that the child has adequate caloric intake. Hospitalization may be indicated with, potentially, referral to child protective services if it appears to be warranted. In younger infants, provision of adequate calories may be associated with prompt weight gain. For older infants and toddlers in whom eating or feeding problems have become more psychologically complex, symptoms remediation may be more challenging. Clinical management should include careful consideration of the degree of malnutrition (e.g., based on ideal body weight, body mass index [BMI], and so forth). Sixty percent of ideal body weight has been suggested as an indicator of severe malnutrition (see Woolston and Hasbani, 2007). Associated physical findings such as low pulse rate or blood pressure can be seen in more severe malnutrition.

For infants who have not been given sufficient nourishment, provision of such nourishment typically results in prompt weight gain and growth. In these cases, the prognosis is good as long as the factors that contributed to the initial difficulty can be addressed. For infants in whom feeding is difficult, some improvement may occur as developmental levels increase. Consultation with speech pathologists and occupational therapists as well as nutritional specialists may be needed around oral-motor issues.

Course and Prognosis

The DSM-IV-TR feeding disorder concept is relatively new. The older literature on FTT suggests a highly variable outcome. Family functioning, psychosocial adversity, parental psychopathology, and parental education are all potential mediating variables. The prognosis is generally worse in the presence of chronic developmental delay and malnutrition.

Factors that impact outcome include age of onset, duration, degree of malnutrition and of growth problems, associated problems in the child (e.g., medical conditions, developmental delays), and risk factors in the parents and family. With infants younger than 1 year of age, absent associated medical conditions, the child either has not been given sufficient caloric intake or has such significant difficulties with feeding that the act of feeding becomes tremendously difficult. Infants are at higher risk for physical abuse and neglect.

Height and head circumference also provide some suggestion of the degree and chronicity of associated malnutrition and can be important prognostic indicators. With provision of treatment, developmental functioning can improve over time.

ANOREXIA NERVOSA AND BULIMIA NERVOSA

It is likely that the first reports of anorexia nervosa are found in the lives of saints, (e.g., many of whom were concerned with weight, purging, and self-starvation; Bell, 1985). By the 19th century, cases were regularly reported. Distinctions between anorexia nervosa and bulimia nervosa began to be made in the late 1970s.

TABLE 14.2

CLINICAL FEATURES OF ANOREXIA NERVOSA AND BULIMIA NERVOSA

Essential Clinical Features	Anorexia Nervosa	Bulimia Nervosa
	Body weight not maintained (weight lost or failure to gain) Fear of being obese Body image distortion or misperception	Binge eating (large amount of food ingested over short period of time; sense of loss of control) Other behaviors designed to prevent weight gain (e.g., exercise, laxatives use) and over preoccupation with body or weight)
Duration	In menstruating women, absence of at least 3 periods	Binges several times a week for several months
Subtypes	Restricting Binge-purging	Purging Nonpurging

Definitions and Clinical Descriptions

Anorexia nervosa and bulimia nervosa are the two most well-known eating disorders, typically with an onset after puberty, although sometimes before. Clinical features for anorexia nervosa and bulimia nervosa are provided in Table 14.2. The four defining features include refusal to maintain body weight at a "minimally normal" weight (for age and height) or failure to make expected weight gain (e.g., during the developmental period); an intense fear of becoming fat; disturbance in body image; and, if applicable, amenorrhea for at least 3 cycles. A distinction is made between two subtypes. In the restricting subtype, the person restricts food or caloric intake but does not binge or purge; in the binge-eating or purging subtype, either of the two behaviors is present.

There can be some difficulties in application of the DSM-IV-TR criteria to children and adolescents. Even when pediatric weight charts are used, there can be disagreements about what the "normal" weight of an adolescent should be. The BMI has the advantage of taking weight and height into account. and typically a BMI below 17.5 is taken as underweight (conversely, a score 25 and 30 typically defines overweight, and a BMI over 30 defines obesity). Sometimes the DSM-IV-TR criterion of intense fear of weight gain is striking, although some patients deny it (even when engaging in behavior consistent with it).

The distortion of body image criterion is often expressed in complicated ways (e.g., the individual may have a preoccupation with a particularly body part). The body image problem also is associated with dysphoric feelings or fears (e.g., of being out of control). In adolescents, menarche may be delayed. Differences in presentation and comorbidities are associated with the two subtypes. Those who engage in binge eating and purging often have associated problems with one or more impulsive behavior problems (e.g., substance abuse, suicide attempts, promiscuity). This group has a higher rate of premorbid obesity, personality problems, and various medical complications Self-mutilation may be noted in this group as well.

The clinical presentation of anorexia nervosa typically includes marked denial of the nature of the problem and intense resistance to treatment. Both present challenges for assessment and intervention. Although patients may deny intense preoccupations with weight or weight gain and body image, their behavior may convey the intensity of their preoccupation. Often, concerns with food and worries about obesity are dramatic. The individual may be so preoccupied with food that eating a meal takes an inordinately long time (e.g., the food may have to be presented or consumed in a very specific way). There may be intense preoccupation with appearance (e.g., with constant checking in the mirror). There may be associated obsessive-compulsive symptomatology (e.g., preoccupation with cleanliness).

For bulimia nervosa, several features must be present (see Table 14.2). These include recurrent binge eating (although the issue of how much binge eating must be present is left to the clinician's judgment). Patients do characteristically report a sense of being out of control. Recurrent behaviors designed to avoid weight gain are present, typically self-induced vomiting but potentially misuse of laxatives, diuretics, or even excessive exercise may qualify. As specified in the DSM-IV-TR, a minimal frequency of binge eating and compensatory behaviors must be present (at least twice a week for at least 3 months). As in anorexia nervosa, the patient is overly preoccupied with weight and body shape. By definition, in the DSM-IV-TR, the condition does not occur only during episodes of anorexia nervosa; a distinction is also made between purging and nonpurging subtypes. In the latter, self-induced vomiting or (e.g., laxatives) are not used. The latter group of patients appear to have a lesser degree of body image problems (see Halmi, 2007).

Typically, patients with bulimia nervosa are not below 15% of normal weight and can actually be overweight. Patients with binge-purge anorexia nervosa are more likely to be below the 15th percentile. Binge eating is often associated with a sense of loss of control. Episodes of binge eating may be terminated by abdominal discomfort or self-induced vomiting; termination of the episode is often associated with feelings of depression and disgust. There may be a marked fear of not being able to stop eating, which can lead to fasting followed by profound hunger and loss of control. Typically, high-calorie foods are consumed during a binge. In contrast to anorexia nervosa, severe weight loss may not be present in bulimic patients who, in a minority of cases, have previous anorexia nervosa. Depression is a frequent comorbid condition as are anxiety disorders and high levels of compulsive behavior. Substance abuse is frequent (e.g., with use of appetite suppressing drugs such as amphetamines). In both disorders, dental problems are frequent. Some of the other medical complications associated with binging and purging include cardiomyopathy, renal failure, seizures, metabolic alkalosis with hypokalemia, and cardiac arrhythmia, among others (see Halmi, 2005).

The DSM-IV-TR also provides for eating disorder "not otherwise specified" for individuals who fail, for various reasons, to meet the inclusion criteria for anorexia nervosa or bulimia nervosa (e.g., binge eating can occur in the absence of other features of bulimia nervosa or some patients may have some features of anorexia nervosa or bulimia nervosa but manage to maintain normal body weight).

Case Report: Anorexia Nervosa

Linda, a 16-year-old high school sophomore, was evaluated at the insistence of her parents, who were concerned about her high levels of exercise and weight loss. Although 5 feet 6 inches tall her greatest weight, of 105 lb, had been achieved 1 year ago. At that time, a friend had commented unfavorably on her weight, and Linda began a program of diet and exercise. Over the next 6 months, she lost 25 lb through vigorous exercise. She became obsessed with food, spending much time planning elaborate meals, which she barely ate. She became more irritable, and her grades began to suffer. Even with her weight loss, she remained unsatisfied with her appearance and believed she needed to lose more weight. She had stopped having her period several months previously.

A multimodal treatment program was begun that included education and cognitive behavior therapy as well as treatment with a selective serotonin reuptake inhibitor and program designed to help her achieve a reasonable weight. Although her initial course was rocky, she was able to achieve what she, her family, and her therapists agreed was a reasonable goal weight.

Epidemiology and Demographics

Although epidemiologic data are somewhat limited (Halmi, 2007), it does appear that rates have increased over the past 50 years. Rates vary, but probably about one in 5000 has anorexia nervosa and perhaps one in 10,000 has bulimia nervosa. Females are much more likely to have the disorder than males; generally, they outnumber them between 10 and 20 to one. The onset is typically in young adulthood, although adolescent onset is not uncommon. Most individuals develop the condition between ages 13 and 20 years of age.

Etiology

Various factors appear to be involved etiologically. These range from societal to familial to individual ones. Weight loss may initially be perceived very positively by peers or even parents. Psychologically, issues of control and relief of anxiety are frequently observed.

Social and cultural issues can be prominent. Anorexia and bulimia nervosa are generally "Western" disorders (e.g., they are rare in poorly industrialized countries, and in countries such as Japan they have increased markedly with industrialization). Studies of immigrants from less developed countries who move to more developed ones generally show increased rates of these disorders.

Some ethnic differences have also been noted, although they may predominately reflect socioeconomic status issues. Some authors have focused on the overvaluation of cultural ideals of beauty in relation to self-esteem. Peer influences are also important. Western media also tends to value certain stereotyped views of women and thinness, underscoring the importance of sociocultural factors.

In some cases, stressful life events may play an important role. Precipitants for eating problems include menarche, moving from the family home to college, or developing new relationships. Several studies have noted increased rates of anorexia nervosa and bulimia nervosa in first-degree relatives of anorexia nervosa and bulimia nervosa patients. Twin studies similarly have suggested a potential genetic contribution. Neuroendocrine changes appear to directly relate to decreased caloric intake and weight loss and return to normal levels after usual eating is resumed. The role of the neurotransmitter serotonin has been examined, although results are contradictory. Another line of work has centered on abnormalities in the dopaminergic system in relations to abnormal pleasure–reward responses to food.

Although complicated to interpret, studies of psychological functioning suggest high levels of perfectionism and obsessive-compulsive features. Family factors have also been studied, although the degree to which they contribute to the condition remains the topic of much debate.

Differential Diagnosis and Assessment

In assessing a patient with an eating disorder, it is important to search for medical conditions that might result in weight loss. In addition to the weight loss requirement, other features of anorexia nervosa should be present if that diagnosis is made. Weight loss can be seen in other psychiatric disorders, and there is some potential for confusion if an agitated depression is present. Usually, however, the characteristic features of anorexia nervosa will alert the clinician to the correct diagnosis (e.g., preoccupations with food, exercise, bodily appearance). Occasionally, delusions regarding food are seen in schizophrenia, although other features of that disorder should also be present.

In anorexia nervosa, physiological differences emerge in relation to the degree of malnutrition or as a function of purging. For patients who induce vomiting or who abuse laxatives and diuretics, there may be development of a hypokalemic alkalosis associated with weakness, lethargy, and cardiac arrhythmia. There can be sudden death in patients, particularly those

Case Report: Bulimia Nervosa

Nancy, an 18-year-old senior in high school, was referred for evaluation by her parents because of binge eating. She had begun to binge periodically in her junior year, often when she was anxious and studying for her classes. She had been urged by her parents to take a challenging course load in hopes of getting her into the most advanced advanced placement classes this year. The binges included a range of what she called "junk food" (typically, she consumed high-calorie foods). At these times, she described herself as having lost control over eating, and she would feel disgusted with herself afterward. As her weight started to increase, she began to self-induce vomiting and used laxatives in an attempt to keep her weight down. At the time of this referral, she was not overweight, although her recurrent vomiting had begun to cause some dental problems. The parents had been largely unaware of these behaviors until the dentist spoke with them about his concern. At the time of referral, Nancy reported that she was typically vomiting several times a week and had been doing so for most of the past year. On examination, Nancy was noted to be depressed and somewhat anxious. Intervention included a number of different components, including work with the family, individual work with Nancy, careful monitoring of her eating, and an explicit focus on the link between anxiety and depression and her eating.

who purge. Liver enzymes may be elevated both in the anorectic phase and during refeeding. Frequent laboratory findings observed in anorexia nervosa are listed in Table 14.3, and findings associated with binging and purging behavior are provided Table 14.4.

Treatment

Several excellent guidelines to treatment now exist (see Halmi, 2007, for a review). In general, outpatient treatment is preferred, although not always possible. Inpatient treatment is typically reserved for the most concerning cases and should be conducted by individuals experienced in the care of patients with eating disorders. The focus should include the family as well as the patient.

Treatments of anorexia nervosa and bulimia nervosa share some similarities and differences. For anorexia nervosa, relatively few well-controlled treatment studies with random assignment are available. Typically, treatment includes multiple components, including patient education, medical management, and individual psychotherapy using behavioral as well as cognitive behavioral principles. Outpatient treatment is most successful if begun early in the course of the illness and if patients do not have vomiting and binging and have a supportive family who participate in the treatment program.

Pharmacologic interventions are sometimes used, although well-controlled studies of these interventions are sparse. Chlorpromazine has been frequently used in Europe, particularly if the patient is highly preoccupied; treatment is typically started at low doses and gradually increased (see Halmi, 2007). Other medications evaluated have included olanzapine and cyproheptadine. The latter was helpful in reducing symptoms of depression. Fluoxetine has also been used. As part of medical management, a nutritional program should establish a target weight and specific goals for weekly weight gain. Ongoing medical assessment includes monitoring for signs of behavioral relapse as well as of vital signs, electrolytes (plus phosphorous), and weight gain. Patients should be observed for complications if rapid weight gain and fluid overload occur. In life-threatening situations, nasal-gastric feeding may be indicated.

For bulimia nervosa, cognitive behavior therapy (CBT) has been found to be effective in many well-controlled studies. Typically, treatment programs lasts 16 to 20 weeks, and about

---

TABLE 14.3

COMMON LABORATORY FINDINGS IN EMACIATED ANOREXIA NERVOSA

1. Hematologic
   Anemia
   Leukopenia with relative lymphocytosis
2. Serum and plasma
   Hypercarotenemia
   Hypoproteinemia
   Hypercholesterolemia
3. Endocrine
   Decreased estrogens
   Decreased testosterone (in males)
   Immature secretion pattern of luteinizing hormone
   Decreased or blunted luteinizing hormone–releasing
     hormone
   Decreased triiodothyronine
   Increased corticotropin-releasing hormone
   Increased fasting and impaired growth hormone secretion
     responses
   Blunted diurnal cortisol levels
   Uncoupled vasopressin secretion from osmotic challenge
   Low basal metabolic rate
   Reduced bone density

Reprinted from Halmi, K. A. (2007). Anorexia nervosa and bulimia nervosa. In A. Martin & F. Volkmar (Eds.), *Lewis's Child and Adolescent Psychiatry: A Comprehensive Textbook*, 4th edition, p. 595. Philadelphia: Lippincott Williams & Wilkins.

half of patients are able to stop binging and purging. In most cases, these behaviors are significantly reduced even when not eliminated (Halmi, 2007). Goals of treatment include interruption of the binge–purge cycle and helping change the patient's view of food, body image, weight, and so forth. Therapists need special training in these methods (see Wilson & Fairburn, 1993). A family component is typically included in treatment. A number of different medications have been evaluated in patients with bulimia nervosa, including various antidepressants and selective serotonin inhibitors. The latter are often preferred because of more favorable side effect profiles. These agents were significantly better than placebo in multiple areas, including

---

TABLE 14.4

COMMON LABORATORY FINDINGS WITH BINGEING AND PURGING BEHAVIOR

Hypokalemia
Hypochloremic alkalosis
Elevated serum amylase
Electrocardiography: QT and T-wave changes
Photon absorptiometry: reduced bone density

Adapted from Halmi, K. A. (2007). Anorexia nervosa and bulimia nervosa. In A. Martin & F. Volkmar (Eds.), *Lewis's Child and Adolescent Psychiatry: A Comprehensive Textbook*, 4th edition, p. 595. Philadelphia: Lippincott Williams & Wilkins.

reduced frequency of binges, improved mood, and decreased preoccupation with weight and body image. Unfortunately, total abstinence from binging and purging was seen only in about 25% of cases (see Mitchell & DeZwaan, 1993). Some authorities have advocated combining drug treatment with CBT. Topiramate has been used in a 10-week randomized controlled trial and was more effective than placebo. Some clinicians combine CBT with group treatment approaches; this has been particularly helpful for college students. CBT has been used with older children and adolescents as well as in adults.

Course and Prognosis

In general, long term follow-up studies note ongoing problems in most patients with anorexia nervosa. Typically, about 25% recover and 25% remain chronically ill, with the remainder having ongoing problems. There is a potential for serious long-term medical problems and death. In younger patients with anorexia nervosa, positive predictors include the purging type presentation (a different pattern than in adult-onset cases). Adolescents who are more isolated and less social and who engage in compulsive exercise also do less well. For anorexia nervosa, other predictors of outcome include younger onset (better outcome). Later onset (after age 18 years), repeated hospital stays, and low initial weight are associated with worse outcome.

In bulimia nervosa, the overall mortality rate is lower than in anorexia nervosa. Follow-up studies suggest that about half of patients will be fully recovered over time, and perhaps 20% will continue to meet criteria for the condition. There is potential for relapse. In bulimia nervosa, difficulties with impulse control are associated with worse outcomes.

OBESITY

Although technically not (at least at present) a psychiatric disorder, obesity is an important public health problem that, in some sense, should be considered in the context of other problems in eating or feeding. Various approaches to the definition of obesity and overweight exist, although, in practice, computation of the BMI presents the simplest method (BMI = Weight in kilograms/Height in meters squared). This has become the most widely accepted weight–height index in children and adolescents. In general, it is a good approximation to percent body fat for most individuals. Typically, the BMI increases in the first few months of life and then declines until about 6 to 8 years of age (Figure 14.1) when it again increases and continues to do so through adolescence, In boys, the adolescence increase is primarily attributable to an increase in fat-free mass; in girls, the percent body fat actually increases. Birth weight has a very modest power to predict adult weight, but the correlation of childhood to adult BMI gradually increases during childhood and adolescence. Childhood obesity often persists into adulthood, particularly if parents are also obese (Figure 14.2).

In adults, BMI cutoffs for overweight (BMI >25), obesity (BMI >30), and extreme obesity (BMI >40) have been identified. The issue of definition in children and adolescents is more controversial. Over time, at least in the industrialized world, average height and BMI have both increased, and the mean onset of puberty has decreased, although some plateauing of this effect has recently occurred. The "outbreak" of obesity is a relatively recent historical phenomenon (see Fairburn & Brownell, 2002) with about two-thirds of U.S. adults now being classified as overweight. This phenomenon is not, unfortunately, confined to adults. As a group, children and adolescents have experienced a fourfold increase in overweight (in children ages 6 to 11 years) and a threefold increase in adolescents ages 12 to 19 years over about the past 3 decades (Hebebrand, 2007). Within the United States, children who are black or Hispanic are particularly vulnerable.

Various medical problems are associated with overweight and obesity, including hypertension, type 2 diabetes mellitus, dyslipidemia, and metabolic syndrome, among others. As with other eating or feeding problems, the causes of obesity are complex and multifactorial. These

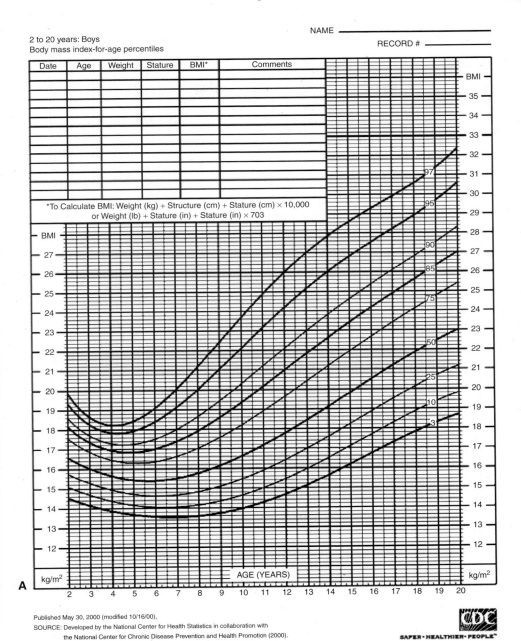

2 to 20 years: Boys
Body mass index-for-age percentiles

NAME _____

RECORD # _____

Date	Age	Weight	Stature	BMI*	Comments

*To Calculate BMI: Weight (kg) + Structure (cm) + Stature (cm) × 10,000
or Weight (lb) + Stature (in) + Stature (in) × 703

AGE (YEARS)

A

Published May 30, 2000 (modified 10/16/00),
SOURCE: Developed by the National Center for Health Statistics in collaboration with
the National Center for Chronic Disease Prevention and Health Promotion (2000).
http://www.cdc.gov/growthcharts

SAFER · HEALTHIER · PEOPLE™

FIGURE 14.1. Body mass index-for-age percentiles for boys (A) and girls (B) for the U.S. population. (From http://www.cdc.gov/growthcharts.)

2 to 20 years: Girls
Body mass index-for-age percentiles

NAME _____

RECORD # _____

Date	Age	Weight	Stature	BMI*	Comments

*To Calculate BMI: Weight (kg) + Structure (cm) + Stature (cm) × 10,000
or Weight (lb) + Stature (in) + Stature (in) × 703

B

AGE (YEARS)

kg/m²   kg/m²

Published May 30, 2000 (modified 10/16/00),
SOURCE: Developed by the National Center for Health Statistics in collaboration with
the National Center for Chronic Disease Prevention and Health Promotion (2000).
http://www.cdc.gov/growthcharts

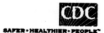

FIGURE 14.1. (Continued)

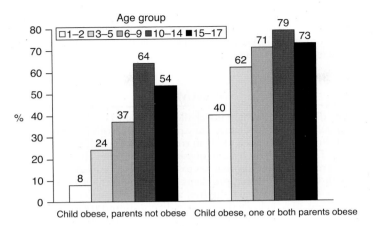

FIGURE 14.2. Risk of persistence of childhood obesity into adulthood. Obesity in childhood and young adulthood (21–29 years of age) was defined via a body mass index (BMI) at the 85th percentile or above for age and sex and a BMI at or above 27.8 for men and 27.3 for women. (From Whitaker, R. C., Wright, J. A., Pepe, M. S., Seidel, K. D., & Dietz, W. H. (1997). Predicting obesity in young adulthood from childhood and parental obesity. *New England Journal of Medicine, 337,* 869–873.)

range from psychosocial and cultural to genetic. As noted previously, the discovery of the leptin gene was a major advance in the field. Recent work has focused on examination of environmental, metabolic and genetic factors.

Parental obesity is clearly the strongest risk factor for obesity in children and adolescents. Maternal obesity appears to be a stronger predictor than paternal obesity. Twin studies have also supported a strong genetic component. Epigenetic factors may also be important (e.g., methylation patterns of specific genes might impact obesity risk). Clearly, rare mutations in the genes for leptin and related compounds can lead to early-onset, extreme obesity. Interestingly, in contrast to other genes, such as those involved in Prader-Wili syndrome (see Chapter 5), these genes do not produce intellectual deficiency. However, the effect sizes of most gene involved in predisposition to overweight and obesity are small.

Environmental factors are also important (e.g., changes in caloric intake and expenditure), although the effects have been, in many ways, less than expected (e.g., TV viewing and inactivity have been thought to relate to levels of overweight and obesity). Other issues include changes in caloric intake and portion size. Interestingly, maternal effects have included an association of maternal smoking with increased risk and an association of breastfeeding with decreased risk of obesity. Psychiatric predictors include depressive symptoms and various psychoactive medications (e.g., atypical antipsychotics and some of the mood-stabilizing medications).

In addition to its medical risk, obesity and overweight also entail a significant psychological burden for children and adolescents. Overweight and obesity take a toll on peer relations, peer popularity, and self-esteem, and they increase the risk for other mental health problems (e.g., mood and anxiety disorders in some samples).

There are significant challenges for developing effective intervention programs. Expectations of children and parents can be unrealistic. Treatment effects tend to be relatively modest, and ongoing work is required to maintain weight loss. High dropout rates from intervention programs are also typical. Interventions have focused both on modification of lifestyle and medication development. Unfortunately, it is often the case that initial positive results are not maintained. Given these issues, it is not surprising that bariatric surgery is increasingly available to morbidly obese adolescents.

Studies aimed at prevention have targeted preschool- as well as school-aged children, often combining some aspects of education, relative to diet, with physical fitness activities. Although results have been somewhat mixed, the studies generally demonstrated improved diet and activity. Existing data suggest the importance of early treatment.

SUMMARY

Eating and feeding disorders present many challenges. From a clinical standpoint, they exist at the interface of psychiatry and medicine. They present numerous challenges for collaboration and management. Progress has been made in treatment, although additional, well-controlled studies are needed. The marked increase in obesity presents other challenges for the health care system. In terms of research, new approaches to diagnostic classification are a priority because many patients with significant eating problems do not precisely fit the current (DSM-IV-TR) system. This is true for both younger children as well as for adolescents. Greater public and professional awareness may help facilitate early diagnosis and treatment. Given the existing data on outcome, treatment should be started as early as possible. In anorexia nervosa and bulimia nervosa, there are several important areas in need of additional research. Our understanding of potential genetic contributions to these conditions remains limited. Although many treatment studies have been done, the development of more effective treatments remain a high priority, particularly given the difficulties of conducting research in this population. High dropout rates in treatment studies typically argue for the need for more effective short-term treatments that can engage the patient and family to help treatment continue.

Selected Readings

Attia, E., & Walsh, B. T. (2009). Behavioral management for Anorexia nervosa. *New England Journal of Medicine*, 360(5), 500–506.

Bell, R. M. (1985). *Holy Anorexia*. Chicago: University of Chicago Press.

Brownley, K. A., Berkman, N. D., Sedway, J. A., Lohr, K. N., & Bulik, C. M. (2007). Binge eating disorder treatment: a systematic review of randomized controlled trials. *International Journal of Eating Disorders*, 40(4), 337–348.

Bulik, C. M., Berkman, N. D., Brownley, K. A., Sedway, J. A., & Lohr, K. N. (2007). Anorexia nervosa treatment: a systematic review of randomized controlled trials. *International Journal of Eating Disorders*, 40(4), 310–320.

Capasso, A., Petrella, C., & Milano, W. (2009). Pharmacological profile of SSRIs and SNRIs in the treatment of eating disorders. *Current Clinical Pharmacology*, 4(1), 78–83.

Chatoor, I., Ganiban, J., Colin, V., Plummer, N., & Harmon, M. J. (1998a). Attachment and Feeding Problems: A reexamination of nonorganic failure to thrive and attachment insecurity. *Journal of the American Academy of Child and Adolescent Psychiatry*, 37, 1217–1224.

Chatoor, I., Hirsch, R., Ganban, J., Persinger, M., & Hamburger, E. (1998b). Diagnosing infantile anorexia: The observation of mother-infant interactions. *Journal of the American Academy of Child and Adolescent Psychiatry*, 37, 959–967.

Drotar, D., & Sturm, L. (1998). Prediction of intellectual development in young children with early histories of nonorganic failure to thrive. *Journal of Developmental and Behavioral Pediatrics*, 13, 281–296.

Fairburn, C. G., & Brownell, K. D. (2002). *Eating Disorders and Obesity: A Comprehensive Textbook*, 2nd edition. New York: Guilford.

Godart, N. T., Perdereau, F., Rein, Z., Berthoz, S., Wallier, J., Jeammet, P., & Flament, M. (2007). Comorbidity studies of eating disorders and mood disorders. Critical review of the literature. *Journal of Affective Disorders*, 97(1–3), 37–49.

Gonyea, J. (2007). Pica—Do you know what your patients are eating? *Nephrology Nursing Journal: Journal of the American Nephrology Nurses' Association*, 34(2), 230–231.

Halmi, K. A. (2007). Anorexia nervosa and bulimia nervosa. In A. Martin & F. Volkmar (Eds.), *Lewis's Child and Adolescent Psychiatry: A Comprehensive Textbook*, 4th edition, pp. 592–602. Philadelphia: Lippincott Williams & Wilkins.

Halmi, K. A. (2009). Anorexia nervosa: an increasing problem in children and adolescents. *Dialogues in Clinical Neuroscience*, 11(1), 100–103.

Hebebrand, J. (2007). Obesity. In A. Martin & F. Volkmar (Eds.), *Lewis's Child and Adolescent Psychiatry: A Comprehensive Textbook*, 4th edition, pp. 592–614. Philadelphia: Lippincott Williams & Wilkins.

Hedges, D. W., Renhert, F. W., Hoops, S. P., Rosenthal, N. R., Kamin, M., Kamin, R, & Capece, J. (2003). Treatment of bulimia nervosa with topiramate in a randomized-double-blind, placebo-controlled trial, part 2: Improvements in psychiatric measures. *Journal of Clinical Psychiatry*, 64, 1449–1454.

Herguner, S., Ozyildirim, I., & Cansaran, T. (2008). Is pica an eating disorder or an obsessive-compulsive spectrum disorder? *Progress in Neuro-Psychopharmacology & Biological Psychiatry*, 32(8), 2010–2011.

Herpertz-Dahlmann, B., & Salbach-Andrae, H. (2009). Overview of treatment modalities in adolescent anorexia nervosa. *Child & Adolescent Psychiatric Clinics of North America, 18*(1), 131–145.

Kettaneh, A., Eclache, V., Fain, O., Sontag, C., Uzan, M., Carbillon, L., Stirnemann, J., & Thomas, M. (2005). Pica and food craving in patients with iron-deficiency anemia: a case-control study in France. *American Journal of Medicine, 118*(2), 185–188.

Lacey, E. P. (1993). Phenomenology of pica. In J. L. Woolston (Ed.), *Child and Adolescent Psychiatric Clinics of North America. Vol 2: Eating and Growth Disorders*, pp. 75–91. Philadelphia: Saunders.

McAdam, D. B., Sherman, J. A., Sheldon, J. B., & Napolitano, D. A. (2004). Behavioral interventions to reduce the pica of persons with developmental disabilities. *Behavior Modification, 28*(1), 45–72.

Mitchell, J. E., & DeZwaan, M. (1993). Pharmacological treatments of binge eating. In C. G. Fairburn & G. T. Wilson (Eds.), *Binge Eating: Nature, Assessment and Treatment*. New York: Guilford Press.

Nicholls, D., & Bryant-Waugh, R. (2009). Eating disorders of infancy and childhood: definition, symptomatology, epidemiology, and comorbidity. *Child & Adolescent Psychiatric Clinics of North America, 18*(1), 17–30.

Shah, M. D. (2002). Failure to thrive in children. *Journal of Clinical Gastroenterology, 35*, 371–374.

Shapiro, J. R., Berkman, N. D., Brownley, K. A., Sedway, J. A., Lohr, K. N., & Bulik, C. M. (2007). Bulimia nervosa treatment: a systematic review of randomized controlled trials. *International Journal of Eating Disorders, 40*(4), 321–336.

Signorini, A., De Filippo, E., Panico, S., De Caprio, C., Pasanisi, F., & Contaldo, F. (2007). Long-term mortality in Anorexia nervosa: a report after an 8-year follow-up and a review of the most recent literature. *European Journal of Clinical Nutrition, 61*(1), 119–122.

Singer, L. T., Ambuel, B., Wade, S., & Jaffe, A. C. (1992). Cognitive-behavioral treatment of health-impairing food phobias in children. *Journal of the American Academy of Child and Adolescent Psychiatry, 31*, 847–852.

Skarderud, F. (2007). Eating one's words: Part III. Mentalisation-based psychotherapy for anorexia nervosa—An outline for a treatment and training manual. *European Eating Disorders Review, 15*(5), 323–339.

Stefano, S. C., Bacaltchuk, J., Blay, S. L., & Appolinario, J. C. (2008). Antidepressants in short-term treatment of binge eating disorder: Systematic review and meta-analysis. *Eating Behaviors, 9*(2), 129–136.

Stiegler, L. N. (2005). Understanding pica behavior: A review for clinical and education professionals. *Focus on Autism and Other Developmental Disabilities, 20*, 27–38.

Stokes, T. (2006). The earth-eaters. *Nature, 444*(7119), 543–544.

Wilfley, D. E., Bishop, M. E., Wilson, G. T., & Agras, W. S. (2007). Classification of eating disorders: Toward DSM-V. *International Journal of Eating Disorders, 40*(suppl), S123–S129.

Wilson, C. G., & Fairburn, C. G. (1993). Cognitive treatment for treating eating disorders. *Journal of Consulting and Clinical Psychology, 61*, 261–269.

Woods, A. J., & Stock, M. J. (1996). Leptin activation in hypothalamus. *Nature, 381*, 745.

Woolston, J. L., & Hasbani, S. M. (2007). Eating and growth disorders in infants and children. In A. Martin & F. Volkmar (Eds.), *Lewis's Child and Adolescent Psychiatry: A Comprehensive Textbook*, 4th edition, pp. 583–592. Philadelphia: Lippincott Williams & Wilkins.

CHAPTER 15 ■ SUBSTANCE ABUSE DISORDERS

Use and abuse of alcohol and narcotics have occurred throughout history. Indeed, until recently their use to alleviate pain was one of the few effective medical therapies. Advances in chemistry led, particularly during the 19th and 20th centuries, to the formulation of more potent preparations as active ingredients were identified and then used to search for other agents. At one time, cocaine and the opiates were widely prescribed and readily available, often being included in various elixirs and tonics. By 1924, an awareness of the potential for abuse led to federal regulation so that opiates and cocaine could only be prescribed by physicians. Similarly, the advent of Prohibition meant that alcohol was no longer freely available; as a result (until repeal in 1933), there was an extensive black market in alcohol as there now is other substances (see Musto, 1999, for an historical review). Over time, the federal government has taken an increasingly active role in the regulation of medications and substances with abuse potential. State governments do, however, continue to be the primary regulators in some areas, e.g., for alcohol sales.

Advances in understanding the pharmacology and mechanisms of action (e.g. using animal models) have advanced our knowledge of brain processes and the mechanisms that may underlie substance abuse. Until recently, most of the work on substance abuse and substance dependence has come from work with adults. There has been less research on children and adolescents. Clearly, adolescents who abuse drugs or alcohol have sure risk for developing dependence in adulthood. Among adolescents, substance abuse is significantly more common than dependence (probably by about two to one), and abuse of multiple substances is fairly common. There is some suggestion (Hopfer & Riggs, 2007) that in contrast to adults, the distinction currently made between abuse and dependency may be more artificial in adolescents.

DEFINITIONS

The *Diagnostic and Statistical Manual of Mental Disorder* (DSM-IV-TR) (2004) provides diagnostic codes for a host of substance related disorders. Substances of potential abuse include alcohol, amphetamines, caffeine, cannabis, cocaine, hallucinogens, inhalants, nicotine, opioids, phencyclidine, and sedative-hypnotic categories. Other codes provide for polysubstance or unknown substance use/abuse. As a practical matter, in children and adolescents, substance abuse and substance dependence are more frequently encountered (e.g., rather than withdrawal syndromes).

Substance abuse is usually considered a less severe syndrome than substance dependence (the diagnosis of the former is not met if the latter is present). Whereas substance abuse entails impairment of clinical significance caused by use of a substance, dependence involves a number of symptoms reflecting persistent use even in the face of negative consequences. For example, substance abuse involves recurrent use associated with some degree of interference or use in situations in which some danger is involved but without tolerance, withdrawal, and major life impact present. Substance abuse does not entail the same degree of preoccupation with the substance (e.g., worrying where one's next drink will come from) nor are physiological related to withdrawal present. If the individual meets criteria for tolerance or withdrawal in regard to the substance being abused, physiological dependence is noted as a qualifier.

The various substances of abuse share some similarities as well as many differences in terms of their physiological effects and potential for addiction. Individual factors as well as route of administration all can be important. For some substances (e.g., cocaine), rapid development of dependency may occur. Alcohol is often the first substance adolescents use and accounts for much of adolescent substance use and abuse. In one large national survey, 6% of adolescents met criteria for alcohol abuse or dependence in the previous year. Acute alcohol intoxication is characterized by sedation, slurred speech, decreased heart rate, poor coordination, and reduced blood pressure. Repeated drinking can lead to tolerance and, occasionally, adolescents can even experience alcohol withdrawal states. As with adults, alcohol withdrawal may require emergency medical management. Severe alcohol intoxication can also be an emergent medical problem (e.g., group drinking at parties) and can lead to death at high levels. Impaired judgment and coordination also contribute to accidental death and injuries.

Nicotine in tobacco products can produce dependence and is associated with a number of medical problems. One of the major concerns about tobacco use is its potential for serving as an entry to use of other substances. The effects of nicotine are prompt after inhalation or ingestion (e.g., from chewing) and include central nervous system (CNS) stimulation followed by symptoms of withdrawal. The mechanism of nicotine on acetylcholine receptors is well known. With a half-life of several hours, nicotine can accumulate in the body over the course of the day. Cessation of use can result in irritability, characteristic craving, and problems in mood and concentration.

The most frequently used illicit drug in adolescents is marijuana, and dependence is most frequently cited as the reason for adolescent admissions to substance abuse treatment. About 4% of adolescents meet criteria for use or dependence within the past year. The mechanisms of action of the active ingredients Δ-9 tetrahydrocannabinol (THC), has been increasingly studied. This agent binds to the CNR1 receptor which is widely distributed in the brain. Effects on anxiety, appetite, pain are reported as are analgesic effects and enhancement of appetite. Hallucinogenic effects can also be noted. Although the DSM-IV-TR does not recognize a withdrawal syndrome, there is some suggestion that one, in fact, does exist. There is also some suggestion that repeated use may increase the risk for psychosis and other psychiatric problems.

Abuse of heroin and prescription opiates has increased over the past decade and has become the source of increasing concern. One survey suggests that as many as one in 20 high school 12th graders had reported using OxyContin illicitly. The use of various routes of administration of purer heroin, including smoking and snorting, have probably contributed to this increase. Heroin has very significant potential for addiction, and its use is associated with a range of problems impacting adolescents at home and in school.

Cocaine has various psychological effects, including a sense of mental clarity and lack of fatigue. Physical effects include increased heart rate, temperature, and blood pressure as well as dilated pupils. The route of administration leads to major differences in duration of its effects (e.g. smoking leads to a more intense but shorter high than snorting). About 6% of users become dependent within 1 year (Hopfer & Riggs, 2007).

Amphetamines have a long history of legitimate use in medicine, including in the treatment of attention-deficit disorders. About 2% of adolescents report use of a stimulant illicitly.

Various street names for methamphetamine including *ice, speed, crystal, glass,* and *crank.* This agent can be used in a host of ways, including injection, inhalation, and smoking. Similar to cocaine, dependence can develop quickly and be associated with a rapid decrement in functioning. Associated effects can include psychotic behavior; aggression; and various neuropsychological deficits, including memory loss. Appetite suppression is common as is decreased need for sleep. Euphoria is often noted. Physical effects include hyperthermia, increased respiration, and increased risk for seizures.

MDMA (3,4-methylenedioxymethamphetamine) ("Ecstasy") is another frequently abused agent with both stimulant and psychedelic effects. Slightly more than 1% of adolescence report using it over the course of a year. Taken orally, the psychedelic effects of the agent last for several hours. Mental status changes can include anxiety, paranoia, depression, and sleepless. Physical symptoms can include blurred version, a sense of muscle/body tension, nausea, and sweating; occasionally, severe hyperthermia develops. Available data suggest that most users stop use of the agent in young adulthood, although some who become dependent continue.

GHB (γ-hydroxybutyrate) is known on the street as *G, grievous bodily harm,* or *liquid Ecstasy.* This drug was originally used as a muscle growth agent and sold in health food stores before its CNS effects were recognized. A CNS depressant, many of the effects of GHB are similar to those of alcohol. Effects last for several hours. Dependence can develop along with a withdrawal syndrome similar to that sometimes seen with benzodiazepines. About 2% of high school seniors report use of this agent in the previous year (Hopfer & Riggs, 2007).

Although many (about one in six) adolescents will have tried inhalants on at least one occasion, actual rates of abuse or dependence are much lower, around 0.1% (Sakai et al., 2004). These organic fumes and gases are more frequently abused in younger adolescents probably because of greater accessibility. These compounds can be sprayed into the mouth or inhaled either through putting the material into a cloth and inhaling it ("huffed") or by inhaling via a bag ("bagged"). Psychological effects include euphoria and disorientation. A period of drowsiness or confusion may follow. A variety of materials are inhaled. They have the potential for causing relatively rapid neurological features and changes in cognition. Their continued use can lead to neurotoxicity, making detection and treatment important public health problems.

Anabolic steroid abuse has become relatively common, with about 3% of male adolescents in the United States reporting use in the prior year. The main goal for abuse of steroid is building muscle mass, so intrinsically, abuse of these agents differs from other substances of abuse in which the effect has more to do with immediate psychological changes. There are many different medical and psychological sequelae, including stopping growth prematurely and testicular shrinkage. Psychological problems can include pronounced mood swings and even psychosis (Brown, 2005).

EPIDEMIOLOGY AND DEMOGRAPHICS

There have been major changes in the use of drugs over the past decade in adolescents in the United States. As noted in Figure 15.1, there have been some fluctuations in patterns of substance abuse, although the most consistently used substances in adolescents have included alcohol, tobacco, and marijuana. About one-third of high school seniors report use of some illegal substance (apart from marijuana) at some point in their lives. Variations in patterns of substance abuse are noteworthy but not always well understood. There has been a noteworthy increase in the use of hydrocodone in adolescents.

Age-related data from publicly funded substance abuse treatment programs are presented in Table 15.1. For younger adolescents, marijuana is most frequently cited as the primary substance of abuse, but for the oldest adolescents and young adults, marijuana combined with alcohol continues to be a major problem along with a variety of other substances. There is a steady increase in prevalence of substance use and disorders of substance use over the course of adolescence with about 25% of older adolescents meeting criteria for abuse and 20% for disorder.

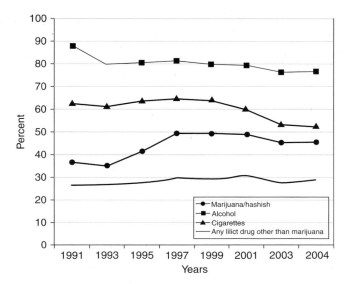

FIGURE 15.1. Trends in prevalence of twelfth grade lifetime drug use. (Adapted from Johnson, L. D., O'Malley, P. M., Bachman, J. G., & Schulenberg, J. E. (2005). *Monitoring the Future: National Survey Results on Drug Use, 1975–2004. Volume 1: Secondary School Students.* Bethesda, MD: National Institute on Drug Abuse; 680. NIH Publication No. 05-5727.)

Boys and young men are more likely to engage in substance abuse and also are more likely to meet criteria for dependence in late adolescence, particularly for alcohol and marijuana. Girls and young women are more likely to report nicotine dependence. Rates of substance use disorders are high in a mental health setting and even more so in juvenile justice setting, where a majority of individuals meet lifetime criteria for substance use disorders.

Risk appears to increase with early onset of substance use. It remains unclear why this is so, although animal studies have suggested greater potential for vulnerability to drug sensitization during the adolescent period. It may also be that early use of substances arises as a result of more general risk factors.

ETIOLOGY

Various risk factors are associates with substance abuse disorders in adolescents (see Whitmore & Riggs, 2006). Obviously, development of these disorders depends on ready access to substances of abuse. However, even when these substances are widely available, only a small number of adolescents develop substance use disorders. Attempts have been made to understand genetic and environmental factors using twin and adoption studies. Genetic factors become more apparent if environments support their expression. Genetic mechanisms can be complex (e.g., there may be a direct impact on the ability to metabolize or react to substances). Effects may also be more indirect (e.g., by impacting other aspects of development or behavior). It is clear that family history of substance abuse or dependence is a powerful predictor of risk.

Risk for substance and abuse and dependence is increased in association with a number of other conditions. For example, the various externalizing disorders are a major risk factor (Crowley & Riggs, 1995). Because of their frequent association with each other, disentangling contributions of these conditions is complicated, but it is clear that conduct disorder is a major risk factor and the less severe oppositional defiant disorder (ODD) and even attention-deficit/hyperactivity disorder (ADHD) also appear to increase risk.

TABLE 15.1

PRIMARY ADMITTING SUBSTANCE OF ABUSE (% OF TOTAL ADMISSIONS), BY AGE FROM THE TREATMENT EPISODE DATA SET

Substance	Age (years)		
	12–14 %	15–17 %	18–20 %
None	8.3	2.2	0.9
Alcohol	17.7	19.9	30.6
Crack or cocaine	1.2	2.4	6.3
Marijuana or hashish	66.7	66.9	37.9
Heroin	0.2	1.2	9.8
Nonprescription methadone	0	0	0.1
Other opiates and synthetics	0.4	0.6	2.5
PCP	0.1	0.1	0.4
Hallucinogens	0.1	0.3	0.4
Methamphetamine	2.1	4	8.4
Other amphetamines	0.6	0.9	1.4
Other stimulants	0.2	0.1	0.1
Benzodiazepines	0.2	0.2	0.4
Other tranquilizers	0.1	0.1	0
Barbiturates	0	0	0
Other sedatives or hypnotics	0.2	0.1	0.2
Inhalants	0.9	0.2	0.1
Over-the-counter medications	0.2	0.2	0.1
Other	0.9	0.6	0.5
Total percent	100	100	100
(Total N)	(24,911)	(123,496)	(119,138)

PCP, phencyclidine.
From TEDS: Treatment Episode Data Set. (2003). *Highlights. National Admissions to Substance Abuse Treatment Services, DASIS Series: S-27.* Rockville, MD: Services DoHaH. DHHS Publication No. SMA 05-4043, with permission.

Various models have been developed to understand the pattern and progression of substance abuse. Stage theory suggests that alcohol or tobacco is first used followed by marijuana before the adolescent goes on to use other substances (Kandel et al., 1992). A similar notion, the "gateway hypothesis," views marijuana as a key to the adolescent's going on to use of other drugs. Various explanations have been used to account for this mechanism (Lynskey, 2005).

The aggregation of substance use or abuse in families has genetic and environmental components. Clearly, use or abuse of substances by parents or older siblings increases risk. Peer effects are also important, although the notion that "peer pressure" leads straightforwardly to substance abuse is overly simplistic.

Animal studies have demonstrated chronic behavioral, neurobiological, and physiological effects of substance use and abuse. Loss of the substance leads the dependent animal into a pattern of craving and dysphoria similar to that seen in humans.

DIFFERENTIAL DIAGNOSIS AND ASSESSMENT

Typically, information is obtained through direct interview of the adolescent as well as through parents, teachers, and other sources. The adolescent with a substance abuse problem often minimizes it. In general, the clinician should try to foster rapport with the patient using a nonjudgmental, empathetic but honest approach designed to build a therapeutic relationship. The clinician should be clear about confidentiality and its limits. The adolescent should understand that, within certain limits, rules of confidentiality do apply with important exceptions relating to dangerous behaviors (see Hopfer & Riggs, 2007). Assuring the adolescent of confidentiality (within stated limited) generally encourages honest reporting of substance abuse problems. Relevant information from the adolescent will include the nature and extent of substance use or abuse, its onset and persistent, and association with other relevant factors in the adolescent's life (e.g., relation to stress, depression, impulse control problems). Often, the initial interview is best done with both the adolescent and parents present so that rules for the evaluation can be heard by all parties concerned.

The interview with parents should complement the interview with the adolescence to understand relevant factors from history and current functioning of the child and family. The

---

Case Study: Adolescent Substance Abuse

Timmy, a 15-year-old boy, was seen for evaluation at the request of his parents, who were concerned about a noteworthy decline in academic skills over the past months (since starting high school) associated with increasing difficulties at home. The latter took the form of an apparent lack of engagement alternating, at times, with angry confrontations with parents and family members. Until about 1 year previously, he had been reported to be a solid academic student who was deeply engaged in several sports. On moving into high school (in the sophomore year), he had become involved with a new group of friends. His mother suspected that he had been drinking on several occasions when he came home late; she also discovered cigarettes and, recently, found a joint of marijuana in his clothing. When confronted about this, Timmy denied any problems and complained his parents were hounding him. He reported that school was now boring. In the interview with his parents, it appeared that several stresses had contributed to both parents being less involved with Timmy over the past several year; this included a serious medical illness in a younger sibling and the onset of marital problem partly related to the younger sibling's repeated hospitalizations. They also noted that several relatives had a strong history of substance abuse, mostly involving alcohol.

On interview, Timmy inquired about confidentiality. Although seemingly at first disinterested, he became more involved in the interview and disclosed a history of polysubstance abuse extending back over about 18 months, starting with cigarettes and an occasional beer and progressing to marijuana use. He had recently moved on to try a range of other street drugs, including amphetamines. Several of his new friends at school used drugs extensively. It appeared that with the onset of high school and a heavier academic demand and increased demands by coaches, he began to use substances in combination, often drinking and smoking pot. As he became more engaged in the assessment, both significant anxiety and depression were noted. Treatment included family support; cognitive behavior therapy; examination of his school program (and provision of some supports); and eventually, treatment with selective serotonin reuptake inhibitor. On follow-up 1 year later, he was doing well.

Comment: This case illustrates several features relatively typical in adolescents with substance abuse problems. Timmy began to use nicotine and alcohol, gradually adding other substances. Family stress and lack of supervision combined with stresses and some degree of depression with regard to both his family situation and school demands also contributed to his problems. As is often the case, treatment was multimodal. It is somewhat less typical for adolescents to have depression and anxiety problems; externalizing difficulties (in this case possibly including the angry outbursts) are more frequent.

TABLE 15.2

TYPICAL URINE DETECTION PERIODS FOR VARIOUS SUBSTANCES

Substance	Urine Detection Time
Alcohol	After absorption, decreases by -0.02 g%/hr
Amphetamine	24–72 hours
Barbiturates	1–2 days
Benzodiazepines	3 days for therapeutic dose
Cannabis (single use)	1–3 days
Cannabis (moderate use)	3–5 days
Cannabis (heavy use)	10 days
Cocaine	24–96 hours
Codeine or morphine	24–72 hours
Heroin	24–72 hours
Methamphetamine	24–72 hours
PCP	14–30 days
LSD	1.5–5 days

LSD, lysergic acid diethylamide; PCP, phencyclidine.
Reprinted from Hopfer, C., & Riggs, P. (2007). Substance use disorders. In A. Martin & F. Volkmar (Eds.), *Lewis's Child and Adolescent Psychiatry: A Comprehensive Textbook*, 4th edition, p. 619. Philadelphia: Lippincott Williams & Wilkins.

interview with the adolescent can then follow. As is often true with adolescents, beginning the interview with more affectively neutral topics (e.g. developmental history) before moving to more sensitive ones often is helpful.

As noted previously, the differential diagnosis is complicated by significant potential for comorbidity to be present; in adolescents, this is true more than half the time and, in at least one study, almost 75% of the time. In addition, the clinician must determine whether substance abuse or substance dependence is present. Both externalizing disorder (ODD, conduct, ADHD) and internalizing disorders (anxiety, mood disorders) can be present, although it is somewhat more likely for the externalizing disorders to coexist with substance abuse problems.

Laboratory studies, particularly urine toxicology screening, have assumed increased importance in screening for substance abuse. It is important, however, to realize that some substances are more readily detected or are only detectable for brief periods (e.g., inhalants are difficult to detect in urine, and alcohol is quickly eliminated). In most clinical settings, a standard panel of tests is available focused on the most commonly used substance. Alcohol levels can be done using breathalyzer, and a specialized test can be used if inhalants are suspected. For the hallucinogens, MDMA, and GHB, specific tests are required. Detection times are summarized in Table 15.2.

TREATMENT

Given the complex nature of substance abuse problems and frequent associations with other conditions, treatment planning should be flexible and be based on an awareness of the chronicity of these conditions and the potential for relapse. Often, the adolescent is not the person complaining, and motivation, or lack thereof, for treatment is important to assess. Initial efforts typically focus on eliminating or reducing substance use, addressing the various needs of the adolescence, and preventing relapse. Various evidence based treatment approaches are

TABLE 15.3

COMMON COMORBID DISORDERS: PHARMACOTHERAPY FOR ADOLESCENTS WITH SUBSTANCE USE DISORDERS

Comorbid Disorder	Effective Treatment for Adolescents without Substance Use Disorder	Impact of Treatment on Adolescents with Substance Use Disorders
Attention-deficit/ hyperactivity disorder (ADHD)	First-line pharmacotherapy: generally psychostimulants Medication options with low abuse potential: pemoline, bupropion, atomoxetine	One controlled trial of pemoline (Riggs et al., 2005; $n = 69$) suggests: ■ Efficacy for ADHD despite non-abstinence ■ Good safety profile in 12-week trial; potential for hepatotoxicity; relative contraindication for pemoline ■ No decrease (or increase) in drug use in the absence of specific behavioral intervention for substance abuse disorders ■ Potential for hepatoxicity relative contraindication for pemoline given other current options ■ Clonidine relatively contraindicated
Bipolar disorder	First-line pharmacotherapy: mood stabilizers (lithium, valproic acid, carbamazepine)	One randomized controlled trial of lithium in adolescents with substance abuse disorders and comorbid bipolar disorder (Geller et al., 1998; $n = 25$) suggests: ■ Efficacy and reasonable safety for bipolar disorder despite non-abstinence ■ Not adequate as an effective treatment for substance abuse disorder in the absence of specific behavioral treatment for substance abuse disorder
Depression	First-line therapy: combined pharmacotherapy and psychotherapy Pharmacotherapy: SSRIs (greater support, fluoxetine) in adolescents without substance abuse disorders Psychotherapy: CBT and interpersonal psychotherapy combined with medication for severe depression, fuoxetine + CBT has greater efficacy than either alone (TADS study March, 2005)	One randomized controlled trial of fluoxetine in adolescents with substance abuse disorder and comorbid MDD + CBT for substance abuse disorder (Riggs et al., 2005; $n = 126$) suggests: ■ Efficacy for depression despite non-abstinence (16-week trial) ■ Good safety profile for fluoxetine (possibly other SSRIs) ■ High rate of depression remission in both fluoxetine- and placebo-treated subjects suggests that CBT also has an impact on depression despite focus on drug abuse, not depression ■ Remission of depression, regardless of medication assignment, was a more important predictor of decreased drug use than fluoxetine vs. placebo ■ Remitters drug use decreased significantly; non-remitters had no change in drug use ■ TCAs are relatively contraindicated in adolescents with substance abuse disorder (e.g., arrhythmias, anticholinergic adverse effects)

(continued)

TABLE 15.3
(CONTINUED)

Comorbid Disorder	Effective Treatment for Adolescents without Substance Use Disorder	Impact of Treatment on Adolescents with Substance Use Disorders
Anxiety disorder (often comorbid with depressive disorders)	First-line therapy: combined psychotherapy (CBT) and pharmacotherapy (greater evidence, SSRIs)	40% of adolescents in aforementioned controlled trial of fluoxetine for MDD in adolescents with substance abuse disorders (Riggs et al., 2005) suggests: ■ Fluoxetine (possibly other SSRIs) showed efficacy and safety in reducing symptoms of anxiety in depressed, substance-dependent adolescents with significant anxiety symptoms or anxiety disorders (GAD, social anxiety disorder, PTSD) ■ No difference in depression and drug use outcomes comparing those with and without anxiety disorders

CBT, cognitive behavioral therapy; GAD, generalized anxiety disorder; MDD, major depressive disorder; PTSD, posttraumatic stress disorder; SSRI, selective serotonin reuptake inhibitor; TADS, Treatment for Adolescents with Depression Study; TCA, tricyclic antidepressant.
Adapted and reprinted from Hopfer, C., & Riggs, P. (2007). Substance use disorders. In A. Martin & F. Volkmar (Eds.), *Lewis's Child and Adolescent Psychiatry: A Comprehensive Textbook*, 4th edition, p. 622. Philadelphia: Lippincott Williams & Wilkins.

now available. In selected cases, the judicious use of psychopharmacological interventions (e.g. to address comorbid problems) may be useful (Hopfer & Riggs, 2007).

Motivational enhancement techniques help establish a treatment alliance and initial engagement. This set of empirically based techniques increases motivation to change by systematically focusing on "change talk" and behavioral changes. These techniques can be particularly useful for adolescents, who often have, at best, ambivalence about treatment. These methods can also be combined with family or other individual treatment approaches.

Cognitive behavior therapy (CBT) has also been systematically studied. Both individual and group-based CBT methods appear effective. These manualized treatments can are usually time limited, lasting from 5 to 16 weeks. The focus is on cognitive distortions and learned behaviors associated with substance abuse combined with methods to teach more effective coping strategies (e.g., in dealing with stress and drug cravings). These methods also focus on social and communication skills. Riggs et al. (2005) conducted a randomized controlled trial in adolescents with substance abuse disorders and depression and noted a high rate of compliance and retention as well as good response for both depression and substance abuse. This study also underscored the importance of removing barriers to treatment.

Various family-based treatment approaches have been used in management of adolescents with substance abuse problems. These treatments have the advantages of focusing more broadly on the context of the substance abuse and have demonstrated efficacy. Multisystemic therapy uses frequent home visits and ready accessibility to therapists and has been highly effective in ensuring that adolescents remain in treatment. Less intensive approaches include brief strategic family therapy and multidimensional family therapy. Another approach, community reinforcement therapy, focuses on skill building and encouraging adaptive coping. Both parents and youths are engaged in and can profit from this manualized approach.

When comorbid conditions are present, pharmacotherapy may be a relevant consideration. See Tables 15.3 and 15.4 for a summary.

TABLE 15.4

PHARMACOTHERAPIES FOR ADOLESCENT SUBSTANCE USE DISORDER

Substance	Medication	Dose	Comments
Alcohol	Disulfiram	250 mg PO QD or 500 mg PO QOD	FDA approved for alcohol dependence in adults Carroll et al. (2000) showed that in adults, it was also effective for cocaine dependence when alcohol involved
	Acamprosate	1–4 g per day given in a TID dosing schedule	FDA approved for alcohol dependence in adults One study (Niederhofer & Steffan, 2003; $n = 26$) suggests similar efficacy in adolescents as for adults
	Naltrexone	50 mg PO QD also available in injection form	FDA approved for alcohol dependence in adults Deas et al. (2005) showed in open-label trial ($n = 5$) that it was safe and well tolerated
	Topiramate	25–300 mg PO QD	Not yet FDA approved; review by Johnson (2005) indicates effectiveness for adults
Nicotine	Bupropion	100–300 mg PO QD	FDA approved for smoking cessation in adults
	Nicotine patch	Varies depending on product	
Opiates	Methadone	Varies	For adolescents younger than 18 years of age, must have two documented failures at drug-free detoxification Needs to be prescribed at a certified clinic; see Hopfer et al. (2003)
	Buprenorphine	Varies	Marsch et al. (2005) showed effectiveness for adolescent detoxification in first randomized controlled trial
	Naltrexone	50 mg PO QD	Low compliance without monitoring; an injectable form was recently approved and is available

FDA, Food and Drug Administration; PO, orally; QD, every day; QOD, every other day; TID, three times a day.
Adapted and reprinted from Hopfer, C., & Riggs, P. (2007). Substance use disorders. In A. Martin & F. Volkmar (Eds.), *Lewis's Child and Adolescent Psychiatry: A Comprehensive Textbook*, 4th edition, p. 623. Philadelphia: Lippincott Williams & Wilkins.

COURSE

The prognosis of substance abuse disorders depends on the nature of the substance used, the severity of the problem, and the presence of comorbid condition. In general, earlier onset is associated with more severe difficulties and comorbidity and a worse outcome. Unfortunately, substance abuse problems are often chronic with periods of better control followed by relapse.

SUMMARY

Adolescents, and sometimes children, who abuse substances present important challenges for mental and public health. In adolescents, abuse, rather than dependence, is more frequently encountered. A range of different substances are abused often in combination with each other. Adolescent substance abuse can lead to substance dependence in adulthood. Particularly in juvenile justice and mental health settings, substance use problems are frequent. Adolescents who abuse substances of various types often have associated psychopathology, particularly the externalizing disorders.

Selected Readings

Alouf, B., Feinson, J. A., & Chidekel, A. S. (2006). Preventing and treating nicotine addiction: a review with emphasis on adolescent health. *Delaware Medical Journal, 78*(7), 249–256.

Becker, S. J., & Curry, J. F. (2008). Outpatient interventions for adolescent substance abuse: A quality of evidence review. *Journal of Consulting & Clinical Psychology, 76*(4), 531–543.

Briones, D. F., Wilcox, J. A., Mateus, B., & Boudjenah, D. (2006). Risk factors and prevention in adolescent substance abuse: a biopsychosocial approach. *Adolescent Medicine Clinics, 17*(2), 335–352.

Brown, J. T. (2005). Anabolic steroids: What should the emergency physician know? *Emergency Medicine Clinics of North America, 23*, 815–826, ix–x.

Carroll, K. M., Nich, C., Ball, S. A., McCance, E., Frankforter, T. L., Rounsaville, B. J. (2000). One-year follow-up of disulfiram and psychotherapy for cocaine-alcohol users: sustained effects of treatment. *Addiction, 95*, 1335–1349.

Crews, F., He, J., & Hodge, C. (2007). Adolescent cortical development: a critical period of vulnerability for addiction. *Pharmacology, Biochemistry & Behavior, 86*(2), 189–199.

Crowley, T. J., Riggs, P. D. (1995). Adolescent substance use disorder with conduct disorder and comorbid conditions. *NIDA Res Monogr, 156*, 49–111.

Deas, D. (2006). Adolescent substance abuse and psychiatric comorbidities. *Journal of Clinical Psychiatry, 67*(suppl 7), 18–23.

Deas, D., May, M. P., Randall, C., Johnson, N., Anton, R. (2005). Naltrexone treatment of adolescent alcoholics: an open-label pilot study. *J Child Adolescent Psychopharmacol, 15*, 723–728.

Foley, J. D. (2006). Adolescent use and misuse of marijuana. *Adolescent Medicine Clinics, 17*(2), 319–334.

Fournier, M. E., & Levy, S. (2006). Recent trends in adolescent substance use, primary care screening, and updates in treatment options. *Current Opinion in Pediatrics, 18*(4), 352–358.

Galanter, M., Glickman, L., & Singer, D. (2007). An overview of outpatient treatment of adolescent substance abuse. *Substance Abuse, 28*(2), 51–58.

Griswold, K. S., Aronoff, H., Kernan, J. B., & Kahn, L.S. (2008). Adolescent substance use and abuse: recognition and management. *American Family Physician, 77*(3), 331–336.

Hall, W. D., & Lynskey, M. (2005). Is cannabis a gateway drug? Testing hypotheses about the relationship between cannabis use and the use of other illicit drugs. *Drug Alcohol Review, 24*, 39–48.

Hopfer, C., & Riggs, P. (2007). Substance use disorders. In A. Martin & F. Volkmar (Eds.), *Lewis's Child and Adolescent Psychiatry: A Comprehensive Textbook*, 4th edition, pp. 615–624. Philadelphia: Lippincott Williams & Wilkins.

Hopfer, C. J., Crowley, T. J., Hewitt, J. K. (2003). Review of twin and adoption studies of adolescent substance use. *J Am Acad Child Adolesc Psychiatry, 42*, 710–719.

Johnson, L. D., O'Malley, P. M., Bachman, J. G., & Schulenberg, J. E. (2005). *Monitoring the Future: National Survey Results on Drug Use, 1975–2004. Volume 1: Secondary School Students*. Bethesda, MD: National Institute on Drug Abuse; 680. NIH Publication No. 05-5727.

Kandel, D. B., Yamaguchi, K., & Chen, K. (1992). Stages of progression in drug involvement from adolescence to adulthood: Further evidence for the gateway theory. *Journal of the Study of Alcohol, 53*, 447–457.

Lynsky, M. T., Glowinski, A. L., Todorov, A. A., et al. (2004). Major depressive disorder, suicidal ideation, and suicide attempts in twins discordant for cannabis dependence and early-onset cannabis use. *Archives of General Psychiatry, 61*, 1026–1032.

Marsch, L. A., Bickel, W. K., Badger, G. J., et al. (2005). Comparison of pharmacological treatments for opioid-dependent adolescents: a randomized controlled trial. *Arch Gen Psychiatry, 62*, 1157–1164.

Musto, D. F. (1999). *The American Disease: Origins of Narcotic Control*, 3rd edition. New York: Oxford University Press.

Nanda, S., & Konnur, N. (2006). Adolescent drug & alcohol use in the 21st century. *Pediatric Annals, 35*(3), 193–199.

Niederhofer, H., Staffen, W. (2003). Acamprosate and its efficacy in treating alcohol dependent adolescents. *Eur Child Adolesc Psychiatry, 12,* 144–148.

Perepletchikova, F., Krystal, J. H., & Kaufman, J. (2008). Practitioner review: Adolescent alcohol use disorders: Assessment and treatment issues. *Journal of Child Psychology & Psychiatry & Allied Disciplines, 49*(11), 1131–1154.

Riggs, P. D., Lohman, M., Davies, R., et al. (2005). *Randomized Controlled Trial of Fluoxetine/Placebo and CBT in Depressed Adolescents with Substance Use Disorders*. Paper presented at the 2005 Annual Meeting of the American Academy Addiction Psychiatry, Scottsdale, AZ.

Sakai, J. T., Hall, S. K., Mikulich-Gilbertson, S. K., & Crowley, T. J. (2004). Inhalant use, abuse, and dependence among adolescent patients: Commonly comorbid problems. *Journal of the American Academy of Child and Adolescent Psychiatry, 43,* 1080–1088.

Schepis, T. S., Adinoff, B., & Rao, U. (2008). Neurobiological processes in adolescent addictive disorders. *American Journal on Addictions, 17*(1), 6–23.

Ziedonis, D., Haberstroh, S., Hanos Zimmermann, M., Miceli, M., & Foulds, J. (2006). Adolescent tobacco use and dependence: assessment and treatment strategies. *Adolescent Medicine Clinics, 17*(2), 381–410.

Zimmermann, U. S., Blomeyer, D., Laucht, M., & Mann, K. F. (2007). How gene-stress-behavior interactions can promote adolescent alcohol use: The roles of predrinking allostatic load and childhood behavior disorders. *Pharmacology, Biochemistry & Behavior, 86*(2), 246–262.

CHAPTER 16 ■ SLEEP AND SLEEP DISORDERS

BACKGROUND

There have been major advances in understanding sleep and sleep problems in both children and adults over the past several decades. This began with the advent of polysomnographic (PSG) sleep recording in the 1950s and the description of rapid eye movement (REM) and non–rapid eye movement (NREM) sleep. Consensus on nosology and classification and the development of both sleep laboratories and clinical training programs have advanced the field. Sleep disorders medicine has now been recognized and includes a pediatric section (see Anders, 2007, for detailed discussion).

THE ORGANIZATION OF SLEEP: DEVELOPMENTAL ASPECTS

The organization of sleep–wake patterns has marked developmental aspects. Adults spend about 80% of their sleep time in NREM sleep and 20% in REM. In contrast, newborn infants spend about half of their time in REM sleep. Other differences include the duration of sleep and the length of the average sleep cycles. By adolescence, individuals archive the pattern of sleep organization seen in adults (Table 16.1). Other differences include the pattern of sleep. When adults begin to sleep, they typically start in stage 4 of NREM sleep and spend a considerable initial period in this sleep stage before the REM–NREM cycles recur, at intervals of about 90 minutes, during the night. Proportionally, most of the REM sleep occurs in the latter part of the sleep cycle in adults. Interestingly, infants have sleep patterns associated with an initial REM period and with REM and NREM sleep alternating through much of the night. The gradual reorganization of the sleep cycles begins early in life as central timing mechanisms become more active.

For developing infants (and for the parents), the regulation of sleep–wake cycles and the ability to sleep through the night are important tasks that provide important opportunities for interaction and set the stage for other aspects of self-regulation. Difficulties in this process thus typically require some assessment of psychosocial and parent–child issues that might be having an impact. Factors important in this regard include the physical and mental health of the caregivers, their own history of being parents and experiences of sleep, social and family support and resources, and the infant's own temperament (see Chapter 2). The latter has

TABLE 16.1

SLEEP–WAKE STATE CHANGES WITH AGE

	Infants	Adults
REM/NREM %	50/50	20/80
Ultradian cycle	50–60 min	90 min
Circadian cycle	Polyphasic	Diurnal
Temporal	Equidistributed	Fast third, last third
Sleep stages	States only	Four stages of NREM

NREM, non–rapid eye movement; REM, rapid eye movement.
From Anders, T. F. (2007). Sleep disorders. In A. Martin & F. Volkmar (Eds.), *Lewis's Child and Adolescent Psychiatry: A Comprehensive Textbook*, 4th edition (pp. 625). Philadelphia: Lippincott Williams & Wilkins.

increasingly been recognized as a critical aspect of the situation. Cultural, family, and other environmental influences may be important as are other potential variables such as the physical conditions of the infant and mother. There are frequently complicated interactions between the infant's sleep pattern and the entire family's ability to sleep through the night. In clinical practice, all possible permutations and combinations are seen (e.g., some infants may sleep or nap at day care but not at home or an infant may be more readily put to bed by a nanny or other caretaker than the parents). Occasionally, infants sleep better for one parent or the other (a particularly complex family dynamic). Figures 16.1 and 16.2 illustrate idealized sleep–wake patterns in newborns and one year olds, respectively, and Figure 16.3 provides a schematic of the context in which sleep problems emerge.

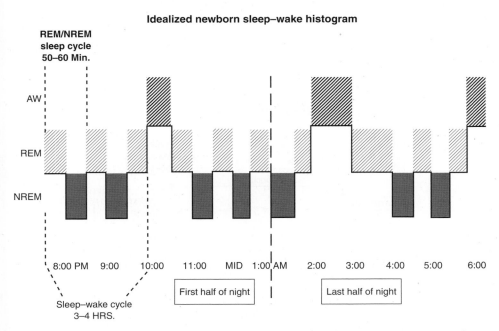

FIGURE 16.1. Note the regular distribution (~50:50) between rapid eye movement (REM) and non–rapid eye movement (NREM) sleep throughout the sleep cycle and the initial REM sleep period at sleep onset. (From Anders, T. F. (2007). Sleep disorders. In A. Martin & F. Volkmar (Eds.), *Lewis's Child and Adolescent Psychiatry: A Comprehensive Textbook*, 4th edition (p. 626). Philadelphia: Lippincott Williams & Wilkins.)

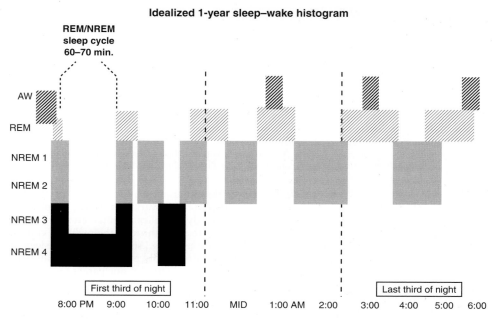

Idealized 1-year sleep–wake histogram

REM/NREM sleep cycle 60–70 min.

AW

REM

NREM 1

NREM 2

NREM 3

NREM 4

First third of night

Last third of night

8:00 PM   9:00   10:00   11:00   MID   1:00 AM   2:00   3:00   4:00   5:00   6:00

FIGURE 16.2. Note that the majority of non–rapid eye movement (NREM) 3 and 4 occurs during the first third of the night and that rapid eye movement (REM) periods progressively lengthen during the middle and last third of the sleep cycle. The initial REM sleep bout is brief and sometimes absent. The descent to NREM stages 3 to 4 is rapid. (From Anders, T. F. (2007). Sleep disorders. In A. Martin & F. Volkmar (Eds.), *Lewis's Child and Adolescent Psychiatry: A Comprehensive Textbook*, 4th edition (p. 626). Philadelphia: Lippincott Williams & Wilkins.)

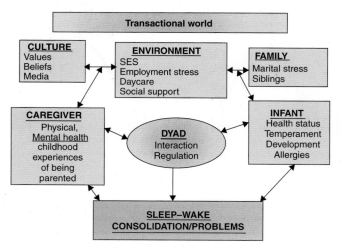

FIGURE 16.3. Transactional world. (From Anders, T. F. (2007). Sleep disorders. In A. Martin & F. Volkmar (Eds.), *Lewis's Child and Adolescent Psychiatry: A Comprehensive Textbook*, 4th edition (p. 627). Philadelphia: Lippincott Williams & Wilkins.)

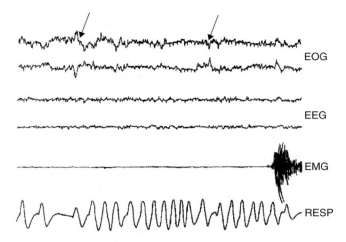

FIGURE 16.4. Polygraphic recording of rapid eye movement (REM) sleep. An epoch of REM sleep in a newborn infant characterized by a low-voltage, fast electroencephalogram; active rapid eye movements (*arrows*); an inhibited electromyograph; and rapid irregular respirations. (From Anders, T. F. (2007). Sleep disorders. In A. Martin & F. Volkmar (Eds.), *Lewis's Child and Adolescent Psychiatry: A Comprehensive Textbook*, 4th edition (pp. 630). Philadelphia: Lippincott Williams & Wilkins.

The typical sleep laboratory usually obtains a variety of measures during a sleep study. These include measures of peripheral muscle tone and eye movements and an electroencephalogram (EEG) as well as other measures of cardiac, respiratory, and peripheral motor activity. Typically, these measures are obtained from nighttime recordings in a sleep laboratory, although sometimes several nights of recording are required, particularly for children, given the potential for the various sensors and unfamiliar setting to disrupt usual sleep patterns. Increasingly, there is potential for both home-based and 24-hour recording approaches, which have particularly value for children. Figures 16.4 and 16.5 present the differences in records of REM and NREM sleep in newborns and one year olds.

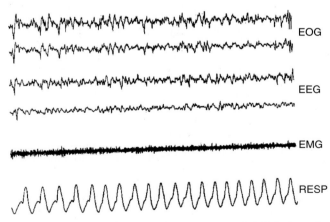

FIGURE 16.5. Polygraphic recording of non–rapid eye movement (NREM) sleep. An epoch of NREM sleep characterized by high-voltage, slow waves on the electroencephalogram; an absence of rapid eye movements; a tonic electromyograph pattern; and slowed, regular respirations. (From Anders, T. F. (2007). Sleep disorders. In A. Martin & F. Volkmar (Eds.), *Lewis's Child and Adolescent Psychiatry: A Comprehensive Textbook*, 4th edition (pp. 630). Philadelphia: Lippincott Williams & Wilkins.)

The EEG pattern during REM sleep is characterized by fast, low-voltage activity similar to that observed while the individual is awake. During REM sleep, there are bursts of eye movements and rapid, irregular breathing and heart rate patterns. Dreams are reported during REM sleep. Thus, although the individual appears to be sleeping, and is, significant central nervous system activity is noted. This is observed in infants as well, in whom it is sometimes referred to as *active sleep*. In contrast to the apparent activation during REM sleep, the pattern during NREM sleep is one associated with inhibition (e.g., slow and regular heart and breathing rate with EEG activity showing slower frequencies). In babies this stage is also referred to as *quiet sleep*.

CLASSIFICATION OF CHILDHOOD SLEEP DISORDERS

Various nosologies for classifying pediatric sleep disorders are available (see Anders, 2007, for a review), but none is totally adequate. Table 16.2 provides an overview of the *Diagnostic and Statistical Manual of Mental Disorder* (DSM-IV-TR) approach.

In the DSM-IV-TR, the dyssomnia (disruptions of REM–NREM patterns) include primary insomnia, primary hypersomnia, narcolepsy, and breathing-related sleep disorder as well as circadian rhythm sleep disorder (formerly referred to as *sleep–wake schedule disorder*) and an unspecified type. The parasomnias include nightmare disorder (formerly *dream anxiety disorder*), sleep terror disorder, and sleep walking disorder. In the parasomnias, there are intrusions of events in an otherwise normally organized sleep–wake process. Criteria for these conditions differ in the International Classification of Sleep Disorders: Diagnostic and Coding Manual, 2nd ed. (ICSF-DCM2) system in some respects (see Anders, 2007), but the DSM-IV-TR diagnostic criteria for dyssomnias in young children have been particularly criticized for being overly stringent.

In addition, sleep problems can be noted in association with other medical, psychiatric, or substance-induced difficulties. As a practical matter, several complaints about sleep are likely to arise in clinical practice.

INSOMNIA AND ESTABLISHING A SLEEP PATTERN

Parents frequently complain that their infants do not sleep through the night. There are wide variations in when this landmark is achieved developmentally; some infants do it very early in life but others not until much later. Sometimes the difficulties center around the child's falling to sleep (e.g., needing a long period of rocking or nursing). As children become slightly older, sleep issues may revolve around problems or wakening during the night and the ability to return (or not) to sleep independently. At times, these issues have significant impact on the family and become a source of parental disagreement. In reality, various issues impact this process. Particularly today when parents may work, the time preschoolers have at home with parents may be very highly valued by the preschooler. Parents may also engage in energizing activities having missed the child during the day. Various other factors, including potential overstimulation from television and other sources and lack of physical activity, may delay bedtime or be the source of arousal. Separation issues also can be important.

For many children, the use of familiar routine and of a transitional object (see Chapter 2) and the presence of a parent may help the child fall asleep. Establishing good sleep habits and use of a familiar (quieting) routine can also be helpful. Children with developmental vulnerabilities can be particularly prone to developing poor sleep patterns. For both typically developing and children with developmental disorders, several resources are available (see Selected Readings). In severe cases, pharmacological and behavioral methods (including cognitive behavior therapy) can be useful.

For older children and adolescents, sources of insomnia can include stress, substance abuse, and co-occurring mental illness (e.g., in bipolar disorder, the adolescent may remain awake through much of the night).

TABLE 16.2

AN OVERVIEW OF DSM-IV SLEEP DISORDERS MOST RELEVANT TO CHILDREN AND ADOLESCENTS[1]

Disorder (Type or Condition)	Clinical Description
Dyssomnias	Disruption of REM–NREM patterns with early wakening and disrupted sleep with too much or too little sleep or disturbed daily sleep rhythm pattern
Primary insomnia	More frequent in adults but can occur in children with stress or in association with other disorders (e.g., depression); for children, establishing good sleep patterns and regular routine is important
Primary hypersomnia	Long sleep periods after which the individual does not feel refreshed; may be associated with some medical conditions (e.g., Klein-Levin syndrome), related to insufficient sleep or substance abuse, or be idiopathic
Narcolepsy	Often associated with cataplexy, excessive daytime sleepiness, sleep paralysis, and hypnagogic hallucinations; REM sleep occurs quickly after onset of sleep and in daytime naps; sometimes seen without cataplexy; narcolepsy may also be associated with various medical conditions (e.g., Prader-Willi syndrome)
Breathing-related sleep disorder	Although not common in children, this can be observed in premature infants and those with congenital abnormalities or partial airway obstruction
Circadian rhythm sleep disorder	The usual sleep–wake cycle is disturbed; some developmentally delayed children have difficulty in adopting the usual sleep–wake cycle; may also be associated with substance abuse, jet lag, and so on
Parasomnias	Sleep is disrupted by partial arousal (e.g., movements, behaviors, affective states, dreams)
Nightmare disorder	Occurs during REM sleep; much more common in children than adults; may be associated with stress; can lead to insomnia and poor sleep habits
Sleepwalking disorder	Usually occurs during slow-wave sleep (NREM); individual may sit up or ambulate; exacerbated by sleep deprivation; when awake, the person is confused; occasionally a source of danger; frequent in children between ages of 4 and 8 years; typically diminishes with age
Sleep terror disorder	Child arouses suddenly with intense anxiety (including autonomic symptoms) but is difficult to awake with no recollection of the experience in the morning; events are associated with no or minimal mental content (i.e., no apparent nightmares); usually resolves without treatment

[1]Sleep problems may also be associated with a variety of medical conditions, substance abuse problems, and so forth.
NREM, non–rapid eye movement; REM, rapid eye movement.

Case Report: Night Terrors

Tommy, age 4 years, was brought to his pediatrician by his mother because she was concerned about what she thought might be seizures. Over the past months, he had experienced a number of episodes of awakening at night. At these times, he was fearful and cried but was hard to arouse (the reason the mother was concerned about seizures). These episodes were brief, lasting perhaps 10 minutes. During these episodes, Tommy appeared to be highly aroused, but he could not remember any bad dreams and indeed had no recollection of the event the next morning. These episodes came sporadically and apparently unpredictably over the past month but usually seemed to happen about 90 minutes after he had fallen to sleep. The parents had taken several steps to give him a more stable bedtime routine but with no apparent impact on these episodes, which now occurred at least once every week. The physical examination (including neurological examination) results were normal, and Tommy appeared to be developing appropriately.

The pediatrician suspected night terrors and provided the mother with information and reassurance. She was urged to be sure he was safe and comfort him but not attempt to waken him. Over the next several months, these episodes began to diminish.

Comment: Unlike nightmares, night terrors typically occur early in the night's sleep. The child is difficult to arouse and has no recollection of the event in the morning. Typically, these disappear by adolescence, and no specific treatment is indicated.

Nightmares and Night Terrors

Toddlers often start to report dreaming by the time they are around 3 years of age, and nightmares follow shortly thereafter. These occur during REM sleep and thus tend to be noted in the last part of the night. In contrast to night terrors, these have content, often involving issues of injury or separation, monsters, and so forth. Nightmares become more frequent in children who experience the effects of stress.

In night terrors, there is a period of marked arousal and agitation with limited responsiveness. Sleep studies reveal high-voltage delta waves on the EEG typical of NREM stage 4 sleep associated with marked autonomic arousal. These episodes are dramatic and a source of parental anxiety; however, they are typically brief (3 to 5 minutes) but sometimes longer. Parents can awaken the child who will, however, typically be confused and disoriented. The child is amnesic for the episode. These events often occur just before a transition to REM sleep while the child transitions from NREM stage 4 sleep (the deepest stage) of sleep. It is interesting that there is a marked male (six to eight times) predominance and also a strong male familial basis for this condition. In contrast to nightmares, night terrors are *not* associated with vivid dream imagery, are not remembered the following day, and are not associated with mental content. Stress and overexertion may be related to a need for more NREM stage 4 sleep; regular sleep habits are also helpful and a nap after school can also be helpful. In some situations, the problem may lead to difficulties (e.g., with sleeping at a friend's house), and a benzodiazepine medication may be helpful (although not curative of the problem). Sometimes sleep-related seizures can be a source of confusion (particularly in adolescent-onset cases). Because the situation is typically time limited, reassurance and parental support are mainstays of treatment. If there is an issue of seizure activity, a sleep study can help to resolve the diagnosis in some cases.

Obstructive Sleep Apnea

Although more common in adults, obstructive sleep apnea is sometimes seen in young children, particularly those with enlarged tonsils and adenoids. Snoring is usually present. Less commonly, obesity may contribute to the problem and, on occasion, a birth defect can result in narrowing of the airway during sleep. In this condition, periods of brief awakening restore breathing alternating with apneic episodes and produce highly fragmented sleep. This in turn leads to fatigue and sleepiness during the day. Occasionally, this can present as inattention and even hyperactivity as the child copes with his or her somnolence. Sometimes the problem interferes with growth hormone secretion, leading to growth retardation. Treatment varies depending on the age of the child and the clinical circumstances.

Sleep Walking

Similar to night terrors, sleepwalking occurs relatively quickly (1.5 to 2 hours) after sleep onset. The child may sit up and even leave the bed and might be found sleeping in a new spot in the morning with no recollection of having moved. The individual is difficult to arouse but seems confused if awakened. There is some danger of injury, and parents should be careful to attend to safety issues such as securing windows, locking doors, and so forth. The individual may become confused and combative if aroused.

Although popular press reports suggest complex activity, such as driving, is possible, in reality this is very unusual. Similarly, sleep talking is typically confined to NREM stage 4 sleep with short episodes that are usually garbled and unremembered the next morning. Sleep walking is relatively common in children and decreases dramatically, often disappearing during adolescence.

Narcolepsy

Narcolepsy often has an onset in adolescence. It is the only disorder of REM sleep and usually has its onset at this time. This condition is associated with problems in the brainstem mechanisms regulation of sleep–wake cycles. In classic narcolepsy, four symptoms are present. These include attacks of REM sleep that intrude on wakefulness, loss of peripheral muscle tone bilaterally (catalepsy), hypnagogic hallucinations, and sleep paralysis. The condition is lifelong with a peak age at onset in adolescence and young adulthood. A strong role for genetic factors has been suggested, and mechanisms related to cholinergic–dopaminergic interactions are implicated. Adolescents with the condition nap every 3 to 4 hours for short (20- to 40-minute) times but feel refreshed after sleeping (unlike people with other conditions). To make a definitive diagnosis, a sleep study is needed. Treatment is individualized but frequently includes the use of stimulants for sleepiness in the daytime with the use of tricyclics for cataplexy. The latter appear to suppress REM sleep in the daytime; the selective serotonin reuptake inhibitors have been increasingly used given their more favorable side effect profile. Although pharmacological interventions are very useful in this disorder, the clinician should also attend to other issues, including careful monitoring, use of naps, and so forth. The monoamine oxidase inhibitors can be used in the treatment of both cataplexy and REM sleep onset symptoms. A new agent, modafinil (Provigil), may be more effective than traditional stimulants.

Interestingly, one retrospective study of adults suggested high rates of attention-deficit/hyperactivity disorder in adolescence (when treatment with stimulants is frequent). Narcolepsy is relatively rare (on the order of one in 2500 individuals). However, the condition is a source of both social and school problems and is frequent associated with anxiety or mood problems as well as substance abuse. Counseling and other supportive measures are important components of treatment as is encouragement of regular sleep and bedtime patterns. Self-support groups are also helpful.

Circadian Rhythm Sleep Disorder

This condition is more frequent in adolescents, who often accumulate sleep deficits because of late sleep onset and early arousal for school. Often, the adolescent will begin to "sleep

Case Report: Narcolepsy with Cataplexy

Joe, a 16-year-old boy, a junior in high school, complained of trouble with being tired and constantly sleepy for several years. He complained that he often fell asleep in classes, even ones he was interested in. Getting a good night's sleep and taking an afternoon nap had not helped. He was now worried about driving a car because over the past several months, had several episodes of "zoning out" while he was in the car with his parents. The recent observation, during one of these episodes, of slurred speech and what appeared to be motor weakness prompted an evaluation for possible seizures. His parents were also concerned because he told them he sometimes seemed to see things on going to sleep. Neurological and psychiatric examination results were normal apart from the history. Joe reported seeing some unusual visual patterns (typically vivid bright spots or lines) when going to sleep. The neurologist requested a sleep study. This demonstrated noteworthy decreases in sleep latency and the onset of rapid eye movement (REM) sleep. Because of the combination of narcolepsy with cataplexy, he was treated with both a stimulant medication (methylphenidate) and a tricyclic antidepressant (TCA) with considerable improvement. The latter included his academic performance. It is common for individuals with narcolepsy to also exhibit cataplexy.

Subsequently, although Joe did reasonably well academically he still had some difficulties socially. He also became more anxious and began to drink as an apparent result. An increased focus on psychosocial supports, a schedule of regular sleep and naps, and some academic accommodations were very helpful to him.

Comment: Both academic and social difficulties are frequent in patients with the condition. Additional psychiatric difficulties can include anxiety and mood problems and increased risk for substance abuse. Schedules in schoolwork (or occupation) that accommodate the special needs of the individual and provision of psychosocial supports are beneficial.

in" over the weekends, and there is a gradual shift of the sleep cycle away from usual hours. Unfortunately, adolescents need 9 to 10 hours of sleep every evening, and many adolescents fail to achieve this goal. Various interventions have been used for treatment, including use of bright lights to alter the internal biological rhythm. Melatonin has also been used, and a prescription form is available in the United States for treatment of sleep-onset insomnia but is widely used for circadian sleep problems as well. For developmentally delayed children, working to establish a stable day–night cycle is helpful (see Durand, 1997).

Sleep Problems in Psychiatric and Medical Disorders

Although information is relatively limited, it does appear that sleep problems are very frequently associated with other psychiatric and medical conditions. For example, children reared in institutions and with significant developmental problems exhibit a range of sleep difficulties. Although frequently reported in association with a range of psychiatric conditions, the association of sleep problems with other conditions is a topic of controversy. It does appear that although some children with major depression frequently have disturbed sleep patterns, others do not. Similarly, attention-deficit disorder is frequently associated, by parents, with a disturbed sleep patterns, but confirmatory data are limited. Adolescents with substance abuse problems can exhibit either of two sleep problems; there can be decreased REM sleep and generally more disrupted sleep associated with withdrawal from various agents, and intoxication can be associated with prolonged periods of atypical sleep. Various complexities, including issues of dose, differences in substances of abuse, and chronicity of abuse, can impact sleep problems. Although initially increasing sleep, the chronic use of sedatives is associated with sleep, particularly REM sleep, deprivation. Self-medication with alcohol or other agents can occur and frequently complicates clinical assessment (i.e., in the ascertainment of whether the degree of substance use or abuse has caused sleep disruption or whether problems with sleep led to substance abuse). Intervention in these cases depends on the underlying cause of the sleep problem.

OBTAINING A SLEEP HISTORY

The clinician is well advised to take a careful sleep history in children with specific sleep-related complaints and, indeed, in all children with behavior problems. This detailed history includes a thorough review of sleep-related symptoms, a history of sleep problems, and review of sleep difficulties in other members of the family. The sleep history will include a review of the onset of difficulties, their frequency, their stability, and so forth. This history will also include attention to the child's typical sleep habits, a review of sleeping arrangements, and so forth.

The use of a sleep diary or log before evaluation is often helpful. This documents the stability (or variability) of the difficulties. Several instruments, including the Child Sleep Habits Questionnaire (CSHQ) and the Pediatric Sleep Questionnaire (PSQ), are useful in documenting sleep problems and associated difficulties. Some instruments have been adapted for use in younger children, and other screening instruments have now been developed. Various guides designed specifically to help parents deal with sleep problems in both typically developing children and those with disabilities are available (Durand, 1997; Ferber, 1985).

SUMMARY

Considerable progress has been made in our understanding of sleep–wake cycles in children and adolescents. Many sleep disorders can now been treated. In some areas, knowledge remains limited. Clearly, sleep problems can have important negative effects on growing children. Available research on sleep disorders in preschool children is limited, and the nature of sleep problems in relation to both general medical and psychiatric donations remains controversial. Larger scale treatment studies are needed to establish the efficacy of commonly recommended treatments, although increasingly effective treatments are available.

Selected Readings

American Academy of Sleep Medicine. (2005). *The International Classification of Sleep Disorders, Diagnostic and Coding Manual (ICSD)*, 2nd edition. Westchester, IL: American Academy of Sleep Medicine.

American Psychiatric Association. (2004). *Diagnostic and Statistical Manual of Mental Disorders-TR*, 4th edition. Washington, DC: Author.

Anders, T., & Dahl, R. (2006). Classifying sleep disorders in infants and toddlers. In I. Chatoor & D. Pine. (Eds.), *A Research Agenda for DSM-V*. Washington DC: American Psychiatric Association.

Anders, T. F. (2007). Sleep disorders. In A. Martin & F. Volkmar (Eds.), *Lewis's Child and Adolescent Psychiatry: A Comprehensive Textbook*, 4th edition, pp. 623–632. Philadelphia: Lippincott Williams & Wilkins.

Broughton, R. J. (2000). The treatment of narcolepsy. *Supplement to Clinical Neurophysiology*, 53, 371–374.

Chemelli, R., Willie, J., Sinton, C., et al. (1999). Narcolepsy in orexin knockout mice: Molecular genetics of sleep regulation. *Cell 98*, 47–51.

Chervin, R. D., Aldrich, M. S., Pickett, R., & Guilleminault, C. (1997). Comparison of the results of the Epworth Sleepiness Scale and the Multiple Sleep Latency Test. *Journal of Psychosomatic Research*, 42, 145–155.

Carskadon, M., & Dement, W. (1987). Sleepiness in normal adolescents. In C. Guilleminault (Ed.), *Sleep and Its Disorders in Children*, pp. 53–66. New York: Raven.

Dahl, R., & Puig-Antich, J. (1990). Sleep disturbances in child and adolescent psychiatric disorders. *Pediatrician 17*, 32–37.

Durand, V. M. (1997). *Sleep Better: A Guide to Improving Sleep for Children with Special Needs*. Baltimore, MD: Brooks Publishing.

Ferber, R. (1985). *Solve Your Child's Sleep Problems*. New York: Simon & Schuster.

Gromov, I., & Gromov, D. (2009). Sleep and substance use and abuse in adolescents. *Child & Adolescent Psychiatric Clinics of North America*, 18(4), 929–946.

Hoban, T. F. (2010). Sleep disorders in children. *Annals of the New York Academy of Sciences, 1184*, 1–14.

Ivanenko, A., & Gururaj, B. R. (2009). Classification and epidemiology of sleep disorders. *Child & Adolescent Psychiatric Clinics of North America, 18*(4), 839–848.

O'Brien, L. M. (2009). The neurocognitive effects of sleep disruption in children and adolescents. *Child & Adolescent Psychiatric Clinics of North America, 18*(4), 813–823.

Owens, J., Maxim, R., Nobile, C., McGuinn, M., & Msall, M. (2000). Parental and self-report of sleep in children with attention-deficit/hyperactivity disorder. *Archives of Pediatric and Adolescent Medicine, 154*, 549–555.

Owens, J. A., & Moturi, S. (2009). Pharmacologic treatment of pediatric insomnia. *Child & Adolescent Psychiatric Clinics of North America, 18*(4), 1001–1016.

Powell, S., Kubba, H., O'Brien, C., & Tremlett, M. (2010). Paediatric obstructive sleep apnoea. *BMJ, 340*:c1018–1023.

Stores, G., & Wiggs, L. (Eds.). (2001). *Sleep Disturbance in Children and Adolescents with Disorders of Development: Its Significance and Management. Clinics in Developmental Medicine*, p. 155. London: Mac Keith Press.

CHAPTER 17 ■ SOMATOFORM DISORDERS

The somatoform disorders present important challenges in relation to medical and psychiatric systems of care. The child or adolescent may present with dramatic or painful somatic symptoms even when no pathological process is demonstrable. These symptoms challenge the model of medicine practiced in the United States and other developed countries, where distinctions between physical and mental illnesses tend to be drawn rather sharply and where differences in conceptualization (i.e., of mental and physical illness) may make for major differences in both treatment and reimbursement of care. Child and adolescents with what appear to be "functional" problems tend to be viewed with suspicion and distrust. The original concept of neurosis, as developed by Freud and others, particularly Freud's conceptualization of hysteria, underscored the attempt to understand physical symptoms in the apparent absence of medical disease. Developmental issues are important, as anyone who has dealt with young children is very much aware, given the potential anxiety related to bodily experiences in this age group.

DEFINITION AND CLINICAL FEATURES

The *Diagnostic and Statistical Manual of Mental Disorder* (DSM-IV-TR) recognizes several conditions in which symptoms suggest a physical disorder but are not adequately explained by the presence of an associated general medical condition. These include *somatization disorder, undifferentiated somatoform disorder, conversion disorder, pain disorder, hypochondriasis, body dysmorphic disorder (BDD),* and *somatoform disorder not otherwise specified (NOS).* These diagnoses require clinical judgment about the extent to which a particularly symptom does or does not arise from a general medical condition and whether that disorder, if present, is sufficient to account for the patient's difficulties. By definition, these disorders do not represent conscious falsification or malingering. They are also distinguished from *psychological factors affecting medical conditions.* Given the potential of children to experience somatic symptoms with a range of problems, notably anxiety disorders, a clinical judgment must be made about whether the somatic symptoms are most appropriately ("better") explained by a different condition. As a result of all these factors, these diagnoses may be among the least reliable ones made in child psychiatry. It is particularly important for the clinician to be supportive and not to rush to premature judgment because sometimes the true nature of difficulties will only become apparent over time. On the other hand, if findings are negative and the child or adolescent's functioning is significantly impacted, it is important that plans for treatment and

TABLE 17.1

THE SOMATOFORM DISORDERS: AN OVERVIEW

Condition	Diagnostic Features	Other Information
Somatoform disorder	Multiple symptoms, including pain (multiple sites); GI (at least two symptoms); and some sexual, reproductive, or other (nonpain) symptoms	Diagnosis is unusual in children (partly because of the definition); concept has its origins in Briquet's description (he noted that symptoms typically began before adulthood)
Undifferentiated somatoform disorder	Multiple somatic complaints, various body systems or locations, lasting at least 6 months	Children are more likely to qualify for this diagnosis
Conversion disorder	One or more symptoms in voluntary motor or sensory system suggesting neurological or other medical condition, but symptoms appear to have a psychological basis (e.g., might arise after stress, family model of illness) and often the child is not particularly disturbed by the symptom (*la belle indifference*)	In children and adolescents, apparent seizures, paralysis, sensory symptom(s), or gait problems are most common; various subtypes proposed based on symptom nature (motor, sensory, seizures, mixed motor and sensory)
Pain disorder	Pain in one (or more) sites causing clinical attention and distress or impairment	Subtypes include association with psychological factors, medical condition, or both
Hypochondriasis	Persistent fear or belief that a child or adolescent has a physical disease; must last at least 6 months	Issues of overlap with anxiety disorders, and OCD in particular has been noted
Body dysmorphic disorder	Either a slight or imagined body defect becomes preoccupation, causing distress or impairment	Limited information in children and adolescents is available, but the condition clearly starts during this time in some cases; skin concerns are most common; possible relationship to OCD
Somatoform disorder not otherwise specified	A residual category used when an individual does not meet specific criteria for one of the somatoform disorders but symptoms are present	This category would be used, for example, in cases not yet meeting time or duration criteria

GI, gastrointestinal; OCD, obsessive-compulsive disorder.

intervention move forward. Various alternatives to the current approach have been considered and it is likely that changes will be made in these categories and their definitions in the future (Campo & Fritz, 2005). Table 17.1 provides an overview of these disorders.

In *somatization disorder*, various, multiple somatic complaints are present in association with requests for medical treatment or some significant impairment. These complaints must have their onset before age 30 years. The DSM-IV-TR required multiple (at least four) pain symptoms in various part of the body or /bodily functions, at least two gastrointestinal (GI), one sexual, and one apparently neurological symptoms. By definition, these difficulties have not been explained after reasonably medical assessment or, if a medical condition is present, the degree of impairment or complaint is excessive. By definition, the disorder cannot be one that is consciously produced (in such a situation malingering or "factitious" disorder) would be diagnosed. In undifferentiated somatoform disorder, the patient has ether one or more physical complaints, which again, do not appear to be explained adequately by a medical condition or use of a drug or medication or, if such a condition were present, the impairment or complaint is greater than would be expected.

The notion of somatoform disorder has its roots in the notions of hysteria or, as it is sometimes termed, *Briquet's syndrome*. Briquet noted that the onset was often in childhood or adolescence and that early onset seemed to prefigure worse outcome. The DSM-IV-TR criteria are somewhat detailed and arbitrary and require some sexual symptoms, which makes the diagnosis somewhat more difficult (but not impossible to make) in children. Children and adolescents with complaints in various locations who do not meet criteria for somatization disorder often do meet criteria for *undifferentiated somatoform disorder*, although this requires a minimum duration of 6 months. This term roughly corresponds to an old term, *neurasthenia*, which is no longer recognized in the DSM-IV.

The diagnosis of conversion disorder is made when there is a disturbance in voluntary motor or sensory functions suggesting a specific medical or neurological disorder but when psychological factors appear to play a major role (e.g., stress, conflict, or bereavement). Frequent presenting symptoms include the onset of paralysis, a movement problem, or other muscular or sensory disturbance after some stress. Typically, the child or adolescent is much less concerned about the symptom than either parents or physicians; the term *la belle indifference* has been used to refer to this phenomenon. Symptoms may also take the form of sensory symptoms or apparent seizures, gait disturbance, or paralysis. Although usually self-limited, these symptoms can occasionally result in long-term disability. The DSM-IV-TR makes various distinctions between subtypes based on the nature of the symptoms present (e.g., motor, sensory, seizures, mixed). The condition is unusual in that psychological factors are thought to be clearly associated with the symptom or disturbance, which must be a source of distress or impairment. The diagnosis is not made if the condition is factious or if the problem is limited to pain or sexual dysfunction.

In pain disorder, pain is present in one or multiple sites and is sufficient to warrant attention and cause distress or impairment. The subtypes of this disorder reflect the degree to which the difficulties are associated with a medical condition, a psychological factor, or some combination of the two. A further distinction is made based on chronicity (shorter vs. longer than 6 months' duration).

In hypochondrias, the child or adolescent fears or indeed believes that he or she has a significant medical condition, and this fear persists for at least 6 months even when medical reassurance is provided. The term *somatosensory amplification* refers to the misinterpretation or experience of excessive concern related to one or more physical sensations. The condition must be differentiated from delusional disorder; in the latter, the concern is of delusional proportion. The condition is not diagnosed if the preoccupation or belief is related to some perceived body defect; in such cases, BDD (described subsequently) is the more appropriate diagnosis. Differentiation from other conditions (e.g., obsessive-compulsive disorder [OCD]) can be a challenge at times, and in some ways, hypochondria might just as appropriately be viewed as an anxiety disorder.

In BDD, there is preoccupation with either a real, although slight, or imagined defect in physical appearance. This must be the source of significant distress or impairment. Although the literature on this topic in children is very limited, it does appear that in perhaps 10% of cases the onset is in childhood or adolescence. Any body area or part can be the focus of the preoccupation, although skin concerns (scars, facial acne, other blemishes) are most common. BDD is one of the easier diagnoses to miss because it often the focus of much shame, and attempts are made to conceal it. Furthermore, the condition may present more in dermatologic or surgical settings, where an awareness of real lesions (even if self-inflicted) may lead to the impression of a significant medical problem and to treatment. Efforts to conceal the presumed defect may be considerable. In many ways, this condition is closely related to OCD.

A final category, *somatoform disorder NOS*, is made when symptoms consistent with a diagnosis in this group of disorders are present but the individual fails to meet specific guidelines for one of the other, better defined, disorders.

EPIDEMIOLOGY AND DEMOGRAPHICS

As any pediatrician or primary care provider can attest, it is very common for children (and or their parents) to present with physical symptoms without an apparent medical etiology. Available research on the topic is complicated by many factors (e.g., changes in definition, problems in case finding and sample selection, overreliance on a single informant, or a selective focus on some symptoms to the exclusion of others). A major problem arises relative to the issue of a symptom's being medically "unexplained." Sometimes early in the course of an illness, the child or adolescent may present with vague symptoms without having, as yet, developed characteristic physical findings, and it is important that the clinician keep this in mind before "writing off" patients with unexplained pain or physical complaints. A failure to include careful medical examination at the time and at follow-up is another limitation of much of the available case report literature.

About 50% of preschool- and school-age children will report at least one functional somatic symptom. Often, more than one complaint is present. One study (Offord et al, 1987) found recurrent, but distressing, symptoms in 4% of boys and 11% of girls (ages 12 to 16 years of age). It is common for multiple complaints and symptoms to cluster together. Similarly, chronic pain is a relatively frequent complaint in children and adolescents with a prevalence of perhaps 25%. Medications for pain are frequently given, and medical evaluations are common. Headache is the most frequently reported pain symptom in children and adolescents and probably accounts for 1 to 2% of all outpatient pediatric visits. Other frequent complaints include functional abdominal pain frequently associated with other GI symptoms. Complaints of chest pain are also relatively frequent. Other functional difficulties may include chronic fatigue, musculoskeletal aches and pains, and fatigue. The latter is more frequent in adolescents, and GI complaints are more common in preschool children (Abu-Arafeh & Russell, 1995).

Conversion symptoms are most frequently seen in specialized centers, at least within Western cultures, typically because of concern for possible seizure. Important cultural and societal influences have been noted (e.g., conversion symptoms are more frequently observed in non-Western settings). One prospective study conducted in Europe found the prevalence of somatoform disorders and symptoms to be about 3% with as many as 10% of individuals reporting difficulties that did not meet threshold for a specific diagnosis. Pain disorder was the most frequent specific diagnosis; diagnoses of other conditions were much less common. For individuals with somatic complaints, these did, however, tend to persist over time with some fluctuation

---

Headache

Distinctions have traditionally been made between *migraine* and *tension-type headache (TTH)*. In migraine headache, the child or adolescent has recurrent headache attacks lasting from 1 hour to several days; in contrast to tension headaches, migraines usually have moderate to severe pain, are located unilaterally, often have a pulsatile quality, and can be aggravated by activity. These may be associated with nausea, vomiting, or photophobia. An aura, including sensory or motor symptoms, may precede the headache. In contrast TTHs are usually bilateral, nonpulsatile, not worsened by activity, and have mild to moderate levels of intensity.

in presentation. Girls are more likely than boys to complain of somatoform illness, particularly in later childhood and adolescence, with lower socioeconomic status, and after specific stressful events. Sexual trauma or other traumatic events were also associated with higher rates of somatoform disorder. Frequently associated conditions included anxiety or mood disorder and substance abuse problems. Estimates of BDD have varied from about 1% to 2%.

As noted previously, age has an important influence on the expression of these conditions. Whereas younger children are more likely to complain of GI symptoms, adolescents may complain of fatigue. Headache is more evenly distributed as a complaint across children and adolescents. With adolescence, the complexity of the presentation often increases, with multiple body areas and presenting symptoms. Conversion disorder and BDD become more common during adolescence. Cultural factors may also be important in the clinical presentation.

ETIOLOGY

A family history of medically unexplained physical symptoms is frequently observed in these conditions. Both difficulties with chronic fatigue and somatization disorder tend to cluster within families. Parental illness is also a risk factor as is the presence of functional symptoms in parents. The nature of etiological mechanisms is unclear (e.g., exposure to parents with high levels of anxiety about health or high use of health care providers may be important as a model for ways to cope with anxiety and stress). Other family influences may also be operative (e.g., in diverting parents from marital problems). Risk factors in children include behavioral inhibition and patterns of chronic worry or anxiety or mood problems. There is also some suggestion of a heritable component (i.e., apart from modeling), and most investigators assume that an interplay of genetic and environmental factors is important in pathogenesis.

Traumatic experiences and other stressful life events have also been implicated in the pathogenesis. Since the time of Freud, sexual maltreatment has been related to specific somatic symptoms and somatoform disorders. Other stresses identified as risk factors include parental neglect and abuse as well as other trauma (e.g., accidents).

DIFFERENTIAL DIAGNOSIS AND EVALUATION

As noted previously, individuals with somatoform disorders have high rates of psychiatric symptoms and disorders. Risk is particularly high for anxiety and depressive symptoms in children with complaints of chronic pain or fatigue. The presence of these difficulties can further increase levels of functional impairment (e.g., with significant impact on school attendance and performance). Other conditions associated with functional symptoms include substance abuse, eating disorders, and attention-deficit/hyperactivity disorder.

Assessment must be individualized. It is frequently the case that the child or adolescent will have been seen by many different health care professionals before psychiatric consultation. The latter is sometimes viewed as the "last resort" when sometimes very extensive medical evaluations have failed to reveal a specific medical etiology. Unfortunately, even in such circumstances, it can be difficult to be sure that an associated medical condition is not present. In addition, the referral for mental health consultation is often taken by the child and parents as having the difficulties "written off." In this regard, it is important to note that the child's distress, pain, and impairment are very real, and an acknowledgment of this and of the family's understandable concern is indicated.

Depending on the history, families and the child may have developed an adversarial relationship with health care providers. The patient and family should be helped to view the mental health professional's concern as genuine. Attempts to dismiss or diminish the degree of difficulty will usually not succeed. Rather, an attempt should be made to develop a working therapeutic alliance. Ideally, this is done within a consultation model in which the primary care provider can be viewed as important and relevant part of the assessment and treatment.

In taking the history, a careful exploration of the development of the symptom(s), associated stressful event, intended and unintended consequence of the "sick role," and other issues

Case Report: Conversion Disorder

A.L., a 9-year-old girl, was brought to an emergency department after an episode of unresponsiveness and paralysis. A good student with no history of behavioral problems, A.L. lived with her maternal grandmother and two older sisters in a public housing project.

After a mild reprimand from a teacher over an argument with a peer, A.L. returned home from school complaining of dizziness and stomach pain. After falling off a sofa, she was found limp and unresponsive by her grandmother. After a few minutes, A.L. was able to open her eyes but could not move or speak. She was transported by ambulance to the hospital. Within 2 hours of arrival, she was able to move all of her limbs. The next day, she regained the ability to speak but had no memory of the episode. There was no personal or family history of seizure disorder. She was hospitalized for 4 days for diagnostic testing. Physical examination, computed tomography scan, toxicology screen, and electroencephalography results were all normal.

A psychiatric interview revealed that, 2 years before, A.L. had witnessed her mother's fatal stabbing by a female neighbor during an argument. The argument had escalated from a dispute between the other woman's child and A.L. At age 7 years, A.L. was a key witness in the murder trial, where she testified in the judge's chambers. The case was now up for appeal, and A.L. soon would be expected to testify in court.

A.L. recounted the details of her mother's death in a dramatic and emotionally detached manner. Aside from this inappropriate affect, the mental status examination results were entirely normal. A.L. and her grandmother were given an explanation of the psychological origin of the episode of unresponsiveness. They were reassured that no general medical problem was found. Psychiatric treatment was recommended, and they were referred to a local children's guidance center. No appointments were kept, and the family was lost to follow-up.

Comment: A.L. was unable to openly express her fears about having to testify in court and confront her mother's murderer. In addition, the teacher's reprimand may have reactivated guilt feelings that she indirectly caused her mother's death by arguing with the murderer's child. The choice of symptoms–dizziness, abdominal pain, becoming limp and unresponsive–may have been a reenactment of the memory of her mother's injury and death. The inability to speak may have related to her ambivalence about testifying in court.

Without psychotherapy to help this child deal with her unresolved grief and guilt surrounding her mother's death, she is at high risk for a recurrence of conversion symptoms or the development of other psychiatric disorders.

Case reprinted from Nemzer, E. D. (1996). Somatoform disorders. In M. Lewis (Ed.), *Child and Adolescent Psychiatry: A Comprehensive Textbook*, p. 701. Baltimore: Williams & Wilkins.

should be carefully explored. As with other areas in child psychiatry, use of multiple informants, including parents, teachers, and health care providers, can be very informative. The clinician should be alert to the potential for undiagnosed physical disease. Sometimes medically unexplained symptoms are just that. In general, a balanced approach should be used with, as much as possible, a thorough physical workup being weighed relative to risks of additional tests. Risks of additional tests include prolongation of the child in the "sick role" as well as of facilitating the maintenance of somatoform illness. A reasonable balance must be achieved between having a thoughtful search for unrecognized disease and the risk of fostering continued difficulties by additional testing or evaluation. Unfortunately, it is sometimes the case that functional difficulties can be superimposed on top of physical illness or after an accident or other traumatic event, thus making efforts to disentangle functional and nonfunctional complaints difficult.

The diagnosis of a somatoform disorder should be one based on positive findings (i.e., not just an apparent absence of physical disease). Factors that suggest a somatoform diagnosis include association with psychosocial stresses; models for the symptoms; and some symbolic nature of the symptoms or apparent secondary gain to the patient (in terms of family, personal, social, or some other function), particularly if apparently associated with a lack of distress (*la belle indifference*). Symptoms that relate to perceived rather than anatomic patterns of dysfunction (anesthesia or movement problems that do not correspond to neural pathways) are suggestive. A strong response to suggestion may also be present. By itself, one of these features is not necessarily diagnostic. In their review of 30 cases of conversion disorder, Volkmar and colleagues (1984) noted that the most frequently presenting complaints were neurological problems, including seizure or movement problems (43% of cases), sensory issues (13%) or paralysis (13%), or pain (7%), and the chief complaints of school-related issues (13%) or mood or behavior problems (7%) were less common. In addition to their chief complaints, patients in the conversion disorder group also had a wide range of other symptoms and were significantly more likely than a comparison group to have had prior psychiatric treatment and a history of a "model" illness in family members.

It is important to distinguish factitious disorders and malingering from functional disorders. In the former, symptoms are deliberate and intentionally produced. Malingering may occur when the child desires to avoid an activity or is in conscious pursuit of a specific goal. Frequently, some inconsistencies in the history of examination are noted. Patients may even supply copies of their medical records, which may not necessarily be accurate. Any family history of illness, disability, or overt psychiatric disorder should be reviewed in detail. Similarly, factors in the child that might have let to a presumption of weakness or vulnerability should be noted (e.g., history of prematurity or previous serious illness). Stresses, marital problems, and other potential contributors should be noted. Conversion symptoms may also occur in the context of abuse, including sexual abuse, so complaints involving the genitourinary tract or involving multiple somatic complaints should prompt consideration of this issue.

TREATMENT

The diversity of clinical presentations and frequent associations with other conditions, particularly mood and anxiety disorders, complicates the management of children and youth with somatoform disorders. A further complication is the relative lack of research, particularly well-controlled treatment studies. Campo and Fritz (2007) have outlined several "core principles" in management with a straightforward discussion of diagnosis and supportive treatment planning. The diagnosis should be reviewed nonjudgementaly and discussed with the family and patient. This can include a review of the history, symptom profile, relevant aspects of history, and findings on examination. When the diagnosis is not clear, as sometimes is the case, this should also be discussed. If there is relative certainty of the diagnosis, additional medical studies are typically to be avoided unless new information comes to light or if the risk-to-benefit ratio supports such studies. In discussing these issues, the clinician should avoid communicating anxiety or embarrassment; rather, the emphasis should be helping the patient and family orient in a positive direction toward problem solving and treatment. Clarification of the frequently made false dichotomy of mind and body may be helpful as can be a discussion of the nature of pain and the considerable individual variation in the experience of pain.

In developing a treatment plan, the emphasis should be on a collaborative treatment model aimed at helping achieve shared functional goals for the patient and family. Treatment should be individualized. Parents should be discouraged from "doctor shopping" and, as much as possible, be actively engaged in the treatment plan. Given the strong somatic presentation, there may be resistance to mental health involvement even though this is often critical. Several different factors or issues are typically addressed in treatment. These include helping the

Case Study: Somatization Disorder

B.H., a 15-year-old girl, was admitted to a children's hospital neurology service because of severe intractable headaches. A complete workup, including a computed tomography scan, spinal tap, magnetic resonance imaging, and electroencephalography, found no general medical problems other than mild scoliosis. A psychiatric consultation was requested.

Further history revealed that B.H. had frequent school absences because of illness every year since kindergarten. These illnesses included colds and ear infections, mild asthma, nausea and vomiting, headaches, and menstrual cramps. She often requested to leave school early because of "not feeling well." B.H. was a capable student, but her grades were barely passing because of her frequent absences. She had only one friend.

Her father was a large, domineering, and authoritarian man; he was disabled because of back problems. Her mother had frequent headaches, was chronically depressed, and looked to her daughter for emotional support. The marital relationship was poor.

In the initial consultation, B.H. appeared depressed and tearful. She complained of sleep and appetite problems of 2 months' duration. She expressed anger at her parents for being strict and overprotective and allowing her very little freedom or privacy. She was intimidated by her father's "violent temper." She felt helpless about the situation, saying: "It's no use. They never listen to me."

The diagnoses of major depression and probable somatization disorder were made, and she was referred for further psychiatric treatment. After 3 weeks on antidepressant medication, B.H.'s mood improved, and her headaches became less frequent, although other somatic problems continued. She still did not return to regular school attendance and received home tutoring at her parents' insistence. The parents abruptly withdrew B.H. from treatment after they were confronted about family issues.

B.H. made a suicide attempt several months later, and the family resumed treatment with another psychiatrist, who was able to establish a therapeutic relationship with both B.H. and her parents. B.H.'s somatic symptoms decreased, and her school attendance improved.

Comment: This case illustrates a number of points regarding somatization disorder. At 15 years of age, B.H. did not meet *Diagnostic and Statistical Manual of Mental Disorders* (DSM-IV) criteria for somatization disorder. However, it is likely that she would, eventually, if this pattern continued for several years. Somatizing families such as this often have difficulty using psychotherapy and are often resistant to therapeutic interventions. B.H. had difficulty communicating openly with her parents. Both parents had health problems that provided ample models for use of somatic symptoms. By being overly solicitous of her health and safety, they rewarded dependency and discouraged attempts toward normal adolescent strivings for autonomy.

Case reprinted from Nemzer, E. D. (1996). Somatoform disorders. In M. Lewis (Ed.), *Child and Adolescent Psychiatry: A Comprehensive Textbook*, p. 701. Baltimore: Williams & Wilkins.

patient understand connections between the various factors involved in symptom formation, reassurance about the ability to improve, and so forth. Parents should be helped to understand that the patient's difficulties are associated with real distress but not somatic damage. In cases in which hypochondrial fears and obsessional worries are prominent, reassurance is less helpful than an active treatment plan.

In general, the emphasis of treatment focuses on a rehabilitative approach with a return to activities (even in the face of persistent symptoms), encourages positive coping, and discourages less adaptive behaviors. This approach has the potential advantages of engaging the patient and family in a more direct way in management. It also undercuts the idea that the symptom(s) must be resolved before the child can return to his or her usual activities and interests. This approach also should emphasize the child's areas of strength and positive coping capacities. School attendance and academic performance can serve as important metrics for success. Homebound instruction should be discouraged. Parents should be helped to view the efforts to facilitate the child's return to normal activities as an important positive step not, for example, as punishment. Various approaches based on aspects of cognitive behavior therapy have been used in treatment of children with somatoform disorders (see Selected Readings). Although studies have been few in number and often limited by small sample sizes, initial results have been encouraging with greater levels of improvement and lower levels of relapse in treated patients. The emphasis of these programs is on encouraging positive coping, teaching self-monitoring strategies, coping with anxiety and stress, and so forth.

Behavioral methods may also be used, although such methods have been less frequently studied. These approaches generally emphasized a thoughtful analysis of desired adaptive behaviors and behaviors to be reduced or eliminated (e.g., behaviors that relate to healthy coping and adaption are encouraged, and those related to sick role behaviors are discouraged). Other approaches used have included self-management training, hypnosis, and biofeedback. Family-based interventions may also be part of the treatment program but have been much less frequently studied. The use of these methods may be particularly important when the parents have been important in encouraging or maintaining the sick role.

Pharmacological treatments have been uncommonly studied in this population, and practice in this area has been shaped, in large part, by experience with adults. Drug treatments are most frequently considered when obvious comorbid conditions (anxiety, depressive disorders, OCD) are present as well. They are also frequently considered when the results of behavioral and psychotherapeutic treatments appear to have been maximized. Adults with somatoform disorders, including pain syndromes, BDD, and other difficulties, have been reported to benefit from antidepressants; Selective serotonin reuptake inhibitors (SSRIs) have also been used. The adult literature suggests that the presence of significant comorbid mood or anxiety problems may be an indicated for drug treatments. Campo and Fritz (2007) advocate the use of SSRIs for functional pain syndromes and note that anxiolytics may sometimes be helpful when physical symptoms are strongly associated with anxiety. The lack of large, well-controlled studies in this area is unfortunate.

COURSE AND PROGNOSIS

Unfortunately, functional somatic complaints are often very persistent. Between one-third and half of children with functional abdominal pain continue to have difficulties in adulthood. In addition, these individuals have increased risk for other conditions, particularly anxiety and depressive disorders. Adults with functional symptoms frequently report that their onset was early in life.

SUMMARY

Children and adolescents with these conditions represent an important public health problem. These children suffer and are viewed as more at risk by their parents and others. They also can experience considerable functional impairment and can consume important health care resources. Extensive medical investigations can also put the child at some risk. The diagnosis of a "functional" problem may also be misconstrued as meaning "there is nothing wrong."

The assessment and management of somatoform disorders in children and adolescents raise many challenges for the health care system. If treatment is to be successful, the clinician should be aware of the importance of a broad-based intervention program that encourages good collaboration with all those involved in the child's care, both in the medical and educational areas. The involvement and support of primary care providers is critical as is a good working relationship with the patient and family. Encouraging positive coping and rehabilitation with a return to typical levels of functioning is the treatment goal. Many different strategies, including behavioral, cognitive-behavioral, and pharmacological, can be used to this end. The emphasis in treatment should be on the development of an individualized, collaborative model aimed at helping achieve shared functional goals for the patient and family.

Study of these conditions has been hindered by their existence at the interface of general medicine and psychiatry. Symptoms may be expressed overtly in one domain but lead to major disruptions of the child's life in many other areas. Critical areas for future work include longitudinal studies of children with these conditions, better (large and well-controlled) treatment studies, and issues of comorbidity and symptom overlap with other conditions.

Selected Readings

Abu-Arafeh, I., & Russell, G. (1995). Prevalence and clinical features of abdominal migraine compared with those of migraine headache. *Archives of Disease in Childhood, 72*(5), 413–417.

American Psychiatric Association. (1994). *Diagnostic and Statistical Manual of Mental Disorders*, 4th edition. Washington, DC: Author.

Apley, J., & Naish, N. (1958). Recurrent abdominal pains: A field study of 1,000 school children. *Archives of Disease in Childhood, 33*, 165–170.

Beck, J. E. (2008). A developmental perspective on functional somatic symptoms. *Journal of Pediatric Psychology, 33*(5), 547–562.

Campo, J., & Fritz, G. (2001). A management model for pediatric somatization. *Psychosomatics, 42*, 467–476.

Campo, J. V., Bridge, J., Ehmann, M., Altman, S, Lucas, A., Birmaher, B., Di Lorenzo, C., Iyengar, S., & Brent, D. A. (2004). Recurrent abdominal pain, anxiety, and depression in primary care. *Pediatrics, 113*(4), 817–824.

Campo, J. V., Shafer, S., Strohm, J., Lucas, A., Cassesse, C. G., Shaeffer, D., & Altman, H. (2005). Managing pediatric mental disorders in primary care: A stepped collaborative care model. *Journal of the American Psychiatric Nurses Association, 11*(5), 1–7.

Davison, I., Faull, C., & Nicol, A. (1986). Research note: Temperament and behaviour in six-year-olds with recurrent abdominal pain: A follow up. *Journal of Child Psychology and Psychiatry, 27*(4), 539–544.

Fabrega, H. (1990). The concept of somatization as a cultural and historical product of Western medicine. *Psychosomatic Medicine, 52*, 653–672.

Fallon, B. (2004). Pharmacotherapy of somatoform disorders. *Journal of Psychosomatic Research, 56*, 455–460.

Fritz, G., Fritsch, S., & Hagino, O. (1997). Somatoform disorders in children and adolescents: A review of the past 10 years. *Journal of the American Academy of Child & Adolescent Psychiatry, 36*(10), 1329–1338.

Garralda, M. (1992). A selective review of child psychiatric syndromes with a somatic presentation. *British Journal of Psychiatry, 161*, 759–773.

Garralda, M. E., & Chalder, T. (2005). Practitioner review: Chronic fatigue syndrome in childhood. *Journal of Child Psychology and Psychiatry, 46*, 1143–1151.

Green, M., & Solnit, A. (1964). Reactions to the threatened loss of a child: A vulnerable child syndrome. *Pediatrics, 34*, 58–66.

Leslie, S. (1988). Diagnosis and treatment of hysterical conversion reactions. *Archives of Disease in Childhood, 63*, 506–511.

Maisami, M., & Freeman, J. (1987). Conversion reactions in children as body language: A combined child psychiatry/neurology team approach to the management of functional neurologic disorders in children. *Pediatrics, 80*, 46–52.

Mayville, S., Katz, R., Gipson, M., & Cabral, K. (1999). Assessing the prevalence of body dysmorphic disorder in an ethnically diverse group of adolescents. *Journal of Child and Family, 8*, 357–362.

Offord, D., Boyle, M., Szatmari, P., Rae-Grant, N. I., Links, P. S., Cadman, D. T., Byles, J. A., Crawford, J. W., Blum, H. M, Byrne, C., Thomas, H., & Woodward, C. A. (1987). Ontario Child Health Study. II. Six-month prevalence of disorder and rates of service utilization. *Archives of General Psychiatry, 44*(9), 832–836.

Phillips, K., Menard, W., Fay, C., & Weisberg, R. (2005). Demographic characteristics, phenomenology, comorbidity and family history in 200 individuals with body dysmorphic disorder. *Psychosomatics, 46*, 317–325.

Spratt, E. G., & Thomas, S. G. (2008). Pediatric case study and review: Is it a conversion disorder? *International Journal of Psychiatry Medicine, 38*(2), 185–193.

Stone, J., Smyth, R., Carson, A., Lewis, S., Prescott, R., Warlow, C., & Sharpe, M. (2005). Systematic review of misdiagnosis of conversion symptoms and "hysteria." *British Medical Journal, 331*(7523), 989.

Veale, D. (1984). Body dysmorphic disorder. *Postgraduate Medical Journal, 80*, 67–71.

Volkmar, R., Poll, J., & Lewis, M. (1984). Conversion reactions in children and adolescents. *Journal of the American Academy of Child and Adolescent Psychiatry, 23*, 424–430.

CHAPTER 18 ■ ELIMINATION DISORDERS: ENURESIS AND ENCOPRESIS

BACKGROUND

In Western countries, toilet training is a process that is typically completed in toddlerhood. In the United States, this typically starts between the ages of 18 months and 3 years, with boys usually being trained slightly later than girls. Some cultures encourage earlier and others later toilet training. Toilet training goes most smoothly when there is consistency in approach and emphasis on positive reinforcement. The process is facilitated by several other factors, including, the required motor abilities of the child, the child's cognitive ability to understand what is desired, and a desire to please the parents or caregivers. The absence of any one of these can lead to difficulties. As Piaget noted, the child's understanding of what it means for things to be living may be a further complication (young children tend to assume that anything that comes from a living thing must be alive, a potential source of confusion for toilet training). Complications can also arise because of inconsistency in approach on the part of parents or through use of a harsh or punitive approach. Parents have been preoccupied with the best ways to achieve toilet training for thousands of years.

ENURESIS

Definition and Clinical Description

Primary enuresis occurs when the child has never been fully toilet trained for urine; in secondary enuresis, this was once achieved (for at least a year). Daytime wetting (diurnal enuresis) is less common as an isolated phenomenon than night wetting (nocturnal enuresis). As defined in the *Diagnostic and Statistical Manual of Mental Disorders* (DSM-IV-TR), functional enuresis is defined by "repeated voiding" into bed or clothes (in either day or night) and must be "clinically significant," meaning either because of its frequency (several times a week for multiple consecutive months) or because it is the source of distress or impairment. The child must have an age (or developmental level) of 5 years, and the condition is not solely attributable to a general medical condition or substance. The type (nocturnal, diurnal, or both) can also be specified. A distinction between primary and secondary enuresis is also made, although the definition is somewhat imprecise, indicating that the secondary form develops only after a period of established urinary continence. Typically, the secondary form develops between ages 5 and 7 years.

Epidemiology and Demography

Several different longitudinal studies have yielded rather similar findings on the prevalence of enuresis by age group. Boys are more likely than girls to exhibit enuresis. By age 6 years, about 90% of children are dry at night. There is a continued decrease in bed wetting with age so that, for example, by age 14 years, about 1% of boys and 0.5% of girls have enuretic episodes at least once a week. In addition to particular vulnerabilities within the child, psychosocial stress and socioeconomic disadvantage also contribute to increased risk. The condition also tends to run in families.

Etiology

Many different theories have been proposed to account for enuresis. Some have focused on anatomical abnormalities, others on neuropsychological or neurological immaturities, and still others on psychogenic or psychodynamic explanations. There is clearly a relationship between delayed development and later toilet training, and there is some suggestion of a complex interaction of factors (e.g., children with smaller bladders may be more likely to have both developmental and behavioral problems). Other work has been consistent with a notion of general neurophysiologic immaturity. Physical factors (e.g., bladder infections or structural abnormalities) can also contribute. Nocturnal enuresis has also led to a series of sleep studies (e.g., in which stage of sleep has been related to enuretic events). Correlations with psychosocial stressors suggest an important role for psychological factors to contribute, and such theories exist but have proven difficult to experimentally verify. The interrelationships of behavioral and developmental difficulties with enuresis have been difficult to disentangle, although it does appear that, at least in some cases, a strong genetic component is present, and efforts to identify specific genes potentially involved are underway.

Differential Diagnosis and Assessment

Urinalysis is an obvious first step in evaluation of enuresis (e.g., to rule out urinary tract infection as a cause). In general, invasive laboratory studies do not have a particularly high yield and would not be indicated unless other indications were present. Children who have problems in both the nighttime *and* daytime may be more likely to exhibit structural or other problems of the urinary tract. Ultrasound evaluation is less invasive than past procedures.

At time, enuresis may arise after other medical problems (e.g., hyperthyroidism), although this is infrequent. A physical examination should look for potentially treatable underlying conditions. Associations with other factors (e.g., nocturnal enuresis that occurs after administration of a new medication) should be explored as relevant.

Treatment

Historically, two rather different treatments have been used with greatest success in treatment of enuresis: behavioral and pharmacological approaches. Behavioral treatments have a long history and have the important advantage of avoiding potential side effects of pharmacological ones. It is important to note that there is some potential for the parents or the child to view use of behavioral techniques as somehow suggesting that the condition is, at least in part, volitional. The bell and pad method has a long history of use and, essentially, combines principles of both classical and operant condition in helping the child learn to avoid nighttime awakening. In this approach, the child sleeps on a pad that, when wet, rings a bell, arousing the child from sleep. This method has a reasonably high success rate (as many as two-thirds of children will respond), and response is maintained in many (>50% of cases) after the treatment is discontinued. Lower levels of family stress and an absence of other psychiatric problems in the child are associated with higher success rates. Some studies have investigated the impact of bladder capacity and response to this treatment. New behavioral approaches continue to be developed (e.g., using an alarm clock to wake the child at a predetermined time during the night or using an ultrasonic monitor attached to the abdomen to awaken the child when a specific bladder volume has been reached).

These treatments have also been combined with pharmacological ones. Drug treatments include the use of impramine and, more recently, desmopressin acetate (DDAVP). The tricyclic antidepressant impramine has been used for treatment of nighttime bed wetting for many decades, and a series of double-blind studies have confirmed its usefulness. It is usual to begin with 25 mg and then gradually increase it, adding 25 mg every week. Usual effective doses are between 75 and 125 mg a day. Some children respond to smaller doses. The maximum dose should be no more than 5 mg/kg/day. Electrocardiography should be obtained at baseline, and continued monitoring is needed at doses greater than 3.5 mg/kg. Given the high rate of remission, regular attempts should be made to evaluate the continued need for medication (e.g., a slow taper every 3 to 4 months allows the medication to be increased if wetting returns). Some children have a transient response to impramine even when the dose is increased. For these individuals, the periodic use of the agent (e.g., at summer camp) may be an option. Given the potential for side effects of this agent, careful education of child and parents is needed (e.g., to avoid a child's taking "extra" medication). There appears to be some correlation between blood level and therapeutic effect, although as a practical matter, side effects such as dry mouth may be a more practical way to be sure that an adequate level has been obtained. The mechanism of action of this agent remains unclear, but it does not simply appear to relate to its antidepressant properties.

Recent interest has centered on the use of DDAVP, a synthetic analogue of the pituitary hormone 8-arginine vasopressin (ADH), which affects renal water conservation. A large number of patients have been enrolled in a series of well-controlled studies. Most of the patients had not responded to previous treatments, and most did respond to DDAVP. The mechanism of action is presumed to be decreased output. Wetting typically returns if the medication is discontinued. The usual dose is 200 to 400 μg given orally (a nasal spray was previously available, but the Food and Drug Administration has recommended against its use for enuresis); there is some suggestion that even lower dose may be effective. The most frequent side effects include headache, flushing, and abdominal pain. The medication should not be used to treat enuresis resulting from a specific medical condition causing increased urination. The most serious complications include hyponatremia and hyponatremic seizures with intranasal use of DDAVP.

In the past, psychotherapy was a mainstay of treatment but is now viewed as being indicated only for associated behavioral problems rather than having a primary impact on enuresis itself. Rates of spontaneous remission are high (as much as 20% of cases), complicating studies attempting to evaluate such interventions. On the other hand, development of enuresis after a stressful event or chronic familial conflict may provide an indication for psychotherapy. Similarly, negative self-image and self-esteem problems associated with nocturnal enuresis may be helped with psychotherapy. Table 18.1 summarizes factors to consider in treatment planning.

Outcome and Follow-up

As noted previously, spontaneous remission of bed wetting is common, particularly between the ages of 5 and 7 years and again in adolescence. In a given year, about 15% of children will experience a spontaneous remission of the condition. One major follow-up study compared

TABLE 18.1

FACTORS TO CONSIDER WHEN CONSTRUCTING A TREATMENT ALGORITHM FOR PRIMARY NOCTURNAL ENURESIS

- Age of child
- Medical cause has been ruled out
- Rate of spontaneous remission (~14%–16% per year)
- Behavioral conditioning with bell and pad or similar methodology
  - Equally effective as pharmacological treatment
  - Lower rate of relapse than with pharmacological treatment
  - Safer than pharmacological treatment
- Most commonly used pharmacological intervention is DDAVP
  - Most serious side effect (rare) is hyponatremia, leading to seizures
- Imipramine is no longer first-line choice for pharmacological treatment but can be used for refractory enuresis
- Combination of behavioral and pharmacological treatment can be considered for refractory enuresis

DDAVP, desmopressin acetate.
Reprinted from Mikkelson, E. (2007). Elimination disorders: Enuresis and encopresis. In A. Martin & F. Volkmar (Eds.), *Lewis's Child and Adolescent Psychiatry: A Comprehensive Textbook*, 4th edition, p. 59. Philadelphia: Lippincott Williams & Wilkins.

Case Report: Enuresis

Tyler, a $7\frac{1}{2}$-year-old boy, had never been fully toilet trained at night. He sometimes wet the bed once a week, more typically 2 or 3 nights a week. His parents had expressed concern to the pediatrician when he was 5 years old, but a medical evaluation had failed to show any medical condition that might account for the problem. His pediatrician had discussed both the "bell and pad" method and medications, but the parents had decided to forgo treatment in hopes that the problem would correct itself over time. Tyler is now frustrated by the problem; he is invited to sleep-overs but almost never goes because of his worry about wetting. His mother reports that his self-image has begun to suffer. Tyler is doing well in school, is popular, and otherwise seems to be developing well.

After some discussion, the parents and Tyler elected a trial of desmopressin acetate (DDAVP). They chose this over the bell and pad method because of a new baby in the home and the general feeling of all concerned that they did not want an alarm going off at night. Tyler responded to relatively small dose and had only the occasional accident. He and his family also restricted his fluid intake before bedtime. After 9 months of treatment, the family and Tyler agreed to taper his medication. At that point, he remained dry and has subsequently.

Comment: This case illustrates the fact that enuresis often resolves over time, but either drug treatment or behavioral intervention may be needed, particularly if the child's self-esteem begins to suffer. In this case, the family elected a pharmacological treatment, although, in general, the bell and pad method is more likely to have last benefit, and the symptom often returns once DDAVP is discontinued.

imipramine, DDAVP, and the bell and pad method along with an observation-only group. Treatment was discontinued after 6 months, and patients were then followed. Six months later, 16% of the observation-only group members were continent compared with 16% of the imipramine-treated group, 10% of the DDAVP group, and 56% of the behavioral treatment group. Accordingly, behavioral treatments should be regarded as the first line of intervention with DDAVP and then imipramine should be made available for children who do not respond to the behavioral intervention.

ENCOPRESIS

Definition and Clinical Description

As defined in the DSM-IV-TR, encopresis is defined "repeated passage of feces into inappropriate places." The soiling must occur at least once a month for 3 months, and the developmental or chronological age of the child must be 4 years. By definition, the condition cannot be diagnosed in the presence of a general medical condition (other than constipation) or be attributable to a physiological effect of a substance (e.g., laxatives). Various distinctions in types of encopresis have been made. The term *primary encopresis* is used if continence has never been achieved, and *secondary encopresis* is used if the behavior occurs after a period of continence had been achieved. The rationale for the current distinction is between children who have fecal leakage related to constipation versus those who are not constipated. The former group is the most common, accounting for about the majority of cases. Primary and secondary encopresis each account for about 50% of cases. Two subtypes are identified based on whether constipation is or is not present.

Encopresis can arise on a voluntary or involuntary basis; some children have bowel control but continue to soil in inappropriate places, and other children may lack the ability to achieve bowel control (e.g., as a result of severe developmental difficulty). For children with the capacity for bowel control, encopresis may have important psychological meaning.

Epidemiology and Demographics

In the Isle of Wight study, Rutter and colleagues (1973, 1989) reported that 1.3% of boys and 0.3% of girls between the ages of 10 and 12 years experienced soiling at least once a month. In younger children, the rate is higher. In one large study in the Netherlands, the prevalence was 4.1% in the 5- to 6-year age range (van der Wal et al., 2005). Encopresis is sometimes observed with daytime enuresis as well as with attention-deficit/hyperactivity disorder and anxiety disorders. Most studies continue to report that boys are more frequently affected than girls.

Etiology

Many factors can lead to encopresis. Chronic constipation is frequent and can itself arise for psychological or physiological reasons. Chronic constipation can contribute to fecal impaction and a diminished sensation and awareness. Stress and trauma can also be associated with encopresis, and various psychodynamic explanations have been formulated.

Primary encopresis is more frequently associated with developmental delays and other forms of psychopathology. In this group, associated enuresis is frequent. Children with secondary encopresis are more likely to have experienced stress and conduct problems.

Differential Diagnosis and Evaluation

Probably only the most severe cases are seen for psychiatric assessment, i.e., primary care providers likely deal with many cases. A careful review of systems and physical examination is indicated. For example, Crohn's disease can lead to diarrhea, and mild cases of aganglionic megacolon may present with soiling. A plain abdominal radiograph may be useful in showing fecal retention.

The history should include a developmental history and review of the nature of the difficulties with parents and child (e.g., frequency, context of the soiling). Children with significant developmental delays (intellectual disability) may present special challenges for toilet training, but various resources, including consultation with a behavior specialist, may be helpful. Associations with other psychiatric problems (e.g., enuresis) should be noted as should associations of the problem with acute or chronic stress.

Treatment

Typically, treatment includes multiple modalities, including education of the child and parent as well as behavioral and psychological approaches. In the situation of chronic constipation, an initial bowel clean out is often undertaken with subsequent interventions designed to assist the child in gaining greater control. This can include modification of diet (with additional fiber), increased exercise and water, and so forth. Behavioral approaches vary depending on the context but might include frequent trips to the bathroom particularly after meals, use of positive reinforcements for success, and so on.

The presence of comorbid conditions and psychopathology or stress may require specific psychotherapeutic treatment. For some children, low self-esteem is an important target for treatment. Parent and family engagement can be particularly helpful. Table 18.2 summarizes approaches to treatment.

Case Report: Encopresis

Shirley was an 8-year-old girl whose parents were going through a bitter divorce and had now separated. The parents had been fighting for well over 1 year. During this time, Shirley was noted to become more anxious and have trouble sleeping. Although previously toilet trained, she had particular trouble in using the bathroom in her father's new home and, eventually, began to have difficulties at her mother's home as well. She had become quite constipated and was regularly having overflow incontinence. This was source of embarrassment to her and a further source of tension with the parents. A medical evaluation revealed significant constipation, but some simple medical interventions and a behavioral reward system instituted by the pediatrician were not successful, partly because the parents fought over this as well. Shirley started to refuse to go to school because of her concern about soiling. A referral was made to a child psychiatrist.

Interviews with the parents focused on their troubled relationship as it related to their inability to parent adequately. Individual sessions with Shirley focused on her anxiety and frustration. In addition to various medical steps taken to reduce constipation, a behavioral program was put into place with both parents agreeing to support it. Although their marriage was ending, they were able to agree to focus on Shirley and her needs and be supportive of each other as parents. Over the course of 3 months of work, tension between the parents significantly decreased, and Shirley was able to reestablish regular bowel control, and her anxiety symptoms lessened.

Comment: Often, simple medical procedures and a behavioral intervention program are sufficient to help children return to being fully continent. However, as in this case, the presence of major psychological problems in the child or family can make this effort more complicated. In this instance, encopresis was one part of a broader array of difficulties. Lessened tension between the parents enabled them to function more effectively and helped Shirley return to continence.

TABLE 18.2
FACTORS TO CONSIDER WHEN CONSTRUCTING A TREATMENT ALGORITHM FOR ENCOPRESIS

- Subtypes of encopresis
  - Retentive (most common)
  - Non-retentive
  - Volitional (least frequent)
- A thorough history is essential that documents the frequency, nature, and circumstances of event
- First line of treatment for retentive subtype usually includes:
  - Education about bowel functioning with both parents and child
  - Physiological treatment with laxatives or mineral oil
  - Behavioral component with time intervals on toilet and positive reinforcement
- Extensive research into biofeedback:
  - Not proven to be more effective than traditional interventions
  - May be a consideration in refractory cases
- Case reports of Impramine in the treatment of non-retentive encopresis
- Psychodynamic assessment for those with volitional encopresis

Reprinted from Mikkelson, E. (2007). Elimination disorders: Enuresis and encopresis. In A. Martin & F. Volkmar (Eds.), *Lewis's Child and Adolescent Psychiatry: A Comprehensive Textbook*, 4th edition, p. 694. Philadelphia: Lippincott Williams & Wilkins.

Outcome and Follow-up Data

About 75% of children respond well to a supportive approach with attention to educational, behavioral, and physiologic aspects. As with enuresis, there is a steady decrease in rates of the condition as children grow older. It is very unusual for the condition to persist after age 16 years.

SUMMARY

Enuresis has been much more extensively studied than encopresis, partly because of the advent of drug treatments. There has long been awareness of a potential role of genetics, and advances in this area may lead to a better understanding of potential subgroups and, hopefully, new treatments. Both enuresis and encopresis provide an opportunity to understand the complex interaction of biological, psychological, and social factors in developmental psychopathology.

Selected Readings

Feehan, M., McGee, R., Stanton, W., & Silva, P. A. (1990). A six-year follow-up of childhood enuresis: Prevalence in adolescence and consequences for mental health. *Journal of Paediatric Child Health, 26*(2), 75–79.

Fritz, G., Rockney, R., Bernet, W., et al. (2004). Practice parameter for the assessment and treatment of children and adolescents with enuresis. *Journal of American Academy of Child Adolescent Psychiatry, 43* (12), 1540–1550.

Matson, J. L., & LoVullo, S. V. (2009). Encopresis, soiling and constipation in children and adults with developmental disability. *Research in Developmental Disabilities, 30*(4), 799–807.

Mikkelsen, E., (2007). Elimination disorders: Encopresis and enuresis. In A. Martin & F. Volkmar (Eds.), *Lewis's Child and Adolescent Psychiatry: A Comprehensive Textbook*, 4th edition, pp. 655–669. Philadelphia: Lippincott Williams & Wilkins.

Moffatt, M. E., Kato, C., & Pless, I. B. (1987). Improvements in self-concept after treatment of nocturnal enuresis: Randomized controlled trial. *Journal of Pediatrics, 110,* 647–652.

Reiner, W. G. (2008). Pharmacotherapy in the management of voiding and storage disorders, including enuresis and encopresis. *Journal of American Academy of Child Adolescent Psychiatry, 47*(5), 491–498.

Robson, W. L. M. (2008). Current management of nocturnal enuresis. *Current Opinion in Urology, 18*(4), 425–430.

Rutter, M. (1989). Isle of Wight revisited: Twenty-five years of child psychiatric epidemiology. *Journal of American Academy of Child Adolescent Psychiatry, 28,* 633–653.

Rutter, M. L., Yule, W., & Graham, P. J. (1973). Enuresis and behavioral deviance: Some epidemiological considerations. *Development of Clinical Medicine, 48*(49), 137–147.

Shaffer, D., Gardner, A., & Hedge, B. (1984). Behavior and bladder disturbance of enuretic children: A rational classification of a common disorder. *Developmental Medicine & Child Neurology, 26,* 781–792.

van der Wal, M. F., Benninga, M. A., & Hirasing, P. A. (2005). The prevalence of encopresis in a multicultural population. *Journal of Pediatric Gastroenterology and Nutrition, 40*(suppl 3), 345–348.

Vande Walle, J., Stockner, M., Raes, A., & Nørgaard, J. P. (2007). Desmopressin 30 years in clinical use: A safety review. *Current Drug Safety, 2*(3), 232–238.

Von Gontard, A., Schaumburg, H., Hollmann, E., Eiberg, H., & Rittig, S. (2001). The genetics of enuresis: A review. *Journal of Urology, 166*(6), 2438–2443.

CHAPTER 19 ■ GENDER IDENTITY DISORDER

Genetic sex is determined at the moment of conception. For typically developing children, an awareness of core gender identity (one's sense of inner sexual identity) begins to develop early in life and is usually firmly in place by age 3 years. Expectations based on sex roles vary depending on cultural, familial, and ethnic expectations along with observation and imitation. The typical preschool child is typically very aware of the differences between the sexes, and this interest can be expressed in play. Since the time of Freud, interest in sexuality and in children's understanding of sexuality and gender has been the focus of considerable attention by psychologists (see Chapter 2 and Martin et al., 2002, for a review).

Research on children with various intersex conditions has made it clear, however, that gender identity is very strongly a function of how the parents perceive the child's external genitalia and consequently assign a sex to the infant and how they subsequently raise the child in the context of social expectations. The work of Money et al. (1957) and others demonstrated that children with intersex conditions can develop secure gender identity if clearly reared as belonging to one gender. On the other hand, studies of sexuality in adults with transsexualism have also made it clear that gender issues are often expressed early in life in these individuals.

DEFINITION AND CLINICAL DESCRIPTION

In the *Diagnostic and Statistical Manual of Mental Disorders* (DSM-IV TR) approach, cross-gender identification must be "strong and persistent" and not simply a result of some presumed advantage to being the other sex. This identification is also associated with continued discomfort about the person's assigned gender or gender role as well as impairment or distress. The condition is not made if a physical intersex condition is present. For children, multiple features of gender identity must be present (e.g., cross-dressing, stated desire, participation in stereotyped activities of other sex, persistent choice of other sex role in play). The DSM system allows for specification of the nature of sexual attraction (male, female, both, neither) in sexually mature individuals and notes that in adolescents, the individual may cross-dress or otherwise engage in activities typical of the other sex.

Typically, the onset of gender identity disorder (GID) is during the first years of life. From the point of the DSM-IV-TR, a critical issue is the degree to which "strong and persistent" signs of cross-gender identification are present and associated with enduring discomfort with the person's gender (or assigned gender). It is not uncommon for features of GID to be present but not of sufficient severity for the diagnosis to be firmly established.

When adolescents present for evaluation of GID, two major subgroups are noted. In one group, the adolescent (both males and females) had a pattern of onset beginning early in childhood and persisting; often, this pattern is associated with a homosexual sexual orientation. In the other group, the adolescent's, almost always male, cross-gender features were not apparently present during childhood (i.e., the condition apparently has its onset in adolescence); these individuals may have various sexual orientations or may be asexual.

Boys with GID are typically preoccupied with, and engage in, activities traditionally viewed as more typically feminine (e.g., dressing in women or girls' clothes, playing games that center on more traditionally "feminine" themes). They may play with dolls and may play more with girls than with boys. They often seem to avoid more stereotypically male activities (e.g., more physical and aggressive play sports, interests, and activities). They may also voice a wish that they had been born a girl or that they truly are a girl. On some occasions, they may report the feeling that their male genitalia are disgusting or pretend, for example, that they do not have a penis.

Similarly, girls with GID typically have strong feelings against engaging in more stereotypically female activities. They may voice the wish to be a boy, may dress in boy's clothes, and may try to appear to look more like a boy. There play often is more focused on activities with boys with more stereotypically male play activities, fantasy figures, and so forth. Often, they have little interest in more sex stereotyped activities of other girls with little interest in dolls or taking feminine roles in play. The girl may claim that she will develop a penis and may voice aversion to bodily changes associated with adolescence. Fantasies and play typically revolve around opposite-sex themes.

Adults with GID may be very uncomfortable with their assigned sex or physical appearance and may seek to change this either through hormonal or surgical means. Often, these individuals adapt, to some degree, clothing and mannerisms typical of the other sex. Sometimes they are highly successful in assuming the role of the other sex.

Sometimes the diagnosis is difficult to make in children and adolescents and becomes clear only over time. Particularly in our society, where sex roles and their perception have changed

Case Study: Gender Identity Issues in a Boy

The parents of Bob, a 6½-year-old boy, sought consultation because of his apparent preoccupation with feminine activities. He had long expressed an interest in cross-dressing and more stereotypically "girl" activities. He avoided rough and tumble play. His father was often absent from the home, and his mother described herself as "at a loss as to how to raise a boy." The mother overtly expressed the wish that Bob had been born a girl and that she had picked out another name for him (Roberta) before his birth.

At the time of his initial assessment, Bob expressed, both in play and drawings, an interest in being a girl. At school, he tended to play only with girls. Interestingly, his parents had described a pattern of odd interests and social interaction early in life, along with speech delay, that had led to an earlier diagnosis of pervasive development disorder not otherwise specified. Part of the stimulus for the present assessment had been the growing concern on the part of parents and teachers about Bob's relative social isolation, which only seemed to increase over time even though social skills training and other educational interventions had appeared to be of significant benefit for his social problems.

Over time, Bob became a somewhat eccentric and reclusive adolescent. He never had strong sexual feelings and as a young adult continued to live with his parents and was asexual with few friends and social interactions other than with colleagues at work and with family members.

Case Report: Gender Identity Issues in a Girl

Kara came for assessment at 12 years of age. She had a long history of being unhappy with her gender. She typically related better to boys than girls and was more likely to play with boys. Her parents had thought of her as a "tomboy" from early on. They became more concerned as adolescence approached and she refused to talk to her mother about menarche, almost never was willing to wear a dress or put on makeup, and so forth. Part of the parental concern, as well, was the worry that she might have a lesbian sexual orientation.

At the time of her initial assessment, Kara expressed a strong feeling that she was really a boy trapped in the body of a girl. She expressed disgust with her developing secondary sex characteristics.

Feelings of gender dysphoria persisted during adolescence and adulthood, and Kara sought surgical procedures as she more actively and overtly assumed a male name and identity.

markedly in recent decades, children and adolescents may assume aspects of more stereotypically "female" or "male" presentations, and this clearly does not, of itself, necessarily qualify as pathological. Indeed, it can be an important aspect of identity consolidation for the adolescent (e.g., a teenage boy who is interested in caretaking other children or a girl who engages in highly competitive sports).

For both children and adolescents, referral may come about if the behavior causes concern to parents or results in social isolation or rejection on the part of peers. Care should be taken in making the diagnosis. Some degree of distress should be present. This may vary in severity and form over childhood.

Epidemiology and Demographics

Epidemiological studies of GID are difficult to conduct, and data must be viewed with caution. In adults, transsexualism is relatively rare, perhaps one in 11,000 men and about a third as common in women (see Zucker, 2005). If questionnaire data are used, only a small group of children are reported to either behave like or wish to be the opposite sex (Achenbach & Edelbrock, 1981). In one study of Dutch twins, the number of children wishing to be the opposite sex was also, low with about 1% of 10-year-old boys and girls reporting wishes to be the opposite sex.

Among preschool- and school-age children, boys are several times more commonly referred for gender identity concerns than girls, but by adolescence, this disparity decreases. Several different possibilities may account for this change, including societal pressures and acceptance by parents and teachers. There is some suggestion that for girls to be referred, more features may be need to be present to prompt referral. Cultural factors may also play a role (see Zucker, 2007).

ETIOLOGY

The vast majority of children with gender issues do not exhibit physical intersex conditions. Speculation has centered on various factors, including prenatal hormonal effects, genetic effects, and environmental factors. It does appear that cross-gender behavior does have a significant genetic component, although studies have identified both shared and nonshared environmental factors. Interestingly, there is some suggestion of early differences in one aspect of temperament and activity level, so that boys with GID exhibit lower activity levels than control boys; similarly, girls with GID have higher levels than control girls (Zucker & Bradley,

1995). There is some suggestion that boys with GID are more likely than control subjects to exhibit lefthandedness. There is also some suggestion that boys with GID may come from later pregnancies within the context of larger families, perhaps suggesting a possible biological mechanism (Zucker, 2005).

Assessment of the role of psychological factors in the etiology of GID is complex. Clearly, for such factors to be operative, they must do so from early in life. Apart from some rare intersex conditions, assignment of sex is typically apparent at birth, and this is true for the vast majority of individuals with GID as well. If parents have a strong preference for one sex over the other, they are, clearly, bound to be disappointed in half of births. The question of whether strong parental preference for an opposite sex child plays a role in the pathogenesis of GID has been addressed in the research literature and, at least relative to mothers of boys with GID, the answer is, in general, no.

Clearly, parental response to early GID behaviors can range from strongly negative to neutral or even encouraging. Green (1974) has emphasized the importance of a lack of discouragement in development of GID. There are various reasons why parents might either passively tolerate or actively encourage cross-gender behaviors. In a small group of cases of boys with GID, a very strong maternal desire for a girl, rather than a boy, may play a role. Studies on the role of psychopathology in parents as a potential contributor to GID are limited almost entirely to mothers of boys with the condition. There is some suggestion that mothers in this group do exhibit higher rates of various conditions, including depression and features of borderline personality disorder, than are present in the general population. The issue of the specificity of these effects remains to be clarified (i.e., it is possible that this is amore general risk factor; this is an active area of research). Studies of boys with GID do suggest high rates of separation anxiety, but the nature of this risk factor similarly is unclear (i.e., most boys with separation anxiety do not go on to have GID).

DIFFERENTIAL DIAGNOSIS AND ASSESSMENT

Laboratory study results are typically normal, although children with children with intersex conditions may be at increased risk for difficulties. Such conditions are usually identified in advance of psychiatric referral. Various measures can be used as part of the assessment of the child or adolescent with gender identity issues (see Zucker, 2005). The diagnosis of GID is, of course, simplest when all required features are present. There appears to be a spectrum of gender identity issues, and in reality, diagnosis can sometimes be difficult. A diagnosis of GID not otherwise specified can be used as a justification for intervention.

GID has been reported to co-occur more frequently with various disorders. Although it might initially seem unlikely, co-occurrence of GID with pervasive developmental disorders has been noted, possibly reflecting some of the core difficulties with social interaction and development associated with these conditions. Studies using parent-report measures, such as the CBCL (see Chapter 3 reading list), consistently suggest that children with GID at are increased risk for a range of difficulties. Boys with GID are more likely to exhibit internalizing problems on the CBCL. Behavior problems often increase as children become older, perhaps reflecting social isolation and peer difficulties (Zucker, 2005).

TREATMENT

Outcome data do suggest that earlier, childhood-onset GID has a range of outcomes and may be responsive to intervention. For later (adolescent) onset, GID this appears less likely to be the case, and for that group, biomedical interventions are more frequently considered. One of the difficulties in the area is the ongoing debate about how best to consider differences in sexual identity and orientation. Terms such as *gender variant* have been proposed and would tend to be less likely associated with more proactive interventions, focusing instead on supporting the child's identity whatever it is. One potential outcome of this view is explicit encouragement of children to foster cross-gender identity from an early age.

For situations in which treatment of GID is considered, a range of approaches are available, including behavioral and psychotherapy, family and group treatment, and various combinations of all of these approaches. Unfortunately, data that would help establish the efficacy and effectiveness of these treatments are limited. The issue of adolescents who express a desire for sex reassignment surgery is complex and controversial. This desire may increase as an awareness of homosexual feelings grows. Individual and group treatment approaches may be helpful. Surgical procedures are not typically available to adolescents, although some work using hormonal treatments has been conducted (Meyer et al., 2001).

COURSE AND PROGNOSIS

Several follow-up studies of children with GID are available (see Zucker, 2005, 2007). Green (1987) studied a large group of boys, most of whom probably would have meet current DSM-IV-TR criteria for GID. In his follow-up study of these behaviorally feminine boys at a mean age of almost 19 years, about 75% of them had either a bisexual or homosexual orientation. Zucker and Bradley (1995) reviewed a series of other follow-up studies and noted slightly higher rates of persistent GID but slightly lower rates of homosexuality. In their own sample, Zucker and Bradley (1995) noted that about 22% were heterosexual in sexual orientation at follow-up, about 50% were asexual and, the remainder were primarily bisexual or homosexual. The degree to which gender dysphoria persists into adulthood is somewhat less clear.

Unfortunately, long-term follow-up information for girls is relatively limited. In one report, persistent GID was noted in 12% of a relatively small sample with a small number having a homosexual orientation or reporting no sexual relationship. For most children, GID does not persist into young adulthood. This may reflect issues of sampling and referral bias, effects of treatment, family and societal pressures, and so forth. It is also possible that with the onset of puberty and adolescence, younger children with GID can develop a greater sense of gender identity; this would also be consistent with the observation that when GID has its onset in adolescence, it is more persistent and more likely to be associated with sexual reassignment surgery.

SUMMARY

Children typically acquire a strong sense of gender identity early in life. Cultural, family, biological and other influences play a significant role in this process. The study of children with unusual conditions (e.g., intersex conditions) has made it clear that both environmental and biological factors are involved. Important clinical differences relate to the age of onset of feelings of gender discomfort or dysphoria. A range of outcomes is noted in adulthood with some individuals achieving some comfort with their overt gender and others seeking surgical or other means to achieve what they experience as a more appropriate gender identity. The appropriateness of classification of the condition as a disorder has been the focus of debate.

Selected Readings

Achenbach, T. M., & Edelbrock, C. S. (1981). Behavioral problems and competencies reported by parents of normal and disturbed children aged four through sixteen. *Monograph of the Society for Research in Child Development, 46* (1, Serial No. 188).

Bailey, J. M., & Zucker, K. J. (1995). Childhood sex-typed behavior and sexual orientation: a conceptual analysis and quantitative review. *Developmental Psychology, 31,* 43–55.

Drummond, K. D. (2006). *A Follow-Up Study of Girls with Gender Identity Disorder.* Unpublished master's thesis, Ontario Institute for Studies in Education of the University of Toronto.

Green, R. (1974). *Sexual Identity Conflict in Children and Adults.* New York: Basic Books.

Green, R. (1987). *The "Sissy Boy Syndrome" and the Development of Homosexuality.* New Haven, CT: Yale University Press.

Martin, C. L., Ruble, D. N., & Szkrybalo, J. (2002). Cognitive theories of early gender development. *Psychological Bulletin, 128,* 903–933.

Meyer, W., Bockting, W., Cohen-Kettenis, P., Coleman, E., DiCeglie, D., Devor, H., Gooren, L. J. G., Hage, J. J., Kirk, S., Kuiper, A. J., Laub, D., Lawrence, A., Menard, Y., Patton, J., Schaefer, L., Webb, A., & Wheeler, C. C. (2001). The Harry Benjamin Gender Dysphoria Association's standards of care for gender identity disorders, sixth version. *Journal of Psychology and Human Sexuality, 13*(1), 1–30.

Money, J., Hampson, J. G., & Hampson, J. L. (1957). Imprinting and the establishment of gender role. *Archives of Neurological Psychiatry, 77,* 333–336.

Van Beijsterveldt, C. E. M., Hudziak, J. J., & Boomsma, D. I. (2006). Genetic and environmental influences on cross gender behavior and relation to behavior problems: A study of Dutch twins at ages 7 and 10 years. *Archives of Sexual Behavior, 35*(6), 647–658.

Zucker, J. J. (2007). *Gender Identity Disorder.* In A. Martin & F. Volkmar (Eds.), *Lewis's Child and Adolescent Psychiatry: A Comprehensive Textbook*, 4th edition, pp. 669–679. Philadelphia: Lippincott Williams & Wilkins.

Zucker, J. J. (2005). Gender identity disorder in children and adolescents. *Annual Review of Clinical Psychology, 1,* 467–492.

Zucker, K. J., & Bradley, S. J. (1995). *Gender Identity Disorder and Psychosexual Problems in Children and Adolescents.* New York: Guilford Press.

CHAPTER 20 ■ ABUSE, NEGLECT, AND THE EFFECTS OF TRAUMA

Children and adolescents who suffer abuse, neglect, or trauma are at increased risk for a range of mental health problems. Children who have been abused physically or sexually may exhibit posttraumatic stress disorder (PTSD), anxiety disorders or mood problems, and aggressive behavior. Children who are severely neglected may exhibit reactive attachment disorders (RADs). Sexual abuse may have special sequela in terms of depresssion, substance abuse, low self-concept, and dissociative states. Neglectful and depriving caregiving environments also increase children's risk for problems in social development and attachment.

Neglect can occur in various forms or combinations of forms, including physical, educational, or emotional. Although poverty and low parental education are risk factors, abuse and neglect are observed in families from all social situations, and clinicians should be constantly alert to the possibility of abuse or neglect. In some instances, the medical system itself becomes involved in the cycle of abuse—in the case of so-called Munchausen by proxy syndrome. Children exposed to trauma within or outside the family are prone to exhibit a range of difficulties, including PTSD.

As an historical phenomenon, child abuse is not new. Abraham's near sacrifice of his son Jacob provides an early reference to potential abuse. Indeed, infanticide was a common phenomenon for religious or economic reasons and continues to the present. Foundling hospitals were equipped to accept infants or children who otherwise would have been abandoned. Only in relatively recent times has child abuse come to be regarded as a medical condition; terms such as *battered child syndrome* and *shaken baby syndrome* came to be used as physicians appreciated the physical findings associated with abuse. Similarly, interest in the response to trauma is also relatively recent.

CHILD ABUSE

Definitions and Clinical Features

Physical abuse entails the intended injury of a child by the caretaker. For infants, this may take the form of shaking or beating, resulting in "shaken baby syndrome." Injury may come from inappropriate or excessive punishment. The term *battered child* is often used to refer to the victims of physical abuse. In sexual abuse, an adult or older child engages in inappropriate

245

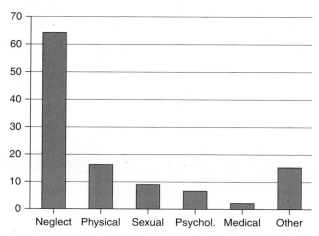

FIGURE 20.1. Data on types of child maltreatment (children can be victims of more than one kind of maltreatment, so numbers can sum to more than 100%). (Data from *Child Maltreatment 2006*. (2008). U.S. Dept. Health Human Services, Administration on Children, Youth, and Families. Washington, DC: US Government Printing Office.)

sexual behavior with a child. Psychological abuse takes the form of repeated threats of abandonment or repeated statements to the child that he or she is unwanted, unloved, or damaged.

The term *neglect* is generally used to refer to situations in which the parent or caretaker does not provide appropriate care of children. This can take the form of failure to provide sufficient food, adequate supervision, or inadequate medical care or education. Physicians and other health care providers are mandated reporters of suspected abuse and neglect. Legal definitions vary from state to state; it is important for health care providers to be aware of the mandates for reporting in their own locations. Unfortunately, the various forms of abuse and neglect frequently co-occur. Figure 20.1 summarizes recent data on abuse types.

Physical abuse should be suspected if a child has injuries that appear to be the result of abuse or when the history provided does not correspond to the findings. A child who was has been abused may look anxious, fearful, depressed, or agitated; older children may be very reticent to reveal the abuse. Marks or bruises (e.g., to the face or head, back or buttocks) may suggest inappropriate punishment; these are often symmetrical (unlike most accidental injuries). Similarly, a belt or rope may leave a characteristic pattern. Burns (e.g., from cigarettes) may be noted. An infant or young child may exhibit multiple and spiral fractures. Severe shaking of an infant can lead to shaken baby syndrome with characteristic retinal hemorrhages. In Munchausen by proxy syndrome (discussed subsequently), there may be a history of repeated emergency department (ED) or hospital visits for treatment of unusual problems.

Child neglect may present to the physician with signs of malnutrition or with signs of lack of care of the child. Such children may be withdrawn and may be indiscriminate in their affection. These children may be more likely to exhibit poor hygiene and be physically small. Occasionally, neglect may present as failure to thrive, although neglect is present in a small minority of such cases.

Sexual abuse is often never revealed or comes to light only after a long pattern of abuse. Uncovering the abuse may be difficult. Obvious indicators are unexpected trauma or sexually transmitted diseases. A young child who is sexually abused may display inappropriate sexual knowledge or preoccupation; behavioral manifestations may include mood problems or aggression. The child may be fearful (e.g., of men if the perpetrator is himself a male). In interviewing the child with suspected child abuse, the examiner should understand that the child may not always be consistent given understandable anxiety. False allegations of sexual abuse do occur, and in many cases, there is not sufficient evidence to substantiate the claim of sexual abuse. Very young children may have great difficulty providing a coherent verbal account of the abuse. The use of play materials can be helpful, but it is important that the interviewer not inappropriately "lead" the child. Incestuous behavior is most common between older male relatives (fathers, brothers, uncles, stepfathers) and girls. Risk factors include poverty, absent or impaired maternal presence, and substance abuse.

All states mandate reporting of possible abuse and neglect on the part of health care providers. Guidelines for evaluation of cases of physical and sexual abuse have appeared (see Selected Readings). It is important for professionals working with children to be aware of specific reporting requirements in their state. Given the high rates of psychiatric sequelae, the possibility of abuse and neglect should be considered in initial evaluations in mental health settings.

Epidemiology and Risk Factors

The Centers for Disease Control and Prevention reports that in 2006, child protective services investigated 3.6 million reports of child abuse or neglect. As noted in Figure 20.1, neglect is the most frequent form of abuse followed by physical and sexual abuse. In 2006 the National Child Abuse and Neglect Data System (NCANDS) reported over 1500 child fatalities from abuse. The children most likely to die as a result of abuse and neglect are mostly babies of less than 1 year (44% of cases) or toddlers from 1 to 3 years of age (34% of cases). It is likely that many child fatalities are not correctly reported as such. Once a case has been reported there is increased risk for subsequent referral. It is typical for the child in protective care to have experienced at least two forms of abuse. Children who suffer from abuse or neglect may exhibit any of several potential risk factors. These include prematurity or physical or cognitive disability or children who are viewed (rightly or wrongly) as demanding, difficult, or overly active. Young age is a major risk factor. Girls are at slightly higher risk than boys.

Although rates remain concerning, it is the case that efforts at prevention and education, as well as prosecution of offenders, have had a major effect. After a peak in 1993, there has been a decline of more than 20%, particularly in the areas of sexual and physical abuse. Sexual abuse in the form of attacks by other children has unfortunately appeared to have increased. Perpetrators have often been abused themselves. Unfortunately, child abuse, spousal abuse, and substance abuse problems tend to co-occur. About 80% of parents who lose their child after investigations for abuse and neglect will have histories of substance abuse, and domestic violence is reported in more than half of cases involved with child protection services.

Course and Prognosis

Neglect and abuse have varied long-term implications for the mental health and life course of victims. Psychiatric problems of sample children who have experienced abuse or neglect have higher rates of PTSD, depression, attachment problem, dissociative symptoms, substance abuse problems, eating disorders, conduct or oppositional disorder, and borderline personality traits. In addition, other problems or issues may be present, including problems with peers and low self-esteem. Academic performance may suffer. In one study, about half the maltreated children had important problems in academic, behavior, and social relationships; fewer than 5% functioned well in all of these domains. In adulthood, these individuals are more likely to be involved in violence with partners and have problems being parents. Although most parents who are abusive have experienced maltreatment themselves, fortunately, overall, only about one in three children who are abused go on to become abusing parents. Inappropriate sexual behaviors are possible indicators of sexual abuse (Table 20.1) but can also be associated with physical abuse, exposure to domestic violence or sexuality, and to mental illness. In the past, it was

Case Study: Child Abuse

Johnny, age 8 months, was brought to the emergency department by ambulance after a frantic call from his mother to 911. His mother had a long history of substance abuse, primarily involving cocaine, and reported that she had left Johnny in the care of her boyfriend only to return and find him left in his crib with the boyfriend nowhere to be found. She reported that Johnny had been a difficult baby "from day 1," and she had to have some time away from him. On examination, Johnny was noted to have retinal hemorrhages with one healing and one new fracture. Evaluation was otherwise negative. The mother denied injuring him but did report that he "may" have fallen a few weeks previously. She had few social supports and was on probation for several theft charges. Child protective services was called, and Johnny was removed from his mother's care. She subsequently returned to prison for violation of probation, and Johnny entered foster care.

Comment: The term *shaken baby syndrome* is often used to refer to a constellation of various injures, ranging from mild to severe, including multiple fractures, retinal hemorrhages, and subdural hematomas. All are warning signs of abuse. In this case, the mother's cocaine habit may have contributed both to some of his early difficulties as well as to her ability to be an effective parent. Infants are more likely than older children to be abused.

believed that fecal soiling was an indicator of sexual abuse, but this has not been shown in recent work.

Most children who are sexually abused do not go on to become abusers, but most sexual offenders have experienced maltreatment in some form. Youth who are sexual abusers often have a history of abuse or maltreatment, and most engage in other antisocial activities. Fortunately, it appears that many youth who engage in sexual offenses do not do so as adults.

Children removed from the parents often enter foster care. The number of children in foster care has increased dramatically over the past several decades. Although many of the more than 500,000 children are able to return home, a large number of them (between 20% and 40%)

TABLE 20.1

DISTINCTIVENESS OF SEXUALIZED BEHAVIORS IN INDICATING ABUSE HISTORY

Moderately Prevalent in Sexually Abused Children and Exceedingly Rare in Psychiatric and Normal Control Subjects	Moderately Prevalent in Sexually Abused Children and Psychiatric Control Subjects and Uncommon in Normal Control Subjects	Moderately Prevalent in Sexually Abused Children, Psychiatric Control Subjects, and Normal Control Subjects
Puts mouth on sex parts Asks to engage in sexual acts Masturbates with an object Inserts objects in vagina or anus	Stands too close to others Hugs adults they do not know well Talks about sexual acts Wants to watch movies that show nudity Knows more about sex than other children their age	Talks flirtatiously Masturbates with hand Touches sex parts at home Tries to look at nude pictures or undressing people

Reprinted from Kaufman, J. (2007). Child abuse and neglect. In A. Martin & F. Volkmar (Eds.), *Lewis's Child and Adolescent Psychiatry: A Comprehensive Textbook*, 4th edition, p. 694. Philadelphia: Lippincott Williams & Wilkins.

reenter the foster care system. Multiple placements are not at all uncommon, and about 5% of children in care have experienced 10 or more placements. Around 100,000 children live in group home or institutional settings. Multiple foster placement significantly increases the risk for subsequent antisocial and violent behavior.

Important moderating variables in mediating the impact of maltreatment and subsequent difficulties have been identified. Caspi and colleagues (2002) identified a genetic risk between child maltreatment and later antisocial behavior, a functional polymorphism of the gene A (MAOA) involved in neurotransmitter metabolism. Children who had been maltreated and who had high levels of MAOA expressed were less likely to develop antisocial problems. This finding has been replicated in other studies. In subsequent work, the same group found that a functional polymorphism in the promoter region of the serotonin transporter (5-HTTLPR) gene was similarly involved in the moderation of maltreatment and life stress on depression.

Other lines of research suggest that support and subsequent positive parenting can modify the effects of child maltreatment. Studies using animal models have shown the potential mitigating effects of support during separation of the young animal from its mother. Similarly, the presence or availability of a supportive caregiver is associated with a better outcome.

Treatment

In many instances, cases with documented maltreatment referred to child protective services receive no support or services after the investigation. Both children and parents have significant needs, which sadly are often not addressed. The failure to provide such services does, of course, increase the likelihood of re-abuse, subsequent placement, and worsened outcome.

Children who have been abused or neglected can present with an unusual range of symptoms and disorders. Compared with children in community samples, those in the child protective service are two to three times more likely to receive psychotropic medications. Behavioral methods, including treatment specific to PTSD (see below), are underused but effective. Given the wide range of potential diagnoses, a comprehensive psychiatric assessment is indicated. Work with this population is more than usually complicated given that not only the child and parent or foster parent but some representative from child protective services will be involved. Given the association of child abuse and neglect with a range of environmental problems and issues, the services of various professional are needed (e.g., to address substance problems in parents, environmental issues and family supports, academic assistance, and mental health support).

The data on the negative effects of multiple and long foster care placements led Congress to enact the Adoption and Safe Families Act in 1997, which mandates that in general, permanency in placement should occur for children in out-of-home care for 15 of the past 22 months. Some states require this if children have been in out-of-home care for only 12 months. There are different routes to permanency, including reunification of the family, adoption, long-term placement with relatives or nonrelatives granted legal guardianship.

Intervention programs must often target parental substance abuse treatment as a priority. This can be accomplished in different ways, including having substance abuse workers in the child welfare program. Various comprehensive programs have been developed.

Various subtypes of abuse have been identified. The next two sections review one particular syndrome of abuse of particular interest to medical professionals. Then the problems in attachment and a specific syndrome resulting from inadequate caretaking and delayed or deviant care are discussed.

MUNCHAUSEN SYNDROME BY PROXY

The term *Münchausen syndrome* was used in the 1950s to describe adults who fabricated symptoms of illness. Named after the a renowned teller of tall tales, the term *Munchausen by proxy syndrome* has now been used to describe a special pattern of child abuse in which parents fabricate illness in a child, often putting the child at risk from various medical procedures and even surgery. It appears that cases of "nonaccidental poisoning" may have represented the first instances of this condition, which was described by Sneed and Bell in 1976 as the *dauphin of Munchausen* and by Meadow in 1977 as *Munchausen by proxy syndrome.*

This condition is listed in the appendix of the *Diagnostic and Statistical Manual of Mental Disorders* (DSM-IV) as a condition requiring further study. It is usually defined by the combination of intentional feigned illness by a parent or caregiver on behalf of a child or someone in his or her care. That individual denies having caused the illness, and there is some psychological gain for the parent or caregiver in assuming, by proxy, the sick role.

The best approach to the definition has been the object of debate. The severity can range from mild to severe. There are other circumstances in which symptoms may be falsified (e.g., in relation to keeping a child out of school or as part of a custody dispute), and these are not typically considered forms of Munchausen syndrome by proxy.

Fortunately, the condition is apparently quite rare. In one study in the United Kingdom and Ireland, the rate was one per 200,000 in children younger than 16 years of age, with most cases reported in the first year of life. A handful of systematic case reviews suggest some commonalities among cases. In addition to the generally expected young age of the children involved, the perpetrator is usually the mother. The mean age of being reported is between 3 and 4 years, although in the British study, the median age was 20 months. Boys and girls are equally as likely to be effected.

The clinical presentation can be highly varied. Usually, the apparent illness seems to be multisystem; at different points in time, the child may appear to have different disorders. In systematic case series reviews, the most common clinical presentations were possible seizures, apnea, diarrhea, and fevers. Many other presentations are reported as well. Various means are used to produce the symptoms or findings (e.g., contamination of intravenous lines or suffocation).

In some cases, the illness is simulated (e.g, by contaminating urine samples), but no damage is done to the child. There may be a history of neglect or of some nonaccidental injury. Siblings may have been the focus of similar reports. In children who present with apnea and when there is a history of sibling death caused by apnea, Munchausen syndrome by proxy should be included in the differential diagnosis. Other warning signs include symptoms only present when one person is with the child and unexplained sibling deaths. At times, the presenting issue may be a complicated, often rare, psychiatric or medical disorder.

Often, the perpetrator, usually the mother, has a long history of involvement in the health care system. Sometimes the mother herself has had a history of extensive medical evaluations. Typically, the staff report that the mother appears to be a model parent and may develop unusual (and inappropriate) relationships with medical staff. At the same time, there may be a vague sense of uneasiness on the part of the staff. Frequently, the mother will seem to hover over the child and never leave the bedside.Interestingly, covert videotaping sometimes reveals a rather different pattern when the mother believes she is not being observed. Rather than be distressed in discussing the child's illness, the mother may seem detached or blandly accepting. The perpetrator may fabricate other information about herself, the child, or family members. Usually, unlike the mother, the father seems largely absent. The marriage relationship may be poor. In contrast to mothers, fathers who are involved as perpetrators are often demanding and unreasonable.

Risk factors include the mother's own experience of abuse as a child, a pathological relationship with the child, and an investment in the interaction with the medical care system. Parent perpetrators also contribute their own, sometimes extensive, psychopathology, with high rates of somatoform or factitious disorders along with substance abuse, depression, and personality disorders. The fabrication of illness is often described as "quasidelusional." There may be an element of disassociation in their presentation as well.

Relatively less is written about the psychiatric aspects of the child who is the victim. For older children, it may be the case that the child is involved the deception. Given the number of intrusive and invasive tests and procedures, children frequently learn to tolerate them rather passively.

Case Study: Munchausen's Syndrome by Proxy

Tammy, a 5-year-old girl, was seen in consultation. She had been hospitalized for 1 week for observation after her mother's report of possible sleep apnea. At the time of admission, the mother reported that the child had a "variant of Rett's syndrome," and she was seeking guidance regarding her school program. Tammy had been born after an uncomplicated pregnancy, labor, and delivery. Her single mother, an LPN, had been worried during the pregnancy about her condition. She was repeatedly reassured by her obstetrician that the pregnancy was progressing normally. After Tammy's birth, the mother reported that she was slow in both talking and walking (although she was doing both by age 18 months). After an episode of asthma, the mother became concerned about Tammy's breathing. She also noted what she believed were staring spells. A pediatric neurologist did an evaluation, including an electroencephalogram, which was within normal limits. The mother found a physician who expressed concern that the combination of breathing problems and staring spells raised the question of Rett's disorder. Her head circumference was, however, at the 50th percentile, as were her height and weight. Another pediatrician recommended specific testing for Rett's disorder but explained to the mother that the clinical picture did not justify it and that the test result was not always positive even in documented cases. On several occasions, the mother had taken the child to the emergency department with complaints of concerns about her breathing. During this hospitalization, two potential apneic episodes had been noted, and on both occasions, the mother had been alone in the room with the child. The mother appeared quite devoted to the child as well as to the hospital staff who were sympathetic to her situation because the mother explained that she had had to stop working to care for her child.

On examination, the child was in the low-average range intellectually with some mild speech articulation difficulties. The neurological examination was not otherwise unusual. Apart from mild asthma, respiratory functions appeared to be normal. One of the staff became suspicious when she saw the mother apparently engaged in some activity with the apnea monitor just before the alarm sounded. The mother then demanded to remove the child from the hospital, and a referral to child protective services was made. Investigation revealed a number of previous evaluations, including two hospitalizations not reported by the mother. The mother herself had a history of multiple unexplained medical symptoms and problems dating back to her childhood.

Comment: Several aspects of this case are relatively typical for Munchausen syndrome by proxy. These include the mother's medical background, the child's age (preschool children are most likely to be involved), multiple medical assessments, a failure to be reassured by the multiple previous assessments, and overengagement with staff.

Management

These cases present a challenge for medical and mental health providers, falling at the intersection of both systems of care. Additional complications for management include the fact that the diagnosis may not be suspected for a long period of time. After it is discovered, the diagnosis itself complicates management given the understandable feelings provoked in staff. Often, there is relatively little insight on the part of the mother or motivation to truly engage in psychotherapy.

Table 20.2 provides a summary of some of the warning signs of Munchausen syndrome by proxy. The child's safety should be the first priority. The medical care provider should act to involve both a mental health consultant and child protective services. An attempt should be made to disentangle the various complaints (e.g., were some things only happening when the

TABLE 20.2

WARNING SIGNS OF MUNCHHAUSEN SYNDROME BY PROXY

Persistent or recurrent illness that cannot be explained
Discrepancies between the history, clinical findings, and general health of the child
Working diagnosis is a rare disorder or experienced clinicians have "never seen a case like it before"
Symptoms and signs occur only in the mother's presence
A mother who is extremely attentive and always in the hospital
A child who is frequently intolerant to treatments
A mother who appears less worried about her child's illness than is the medical staff
Seizures that do not respond to appropriate therapy
Families in which sudden unexplained infant death has occurred
A mother with previous medical or nursing experience or who has an extensive history of illness

Reprinted from Forsyth, B., & Asnes, A. G. (2007). Munchhausen syndrome by proxy. In A. Martin & F. Volkmar (Eds.), *Lewis's Child and Adolescent Psychiatry: A Comprehensive Textbook*, 4th edition, p. 723. Philadelphia: Lippincott Williams & Wilkins, and Meadow, R. (1982). Münchhausen syndrome by proxy. *Archives of Diseases of Childhood, 67*, 92–98.

mother was present? Can independent sources verify history or observations provided by the mother? How does the mother react to the child's illness and the situation?).

Laboratory studies may be helpful (e.g., to determine if blood in urine or stool is the child's or the mother's). Although the rationale for continuous observation by staff is clear, this is usually difficult to actually conduct. Legal guidance should be sought relative to the question of covert video surveillance. After the diagnosis is clear, the mother should be informed and protective service involved. The father and other family members can be involved as appropriate. The consulting psychiatrist can be helpful in multiple regards.

The child psychiatrist can meet with the mother even before the diagnosis is clear. This can usually readily be justified given the seriousness of the child's illness and allows for a discussion of the mother's history and the assessment of potential risk factors. Comments about the child may provide clues relative to motivation, and the interview may also provide information about any overt psychiatric problems in the mother. Having involvement with the psychiatrist before the time she is confronted also gives some potential for building a potentially helpful longer term therapeutic relationship. The psychiatrist can also work with the medical staff around their feelings and be involved in confronting the mother after the diagnosis is clear. Information provided by the psychiatrist may be extremely helpful to child protection services.

Various factors need to be considered in providing treatment for the mother (e.g., the nature of her own psychiatric difficulties, the duration and extent of the abuse, parental perceptions of the child, and willingness to engage in treatment). There have been reports of parents being able to engage in productive psychotherapy.

Course and Outcome

As might be expected, the outcome is variable. Cases in which the condition has been going on for a long period are more challenging as are cases in which severe psychopathology in the mother interferes with treatment. Some activities (e.g., simulating sleep apnea by suffocation) are clearly much more dangerous. In Rosenberg's review (2003), 9% of children in these cases died, and 8% of those surviving had some permanent disfigurement or impairment. Suffocation and poisoning are the most frequent causes of death. As noted previously, a family history of mysterious death is a very worrisome sign. Sometimes outplacement is needed given the potential danger to the child's life.

Relatively little is known about the long-term psychiatric effects on the children involved. A range of difficulties has been described. There is an increased risk for continued fabrication of illness as children become adolescents and adults. More intensive treatments programs may be associated with higher rates of success.

REACTIVE ATTACHMENT DISORDER

Severe neglect, and emotional deprivation, either through parental neglect or institutional rearing, is associated with serious negative effects for children's development. Within the child development literature, there has long been a focus on processes of attachment building on the work of John Bowlby and his colleague Mary Ainsworth (discussed in Bretherton, 1992). Bowlby became interested in attachment after he became aware of the effects of maternal separation in a series of children arrested for theft. Mary Ainsworth worked with him and developed a specific procedure for assessing the quality of young children's attachments. In essence, attachment theory proposed that babies come into the world with an inborn predisposition to develop relationships with caregiving adults.

From the moment of birth, typically developing infants have a strong orientation toward people. By 2 months of age, babies smile socially and become more discriminating, and by around 8 to 9 months, babies become highly attached to their parents and anxious around others (stranger anxiety). As babies are able to move, they maintain physical proximity to their parents and, with the onset of language, an entire range of verbal behaviors enhance the attachment process.

Definitions and Clinical Features

First recognized as a diagnostic entity in the DSM-III, approaches to diagnosis of this condition have changed somewhat over time, and presently several different approaches have been proposed. The DSM-IV approach emphasizes the centrality of severe disturbance in social relatedness in the context of grossly negligent care with an onset in the first 5 years of life (Table 20.3). Two subtypes are specified: an inhibited and disinhibited type. The inhibited type characterizes children, often from institutional settings or who have been severely neglected, who are more passive and disorganized in their approaches to others. The disinhibited type characterizes children in whom the pattern is more one of approach but with many and indiscriminate attachments. The latter may result from situations when care has been provided in group settings or foster care. Some diagnostic systems also recognize a mixed type. By definition, the condition is not diagnosed in the presence of autism or similar disorder, although, as noted subsequently, differentiation can occasionally be a problem.

The clinical presentation varies depending on the age of the child and developmental level, but invariably, the child exhibits severe problems in selective attachment to caregivers and in social interaction. Infants with the condition may, at times, present with failure to thrive or other growth problems. The child may appear poorly nourished and cared for. After appropriate care is provided, the child's physical appearance typically improves. As noted previously, the clinical picture may be one of withdrawal and inhibited responding or one in which the

TABLE 20.3

DIAGNOSTIC FEATURES OF REACTIVE ATTACHMENT DISORDERS

Onset (before age 5 years) of disturbed and inappropriate social relatedness characterized by:
1. Persistent failure to engage because of inhibited or ambivalent interaction or
2. Lack of specificity of attachments

Social difficulties emerge in the context of inappropriately supportive emotional or physical care or with lack of exposure to a stable caregiving environment

Case Study: Reactive Attachment Disorder

Johnny, now 5 years of age (see page 248) was referred for evaluation by his foster parents. Subsequent to removal from his mother's care at 8 months of age, Johnny had been placed in four different foster families. Each had noted difficulties, which had appeared to increase over time. Johnny was difficult to console and seemed to have little empathy for others but was overaffectionate and friendly even with complete strangers. The foster parents complained that, at times, his behavior was disruptive, and they were not sure he could remain with them. He had little evidence of specific attachments to his current foster parents with whom he had resided for 5 months. There had been no contact from the biological mother for 2 years. On examination, he was superficially friendly but overly familiar with the new adult. He appeared to have some mild learning issues and was referred for additional testing prior to school entry.

Comment: Children in foster care can sometimes be in multiple placements, disrupting formation of stable attachment relationships with adults. In this case, the child had an unfortunately early history, and his vulnerabilities may have contributed to the difficulties he subsequently had with remaining in foster placements.

child is inappropriately and indiscriminately friendly. The latter group of children may also exhibit problems with activity and poor attention.

Epidemiology and Demographics

Solid epidemiological data are lacking. In clinics serving very young children, the problem is frequently observed. Children who have been maltreated or abused are clearly more likely to exhibit the condition. One study found that 40% of foster children assessed within 3 months of placement exhibited the condition. Among children in institutional settings, particularly from a young age, rates of 22% to 56% are reported.

Etiology

This disorder and the trauma-related conditions are unique in that the cause is specifically included in the definition of the disorder. Put another way, it would be impossible to make a diagnosis of RAD if appropriate care were provided (in such an instance, an autism spectrum disorder would presumably be more likely). However, Rutter and colleagues have described a small group of children who suffered severe deprivation and presented with continued features suggestive of autism. The degree of social disturbance appeared to correlate with the duration of institutionalization, and the symptoms improved with provision of appropriate care (see O'Connor & Rutter, 2007).

Differential Diagnosis and Assessment

Observation of children in interaction with the caregiver is an important aspect of the assessment of children with RAD. A review of the history and a discussion of the nature and quality of attachment to the caregiver are indicated. There should be careful attention to any history of neglect, repeated changes in caregivers, foster care placement, and so forth. Given the frequent association with a host of other risk factors, including poverty, various other conditions may be seen in this group of patients. There are standard approaches to assessing the quality of attachment using the Ainsworth "strange situation" (a pattern of systematic separation and reunion of the child and mother); modifications of this have been used clinically. It should be emphasized that use of the standard Ainsworth strange situation does not provide a clinical diagnosis and does not substitute for clinical assessment.

In typically developing children, selective attachments are readily observed by 9 months of age. Accordingly, care should be taken in making a diagnosis of RAD in children with severe intellectual deficiency. Usually, children with intellectual abilities above the 9-month level of cognitive ability form attachments (children with autism are a notable exception). As noted, differentiation from autism and related conditions can occasionally be difficult to differentiate from RAD, but usually, social and other gains will be seen in RAD if good caregiving is provided. The most complicated cases are those in which a child may have autism or a related condition *and* has a history of some degree of neglect; fortunately, this situation is not common. Nutritional deficiencies, small size, and growth problems are more typical of children with RAD. Children with RAD who have experienced severe neglect may show stereotyped movements suggestive of autism or a related disorder.

As with other children who have experienced neglect or abuse, a range of additional conditions may be present. These include disruptive behavior disorders, anxiety disorders, and disorders of mood disorders. PTSD may also be observed in children who have experienced abuse.

A developmental assessment should be conducted to document the child's current status and monitor change with provision of a more supportive, nurturing environment. If severe cognitive or other serious developmental delays are noted, a reasonable search for any contributing medical conditions is needed.

Course and Prognosis

When appropriate care is provided, infants usually rapidly develop new attachments. Longitudinal data, particularly past the school years, are limited.

Treatment

Given the importance of stable child–parent relationships it is important, whenever possible, to avoid removal of the child from the home as long, of course, as there is provision of appropriate supports to the family. However, removal to foster care may be the only choice in some cases, and if the new environment is more facilitating, the child may rapidly improve. On the other hand, as a group, children in foster care can be more indiscriminate in their attachments. Children in institutional settings continue to exhibit difficulties. Placement in a supportive family environment is beneficial. For children who are placed in such settings, the inhibited symptoms of attachment disorder are much less persistent that the indiscriminate behaviors. Even when a supportive environment is provided, some difficulties may persist. At times, psychotherapeutic work with the child or parent–child dyad may be indicated. Various models of treatment have been described in the literature. Various alternative approaches to treatment have been proposed with little or no substantive empirical basis; often the notion is to correct early histories of deprivation through holding, rebirthing, and so on.

TRAUMA AND TRAUMA-RELATED DISORDERS

Over the past century and a half, there has been a growing awareness of the negative effects of traumatic experience on psychological functioning. Terms such as *shell shock* and *battle fatigue* began to be used to describe the difficulties experienced by soldiers in war time. Although these problems had, in some ways, been noted for many years (e.g., during the Civil War), they became particularly noteworthy after the protracted, highly stressful trench warfare of World War I. The existence of these difficulties led to a major theoretical problem for

Sigmund Freud—that is, why should there be an apparently nonadaptive repeated remembering of traumatic events? This led him to a major change in his theory of psychological functioning and the postulation of a "death instinct" (see Chapter 1).

Interestingly, the experience of children in London suffering through the blitz in World War II led Freud's daughter, Anna, to consider the nature of traumatic experience in children. In her father's original theories of neurosis, he had speculated on the role of traumatic events in producing neurotic phenomena. Her work was concerned with the impact of stress on children and their potential, in some cases, to find alternative comfort figures and to mitigate the effects of stressful events.

The concept of PTSD was officially recognized in the DSM-III in 1980. Over time, some changes in approaches to the diagnosis, including how it is applied in children and adolescents, have been made. In children and adolescents, violence within the family is the most common source of PTSD, although it can also emerge in the context of natural disaster, accidents, terrorism, war, and other stresses. There may be a single traumatic incident or multiple ones. Research has come from diverse sources and circumstances ranging from the victims of the Chowchilla bus kidnapping to children in Israel living through Scud missiles attacks and children living through the attacks of September 11, 2001.

Definitions and Clinical Features

Various changes have been made in the criteria for PTSD since its inclusion in the DSM-III in 1980. These changes related to emerging data on the duration of symptoms, the level of trauma required, and so forth. Adoption of a minimum duration criterion, (i.e., for symptoms to be present at least 1 month) created some difficulties because a diagnosis and potential intervention were thus delayed. This was dealt with in DSM-IV by including a new acute stress disorder (ASD) category.

For the diagnosis of ASD, the child must exhibit symptoms for at least 2 days up to a maximum of 1 month after the traumatic event; at that time, continued symptoms would require that the diagnosis be changed to PTSD. It is also possible for a child *not* to exhibit an ASD but to develop PTSD some time after the event. For both conditions, exposure to a traumatic event is required (this can experience of a traumatic event personally or witnessing it); the response to the traumatic event includes intense feelings of fear, helplessness, horror, and so on. For ASD, three or more dissociative symptoms (feelings of derealization or depersonalization, absent or detached emotional response, or even amnesia) must be present, and the traumatic event must be reexperienced (e.g., as flashbacks). In PTSD, the traumatic event is reexperienced in some way (e.g., with recurrent recollections or, in children, repetitive play, in dreams, or flashbacks with feelings of reliving the event). In both conditions, avoidance of stimuli that might trigger memories of the event is present (this is more marked in PTSD). Other symptoms in both conditions may include problems with irritability, anxiety, exaggerated startle response, and so on. And in both conditions, significant distress or impairment must be present. The differentiation between the two conditions rests largely on the time course. In ASD, the problems last for at least several days and up to 1 month, but in PTSD, the symptoms have lasted more than 1 month.

Unfortunately it can be difficult for children to provide a detailed description of their response to traumatic events. For both conditions, some reexperiencing, avoidance or dissociation, and hyperarousal symptoms are required. Dissociative symptoms are more frequently required for the ASD responses; they may be fewer or even absent in PTSD. The DSM allows for developmental differences in the presentation of symptoms in children. For example, symptoms might present in children through repetitive play rather than repeated verbalization. The repetitive play may also "count" toward traumatic reexperience (i.e., rather than verbally). Other modifications are made (e.g., relative to nightmares, which need not be specifically trauma focused in children). Similarly, traumatic reenactment may be observed (e.g., inappropriate sexual behavior in sexually abused children). Despite these important changes, problems can arise in making the diagnosis in children, particularly in very young children.

Epidemiology and Demographics

In the National Comorbidity Study, nearly 6,000 individuals (ages 15 to 54 years) were studied. Overall, the prevalence of PTSD was 7.8% with the rate in females (10.4%) twice that seen in males. It appears that rates in children and adolescents are even higher, probably between 25% and 45%. In children exposed to stressful events, between 5% and 45% develop PTSD. The risk is increased by low family income.

Etiology

A growing body of work on stress in adults has identified several important potential biological correlations of stress. These include a range of findings, including reduced volume of the hippocampus, possibly as a potential source of vulnerability, as observed, for example, in studies of twin pairs in which one twin was exposed to trauma.

Animal studies have revealed that high levels of stress can cause specific atrophy in the CA3 region of the hippocampus. Glucocorticoids can also have an impact on dendritic branching and even neurotoxicity. The mechanism appears to be through binding of glutamate to N-methyl-D-aspartate (NMDA) receptors. This phenomenon has not yet been shown in children, although reductions in medial and posterior areas of the corpus callosum have been noted in children with PTSD (see Kaufman et al., 2004, for a review).

Differential Diagnosis and Assessment

Incidents of sexual or physical abuse are frequently denied by parents and children. Domestic violence is the form of violence exposure reported most frequently by parents. There is considerable potential for traumatic exposures to be missed if only one or two sources are relied on for reporting. Several excellent measures are available to help assess childhood trauma. These include semi-structured and structured child interviews as well as several questionnaires (see Stover et al., 2007, for a summary). A number of issues can arise when dealing with assessment of potential trauma in children. As noted previously, data from multiple informants are typically needed. At times, children may deny the experience of a traumatic event that is well document. In such instances, the child should be informed of what is known from other sources and inquiry made regarding PTSD symptoms without necessarily asking for a detailed review of their experience of the event. The discussion can start with items related to overarousal before moving on to the avoidance symptoms and finally to reexperiencing symptoms that are most challenging for children to talk about. Information from parents, teachers, and other can helpfully supplement the information from the child. The clinician should be particularly aware of symptoms that are less likely to be noted by parents, foster parents, or other caregivers ("acting out" or externalizing symptoms are more likely to come to notice than internalizing symptoms).

It is important for clinicians to be aware of other symptoms, in addition to PTSD symptoms, in children exposed to trauma. Comorbid psychiatric difficulties are common over the course of time in individuals with PTSD; additional conditions frequently include major depression and other mood disorders as well as substance abuse. Diagnosis can be complicated because symptoms of both disorders can be simultaneously present. The symptoms of major depression should, for example, include at least some features unique to it rather than to PTSD. Hallucinations are sometimes observed in children who have suffered abuse, but usually other features suggestive of psychotic disorders will be absent. These hallucinations also typically resolve with appropriate intervention. Diagnostic issues in young children are particularly complex. Alternative criteria have been proposed in infants and toddlers (see Stover et al., 2007) given

Case Study: Posttraumatic Stress Disorder

Tammy, an 8-year-old girl, witnessed her father shoot and kill her mother in the family home. The parents had a stormy relationship, and the mother had recently obtained a court order to keep him out of the home. Tammy's older sister was out of the home at the time of the shooting. In the weeks immediately after the event, Tammy appeared to be preoccupied with themes of violence and loss in her play but seemed to be unable to recall many details of the actual event. Her maternal aunt, with whom she now resided, reported that periodically she would be very distressed, becoming highly anxious but being unable to talk about what made her anxious. The aunt's observation was that this often occurred after she watched violent television programs, particularly ones involving shooting. Tammy was reported by her aunt to be more withdrawn. She had difficulties falling asleep and had frequent nightmares; during at least one of the nightmares, she appeared to be talking to her mother. Treatment was instituted 6 weeks after the event, and Tammy appeared to significantly improve but remained somewhat hypervigilant and anxious.

Comment: Posttraumatic stress disorder (PTSD) in children can involve disorganized or agitated behavior. Stress-related symptoms may be seen immediately after the event or sometime later. Acute stress disorder is diagnosed if the condition lasts for at least 2 week for a maximum of 4 weeks and must occur within 4 weeks of the event. PTSD can be diagnosed after that time if other criteria are met.

the major impact of developmental factors and differences in the presentation after traumatic experiences.

Course and Prognosis

Various factors contribute to risk for developing PTSD and its subsequent course. Although the experience of an ASD is one obvious predictor, some children who experience it do not go on to develop PTSD. There appears to be a significant genetic component based on results of twin studies. Other risk factors, including preexisting psychiatric difficulties in the child or family history of psychiatric problems.

The nature of the traumatic experience is also important (e.g., severe, chronic, unexpected traumas are more problematic). The degree to which the psychosocial environment is a supportive one after the event is also a major predictor of response; the absence of such an environment and psychosocial adversity increase risk.

Treatment

Intervention work for PTSD in children has advanced significantly in recent years. A number of treatment models have now been proposed and validated. All share a major initial concern with ensuring the child's safety, providing psychosocial support (including through supporting primary caregivers), and identifying the events that trigger increases in symptoms. Trauma-focused cognitive behavior therapy (Cohen et al., 2004) has been well studied. It includes an emphasis on encouraging expressing feelings, education, stress management techniques, and so on. It provides gradual exposure with joint child–caregiver sessions that support the child's increased ability to confront reminders of the traumatic experience and gain some perspective on the experience. Treatment is usually accomplished over 10 to 18 sessions. This approach has been supported in randomized, controlled trials. Parents as well as children benefit, and the benefits appear to persist over time. Group therapy approaches have been developed, and other models have been proposed in the treatment of younger children.

In adults with PTSD, the selective serotonin reuptake inhibitors have been found to be effective in dealing with the three major areas of difficulty associated with PTSD. These drugs have not been as extensively studied in children with PTSD, although one open-label study suggested some potential benefit (De Bellis, 2005). Some work has also been done with atypical neuroleptics for hyperarousal symptoms.

With increased awareness of the potential negative effects of trauma exposure, new preventive models have been developed. For example, the Child-Development Community Policing Program (CD-CP) (Murphy et al., 2005) is a program pairing mental health and law enforcement professionals now used in a number of communities. Training is provided to allow for emergency consultation and follow-up. This innovative approach aims at engaging police officers, often the "front line" in dealing with traumatic events, to work with mental health workers to prevent the negative effects of trauma.

SUMMARY

Children have suffered from the effects of abuse, neglect, and trauma since antiquity. Over the past century, and with an increasingly rapid pace over the past several decades, advances have been made in recognizing abuse and neglect and trauma and its significant sequelae for children's development. There also has been an increased recognition of the importance of several risk factors, including the major role of psychosocial adversity in increasing risk for the child and family. As a result of studies of children who are neglected and deprived, there has been an increasing recognition of the importance of stable parent-child relationships to foster attachment and long-term development. Advances have been made in recognition of the significant effects of trauma on children and ways these effects can be either prevented or lessened and treated when they occur. Several treatment models have been developed. Challenges remain, including the need for better methods of dealing with underlying psychosocial adversity, models that treat perpetrators and victims (often members of the same family), and more integrated adult–child treatment models.

Selected Readings

AACAP Work Group on Quality Issues. (2005). (Boris, N. W. & Zeanah, C. H., principal authors). Practice parameters for the assessment and treatment of reactive attachment disorder in children and adolescents. *Journal of the American Academy of Child and Adolescent Psychiatry, 44*, 1206–1209.

Bernstein, D., Ahluvalia, T., Pogge, D., & Handelsman, L. (1997). Validity of the childhood trauma questionnaire in an adolescent psychiatric population. *Journal of the American Academy of Child and Adolescent Psychiatry, 3*, 340–348.

Besinger, B. A., Garland, A. F., Litrownik, A. J., & Landsverk, J. A. (1999). Caregiver substance abuse among maltreated children placed in out-of-home care. *Child Welfare, 78*(2), 220–239.

Bretherton, I. (1992). The origins of attachment theory: John Bowlby and Mary Ainsworth. *Developmental Psychology, 28*, 759–775.

Burns, B., Phillip, S., Wagner, H., Barth, R., Kolko, D., Campbell, Y., & Landsverk, J. (2004). Mental health need and access to mental health services by youths involved with child welfare: a national survey. *Journal of the American Academy of Child and Adolescent Psychiatry, 43*(8), 960–970.

Caspi, A., McClay, J., Moffitt, T. E., Mill, J., Martin, J., Craig, I. W., Taylor, A., & Poulton, R. (2002). Role of genotype in the cycle of violence in maltreated children. *Science, 297*(5582), 851–854.

Child Maltreatment 2006. (2008). *U.S. Dept. Health Human Services, Administration on Children, Youth, and Families.* Washington, DC: US Government Printing Office.

Cicchetti, D., & Toth, S. (1995). A developmental psychopathology perspective on child abuse and neglect. *Journal of the American Academy of Child and Adolescent Psychiatry, 34*(5), 541–565.

Cohen, J. A., Deblinger, E., Mannarino, A. P., & Steer, R. A. (2004). A multisite, randomized controlled trial for children with sexual abuse-related PTSD symptoms. *Journal of the American Academy of Child and Adolescent Psychiatry, 43*(4), 393–402.

De Bellis, M. D., Keshavan, M. S., Shifflett, H., Iyengar, S., Beers, S. R., Hall, J., & Moritz, G. (2002). Brain structures in pediatric maltreatment-related posttraumatic stress disorder: A sociodemographically matched study. *Biological Psychiatry, 52*(11), 1066–1078.

De Bellis, M. D., & Van Dillen, T. (2005). Childhood post-traumatic stress disorder: An overview. *Child and Adolescent Psychiatry Clinics of North America, 14*(4), 745–772, ix.

Forsyth, B., & Asnes, A. G. (2007). Munchausen syndrome by proxy. In A. Martin & F. Volkmar (Eds.), *Lewis's Child and Adolescent Psychiatry: A Comprehensive Textbook*, 4th edition, pp. 692–700. Philadelphia: Lippincott Williams & Wilkins.

Gilbertson, M., Shenton, M. E., Ciszewski, A., Kasai, K., Lasko, N., Orr, SP., & Pittman, R. K. (2002). Smaller hippocampal volume predicts pathologic vulnerability to psychological trauma. *Natural Neuroscience, 5,* 1242–1247.

Gleason, M. M., & Zeanah, C. H. (2007). Reactive attachment disorder. In A. Martin & F. Volkmar (Eds.), *Lewis's Child and Adolescent Psychiatry: A Comprehensive Textbook*, 4th edition, pp. 692–700. Philadelphia: Lippincott Williams & Wilkins.

Griego, J. A., Kodituwakku, P. W., Hart, B. L., Escalona, R., & Brooks, W. M. (2002). Reduced hippocampal volume and total white matter volume in posttraumatic stress disorder. *Biological Psychiatry, 52*(2), 119–125.

Jones, L. M., Finkelhor, D., & Halter, S. (2006). Child maltreatment trends in the 1990s: Why does neglect differ from sexual and physical abuse? *Child Maltreatment, 11*(2), 107–120.

Kassam-Adams, N., & Winston, F. K. (2004). Predicting child PTSD: The relationship between acute stress disorder and PTSD in injured children. *Journal of the American Academy of Child and Adolescent Psychiatry, 43*(4), 403–411.

Kaufman, J. (2007). Child abuse and neglect. In A. Martin & F. Volkmar (Eds.), *Lewis's Child and Adolescent Psychiatry: A Comprehensive Textbook*, 4th edition, pp. 692–700. Philadelphia: Lippincott Williams & Wilkins.

Kaufman, J., Aikins, D., & Krystal, J. (2004). Neuroimaging studies in PTSD. In J. Wilson & T. M Keane (Ed.), *Assessing Psychological Trauma and PTSD*, pp. 389–417. New York: Guilford Press.

Kaufman, J. (2000). Exposure to violence and early childhood trauma. In A. Martin & F. Volkmar (Eds.), *Lewis's Child and Adolescent Psychiatry: A Comprehensive Textbook*, 4th edition, pp. 195–207. Philadelphia: Lippincott Williams & Wilkins.

Kaufman, J., Jones, B., Steiglitz, E., Vitulano, L., & Mannarino, A. (1994). The use of multiple informants to assess children's maltreatment experiences. *Journal of Family Violence, 9,* 227–248.

Kessler, R., Sonnega, A., Bromet, E., Hughes, M., & Nelson, C. (1995). Posttraumatic stress disorder in the National Comorbidity Survey. *Archives of General Psychiatry, 52*(12), 1048–1060.

Kilpatrick, D., Ruggiero, K., Acierno, R., Saunders, B., Resnick, H., & Best C. (2003). Violence and risk of PTSD, major depression, substance abuse/dependence, and comorbidity: Results from the National Survey of Adolescents. *Journal of Consulting and Clinical Psychology, 71*(4), 692–700.

Meadow, R. (1977). Münchausen syndrome by proxy: The hinterland of child abuse. *Lancet, 2,* 343–345.

McCloskey, L. A., & Walker, M. (2000). Posttraumatic stress in children exposed to family violence and single-event trauma. *Journal of the American Academy of Child & Adolescent Psychiatry, 39*(1), 108–115.

McClure, R J., Davis, P. M., Meadow, S. R., et al. (1996). Epidemiology of Münchausen syndrome by proxy, non-accidental poisoning, and non-accidental suffocation. *Archives of Diseases of Childhood, 75,* 57–61.

Molnar, B. E., Buka, S. L., & Kessler, R. C. (2001). Child sexual abuse and subsequent psychopathology: Results from the National Comorbidity Survey. *American Journal of Public Health, 91*(5), 753–760.

Murphy, R. A., Rosenheck, R. A., Berkowitz, S. J., & Marans, S. R. (2005). Acute service delivery in a police-mental health program for children exposed to violence and trauma. *Psychiatry Quarterly, 76*(2), 107–120.

Myers, J., Berliner, L., Briere, J., Hendrix, C. T., Jenny, C., & Reid, T. A. (2002). *The APSAC Handbook on Child Maltreatment*. Thousand Oaks, CA: Sage Publications.

O'Connor, T. G., & Rutter, M. (2000). Attachment disorder behavior following early severe deprivation: Extension and longitudinal follow-up. *Journal of the American Academy of Child and Adolescent Psychiatry, 9,* 703–712.

Perez, C. M., & Widom, C. S. (1994). Childhood victimization and long-term intellectual and academic outcomes. *Child Abuse and Neglect, 18*(8), 617–633.

Rosenberg, D. A. (2003). Münchhausen syndrome by proxy: Medical diagnostic criteria. *Child Abuse and Neglect, 27,* 420–430.

Shaw, J. A. (2000). Summary of the practice parameters for the assessment and treatment of children and adolescents who are sexually abusive of others. *Journal of the American Academy of Child and Adolescent Psychiatry, 39*(1), 127–130.

Sheridan, M. S. (2003). The deceit continues: An updated literature review of Münchausen syndrome by proxy. *Child Abuse and Neglect, 27,* 431–451.

Smyke, A. T., Dumitrescu, A., & Zeanah, C. H. (2002). Disturbances of attachment in young children: I. The continuum of caretaking casualty. *Journal of the American Academy of Child and Adolescent Psychiatry, 41,* 972–982.

Stover, C. S., & Berkowitz, S. (2005). Assessing violence exposure and trauma symptoms in young children: a critical review of measures. *Journal of Trauma and Stress, 18*(6), 707–717.

Stover, C. S., Berkowitz, S., Marans, S., & Kaufman, J. (2007). Posttraumatic stress disorder. In A. Martin & F. Volkmar (Eds.), *Lewis's Child and Adolescent Psychiatry: A Comprehensive Textbook*, 4th edition, pp. 701–710. Philadelphia: Lippincott Williams & Wilkins.

Teicher, M. H., Dumont, N. L., Ito, Y., Vaituzis, C., Giedd, J. N., & Andersen, S. L. (2004). Childhood neglect is associated with reduced corpus callosum area. *Biological Psychiatry, 56*(2), 80–85.

Thompson, S. (2005). Accidental or inflicted? *Pediatric Annals, 34*(5), 372–381.

Villarreal, G., Hamilton, D. A., Petropoulosm H., Driscoll, I., Rowland, L. M., et al. (2002). Reduced hippocampal volume and total white matter volume in posttraumatic stress disorder. *Biological Psychiatry, 52*(2), 119–125.

Zeanah, C. H., Scheeringa, M. S., Boris, N. W., Heller, S. S., Smyke, A. T., & Trapani, J. (2004). Reactive attachment disorder in maltreated toddlers. *Child Abuse and Neglect, 28*(8), 877–888.

CHAPTER 21 ▪ PEDIATRIC PSYCHOPHARMACOLOGY

SPECIFIC DRUG TREATMENTS

Stimulants

Clinical Applications and Empirical Support

The stimulants (Table 21.1), especially the short- and long-acting forms of methylphenidate and amphetamine, are first-line treatments for attention-deficit/hyperactivity disorder (ADHD). The most commonly used stimulants for the treatment of patients with ADHD include methylphenidate, dextroamphetamine and the mixed preparation of D,L-amphetamine. Immediate-release methylphenidate has been studied more carefully than the other stimulants and remains the most commonly used agent in clinical practice. Although less well studied, the amphetamine products and extended-release formulations of methylphenidate have short-term efficacy and safety profiles that are comparable to methylphenidate.

The empirical basis for the use of stimulants in children with ADHD rests on findings from hundreds of short-term, randomized, placebo-controlled studies conducted over the past 30 to 40 years. Results from controlled studies over the past decade provide additional information about dose response, similarities and differences in response across stimulant preparations, and the importance of clinical monitoring to achieve optimal response.

To date, only methylphenidate has been evaluated in long-term studies. With its sample size of 576 children, the Multimodal Treatment Study of children with ADHD (MTA) provided convincing evidence for the long-term benefits of methylphenidate. In the MTA study, children were randomly assigned to one of four treatment groups: medication management (primarily methylphenidate administered in a systematic fashion with close monitoring); an intensive behavioral treatment program; combined medication management and the same behavioral treatment program; or community care, which served as the control group. After 14 months of treatment, all four groups showed improvement compared with baseline. Comparisons across the four groups showed that the combined treatment group and the medication management group did significantly better than the community care group and the behavioral treatment only group across a range of outcomes.

A variety of extended-release formulations, both formulated with methylphenidate and with D,L-amphetamine, are available. These longer acting preparations are as effective as the

TABLE 21.1
STIMULANTS AND STIMULANT ALTERNATIVES

Drug	Mechanism of Action	Main Indications and Clinical Uses	Dosage mg/d	Schedule	Adverse Effects	Comments	Select Brand Names and Preparations Available
Methylphenidate		ADHD	15–60 (Ritalin) 18–54 mg/d (Concerta)	BID/TID (MPH); QD (Concerta)	Insomnia, decreased appetite, weight loss, dysphoria/Possible reduction in growth velocity during long term use/Withdrawal and rebound hyper-activity/Unmasking or induction of tics.		Ritalin/Methilyn: 5, 10, 20 mg t; Sustained release t, 20 mg Concerta: 18, 36 mg
Dextroamphet-amine	Dopamine presynaptic release and reuptake blockade		10–40	BID/TID		Longer acting preparations may have lower peak and valley effects and less rebound hyperactivity	Dexedrine: 5, mg t; Sustained release spansules, 5, 10, 15 mg
Amphetamine compound			10–40	QD/BID	Possible induction/ accelaraion of mania/ psychosis.		Adderal: 5, 10, 20, 30 mg; Adderal XR: 5, 10, 15, 20, 25, 30 c
Pemoline			37.5–112.5	QD	Same as other stimu-lants/Abnormal liver function tests and serious hepatotoxicity	Liver monitoring necessary (2/month minimum suggested). Rarely used any more given hepato-toxic concerns	Cylert: 18.75, 37.5, 75 t, 37.5 mg chewable t
Atomoxetine	Selective noradrenergic reuptake inhibitor		10–80	QD/BID	Loss of appetite, dizziness, nausea; rare instances of hepatotoxicity have been reported	Technically an anti-depressant and not a stimulant, but used only in the treatment of ADHD.	Strattera: 10, 18, 25, 40, 60, 80 mg c

Note: Doses are provided as general guidelines only, and are not meant to be definitive.
All doses must be individualized and monitored through the appropriate clinical and/or laboratory means.
Abbreviations: c (capsule), t (tablet)

immediate-release compounds and show similar side effect profiles. The advantage of the long-acting preparations is that children do not need to take a dose in school, which may enhance compliance. The longer duration formulations may minimize the behavioral rebound often seen with immediate-release formulations.

Adverse Effects

Growth retardation, presumed to be secondary to stimulant-induced appetite suppression, has been a common concern among clinicians and families alike. Based on data from a large cohort of clinic cases treated with stimulants, it appears that slowed growth may be temporary and that children with ADHD may be shorter than their age mates before puberty but catch up in adolescence. Height and weight should be monitored regularly in children treated with stimulants and tracked during long-term maintenance.

Other common side effects include sleep disturbance, depressed mood, stomachaches, headaches, overfocusing on details, tics and mannerisms, and picking at skin. Insomnia can be difficult to sort out because many children with ADHD have sleep difficulties before receiving stimulant medications. Thus, the child's sleep history should be documented before treatment and monitored throughout. As noted, it is common practice for the third dose of methylphenidate to be lower than the first two to minimize a possible rebound effect. The administration of clonidine as an aid for sleep has been proposed, but its use is controversial. Data regarding the emergence of tics after stimulant treatment have been contradictory, and the issue remains unresolved. Nonetheless, children with tic disorders should be monitored carefully when treated with stimulants. Dose reduction may be sufficient, but discontinuation may be warranted in some cases.

Antidepressants

The antidepressants include a group of chemically diverse compounds that have been shown to be effective in the treatment of adults with major depression. More recently, several antidepressants have been used in the treatment of adults with a range of other disorders, including obsessive-compulsive disorder (OCD), generalized anxiety disorder, panic disorder, social phobia, and posttraumatic stress disorder. These broader clinical applications are likewise being implemented with increasing frequency in the pediatric population even though the level of empirical support varies widely. Antidepressants can be classified according to (1) chemical similarity (e.g., tricyclic compounds, and within these, secondary and tertiary amines), (2) primary mode of action (e.g., the selective serotonin reuptake inhibitors [SSRIs], selective norepinephrine reuptake inhibitors, or monoamine oxidase inhibitors), and (3) miscellaneous, newer antidepressants (e.g., bupropion, venlafaxine, or mirtazapine). The SSRIs are by far the most extensively used antidepressant class in children and adolescents and the class with the best empirical support. Because of these facts and the recent controversy over their potential association with suicidal thoughts, plans, and self-injurious behavior, the SSRIs are discussed first.

Selective Serotonin Reuptake Inhibitors

The SSRIs are a group of chemically unrelated compounds that potently inhibit the return of serotonin into presynaptic neurons (Table 21.2A). Currently marketed SSRIs include fluoxetine, sertraline, paroxetine, fluvoxamine, citalopram, and escitalopram.

Clinical Applications and Empirical Support

As a group, these medications are generally well tolerated, can typically be given once a day, and do not require blood level monitoring or electrocardiographic (ECG) monitoring. Early clinical trials looked at the use of clomipramine and fluoxetine in children and adolescents. Several large placebo-controlled clinical trials were conducted in pediatric populations with

TABLE 21.2A
SSRI ANTIDEPRESSANTS

A. Selective Serotonin Reuptake Inhibitors (SSRIs)

Drug	Mechanism of Action	Main Indications and Clinical Uses	Dosage mg/d	Schedule	Adverse Effects	Comments	Select Brand Names and Preparations Available
Fluoxetine	Serotonin presynaptic reuptake blockade	Obsessive Compulsive Disorder/Major Depression/ Other Anxiety Disorders	2.5–40	QD/ FLV = BID	Irritability/Akathisia/Insomnia/ Appetite decrease (acute use) or increase (chronic)/ GI symptoms/Headaches/ Dizziness/Flu-like symptoms during discontinuation/ Complex drug interactions. All SSRIs have variable degrees of CYP inhibition (see previous chapter). Higher doses often needed for OCD. Exacerbation or new onset of suicidal ideation was initially reported for paroxetine in 2003; careful monitoring recommendations for *all* antidepressants followed a review of all clinical trials for child and adolescent depression (see text for details).	Only SSRI with FDA approval for the treatment of depression. Longest half life.	Prozac: 10 mg t/c 20 mg t, oral solution 20 mg/ 5 ml
Sertraline			25–200				Zoloft: 25, 50, 100 mg t
Paroxetine			10–30			SSRI originally associated with suicidal ideation; no longer recommended for use in children and adolescents.	Paxil: 10, 20, 30, 40 mg t Oral suspension 10 mg/ 5 ml
Fluvoxamine			12.5–200			Short half-life implies BID dosing and greater likelihood of withdrawal syndrome.	Luvox: 25, 50, 100 mg t
Citalopram			10–40			Most favorable drug interaction profiles among the SSRIs.	Celexa: 20, 40 t
l-Citalopram			10–20				Lexapro: 10, 20 t

sertraline and fluvoxamine in OCD, with fluoxetine and paroxetine in depression, and with fluvoxamine in non-OCD anxiety disorders. In each of these studies, the SSRI was superior to placebo in the primary outcome measure of interest.

Depression. Fluoxetine, sertraline, paroxetine, and citalopram have each been studied for the treatment of depression in children and adolescents. A landmark fluoxetine study in 1999 was the first to show superiority of an antidepressant over placebo for the treatment of depression in children and adolescents and was subsequently followed by a replication study. A randomized clinical trial of citalopram has also shown superiority over placebo.

The largest and most important study to date in this area is the Treatment for Adolescents with Depression Study (TADS). In it, 439 adolescents were randomly assigned to fluoxetine alone, cognitive behavior therapy (CBT) alone, their combination, or pill placebo for 12 weeks in the acute phase and for a 6-month extension. Results of the acute phase showed that combined treatment had the highest rate of positive response (71% for the combined treatment compared with 61% for medication alone, 43% for CBT alone, and 35% for placebo). The combined treatment group also had a slightly lower rate of suicidal ideation compared with the fluoxetine-only group. Fluoxetine alone and fluoxetine with CBT were both superior to placebo. However, combined treatment with fluoxetine and CBT was not significantly better than medication only, and CBT alone was not superior to placebo.

Concerns over the safety of the SSRIs in children and adolescents have become paramount. Extensive review by British and American regulatory agencies eventually led to their removal (in the United Kingdom) and the introduction of a U.S. Food and Drug Administration (FDA)—mandated black box warning (in the United States). A review was commissioned by the FDA of all clinical trials using SSRIs in the treatment of children and adolescents with depression and other indications ($n > 4,400$ subjects across 26 controlled trials). This review showed an increase risk of new-onset suicidal ideation in SSRI-treated individuals versus those treated with placebo (occurring at respective rates of 4% and 2%, for a risk ratio of 1.95; 95% confidence interval, 1.28–2.98). All reported events referred to suicidal *ideation* rather than suicidal acts or completed suicides. It is important to note that data suggest that increasing rates of SSRI use during the past decade may be related to decreases in rates of *completed* suicide, particularly among adolescents and young adults. Taken together, these data support the judicious use of antidepressants in children and adolescents, particularly if other interventions have failed or are not available. When treatment with an SSRI is opted for, fluoxetine may be generally recommended as the first-line agent because of its FDA indication for depression and a lower reported rate of incident suicidal ideation. Guidelines from the FDA and the American Academy of Child and Adolescent Psychiatry call for intensive monitoring during the early phases of treatment: as often as weekly for the first 4 weeks, every other week for the next month, and monthly thereafter.

Obsessive-Compulsive Disorder. Sertraline and fluvoxamine have been evaluated in randomized, multisite, placebo-controlled trials of parallel groups. Using the Children's Yale-Brown Obsessive Compulsive Scales (CYBOCS) as the primary outcome measure, both drugs were superior to placebo in improving obsessive-compulsive symptoms. Sertraline was evaluated in 187 subjects and was associated with at least a 25% improvement in the CYBOCS score in 53% of subjects compared with 37% for placebo. In a separate study of 120 children between the ages of 8 and 17 years, fluvoxamine at a mean daily dose of 165 mg was effective in 42% of children compared with 26% among those treated with placebo. Although these data suggest that the SSRIs are effective for the treatment of OCD in children and adolescents, the magnitude of response may not be large, as has been shown in a meta-analysis of all studies published through 2002.

Adverse Effects. As a group, the SSRIs are generally well tolerated. In addition to their propensity for cytochrome P450–based drug interactions common side effects of the SSRIs in children and adolescents appear to be behavioral activation and gastrointestinal (GI) complaints such as nausea or diarrhea. Signs of behavioral activation include motor restlessness, insomnia, impulsiveness, disinhibited behavior, and garrulousness. The potential for behavioral activation early in treatment underscores the importance of starting at low doses and moving upward slowly. As with other antidepressants, hypomania and mania have been reported, and peripubertal children may be at heightened risk. Other adverse effects include heartburn, decreased appetite, fatigue, and sexual side effects. Suicidal ideation is discussed above

A flu-like syndrome characterized by dizziness, moodiness, nausea, vomiting, myalgia, and fatigue occurring in association with the withdrawal or acute discontinuation of shorter acting SSRIs such as paroxetine, fluvoxamine, and sertraline has been described.

Drug Interactions

The use of combined psychotropic medications seems to be on the rise, underscoring the importance of monitoring drug–drug interactions in clinical practice. SSRIs vary in their potential for such interactions at particular P450 cytochromes. As illustrated previously, inhibition of the P450 cytochrome responsible for metabolizing an additive drug raises its serum level, thereby enhancing its beneficial or deleterious effects.

Tricyclic Antidepressants

Clinical Applications and Empirical Support

Tricyclic antidepressants (TCAs; Table 21.2B) have been used to treat several psychiatric disorders of childhood over the past 3 decades, including depression, ADHD, OCD, separation anxiety disorder, and enuresis. Studies have demonstrated the efficacy of desipramine in children with ADHD and of clomipramine for the treatment of OCD in children and adolescents. Because of concerns over cardiotoxicity associated with desipramine, TCAs are now generally reserved for treatment-resistant cases. TCAs continue to have a limited but important role in the treatment of patients with enuresis and treatment-refractory ADHD and OCD.

Clinical Management

For all of the TCAs, repeat vital signs and ECGs should be obtained during the dose adjustment phase and when the maintenance dose has been achieved. As part of the informed consent process, potential cardiac effects and the reason for repeat ECG monitoring should be discussed with the family and with the child in a developmentally appropriate manner. A corrected QT interval (QTc) above 450 msec, a QRS complex longer than 120 msec, or a PR interval greater than 200 msec warrants dose reduction followed by a repeat ECG. Exceeding these parameters should prompt treatment reevaluation and perhaps discontinuation. For patients showing clinical benefit and persistent ECG abnormalities, consultation with a pediatric cardiologist is in order.

Adverse Effects

The TCAs are associated with a range of adverse effects, including sedation, dizziness, dry mouth, excessive sweating, weight gain, urinary retention, tremor, and agitation. In addition to these largely anticholinergic-based side effects, TCAs can have dose-dependent adverse effects on cardiac conduction (which can be tracked with an expectable dose-dependent prolongation of the QTc) as well as on the seizure threshold. With regard to seizures, clomipramine may have the highest potential to lower the seizure threshold, so its dose and possible drug interactions need to be monitored closely.

OTHER ANTIDEPRESSANT MEDICATIONS (Table 21.2C)

Atomoxetine (Strattera)

Atomoxetine was originally developed for the treatment of depression, but it has never been marketed as an antidepressant. As noted previously, atomoxetine is a selective norepinephrine

TABLE 21.2B
TRICYCLIC ANTIDEPRESSANTS

Drug	Mechanism of Action	Main Indications and Clinical Uses	Dosage mg/d	Schedule	Adverse Effects	Comments	Select Brand Names and Preparations Available
B. Tricyclic Antidepressants (TCAs)							
Imipramine	Norepinephrine >dopamine presynaptic reuptake blockade Anticholinergic, antihistamine,	MDD Enuresis ADHD ADHD+Tic disorders	2.5–5.0 mg/kg/d		Anticholinergic (dry mouth, constipation, blurred vision) Weight gain Cardiovascular (mild blood pressure and ECG conduction parameters with daily doses >3.5 mg/kg) Treatment requires serum levels and ECG monitoring	Serum levels can be useful in adjusting dosage, monitoring potential toxicity, determining metabolizer status	Imipramine hydrochloride: 10, 25, 50 mg t Imipramine pamoate: 75, 100, 125, 150 mg c
Desipramine				QD/BID			Desipramine: 10, 25, 50, 75, 100, 150 mg t Nortriptyline: 10, 25, 50, 75 mg; elixir (?) Clomipramine: 25, 50, 75 t
Nortriptyline	alpha-1 postsynaptic effects	Anxiety disorders	2.0–3.0 mg/kg/d				
Clomipramine	Same as other TCAs Serotonin presynaptic reuptake blockade	Same as other TCAs OCD					

TABLE 21.2C
OTHER ANTIDEPRESSANTS

Drug	Mechanism of Action	Main Indications and Clinical Uses	Dosage mg/d	Schedule	Adverse Effects	Comments	Select Brand Names and Preparations Available
C. Other Antidepressants							
Bupropion	Unknown ?Norepinephrine > dopamine presynaptic reuptake blockade	MDD ADHD	3.0–6.0 mg/kg/d	TID	Irritability Insomnia Drug-induced seizures (in doses >6 mg/kg) Contraindicated in bulimia Seizures associated with >300 mg/day or >150 mg/dose.	Useful alternative to stimulants in ADHD, but exacerbation of tics has been reported	Wellbutrin: 75, 100 mg t Wellbutrin SR: 100, 150 t
Venlafaxine	Serotonin/ norepinephrine presynaptic reuptake blockade	MDD	1.0–3.0 mg/kg/d	BID/TID	Similar to selective serotonin reuptake inhibitors Nausea, sleepiness, dizziness Dose-dependent (?) sustained diastolic hypertension Exacerbation of suicidal ideation highest for venlafaxine; careful monitoring especially warranted with its use. Not recommended for routine use in children and adolescents.	Under 150 mg/d, similar to an SSRI; noradrenergic effects at higher doses	Effexor: 25, 37.5, 50, 75, 100 mg t Effexor XR: 37.5, 75, 150 mg c
Trazodone	Serotonin presynaptic reuptake blockade/5HT2a postsynaptic antagonism	Insomnia	25–200	QHS	Nausea, dry mouth, dizziness, constipation/Orthostatic hypotension/Sedation/Priapism	Although the closely related compound, nefazodone, had less alpha antagonism than trazodone (i.e. less risk of hypotension and priapism), it is no longer used because of concerns over liver toxicity.	Trazodone: 50, 100, 150, 300 mg t
Mirtazapine	Alpha₂ presynaptic and 5HT₂A/3 postsynaptic antagonism	MDD	7.5–30	HS	Drowsiness (greater at low doses?) Appetite/weight gain	Useful alternative to SSRIs leading to activation?	Remeron: 7.5, 15 mg

reuptake inhibitor, a property that it shares with desipramine. Unlike desipramine, however, atomoxetine does not appear to prolong cardiac conduction times. Given the efficacy of desipramine for the treatment of patients with ADHD, atomoxetine was evaluated as a treatment for ADHD. After the completion of several placebo-controlled trials, atomoxetine was approved by FDA as a safe and effective treatment for children and adolescents with ADHD. In fact, it is the only approved, nonstimulant medication for the treatment of ADHD. It may also be useful in the treatment of comorbid oppositional defiant disorder.

Mood Stabilizers (Table 21.3)

Lithium

Clinical Applications and Empirical Support. The efficacy of lithium in the acute and maintenance treatment of and prophylaxis of children and adolescents with classic bipolar disorder has been demonstrated in case reports, open trials, and retrospective naturalistic studies. The first placebo-controlled study of lithium in youngsters included 25 adolescents with various forms of bipolar illness and comorbid substance abuse. Although lithium was associated with improvements in overall functioning and a lower rate of substance abuse relapse, there was no difference between active and placebo groups on measures of manic or depressive symptoms. Taken together with other conflicting studies, currently available published data provide limited support for the use of lithium for the short-term or maintenance treatment of bipolar illness in children and adolescents

Other Clinical Applications

Aggression. A study comparing haloperidol, lithium, and placebo in 61 treatment-resistant aggressive children found that after 4 weeks of inpatient treatment, both haloperidol and lithium were superior to placebo in reducing aggressive behavior; and lithium was associated with fewer side effects.

Clinical Management. Before initiating a trial of lithium, a child should have a physical examination, including screening laboratory tests such as a complete blood count, electrolytes, blood urea nitrogen, creatinine, and thyroid indices. In outpatient settings, dosing may be initiated at 300 mg twice a day for children and 600 mg twice a day for adolescents. For children younger than 12 years of age, doses in the range of 10 to 30 mg/kg per day are typical.

Because of its narrow therapeutic index, lithium levels should be monitored closely. The optimal serum level range is in the range of 0.6 to 1.1 mEq/L. Serum levels should be drawn on average 4 days after a dose adjustment to ensure that a steady state has been achieved and 12 hours after the previous dose to ensure a trough reading. When used to treat patients with bipolar illness, the clinical benefit of lithium may be evident within 10 to 14 days of reaching therapeutic serum level in some cases. Current recommendations include repeat laboratory tests at 6-month intervals. Lithium levels should also be obtained when the patient's clinical status changes, if adverse effects occur, and routinely at 3- to 6-month intervals.

Adverse Effects and Toxicity. Lithium appears to be generally well tolerated in children and adolescents. Common side effects include fatigue, nausea, diarrhea, abdominal distress, tremor, ataxia, aggravation of acne, cognitive dulling, and weight gain. Because lithium is excreted by the kidneys, it is generally not recommended in children with compromised renal function. The risk of glomerular damage with long-term lithium treatment appears to be minimal, but polyuria and polydipsia are relatively common because of lithium's effect on tubular reabsorption. Lithium-induced polyuria can generally be managed conservatively by reducing the total daily dose (when possible), by switching from a short to a long-acting preparation, or by the addition of a low dose of a potassium-sparing diuretic such as amiloride. In a few cases, nephrogenic diabetes insipidus can occur, which may warrant discontinuation of lithium.

TABLE 21.3
MOOD STABILIZERS

Drug	Mechanism of Action	Main Indications and Clinical Uses	Dosage mg/d	Schedule	Adverse Effects	Comments	Select Brand Names and Preparations Available
Lithium	Inhibition of phosphatidyl inositol and protein kinase C signaling pathways Enhancement of serotonergic transmission	Bipolar disorder, manic Prophylaxis of bipolar disorder MDD Aggressive behavior/ Conduct disorder Adjunct treatment in refractory MDD	10–30 mg/kg/d, dose adjusted to serum levels in the range of 0.6–1.1 mEq/l	BID/TID	Polyuria, polydipsia, tremor, ataxia, nausea, diarrhea, weight gain, drowsiness, acne, hair loss/ Possible effects on thyroid and renal functioning with long-term administration/Children prone to dehydration are at higher risk for acute lithium toxicity Lithium levels >2 mEq/L can be life-threatening	Therapy requires monitoring of lithium levels, thyroid and renal function	Lithium carbonate: 150, 300, 600 mg c/ Sustained release forms: Lithobid 300 mg t, Eskalith 450 mg t/Lithium citrate elixir: 8 mEq (300 mg)/5 ml
Divalproex	Inhibition of catabolic enymes of GABA, and of protein kinase C signaling	Bipolar disorder/ Aggressive behavior/Conduct disorder/Seizure disorders	15–60 mg/kg/d, dose adjusted to serum levels in the range of 50–125 mcg/l	BID/TID	Sedation, nausea, liver toxicity (requires baseline and close monitoring) Thrombocytopenia, pancreatitis	Policystic ovarian disorder has been reported during long-term use for seizure control	Depakene (valproic acid): 250 mg; elixir Depakote (divalproex): 125, 250, 500 mg t; sprinkles: 125 mg c
Carbam-azepine	Inhibition of glial steroidogenesis/ Inhibition of alpha 2 receptors/Blocks sodium channels/	Bipolar disorder/ Complex partial seizures	10–20 mg/kg/d, dose adjusted to serum levels in the range of 4–14 mcg/l	BID	Bone marrow suppression (requires baseline and close monitoring of blood counts) Dizziness, drowsiness, rashes, nausea Liver toxicity, especially under 10 years of age.	Potent inductor of CYP3A4, leading to auto-induction requiring periodic dose adjustment	100 mg chewable t; 200 mg/Elixir: 100 mg/5 ml
Ocxarbam-azepine	Blocks glial calcium influx		Maintenance dose of 18.5–48 mg/kg/day, not to exceed 2100 mg/day		No reports of bone marrow suppression, and more benign drug interaction profile compared to carbamazepine. No blood level monitoring necessary.	No empirical data available for children and adolescents.	Trileptal: 150, 300, 600 t; 60 mg/ml suspension

Drug	Mechanism	Indication	Dose	Frequency	Side effects	Notes	Formulations
Lamotrigine	Weak 5HT3 inhibition/ ?Release of Aspartate and Glutamate		75–300	QD	Potentially life-threatening rash/ Stevens Johnson syndrome (dose- [direct] and age- [inverse] related event rates)	Slow dose titration (12.5 mg QOWk) may reduce risk of skin reactions	Lamictal: 25, 100, 150, 200 mg t/ Chewable: 5, 25 mg, t
Gabapentin	Gabapentin is chemically related to GABA, but GABAergic effects unclear	Bipolar Disorder/ Seizure disorders	100–1000+	TID	Sedation, ataxia at high doses/ Very high therapeutic index	Excreted renally unchanged No significant drug interactions	Urontin: 100, 300, 400, 600, 300 mg c
Topiramate	Glutamate release antagonist/ GABA reuptake inhibitor		50–400	BID	Cognitive difficulties (dulling, word retrieval, attention) Dizziness, sedation	Weight loss may be a potentially beneficial side effect	Topamax: 25, 100, 200 mg t

Signs of lithium toxicity can occur even at "normal serum levels." In mild forms, symptoms include nausea, diarrhea, impaired concentration, and muscle weakness. At serum levels above 2.5 mEq/L, multiple organs may be affected, and toxicity may prove fatal. Because dehydration can increase lithium levels and may induce toxicity, parents and children should be educated about the importance of adequate fluid intake. Lithium has been associated with a small increased occurrence of tricuspid valve abnormalities and transient neurodevelopmental deficits in exposed newborns. Contraception should be encouraged in adolescents, and treatment of a pregnant mother with lithium should weigh possible fetal effects against the adverse outcomes of an untreated mood disorder.

Valproate

Clinical Applications and Empirical Support. Valproate (VPA) is an anticonvulsant that has been shown to be an effective mood stabilizer in adults. Clinicians have used VPA in the treatment of a range of problems in children and adolescents, including bipolar illness and aggression associated with conduct disorder or oppositional defiant disorder. There are case reports and open studies that support the use of VPA in youth with conduct disorder, explosive behaviors, and impulsive aggression, and two small randomized clinical trials support VPA efficacy in this population. There is less evidence supporting the use of VPA in acute or maintenance therapy of bipolar disorder in youth; two open studies showed a response rate of 50% to 60%, and a study in teens with mixed mania showed more than a 70% response. Studies involving VPA with AAPs have yielded response rates of 80% or higher for the combination therapy. In conclusion, these emerging data provide a modest level of support for the use of VPA in the treatment of children and adolescents with bipolar disorder.

Adverse Effects and Toxicity. GI complaints, sedation, and (rarely) transient hair loss may accompany the initiation of treatment and may subside with continued dosing. Other adverse effects include increased appetite and weight gain, postural tremor, dizziness, asthenia, and cognitive dullness. Rare idiosyncratic effects may also occur. VPA has also been associated with hepatic failure, and in children younger than 2 years of age, with fatal hepatitis. Early in treatment, there is also a small risk of pancreatitis. Agranulocytosis is extremely rare. In women treated for seizure disorders, there have also been reports of polycystic ovary disease manifested clinically by hyperandrogenism, accelerated weight gain, and menstrual and lipid profile irregularities. VPA toxicity can be life threatening and may begin with increased tremor and confusion. It is associated with hyperammonemia, respiratory depression, and multiorgan failure. Because of significant teratogenicity, a negative pregnancy test result and a reliable method of contraception should be documented before initiating treatment with VPA in sexually active female adolescents.

Antipsychotics

Clinical Applications and Empirical Support

The antipsychotics can be classified according to chemical family, such as phenothiazines or butyrophenones, or according to the relative potency of their dopamine blockade. With the introduction of clozapine and a short list of newer compounds, it is becoming common to classify antipsychotics as typical or atypical. Pediatric uses of antipsychotics include the treatment of psychosis, severe behavioral problems associated with autism and other developmental disorders, aggression, tics, and bipolar disorders and as an adjunctive treatment in OCD.

Atypical Antipsychotics (Table 21.4A)

Clozapine (Clozaril). Clozapine is a dibenzodiazepine derivative and is chemically unrelated to any of the typical antipsychotic drugs. Soon after it was introduced in the 1960s, its effectiveness in treatment-resistant patients with schizophrenia was recognized, but initial enthusiasm waned after the report of fatal agranulocytosis in a series of cases in Europe. Two open studies

TABLE 21.4A

ATYPICAL ANTIPSYCHOTICS

A. Atypical

Drug	Mechanism of Action	Main Indications and Clinical Uses	Dosage mg/d	Schedule	Adverse Effects	Comments	Select Brand Names and Preparations Available
Risperidone	Dopamine and 5HT receptor blockade/Atypical antipsychotics in general have high 5HT2a/D2 affinity ratios: Risperidone 8:1 Olanzapine: 5:1 Quetiapine: 1:1 Aripirazole: 10:1 Clozapine: 30:1	Psychosis: positive and negative symptoms/TS/ Augmentation in OCD/Bipolar Disorder/Autism and PDDs/ Aggression and agitation	0.25–4	QD/BID			Risperdal: 0.25, 0.5, 1, 2, 3, 4 mg t/ Elixir: 1 mg/ml
Olanzapine			2.5–10		Sedation/Appetite increase/ Weight gain/Metabolic syndrome (glucose intolerance, dyslipedemia)		Zyprexa: 2.5, 5, 7.5, 10 mg t
Quetiapine			100–600		Low incidence of extrapyramidal adverse effects/		Seroquel: 25, 100, 200 mg t
Aripiprazole			5–40		Insomnia, mild activation more likley with aripirazole		Abilify: 5, 10, 20 mg t
Ziprasidone			40–160		Low incidence of extrapyramidal adverse effects; does not induce distonia	Monitoring of QTc interval recommended	Geodon 20, 40 c
Clozapine		Treatment-refractory psychosis	50–400	BID/TID	Low risk for tardive dyskinesia/Granulocytopenia/ agranulocytosis (treatment requires constant monitoring of blood count) Higher risk of seizures (dose related)	Weekly blood counts mandatory (monitoring for WBC >3000, ANC >2000). Possibility of going to QOWk monitoring by 6 months, QMonth by 12 months. Seizure prophylaxis (with valproate or gabapentin) recommended at higher doses (>300 mg/d)	Clozaril: 25, 100 mg t

and one controlled comparison with haloperidol have been carried out in pediatric populations. Collectively, these studies included 53 patients from ages 6 to 18 years. Clozapine was effective in 56% of these patients. In the controlled trial, doses ranged from 125 to 525 mg/day given in divided doses. Although there were no reports of extrapyramidal side effects (EPS), several serious adverse effects were observed, most notably seizures, hematopoietic abnormalities, and weight gain.

Risperidone (Risperdal). Risperidone is a benzisoxazole derivative that has some pharmacologic features in common with clozapine, but it has not been associated with agranulocytosis. Large multisite studies in adults with schizophrenia have shown that risperidone is an effective antipsychotic with lower risk of neurological side effects than traditional antipsychotics such as haloperidol. It is associated with an increase in prolactin, suggesting more potent D_2 blockade. At doses above 6 mg/day, the risk of neurological side effects increases in a dose-dependent manner.

To date, risperidone is the best studied AAP in pediatric populations. An emerging body of evidence from short-term, placebo-controlled, randomized clinical trials shows that risperidone is safe and effective for serious behavior problems in children with autism, severe disruptive behavior, and Tourette's disorder. A few studies have also shown that short-term gains endure over the intermediate term.

Aripiprazole (Abilify). Aripiprazole is approved for the treatment of adults with schizophrenia, but very few studies are currently available in children and adolescents. This drug has been described as a *third-generation* antipsychotic because of its novel mechanism of action. Aripiprazole is classified as a partial dopamine agonist. Similar to the other AAPs, aripiprazole has serotonin-blocking properties at 5HT2 receptor sites. It is likely that aripiprazole will be evaluated in pediatric populations for many of the same target symptoms described above for risperidone.

Typical Antipsychotics (Table 21.4B)

Chlorpromazine (Thorazine). Chlorpromazine is an aliphatic agent and was the first antipsychotic used in children with severe behavioral disturbances. With the introduction of newer agents, the use of chlorpromazine has declined, although it is still routinely used for the acute management of agitation or aggression, when it can be administered through either oral or intramuscular (IM) routes. When used IM, careful caution must be paid to vital signs because significant hypotension can occur even at seemingly low doses (e.g., less than 25 mg).

Haloperidol (Haldol). A butyrophenone that is structurally unrelated to the phenothiazines, haloperidol represents the prototype of a high-potency typical antipsychotic. Since its introduction in the early 1960s, it has been used to treat children with psychosis, aggressive behavior, tics, and behavioral dyscontrol associated with autism. Compared with the low-potency antipsychotics, haloperidol is much more likely to cause EPS, but it is less sedating. The dose of haloperidol varies according to the target symptoms. In school-age children with tics or severe behavioral dyscontrol associated with autism, the dose is typically in the range of 0.75 mg to 2.5 mg per day. By contrast, doses in the range of 10 mg may be used to deal with an acute psychotic episode.

Adverse Effects. Neurological side effects such as dystonic reactions, rigidity, and akathisia are more common with the high-potency antipsychotics. In addition to these neurological side effects, adverse effects of the typical antipsychotic drugs in children and adolescents may include cognitive blunting, weight gain, depressed mood, social phobia, and elevated prolactin levels. Drowsiness is a common side effect with the low-potency antipsychotic agents, but it may occur in the high-potency antipsychotics as well. Anticholinergic side effects such as dry mouth, constipation, and blurred vision should be monitored. As noted, thioridazine, pimozide, ziprasidone, and other antipsychotics can prolong cardiac conduction times. Expert

TABLE 21.4B
TRADITIONAL ANTIPSYCHOTICS

Drug	Mechanism of Action	Main Indications and Clinical Uses	Dosage mg/d	Schedule	Adverse Effects	Comments	Select Brand Names and Preparations Available
B. Typical (Traditional), or Neuroleptic							
Phenothiazines: Low Potency						A warning label from the FDA was introduced for thioridazine in 2000, advising against its use as a first-line drug, given concerns over QTc interval prolongation.	
Chlorpromazine	D2 receptor blockade All agents in this family have similar efficacy, but different potency based on the dosage required to achieve a similar effect. 100 mg of chlorpromazine are equivalent to:	Psychosis Mania Aggressive behavior/ Agitation/ Self-injurious behavior/Autism	25–400		Anticholinergic (dry mouth, constipation, blurred vision, hypotension—more common with low potency agents) Weight gain		Chlorpromazine: 10, 25, 50, 100, 200 mg t; elixir; suppositories; injectable
Thioridazine							Thioridazine: 10, 15, 25, 50, 100, 150, 200 mg t; elixir
Phenothiazines: Medium and High Potency			4.0–32.0 (Perphenazine) 0.5–10 (Fluphenazine)	QD/ BID/ TID	Extrapyramidal reactions (dystonia, rigidity, tremor, akathisia, greater risk with higher potency)	// Traditional agents are not as effective in treating the negative or affective symptoms of psychosis/Low potency agents have high anticholinergic profiles (e.g sedation, hypotension), whereas high potency agents are likely to cause extrapyramidal side effects (EPS)	
Perphenazine							Perphenazine: 2, 4, 8, 16 mg t; elixir, injectable
Fluphenazine	Thioridazine: 95 mg Perphenazine: 8 mg Fluphenazine: 2 mg				Drowsiness Risk for tardive dyskinesia with long-term administration Withdrawal dyskinesia Hypotension, especially when administered IM		Fluphenazine: 1, 2.5, 5, 10 mg; elixir, injectable, long acting
Other Traditional Anipsychotics–potency	Haloperidol: 2 mg Thiothixene: 5 mg Molindone: 10 mg Pimozide: 1 mg						

(continued)

275

TABLE 21.4B

CONTINUED

Drug	Mechanism of Action	Main Indications and Clinical Uses	Dosage mg/d	Schedule	Adverse Effects	Comments	Select Brand Names and Preparations Available
Haloperidol–high (*butyro-phenone*)			0.5–10				Haloperidol: 0.5, 1, 2.5, 10, 20 mg t; elixir, injectable, long acting
Thiothixene–medium (*thioxanthene*)			1–20				Thiothixene: 1, 2, 5, 10, 20 mg t; elixir, injectable
Molindone–medium (*indole derivative*)			5–150		Lowest weight gain liability among traditional agents		Molindone: 5, 10, 25, 50, 100 mg t; elixir
Pimozide–high		Same as other antipsychotics/Tourette's disorder	1–4		Cardiac arrhythmias (EKG: elongated QTc) Seizures Extrapyramidal reactions Drowsiness Tardive dyskinesia Withdrawal dyskinesia		Orap: 1, 2 mg t

opinion in published guidelines for the use of antipsychotics in Tourette's syndrome (TS) indicates that when using pimozide or ziprasidone in children and adolescents, an ECG should be obtained before treatment, during the dose adjustment phase, and periodically thereafter.

Although the AAPs are less likely to cause neurological side effects, they are not free of adverse effects. Clozapine is associated with a low risk of agranulocytosis and thus is only used in patients with treatment-resistant schizophrenia. Other adverse effects of clozapine include a lowered seizure threshold and tachycardia. An important adverse effect of the AAPs is increased appetite and weight gain, with several reports in pediatric samples showing that clozapine, olanzapine, quetiapine, and risperidone are associated with excessive weight gain. Based on available data in pediatric populations, the risk of weight gain appears to follow this order: clozapine, olanzapine, quetiapine, and risperidone.

The risk of tardive dyskinesia (TD) increases as a function of dose and duration, but it may occur with brief exposures as well. TD has been reported in pediatric patients, and although it does not appear to be common, it should be monitored for. To minimize TD, dose reductions should be done gradually while evaluating changes in symptom severity. In autism and tic disorders, discontinuation may be considered annually for patients in whom good control has been achieved. If symptoms persist, the maintenance dose of the antipsychotic should be reduced to the lowest possible one sufficient to maintain symptomatic control. Based on the collective experience with clozapine, the newer atypicals may also have a lower risk of TD.

Neuroleptic malignant syndrome is a rare adverse effect of antipsychotics, which is characterized by high fever, autonomic instability, and muscle breakdown. It is potentially life threatening, with a mortality rate as high as 9% in children and adolescents. Discontinuation of the medication is usually all that is required; thus, early identification is critical. In severe cases, intravenous fluids are needed, and some authors have advocated the use of dantrolene or bromocriptine to hasten recovery.

Treatment of Antipsychotic-Associated Adverse Effects

Acute neurological side effects seen with traditional antipsychotics include dystonia, torticollis, and oculogyric crisis. The chronic side effect of parkinsonism is manifested as tremor, rigidity, masklike facies, or a festinant gait. These adverse effects can be prevented or reversed with the judicious use of anticholinergic agents. Given that all of these adverse effects are associated with unchecked D_2 receptor blockade, it follows that they are more common with high-potency traditional agents and less common with low-potency compounds. Although less common with AAPs, the risk of neurological side effects increases at higher dose levels of risperidone, olanzapine, or ziprasidone. In most instances, the anticholinergics discussed here (Table 21.5) are used in combination with high-potency agents, and they should rarely (if at all) be used in combination with lower potency drugs. Not only are the low-potency agents less likely to cause neurological side effects, but the addition of antiparkinsonian medications may also exacerbate the inherent anticholinergic properties of the low-potency antipsychotics. This point is of more than academic interest: the additive effects of combining agents with anticholinergic or antihistaminergic effects can rapidly lead to behavioral toxicity, including paradoxical agitation, confusion, or full-blown delirium.

The two most commonly used anticholinergics are diphenhydramine (Benadryl) and benztropine (Cogentin). The antihistamine diphenhydramine is best used in acute situations given its ready availability and benign side effect profile. However, the sedation induced by diphenhydramine can be intense, so this agent should be used sparingly as a maintenance intervention. Alternatively, such sedation can be exploited therapeutically in acutely agitated patients. Benztropine is preferred for longer term management of neurological side effects because it does not induce somnolence. Diphenhydramine is usually dosed in the 12.5- to 50-mg range (single or repeat dose, administered orally or by IM injection), and benztropine is used in 0.5-, 1-, or 2-mg doses, usually given orally in a twice-daily regimen. The long-term use (longer than1 month) of anticholinergic agents should be avoided if at all possible, particularly in younger children, for whom mouth dryness can lead to widespread cavities.

TABLE 21.5
ANTIHISTAMINE, ANTICHOLINERGIC AGENTS

Drug	Mechanism of Action	Main Indications and Clinical Uses	Dosage mg/d	Schedule	Adverse Effects	Comments	Select Brand Names and Preparations Available
Diphenhydramine	Antihistamine	Sleep disorders Agitation, acute dystonic reactions	12.5–100	TID/QID	Sedation, cognitive impairmaint, antichlolergenic (dry mouth, constipation, blurred vision)		Diphenhydramine: 25, 50 mg t; elixir, injectable
Benztropine	Anticholinergic (muscarinic)	Extrapyramidal reactions (dystonia, rigidity, tremor akathisia)	0.5–3	BID/TID	Delirium (rare, except at higher doses)		Benztropine: 0.5, 1, 1 mg; elixir, injectable

TABLE 21.6
NORADRENERGIC AGENTS

Drug	Mechanism of Action	Main Indications and Clinical Uses	Dosage mg/d	Schedule	Adverse Effects	Comments	Select Brand Names and Preparations Available
Alpha Agonists							
Clonidine	Nonspecific alpha-2 presynaptic agonist	Tourette's disorder ADHD Aggression/self-abuse severe agitation Withdrawal symptoms	0.025–0.4	BID/TID/QID	Sedation (very frequent) Hypotension (rare) Dry mouth Irritability Dysphoria Rebound hypertension Localized irritation with transdermal preparation	Transdermal absorption can be erratic; limited bio-availability	Clonidine: 0.1, 0.2, 0.3 mg t Transdermal patch: Catapres TTS 1, 2, 3 (delivering 0.1, 0.2, 0.3 mg/d/wk)
Guanfacine	Selective alpha-2a agonist	Tourette's disorder ADHD	0.5–4	BID/TID	Same as clonidine Less sedation, hypotension		Tenex: 1, 2 mg t
Beta Blockers							
Propranolol	Post-synaptic beta blockade	Akathisia, Lithium-induced tremor Aggression/self-abuse Severe agitation/ Alternative to neuroleptuics, especially in developmentally delayed individuals	2.0–8.0 mg/kg/d	BID	Similar to clonidine Higher risk for bradycardia and hypotension (dose dependent) and rebound hypertension Bronchospasm (contraindi-cated in asthmatics) Rebound hypertension on abrupt withdrawal Contraindicated in diabetics		Propranolol: 10, 20, 40, 60, 80 mg t Long-acting 60, 80, 120, 160 mg t
Nadolol			20–200				Nadolol: 20, 40, 80, 120, 160 mg t

α_2-Adrenergic Agents

The α_2-adrenergic agents (clonidine and guanfacine; Table 21.6) are only approved for use in adults with hypertension. Beginning with the early studies of clonidine for the treatment of TS, these drugs have become increasingly common in child psychiatry for treating tics, ADHD, and aggressive behavior in children.

Clonidine (Catapres)

Clinical Applications and Empirical Support. Early studies of the use of clonidine in the treatment of tics showed contradictory or inconclusive evidence concerning its efficacy versus placebo. In this context, a study was undertaken by the Tourette Syndrome Study Group called the TACT (Treatment of ADHD in Children with Tourette's Disorder) study. Its results suggest that the combination of clonidine plus methylphenidate provided fuller coverage of ADHD symptoms in this population and may have provided some protection against adverse effects, specifically insomnia.

Guanfacine (Tenex)

Guanfacine is an α_2-agonist that is similar to clonidine and was also developed as an antihypertensive agent. Interest in guanfacine has been prompted by three observations. First, compared with clonidine, it is less sedating. Second, it has a longer half-life than clonidine, which could translate into a need for fewer doses per day and a lower risk of rebound effects. Third, accumulated data from a series of animal studies provide compelling evidence that guanfacine is more specific in action than clonidine. The promising results of several studies, including a placebo-controlled study of guanfacine in 34 children, suggest that guanfacine is a safe and effective treatment for children with ADHD and that it can be beneficial in the reduction of tics. Although not as effective as stimulants, guanfacine should be considered when stimulant treatment has failed or cannot be tolerated.

The adverse effects of clonidine and guanfacine are similar, although guanfacine appears to be better tolerated. The most common side effects include sedation, dizziness, irritability (especially when the medication wears off), and mid-sleep awakening. Hypotension is generally not a problem with either drug in children and adolescents, but it warrants monitoring, particularly in the dose adjustment phase. A related concern with clonidine is the well-documented phenomenon of rebound hypertension after precipitous withdrawal. Thus, abrupt discontinuation of either drug should be avoided. There is incomplete consensus in the field regarding the need for ECGs in children and adolescents treated with the α_2-agonists. A recent statement from the American Heart Association indicates that no cardiovascular monitoring other than blood pressure and pulse is required for those taking clonidine or guanfacine.

Anxiolytics

Although SSRIs remain the only empirically proven pharmacologic intervention for the treatment of pediatric anxiety disorders, the benzodiazepines (Table 21.7) remain widely used. The benzodiazepines are often *misused* in pediatrics (as misguided efforts to treat depression, delirium, or agitation), but they are powerful compounds that can be quite useful, even if the empirical database for their use in very limited in pediatrics. Of the many available benzodiazepines, the three most commonly used are lorazepam (Ativan), alprazolam (Xanax), and clonazepam (Klonopin). These agents have similar efficacy as anxiolytics, although they differ widely in their potency (1 mg of lorazepam being roughly equivalent to 0.5 mg of alprazolam or 0.25 mg of clonazepam) and in their half-lives (shorter for lorazepam and alprazolam; longer for clonazepam). All benzodiazepines can cause drowsiness, disinhibition, agitation, and confusion, and clonazepam in particular can lead to dysphoria or depression. Withdrawal reactions can occur if maintenance doses are not slowly weaned down. These medications do

TABLE 21.7

ANXIOLYTICS

Drug	Mechanism of Action	Main Indications and Clinical Uses	Dosage mg/d	Schedule	Adverse Effects	Comments	Select Brand Names and Preparations Available
High Potency Benzodiazepines							
Clonazepam (long-acting)	Enhancement of GABAergic transmission via binding to a specific benzodiazepine site within the GABAa receptor	Anxiety disorders Adjunct in treatment-refractory psychosis Adjunct in mania	0.25–3	QD/BID	Drowsiness, disinhibition, agitation, confusion Depression Withdrawal reactions Potential risk for abuse and dependence Less risk for rebound and withdrawal reactions		Klonopin: 0.5, 1, 2 mg t
Alprazolam (short-acting)		Severe agitation Severe insomnia MDD + anxiety akathisia	0.25–4	TID			Xanax: 0.25, 0.5, 1, 2 mg t
Lorazepam (short-acting)			0.5–6	TID	Same as other benzodiazepines Higher risk for rebound and withdrawal reactions	Does not go through Phase I reactions: good choice in the context of hepatic failure	Ativan: 0.5, 1, 2 mg t injectable
Atypical Anxiolytic							
Buspirone	Serotonin 1A agonist	Anxiety disorders Adjunct treatment refractory OCD	15–60	TID	Drowsiness, disinhibition	No cross tolerance with benzodiazapines	BuSpar: 5, 10, 15, 30 mg t

TABLE 21.8

ANTIENURETIC AGENTS

Drug	Mechanism of Action	Main Indications and Clinical Uses	Dosage mg/d	Schedule	Adverse Effects	Comments	Select Brand Names and Preparations Available
Desmopresin	Antidiuretic hormone analogue	Eneuresis	10–40 mcg	QHS/BID	Headache/Nausea/Hyponatremia and water intoxication at toxic doses	Can be useful for acute situations (e.g. sleepaways)	DDAVP: 0.1, 0.2 mg t; Nasal spray: 10 mcg/spray
Oxybutynin	Antimuscarinic agents		5.0–15	BID/TID	Anticholinergic side effects		Ditropan: 5 mg t
Tolterodine			1–2	BID	Less anticholinergic effects, less sedation		Detrol: 1 mg t

carry a potential risk for abuse and dependence and need to be prescribed cautiously in the context of personal or family history of substance abuse or dependence.

Clonazepam (Klonopin)

Clonazepam is a long-acting benzodiazepine that is approved as an anticonvulsant. In adults, it is also used to treat anxiety disorders and as an adjunctive treatment for tics. A study of 15 prepubertal children showed that clonazepam can be useful in anxiety disorders in some children, but side effects, including disinhibition, irritability, and drowsiness, were common. Clonazepam should not be used as a first-line agent for the treatment of anxiety disorders in pediatric populations, although it can be useful as an adjunctive intervention, especially on a time-limited basis. Treatment can begin with 0.25 mg in the morning and increased to 0.25 mg twice daily after 3 to 4 days. Thereafter, the dose may be increased slowly to a maximum of 2 mg per day in divided doses. Clonazepam should be tapered gradually when discontinued. Children treated for more than 4 weeks should be tapered when coming off of the drug to limit rebound anxiety or seizures.

Antineuritic Agents

Desmopressin, Oxybutynin, and Tolterodine

Desmopressin (DDAVP) is a synthetic antidiuretic hormone, a powerful inhibitor of the production of urine (Table 21.8). It can be administered orally or via intranasal spray. One review suggested that DDAVP helps approximately 25% of children who use it, with minimal risk of adverse effects. Although DDAVP is usually well tolerated, the beneficial effects often do not endure over time. The most effective treatment for enuresis is the use of behavioral interventions, such as a pad and buzzer or a moisture alarm. However, DDAVP can be a useful short-term adjunct, as in the facilitation of sleepovers or overnight camp stays. For longer term pharmacological management of enuresis, usually in cases unresponsive or only partially responsive to behavioral interventions, antimuscarinic agents can occasionally be useful. Alternatives to the time-tested use of low- (25 to 50 mg HS) or regular-dose imipramine include oxybutynin (Ditropan) or the less sedating tolterodine (Detrol). As is the case of other pharmacologic interventions for enuresis, beneficial effects usually disappear rapidly upon drug discontinuation.

CHAPTER 22 ■ PSYCHOTHERAPIES

The origins of psychotherapy can be traced to diverse sources. Freud attempted to understand the horse phobia of a child (Little Hans) in light of his own theories of development and the unconscious. Early behaviorists noted the important role of learning in fear and fear conditions (e.g., the case described by Mary Jones in 1923). Over time, the field of psychotherapy as it applies to children and adolescents has expanded dramatically. During this period, the predominant mode of scientific inquiry has shifted from the focus on the single clinical case to research methods using groups of children in clinical trials. Modern approaches pay considerable attention to issues of study method and design, use of standard measures, manualization to ensure replicability, and so forth (see Weersing & Dirks, 2007).

EFFICACY OF PSYCHOTHERAPY

An important and immediate issue is the question of whether psychotherapy works. The first review of psychotherapy, now more than 5 decades old, raised important questions about the effectiveness of psychotherapy (i.e., over rates of improvement noted in untreated children and adolescents). This result corresponded, in many ways, to an influential review questioning the efficacy of psychotherapy in adults. Both sets of findings were the source of much debate. Thoughtful consideration of these early efforts identified several important limitations of the then available research. These included nonrandom assignment to treatment, lack of attention to independent evaluations, the need for careful control and comparison groups, and so forth. Recognition of these limitations led to the development of more effective clinical trial research.

A substantive body of research is now available, and it has become possible to conduct meta-analytic reviews in which the results of carefully selected studies can be pooled and analyzed. Results can then be summarized in terms of overall effect size. Typically, a statistic such as the statistic proposed by Cohen's d quickly conveys how different a treatment group is from a comparison in terms of units of standard deviation. For example, a d of 0.2 would usually be termed a small effect size, and a d of 0.8 would be viewed as large.

In the first review of this kind in psychotherapy for children, Casey and Berman (1985) noted a reasonably good effect size (0.71). Subsequent work has generally confirmed that medium to large effect sizes are frequently observed, similar to those reported in adults. Subsequent research has also addressed issues that may moderate treatment outcome (e.g., variables in child, family, and environment). Interestingly, the nature of the child or adolescent's difficulties does not appear to straightforwardly related to the degree of improvement. Children and adolescents with internalizing-type problems (depression, anxiety) are just as likely to profit from intervention as are those with externalizing difficulties (conduct disorder, attentional problems). If appropriate controls are used, adolescent girls are more likely to improve, and behavioral interventions appear to be generally more effective than more traditional psychodynamic approaches. On the other hand, some treatments, such as interpersonal therapy (IPT) for adolescents with depression and multisystemic therapy (MST) for youth with conduct problems, do not easily fit into this simplistic dichotomy. Clearly, some treatment approaches, such as family or group therapy, may also include both more behavioral and more psychodynamic elements (Kazdin & Weiss, 2003).

The movement toward evidence-based treatment has factored heavily in attempts to evaluate psychotherapies. To qualify as *evidence based,* a treatment must have been shown to work in two independent, carefully designed, controlled studies with random assignment to treatment and comparison to either a placebo or comparison treatment group. (Some argue that well-controlled single cases studies could also qualify if these were sufficiently numerous.) The term *probably efficacious* has been used when the study design is less stringent (e.g., through comparison of treated cases to a wait list control). Using these guidelines, a series of psychosocial treatments can be regarded as well established for conduct disorder, enuresis, and phobias; the evidence for anxiety and depressive disorders suggests that treatments for patients with these disorders are probably efficacious. Behavioral treatments have been much more numerous, and accordingly, they are more likely to be identified as evidence based than more traditional psychodynamic ones. In the current climate of concern about health care reform and use of potentially scarce resources, it is not surprising that issues of evidence-based treatments have become the focus of much debate. Even when the efficacy of a specific treatment model has been established, typically in a highly research-oriented setting, important questions of the effectiveness of the treatment in real-world settings must also be addressed. The typical university setting for clinical trials offers many advantages in terms of access (e.g. extensive logistical support, the potential for careful training and monitoring treatment methods over time). If conducted as part of a research project, participation may be free or participants may even be paid for being involved. Unfortunately, only a few studies have actually addressed the issue of treatment effectiveness in more usual treatment settings. In one review, Weisz and others (1992) found a handful of studies of clinic treatment as usual and noted that the mean effect size was near zero. Various attempts have been made to address this problem (e.g., through enhanced service coordination), but results have been disappointing. Thus, there is a major gap between what can be done in research settings and what actually happens in the community.

Attempts have been made, particularly in the areas of depression and anxiety disorders, to address these issues, and initial results are encouraging. Studies have also examined combined treatments (e.g., medication and cognitive behavior therapy [CBT]) suggesting a modest benefit of adding CBT to drug treatment. Other efforts have focused on the effectiveness of work with parents, notably in the area of parent management training (PMT), in which studies evaluating both clinical use and cost effectiveness of this approach have appeared with initial positive results (e.g., in reducing number of arrests). Given the public health and social policy significance of youth conduct problems, these results are particularly encouraging, and the approach has been adapted for other populations, including for substance abuse.

Clearly, psychotherapy can work for children and adolescents. The question of how it works remains an important topic for research and active area of debate. The question is a difficult one to answer for many reasons. Even a highly structured treatment will include multiple components, any of which, or any combination of which, may be most relevant to particular problems. For example, in work on anxiety using CBT, is it the explicit teaching of relaxation that is more important or the education, or is it the exposure to the anxiety-provoking situation or the combination? Further problems arise given our limited understanding of the pathophysiology. Only a few studies have attempted to understand treatment processes. It will be important for future work in this area to develop more relevant measures, that is, beyond the typical child and parent report and observation scales, to more direct measures of behavior or physiology.

PSYCHODYNAMIC PSYCHOTHERAPY

Insight-oriented or psychodynamic psychotherapy is the oldest of the psychotherapies and has its origins in the attempt beginning the 19th century to understand mental activity, the interplay of mind and brain, and symptoms and conditions that could be related to these processes. Sigmund Freud's contribution remains substantial, and modern methods owe a considerable intellectual debt to him (e.g., of the conscious and unconscious mind and the importance of developmental issues in understanding symptoms; see Chapter 1). Freud's case of "Little Hans" provides one of the first reports of attempts to engage in psychotherapy with children. Because of Freud's emphasis on the importance of early experience in the analysis of adults, he and his students had a strong developmental orientation. Several of his early trainees, including his daughter Anna, began direct work with children. From early on, this work noted the importance of an awareness of development, the role of parents, and the special complexities of work with children (e.g., the role of education, the place of play activities). In England, Melanie Klein developed the model of play analysis as the analog of free association in adult psychoanalysis and emphasized interpretation with a focus on core issues. In contrast, Anna Freud, who moved to England with her family shortly before World War II and who had been trained as a teacher, emphasized the "educative" functions of child therapy as well as interpretation. The war in Europe, and increased interest in mental health issues after the war, contributed to an influx of European-trained psychiatrists and analysts in the United States. Their ideas influenced a generation of therapists and had an impact on the approaches to treatment used in child guidance clinics, congregate care programs, and similar settings.

Goals of psychodynamic psychotherapy often involve changing patterns of thought, feeling, or behavior that are partly, or even fully, not in the individual's consciousness. This process also relies on the importance of the relationship with the therapist attempting to help the patient. The notion of *transference* arises in the regard and refers to the tendency of people to treat the therapist in ways they believe they have been treated. In addition, there is a significant "real" relationship with the therapist that may also further the psychotherapeutic process; this is particularly the case in work with children. Usually, the therapist attempts to understand the patient's difficulties in light of his or her early history and experiences as well as in the context of the direct observations and interaction with the patient.

Freud elaborated a complex theory of psychological functioning (see Chapter 1), and at different points in his professional life, he emphasized different features, but his theory was always strongly developmental. He highlighted the interplay of biological factors and psychological ones in both normal development and psychopathology. He emphasized the importance of sexual development and believed that the surface (conscious behaviors, thoughts, and feelings reported by people) could be studied scientifically and was multiply determined and that aspects of unconscious or not fully conscious issues could be inferred based on observation and discussion with the patient. His theory also emphasized the importance of conflict (external or internal) in the formation of difficulties and of various "drives" (sexual or aggressive) that the individual must cope with. As a practical matter, his therapy took the form of talking, or with children, playing, to clarify the nature of *conflicts* and developmental arrests and distortions (i.e., in the various ways, maladaptive and adaptive, that the individual dealt with these). One of the goals was to make conscious operations or response patterns that would otherwise remain unconscious and continue to be acted out or acted upon in some way. This was done as the therapist gathered data over time and could make interpretations. Freud also viewed the tendency of the patient to relieve past relationships within the therapy (transference) as important and noted that the therapist could similarly have feelings about the patient (countertransference) that also provided information.

Freud's theory evolved over time but had a tremendous influence on the development of models of the mind and mental illness in the 20th century. Many aspects of Freud's views have been incorporated into other aspects of psychology and many of his concepts have influenced educational practices and child care. Over time, a myriad of other models and approaches have appeared. For example, one group, the ego psychologists, developed a strong interest in understanding the working of the ego. Many members of this group were interested in children's development and child psychotherapy. Another group developed in response, or counterresponse, to some of Freud's notions about female development and female sexuality. Another school of psychoanalytic thought, object relations theory, has emphasized the centrality of internal representations both of the self and others in typical development and psychopathology. This school has been very much concerned theoretically with the earliest development of the mind and clinically with some of the more challenging patients (e.g., those with borderline personality disorders) and emphasizes issues such as early modulation of aggression and the ability to tolerate affect and develop relationships with parents and others.

Regardless of the specific theoretical orientation of the therapist, psychodynamic psychotherapy is centrally concerned with the therapist-patient relationship both as a lens for viewing the past and understanding how the past colors the present. The therapist also looks at patterns in the patient's relationships and daily life to clarify these issues. In addition, the patient has, to some degree, a "real relationship" with the therapist. For therapists working with children, this "real relationship" is often very much present and provides, at least in theory, a greater potential for learning from new experiences. Accordingly, there is great emphasis on how the therapist conducts him- or herself with the child (or adult) patient. The therapist also models a reflective and thoughtful stance encouraging examination, to the extent possible, of repetitive, maladaptive behaviors. This attitude of respect and concern also has the benefit of encouraging the treatment alliance, which is the commitment of the patient to seek greater self-understanding even in the face of anxiety or unpleasant feelings. The countertransference feelings that the patient elicits in the therapist also provide the therapist with important information that can guide treatment.

Many different aspects of treatment can enter into psychodynamic psychotherapy in engaging in psychotherapy with children and adolescents, including work with the parents or family, some degree of education, use of medications, and other modalities. Goals of individual psychodynamic therapy include developing a reasonably full understanding of all the various influences in the child's or adolescent's life and how past experience and patterns of adaptation continue to be expressed in the present (e.g., as symptoms or problem behaviors). This treatment approach is most typically indicated when present difficulties appear to be related to past problems and when intrapsychic conflict and maladaptive solutions (defense mechanisms) can be identified. In some situations (e.g., in relation to current traumatic events or specific life stresses/transitions), psychodynamic therapy can also be helpful. Contraindications for psychodynamic therapy include difficulties that limit capacities for self-reflection and self observation or cognitive capacities (e.g., in terms of language or symbolic thinking). Because such therapy is typically time consuming, it often is not undertaken if a less intensive approach is available. In this regard, however, it is important to note that in contrast to other forms of psychotherapy, the goals of intensive psychodynamic psychotherapy are not limited solely to symptom reduction or elimination. Rather, the goals have to do with helping the individual child or adolescent (or adult for that matter) assume a more normative developmental path with increased capacities for self-regulation, improved relations with others, and an enhanced ability to take appropriate pleasure in school or work activities.

The opening phase of psychodynamic therapy is usually concerned both with fostering the treatment and engagement of the child as well as clarifying aspects of diagnosis and interpersonal dynamics. Depending on the age of the child, the therapist might meet with the parents or, in the case of adolescents, the child first. For younger children, initial visits with the parents can provide important historical information but also let the parents establish a sense of trust in the therapist that can then be conveyed to the child. For adolescents, issues of autonomy, confidentiality, and trust may have special importance. If the therapist meets with the parents first, there is an opportunity to provide some guidance on how to introduce the topic to the child. For younger children, parents may initially join for some portion of the visit with the therapist, although the goal is usually to help the child meet individually with the therapist as quickly as is reasonable. Meeting with the parents early on also helps clarify some aspects of the therapeutic relationship with them (i.e., in general, the therapist strives to maintain confidentiality for the child and typically refrains from conveying information from sessions to the parents, with certain very specific exceptions related, for example, to thoughts of suicide or aggression; see Chapter 24). Children, particularly younger children, may chose to make use of play materials, toys, games, and other activities. For some adolescents, the use of such activities (e.g., cards or chess) may also provide a structure within which the patient can be more comfortable talking "on the side" with the therapist.

Negotiating the complexities of working with the child and meeting periodically with the parents can be challenging. It is important for the therapist to be aware of these complexities and cope as effectively as possible. In some situations, often in child guidance clinics, parents are seen by a colleague for counseling. Even in such cases, however, parents quite rightly want periodic updates and reports of progress.

The therapist strives to foster the therapeutic alliance in several ways. This includes a respectful, supportive, nonjudgmental stance; insistence on confidentiality; and active engagement with the child or adolescent. To this end, the physical location should be appropriate to the needs of the child with appropriate materials for children and adolescents of different levels. For younger children, this includes a set of play materials that can be relatively simple along with drawing and other creative materials and, for older children and adolescents, a selection of games of various types. Some children may bring special materials to therapy sessions or a therapist may supply a specific material in light of a child's needs. At some point, the issue of limit setting will arise. This may initially occur as the child becomes more aggressive or destructive of materials or if the child has difficulty ending a session at the specified time. Setting ground rules and use of routines (e.g., relative to cleaning up materials at the end of each session or storing play materials or activities in a special place) can be helpful.

An evaluation for intensive psychodynamic therapy (i.e., two or more sessions per week) may come either after other treatments have been tried or, occasionally, as an initial option. Typically, the evaluation includes a series of meetings with the child or adolescent and parents during which the therapist tries to formulate an initial diagnostic impression and treatment plan with a specific focus on the issue of whether the child and parents can be helped by the treatment modality. A meeting with the parents, perhaps including the child or adolescent, is held at the conclusion of the evaluation to present an overview of the therapist's perspectives on the difficulties and recommendations for further treatment. Depending on the situation, even more intensive work might be recommended. In classical psychoanalytic treatment, sessions typically occur four or five times weekly. Specific goals are organized around the individual's needs, but there are some important overarching goals, including the desire to help the patient have greater insight, develop new ways to cope with unpleasant feelings and problematic behaviors, and so forth.

The initial or opening phase has to do with obtaining important information on the child or adolescent and his or her difficulties as well as modeling a new approach for the child in attempting to understand these difficulties. This comes about through both implicit processes (modeling, empathizing) as well as more explicit ones (e.g., interpretation). Interpretation consists of helping the child or adolescent understand, with the therapist's help, a new way to understand his or her thoughts, feelings, or impulses. For younger children, the integrative process begins though ongoing commentary of the therapist to the child's play or about the child's behavior or language. The therapist may draw the child's or adolescent's attention to something by wondering about or questioning something with the overarching goal of helping the child become more consciously aware of defense patterns, impulses, or maladaptive ways of coping. The opening phase of treatment typically lasts for weeks to several months.

After a treatment alliance has been established, the middle phase of the treatment concentrates on helping the child develop new defenses and give up old ones. This period, usually the longest phase of treatment, can last from months to even years. By this time, the child or adolescent is actively engaged in treatment as reflected in his or her ability to make use of the therapist's consistency and nonjudgmental approach. Often, play during this time becomes richer and, with older children and adolescents, some activity may alternate or gradually be replaced by talking. Difficulties in the treatment take the focus of resistance (e.g., the child may actively resist coming to sessions or be silent and "bored" during session or, in some cases, the child may be overly compliant but relatively unengaged and passively resistant). The expected moments of resistance or difficulty in therapy, expressed by a sudden shift in topic, feeling, behavior, or withdrawal, can be important clues for the therapist regarding the child's inner experience. It is during the middle phase of treatment that the transference relationship develops most vividly. Thus, the patient will tend to experience the therapist in very specific and unique ways, reflecting previous experiences, particularly with the parents. Important differences from the adult transference relationship exist because the child continues to live with the parents and has a child-adult relationship with the therapist, and the therapist also exists as a new and real person to the child. As a result, the transference relationship in child patients may be less deep and complex than that observed in adult patients. The transference relationship is only one part of the therapeutic process; increased capacity for self-reflection and mastery is also important.

Work with children and adolescents is more immediate and intense than work with adults in intensive psychotherapy or psychoanalysis. The degree to which interpretation and developmental assistance or intervention help is another important difference (i.e., children and adolescents have more opportunities for development and learning in the context of the ongoing treatment). In intensive, psychodynamic therapy even the child's or adolescent's narrative of an external event has the potential for fruitful work (e.g., relative to the patient's growing ability, with increased cognitive maturity, of seeing more than one side of a situation). The therapist continually must balance all of these factors to help the patient achieve a fuller understanding of her or his own mind and its working. A considerable literature exists on this topic; these interventions can include clarification, defense interpretations (pointing out the operation of some specific defensive process), and reconstructions (an explanation that uses the past to explain current experience). Fostering normative developmental processes is also important.

During the middle phase of treatment, the work with parents includes understanding the parent's fears and beliefs about treatment, their hopes for their child in the future, and their fantasies and unrealistic expectations (e.g., that the child will be rescued). In some situations, the parents can see the therapist as a rival or as the authority figure. As much as possible, the therapist should attempt to form an alliance supporting the parents' positive striving as parents. In some situations, parental referral for individual or marital psychotherapy may be appropriate.

The termination phase of treatment involves both the decision to terminate and the process during which treatment is ended. The decision to end treatment can come from the child, therapist, or parents. Ideally, all agree on the appropriateness of setting an ending date. Sometimes a decision will be made unilaterally because of external factors (e.g., a family move). At other times, it may stem from a unilateral decision (e.g., by a parent who feels threatened or ambivalent about the treatment). The final phase of treatment provides an opportunity for a review and reworking of many of the themes and issues raised earlier in the treatment. The child's or adolescent's fantasies and expectations about termination become important. The therapist should consider various factors in considering termination, including the gains made and the child or adolescent's ability to maintain these gains and the degree to which developmental process have been facilitated. Termination awakens issues of separation and loss for both patient and therapist alike. For the patient, the resolution of much less real transference relationship and giving up the very real therapeutic relationship are typically colored by earlier experiences of separation or loss. In this context, regression may occur, and symptoms not seen for some time may reemerge. Such situations provide the child or adolescent with an opportunity to face and discuss these issues and consolidate the insight and self-awareness that hopefully have emerged over treatment. The child or adolescent's ability to internalize some of the therapist's "observing ego" functions is a hallmark of a successful treatment and facilitates longer term development. As much as possible, the child or adolescent patient should be actively involved in the process of termination. The termination phase will be colored by the patient's life experience and can include fear, anger, aggression, or depression. Depending on the situation, the frequency of visits may be gradually reduced or a set frequency may be maintained until the final session. For child and adolescent patients, natural times for ending are frequent (e.g., around the end of school or beginning of a new school or at a prolonged holiday time); it is important that the therapist not, however, choose a date of convenience if this entails giving the patient insufficient time for dealing with her or his reactions to termination. Depending on the situation, a follow-up plan may be put into place; in any event, the door should be left open for the patient to return if the need arises.

In contrast to other treatments, notably CBT (see below), the quality and quantity of research are limited, and in many respects, psychoanalysis and related psychodynamic psychotherapies face major challenges for the future given the absence of this research. This is unfortunate and, in some respects, paradoxical given the origins of psychodynamic treatment in developmental theory and observation. Challenges for research include the diversity of theoretical approaches, the continued reliance on case reports rather than controlled trials, and the dearth of well-done research studies. Fortunately, some work has appeared based on meta-analyses suggesting important gains associated with treatment (see Ritvo & Ritvo, 2007) with reasonably good effect sizes for general psychiatric difficulties, specific targeted problems, and overall functioning at follow-up. Several ongoing research projects, including a large series of carefully conducted studies based at the Anna Freud Center, have shown similarly impressive results. In this series of studies, differences between who did and did not respond to treatment were noted (e.g., children whose symptoms were more severe or whose development were uneven, particularly if they started treatment at younger ages, did well, but those with disorders such as autism did not). Increasingly, studies are being done prospectively. Such work will clarify important issues of treatment dose, efficacy, and patient subject selection. Recent research on psychodynamic therapy has also used some of the method effectively with other treatments (e.g., manualized treatments, carefully selected subject populations, and so forth; Muratori et al., 2003).

COGNITIVE-BEHAVIORAL THERAPY

CBT is the most frequently used evidence-based treatment at present. The term refers to a number of interventions designed to address both cognitive and behavioral issues that impact mental health problems (see Boettcher & Piacentini, 2007). This set of techniques has its origin in learning principles and has had a very strong research basis. As a method, it has grown considerably over the past decade; this reflects its various advantages. In addition to being strongly data based, these techniques are readily learned; are useful for focused, short-term treatment; and are both patient and clinician friendly. CBT has been used in a wide range of disorders, including anxiety disorders, eating disorders, habit and tic disorders, posttraumatic stress disorder (PTSD), conduct disorders, depression, and attention-deficit/hyperactivity disorder (ADHD). It has also been used in targeting social skills and maladaptive behaviors (including anxiety and depression) in individuals with autism and related disorders.

The behavioral foundations of CBT rest strongly in learning theory and the large body of work on behavioral treatments. This work emphasizes the central role of changing behavior with the latter being examined within a broad context, including both antecedences and consequences. This perspective helps clarify what elicits and maintains the behavior and allows for intervention aimed to disrupt some aspect of this process. It is important to understand factors that maintain the behavior, not just those that initially seem to cause it. This approach draws on aspects of both classical and operant conditioning. The work in the 1920s by Mary Cover Jones in demonstrating the learning of fear responses in children was widely applied in the understanding of phobias in general. In phobias, continued avoidance behavior helps to maintain the phobia by preventing exposure to the fear-inducing situation and thus prevents extinction of the fear response. Aspects of classical conditioning can also be used to understand emotional reactions other than fear as well as other mental health problems, including substance abuse and some psychosomatic disorders. As might be expected, treatments based on this model aim to encourage extinction of the learned behavior. Other techniques (e.g., exposure or response prevention) can be used as well. Operant conditioning is similarly based on analysis of antecedents and consequences. In contrast to classical conditioning, operant conditioning can explain acquisition of new behaviors (i.e., not just ones paired with a specific stimulus). This work, based on the work of learning theorists such as Skinner, understands acquisition of new behaviors through reinforcement (e.g., an association of a behavior with a positive outcome). Removal of the reinforcement would, over time, result in a decrease in the behavior. Within this model, rewards or punishments will increase or decrease the frequency of the target behavior (a process called shaping). Different schedules of reinforcement can have different effects in learning (e.g., periodic or variable reinforcement can be even more effective for long-term learning, but continuous reinforcement may be more effective as a behavior is learned). Aspects of operant conditioning have been well studied and widely used (e.g., in the treatment of children with autism in applied behavior analysis; see Chapter 4) along with PMT for children with behavior or conduct problems as well as for many other conditions. Extinction occurs when reinforcement is no longer provided (e.g., to reduce or totally elimi-nate a behavior). This process may be initially associated with higher levels of the behavior of interest (the so-called "extinction burst") before rates of the behavior decrease. Some of the common techniques derived from operant condition principles are listed in Table 22.1.

In addition to its use of behavior therapy, CBT also focuses more broadly on aspects of thinking, feeling, and behavior that may be relevant to the genesis or maintenance of problem. For example, rather than an overt event, it may be a thought or feeling that serves as an

TABLE 22.1

COMMON THERAPY TECHNIQUES ASSOCIATED WITH PRINCIPLES OF OPERANT CONDITIONING

Type and Technique	Description
Reinforcement to increase behaviors	
Token economy	Reinforcing target behavior with "tokens" (e.g., stickers, points, poker chips) that can then be traded in for reinforcers after multiple tokens have been earned
Differential reinforcement of other behavior	Reinforcing specific appropriate behaviors while ignoring inappropriate behaviors that serve the same function
Shaping	Reinforcing gradual approximations of a behavior
Punishment to decrease behaviors	
Overcorrection	Applied consequence that involves engaging in a series of retribution steps that are related to the inappropriate behavior (e.g., washing soiled clothes after toileting accidents)
Response cost	Removal of previously earned reinforcers as consequence of negative behavior; used especially in conjunction with token economy when "tokens" are removed
Time out	Removing all sources of reinforcement for allotted period of time; typically involves placing the individual in a location where access to reinforcing activities, including social attention, is not available
Decreasing behavior with extinction	Removing previously available reinforcement from an inappropriate behavior to decrease the probability that the behavior will occur in the future

Reprinted from Boettcher, M. A., & Piancentini, J. (2007). Cognitive and behavioral therapies. In A. Martin & F. Volkmar (Eds.), *Lewis's Child and Adolescent Psychiatry: A Comprehensive Textbook*, 4th edition, p. 798. Philadelphia: Lippincott Williams & Wilkins.

important antecedent event (e.g., thinking about a fear-inducing stimulus may elicit anxiety even in the absence of the stimulus itself). Thus, CBT is concerned with both behavioral and cognitive techniques in an effort to put emotional difficulties in a broader context. Much of the work of CBT focuses on understanding why some unpleasant experiences or thoughts persist rather than disappear over time. An individual who spends considerable time avoiding a fear-inducing event might, for example, be inadvertently perpetuating and compounding his or her anxiety because there is not an opportunity for exposure to the event, and the individual may believe that the event has been avoided. An example is a child with obsessive-compulsive disorder (OCD) who, having engaged in a number of ritualistic actions, discovers that his parents' health, which he obsessively worries about, remains fine. Attentional issues have importance in the use of the CBT model. An adolescent who is, for example, anxious and depressed may overly attend to cues that support continued feelings of anxiety. Similarly, thoughts or images may be associated with specific reactions (e.g., a child with OCD who is concerned that angry thoughts about his father increase the probability that he will be hurt). Aspects of memory also play an important role (e.g., a person with an anxiety problem may frequently be reminded of past situations in which he or she was anxious or a child with PTSD may recall the traumatic event in response to some relatively minor stimulus and become highly anxious). An overfocus on past mistakes and failings may similarly perpetuate feelings of depression or poor self-esteem. Preoccupation with past negative events may also make it seem more likely that such events will recur.

Cognitive Behavior Therapy in Children and Adolescents

The approach to patients in CBT is a collaborative one in which the therapist works with the patient to better understand and monitor behaviors and thoughts; develop hypotheses about them; and develop alternate ways of coping, behaving, and thinking. Children present some challenges in that they may have problems in self-monitoring. In addition, parental and family influences may also have a major impact on the child. Thus, it is essential that the therapist work within a developmental framework to tailor the treatment effectively to the child's level of understanding and functioning. Issues of autonomy and degree of support must be carefully balanced. The impact of family members or other systematic issues may be important factors to consider as well because, often unwittingly, schools or parents may help maintain problems. Accordingly, work with parents or other adults significant in the child's life may be indicated. Depending on the contact, this may have important advantages for ensuring generalization of effects as well. Difficulties that children, and sometimes adolescents, have with abstract thinking can require adaption of technique (e.g., explanations may have to be made more concrete or a developmental modification can be used to capture some of the child's symptoms or thinking difficulties in a personified way or the child can be encouraged to adopt a role, such as a detective, in gathering information and testing hypotheses). For very young children, modification of CBT through cognitive behavioral play therapy (CBPT) uses cognitive behavioral strategies integrated in more play-based interactions. Modeling or role playing (e.g., with puppets) can be used both to ensure the child's attention and illustrate concepts or issues. For children with higher language and cognitive levels, after about age 9 years, more traditional cognitive techniques can be used. Issues of the frequency, intensity, and duration of treatment are determined considering the child's developmental level. Sometimes even older children may be more likely to be helped by more play-centered approaches.

Family factors are important. Having parents and others focus on antecedents and consequences of behavior can help them notice accommodations that support and even encourage maladaptive behaviors. Similarly, helping parents change routines and disciplinary practices is often an essential aspect of helping the child change. This is particularly true with younger children, who often need adult support in treatment (e.g., in maintaining a focus on treatment goals and homework). Conversely, with older children, parents may need support in allowing the child or adolescent to have greater responsibility for the treatment. Particularly with younger children, parents may be worked with as well, but for older children and adolescents, the child will often be encouraged to attend sessions independently with parents informed in appropriate ways of session content and homework.

CBT is concerned about generalization of treatment effects in several ways, including across settings and between domains of functioning (i.e., behavior and thinking). There is also a concern over generalization of time (i.e., maintenance). For the child to change, techniques and methods should be applied across settings, in various contexts, and over time (i.e., not only in the setting of therapy). Several different strategies are used, including targeting goals for behavior change that cut across settings over time, considering treatment length in light of desired goals, use of behavioral rehearsal (role playing), and so forth.

Regardless of the individual's age, CBT approaches share some basic features such as active involvement of the patient in developing new strategies, use of homework, use of data to monitor treatment, an explicit focus on symptoms and daily functioning, a focus on generalization, and time-limited treatment. The initial phase of treatment usually focuses on assessment of the presenting problem, development of a working relationship, and preparation of the child for the active phase of treatment. The assessments should address detailed information about the symptoms (i.e., chief complaint) and identification of maintaining factors. Normalization of the patient's problems can be an important therapeutic aspect of the assessment phase, which may lead to immediate symptomatic relief. The goal of this phase should be to develop a cognitive behavioral model of the presenting problem to guide treatment. Thus, the assessment phase gathers data on when symptoms occur and their context (location, antecedents, consequences); the cognitions, behaviors, and emotions associated with the symptoms; and the factors that relieve symptoms or make them worse or help to maintain them. In addition, there is a focus on relevant historical information (e.g., previous treatment history, factors associated with the onset of the symptoms), as well as on the cognitions, beliefs, and other experiences that contribute to them. This is often done by asking for a detailed description of a recent episode in which the therapist can ask highly specific questions that will help in designing homework assignments. Having the patient monitor relevant information about symptoms may be helpful.

As symptomatic difficulties and other relevant variables are identified, a treatment plan is developed that usually starts with a focus on educating the child about symptoms and how these can be understood and treated. The active (middle) phase of treatment focuses on implementing and mastering new CBT strategies; this is done with a combination of regular treatment sessions and assigned homework. This phase includes systematic monitoring with the possibility of adjustment made as needed. Psychoeducation is an important element of CBT given the explicit focus on helping the patient understand and change his or her symptoms, feelings, and behaviors. This can include a focus on understanding physiological symptoms and their cognitive components (e.g., a child with PTSD may be helped to understand that intrusive thoughts are common after a traumatic experience). This effort may also itself relieve some anxiety (e.g., about the potential medical seriousness or some symptom). Helping the child make connections between thoughts and events can help the child question prior assumptions (e.g., for a child with OCD, thinking a bad thought is not the same thing as engaging in a bad behavior).

As symptoms become less problematic, the final phase focuses on generalization and maintenance of techniques and preventing relapse. Usually, visits are less frequent, and the child has greater responsibility for ongoing maintenance. Sometimes "booster sessions" may be needed even after treatment has been completed to facilitate maintenance. Treatment frequency can vary somewhat between in- and outpatient treatment settings. It is important that the child have some time between sessions to practice and complete homework. Therapy typically lasts for between 3 and 6 months.

Cognitive Behavior Therapy Techniques

A number of different techniques are used in CBT (see Boettcher & Piacentini, 2007, for a detailed discussion). These include *cognitive restructuring*, which focuses on understanding the role of cognitive distortions in symptoms and replacing them with more accurate and adaptive

TABLE 22.2

COMMON COGNITIVE ERRORS FOUND IN COGNITIVE RESTRUCTURING

Cognitive Error	Description	Example
Catastrophizing	Placing unrealistic importance on thoughts and events and assuming terrible negative outcomes will occur as a result	"I got a C on my report card, so I will never get into college, and I will fail in life."
Magnifying or minimizing	Placing an inaccurate amount of importance on thoughts, feelings, events, and so on (either too much or too little)	Believing getting caught doing drugs is not important because the implications of having a drug problem are too anxiety provoking (minimizing)
Absolutism (black-and-white thinking)	All events and experiences are thought of in extreme categories rather than moderately	"I will *never* lose any weight because I just ate a cookie."
Personalization	Attributing responsibility for external events to the self with no basis for the attribution	"It is my fault that my parents are getting divorced."
Selective abstraction	Taking information out of context and ignoring relevant details	"My soccer coach hates me" when the child did not get to play even though the child started the last previous games
Arbitrary inference	Making arbitrary conclusions contrary to or without evidence	Believing homework is too hard when in fact the child completed the same work that day in class
Ignoring evidence	Leaving out important information when forming thoughts about events	Believing that werewolves are a danger at night even though multiple adults have told the child they do not exist and all the doors in the house are locked
Overgeneralization	Believing the outcome of one situation applies in many situations when it may not	"All my teachers hate me" when one teacher yelled at the child at school
Attending to negative features of events	Placing greater cognitive importance on negative features of events and ignoring positive features	Focusing on one poor grade when all others were good

Reprinted from Boettcher, M. A., & Piancentini, J. (2007). Cognitive and behavioral therapies. In A. Martin & F. Volkmar (Eds.), *Lewis's Child and Adolescent Psychiatry: A Comprehensive Textbook*, 4th edition, p. 803. Philadelphia: Lippincott Williams & Wilkins.

ones, and *identifying automatic thoughts*, which are spontaneous thoughts or responses to situations that contribute to symptoms (Table 22.2). The method of *Socratic questioning and examining the evidence* is used as an important part of cognitive restructuring and involves questioning the patient to help eliciting automatic thoughts and then raise issues regarding their validity. This is particularly important for children who may not understand that thoughts, worries, and so on are not intrinsically true. This method also helps to *correct misinterpretations*, which may cause individuals (e.g., with depression to consistently misinterpret events, their own experience and the behavior of others.

Behavioral experiments are used, particularly as part of psychoeducation to help clarify the importance of cognitive distortions (e.g., the patient may be asked not to think about a particular topic during a short period of time to illustrate how attempts at thought suppression actually result in an overfocus on the avoided topic or idea). Particularly for patients with anxiety, *modification of imagery* may be used to help patients cope with anxiety-provoking events (e.g., in imagining a positive outcome or learning that their images of an event have specific cognitive distortions that result in exaggerated or misplaced anxiety). Certain core beliefs or cognitive schemas that underlying maladaptive thoughts or symptoms may be identified during treatment (e.g., the fundamental core belief that "I am stupid" may result in various compensatory behaviors that are never totally successful). This can be addressed in a number of ways, although it also can be more challenging, particularly for less developmentally mature and sophisticated children.

A range of *physiological techniques* can also be useful, particularly when anxiety leads to significant physical symptoms and bodily sensations. These methods are less dependent on higher levels of cognition and thus more readily used in children. They can take the form of *regulated breathing* during which breathing exercises help reduce physical tension and the tendency to hyperventilation and have the additional benefit of helping patients be more comfortable coping with bodily experiences and sensations. Similarly, *relaxation training* is a technique in CBT that regulates breathing and systematic and progressive tensing and relaxing of muscle groups; this technique can help with anxiety and anger management.

Another set of techniques addresses cognitive distortions through systematic exposure. These *exposure techniques* are based on the idea that the child's anxious and unrealistic overavoidance only exacerbates response to feared situations. Typically, the child is given a series of gradual, progressive exercise to create or recreate situations associated with anxiety (e.g., this might include thinking about fearful situations or actual gradual exposure). Developmental considerations come into play for younger children but have frequently been used in treatment of fears and phobias. Similarly, in childhood OCD, the compulsive behaviors (thought to prevent something bad from happening) might be appropriate targets for exposure exercises. The exposure method can be effectively used in challenging core beliefs (cognitive response prevention), e.g., giving homework assignments in which the child's behavior is inconsistent with the pathological or problematic beliefs. For a child who is overly compulsive about doing his homework in response, for example, to an underlying fear of being stupid, it might be appropriate to ask the child to have some imperfections in the homework while simultaneously thinking that this planned exercise does not make him stupid.

Self-monitoring can be used in various ways, including for work on habit disorders, modification of eating and exercise in eating disorders, and tracking use of behavioral techniques and relaxation in anxiety disorders. *Self-management procedures* include responsibility for implementation of a specific behavioral plan and similarly can be used in a range of conditions, both in terms of improving desired skills and decreasing undesired behaviors. Another approach, *activity scheduling*, is frequently used in the treatment of patients with depression to help increase the individual's involvement in daily activities and to break the negative cycles of depressed mood, thoughts, and behavior that result in lack of participation in previously pleasurable activities, further contributing to depressed mood. *Behavior modification and applied behavior analysis* techniques are helpful in increasing desired behaviors and decreasing undesirable ones. *Counterconditioning* pairs a maladaptive behavior with an incompatible behavior to reduce and eliminate the maladaptive behavior. *Systematic desensitization* is a frequently used counterconditioning technique in which relaxation training is joined to a specific anxiety hierarchy with the goal of reducing anxiety over time. Imagined or real exposure (or both) can be used. This technique combines aspects of counterconditioning with graduated exposure. Given the cognitive demands of this technique, it is used less frequently in younger children. *Habit reversal training* procedures are most frequently used in the treatment of patients with habit disorders (e.g., trichotillomania, skin picking) and in those with Tourette's disorder and the tic disorders. This approach involves awareness training joined with training in an incompatible competing response; social supports are also provided.

INTERPERSONAL PSYCHOTHERAPY

IPT was originally developed as a brief treatment for adults with nonpsychotic depression. It assumes that social relationships are important mitigating and protective factors in depression. The goals of ITP include education about connections between depression and interpersonal relationships with an aim of improving the latter as an important aspect of treatment. This model has its origins in the work of Adolf Meyer and Harry Stack Sullivan as well as the work of John Bowlby on attachment (see Chapter 2). The approach is concerned with helping patients cope with conflicts and losses. The two major goals of this approach have to do with improving social functioning and diminishing or mitigating depressive symptomatology. A series of specific strategies involves identification of problem area(s), of effective approaches to problem solving and communication and practice, initially within sessions, on use of these approaches. Depression is seen as a function of three different elements: symptom formation, personality, and social functioning. The IPT approach has been used for adolescents (interpersonal psychotherapy for depressed adolescents [IPT-A]) as an active and structured treatment approach that involves a significant psychoeducational aspect. As treatment progresses, the goal is to help the teenager develop more effective, action-oriented approaches to coping. This model is particularly relevant to adolescents, who have the task of becoming increasingly independent and autonomous. Several modifications have been made to make the approach more applicable to adolescents (e.g., dealing with parental difficulties, role transitions). Parents are typically involved to some degree in the treatment. At a minimum, this includes some involvement in the opening phase of treatment when much of the focus is on education. Parents may be involved again as treatment works on specific strategies and, at the end, as part of the process of reviewing treatment progress and future needs. Various other modifications are made for adolescents to help concretize the process and to focus on more basic aspects of social skills and negotiation of parent issues. Other modifications can be made in special circumstances (e.g., around issues of abuse, school refusal, suicidality). Table 22.3 summarizes some of the components of ITP.

A body of work supporting the effectiveness of IPT for adolescence now exists (see Mufson & Young, 2007). The treatment itself is manualized, and it has been studied in multiple randomized controlled trials with different teams demonstrating its effects. Current work is focused on broadening the range of conditions targeted and extending the method into community-based settings (e.g., including youth with comorbid anxiety, attentional, or other disorders). Selection of ITP-A as a treatment modality should encompass an awareness of relevant diagnostic issues, motivation and ability to engage in treatment, and severity and other factors. In addition to motivation, the adolescent should have some degree of insight

TABLE 22.3

INTERPERSONAL PSYCHOTHERAPY: PRIMARY COMPONENTS OF TREATMENT

Education	Affect Identification	Interpersonal Skills Building
Psychoeducation Limited sick role	Labeling emotions Clarification of emotions	Modeling Use of therapeutic relationship as sample of interpersonal interaction
Treatment contract	Facilitating expression of emotions Monitoring emotions	Communication analysis Perspective taking Interpersonal problem solving Role playing

Reprinted from Mufson, L., & Young, J. F. (2007). Interpersonal psychotherapy. In A. Martin & F. Volkmar (Eds.), *Lewis's Child and Adolescent Psychiatry: A Comprehensive Textbook*, 4th edition, p. 821. Philadelphia: Lippincott Williams & Wilkins.

and a family that will support or, minimally, tolerate the treatment. Individuals \
onset depression without active suicidal ideation are better candidates than those with
depression and interpersonal problems. The therapist should feel comfortable that a
limited treatment is sufficient. Active psychotic thinking, substance abuse, and a prin.
diagnosis of bipolar disorder should prompt concern about the need for other approaches.
ITP-A can be used in combination with pharmacological treatments. The initial assessment
should include a thorough history with a focus on current diagnosis (diagnoses) and areas
of interpersonal difficulties that may contribute and an assessment of the range of potential
treatment options available.

The initial phase of IPT-A is primarily concerned with provision of psychoeducation and,
to some degree, of identification of affective contributions. Psychoeducational activities center
on helping the adolescent understand aspects of depression and basic treatment principles of
IPT-A. Depending on the circumstances, parents may be involved in the initial assessment
either by themselves or together, with the child. There is also a focus on helping the adolescent
return to prior levels of social functioning. The therapist provides information on the focus and
structure of treatment and conducts a detailed review of significant relationships, both present
and past, through the "interpersonal inventory," which helps provide a summary of significant
people in the adolescent's life and their emotional valence. This typically includes discussions
of areas of strength and weakness, events that may have contributed to depression, and how
relationships may impact symptoms. Typically, by the end of four sessions, the therapist will
be able to provide a formulation, placing the problem areas in the context of both current and
past relationships. The adolescent then has the opportunity to discuss this formulation and
together with the therapist develop an agenda for the relatively brief treatment period.

The middle phase of treatment (usually sessions five to nine) then focuses on the various
identified problem areas with an emphasis on further understanding of difficulties, development and implementation of effective problem solving and coping strategies. During this time,
the therapist will evaluate the effectiveness of treatment, progress in treatment, involvement of
parents, and the need for additional treatments such as medication. Typically, there is a focus
on specific strategies to deal with interpersonal difficulties. The therapist and patient practice
with role play; both more explicit directive techniques (targeted questioning) and nondirective
methods are used to facilitate discussion and help the adolescent achieve greater understanding of the links between mood and relationships and, ultimately, make interpersonal change.
During this time, the therapist can model various relevant skills to encourage effective communication and decision making. There may be specific work assigned to practice relevant
skills.

Typically, around the ninth session, a termination phase begins, although the initial treatment contract (usually 12 weeks) can be modified. The final phase of ITP-A usually includes an
explicit focus on warning signs of recurrence, the delineation of successful coping strategies,
and areas needing improvement. During the final termination, the therapist identifies changes
the adolescent has made (e.g., in his or her ability to communicate or see another person realistically). The final termination process may involve only the adolescent or, more commonly,
both the adolescent and his or her family. As appropriate additional treatments may be needed
(e.g., when symptoms persist in partial remission). Special issues also arise for adolescents
whose parents are divorced or who live with relatives or in foster homes. Regardless of the
biological relationships, the responsible adults should be helped to support the adolescent and,
if needed, be involved in treatment. Parental mental health issues become particularly relevant
if the parent or responsible adult is him- or herself depressed. In particular, helping this adult
deal with his or her own difficulties may facilitate the adolescent's successful adaption.

The combined use of medication with IPT-A is fairly common, particularly for more severely
depressed adolescents. Use of medications should be considered for less severely depressed
adolescents if symptoms do not remit with treatment. In some instances (e.g., when depression
is chronic, an antidepressant may be considered, even at the outset of treatment). In all work
with adolescents crises are fairly common, and the therapist should be prepared for them in
advance. Depending on the nature of the crisis, appropriate steps should be taken. In some
cases, referral for other treatment models is indicated.

In summary, IPT-A is an evidence-based psychotherapy focused on the interpersonal context of depression. It can readily be taught as a method and has been used successfully in community-based settings.

GROUP PSYCHOTHERAPY

Group therapy has many potential advantages in the treatment of children and adolescents. Peers can be powerful mediators of change, bring different perspectives than those of parents and adult therapists, and may more readily provide useful feedback and information. Group treatments has been around for a long time; in many ways, their origins begin with use of congregate care facilities for children in the juvenile justice system at the end of the 19th century. Over time, groups focused on specific activities or issues have also been developed (e.g., groups for teaching social skills to children with difficulties on the autism spectrum or to support children exposed to trauma). As with other psychotherapies, there has been a movement toward increased standardization and development of specific curricula. Depending on its focus and leadership, a therapy group will typically move through several phases (see Moss et al., 2007).

Groups can be time limited or ongoing. The role of the group leaders varies depending on the purposes and nature of the group (e.g., in highly focused, short-term groups, the leader may have an active role throughout the group's duration). In open-ended groups, the leaders role may be more important in early stages, in helping to ensure effective group functioning, and in helping new group members enter as others leave. The interventions of the group leader vary depending on the nature of the group and its stage of existence.

Various theoretical perspectives have been used in the organization of group treatment programs. Having a specific theoretical orientation can help group leaders in management of the group. An overall theoretical perspective may also be important strategically (e.g., in guiding decisions of when to and when not to intervene). Cognitive behavioral, psychodynamic, and gestalt theoretical orientations are among the more frequently used in group treatments. Bion's (1961) early work on groups has had a major influence in the field and has emphasized the importance of the group as well as group leadership in helping groups be effective. The behavior of specific group members is viewed both in the context of the individual person but also within that of the group as a whole. Ideally, discussion, reformulations, interpretations, and other interventions have relevance to the group and not just to single members. Having a shared group goal or focus is particularly helpful.

Groups for children and adolescents must cope with several important tasks. Depending on the age and developmental level of the participants, play or verbalization may be a major mode of communication. Some groups have a more traditional insight-oriented, psychodynamic orientation; others are briefer and more highly focused. Some groups, such as social skills groups, may aim to increase skills levels. Such groups can include typically developing children as well as those with social vulnerabilities or may be limited only to children with vulnerabilities. Support groups may be primarily concerned with helping the child or adolescent deal with a very specific problem (e.g., substance abuse, loss, or trauma). Groups can be more or less didactic. Members of the group should have a clear sense of the purpose of the group. Activities of the group vary depending on the nature, focus, and developmental levels of participants but are typically divided, to varying degrees, around processes that help the group focus on its specific areas of activity or interest as well as activities that are essential in maintaining the group. Issues that group leaders, and sometimes the group itself, will have to consider include recruiting members into the group and the specific composition of the group (e.g., around a focus on a specific problem or around a specific diagnostic category). Issues of composition encompass issues of diversity (e.g., age, gender) and sensitivity to group composition is important because a person who is or becomes a solitary member representing some specific group or issue can be isolated. The size of the group and its duration are other considerations. In general, there should be an effort to achieve a balance sufficient to lead to productive group as well as dyadic activities and process without sacrificing a sense of group community and intimacy. Issues of gender can arise in some contexts (e.g., around issues related to sexuality or aggression), although more typically, groups are not confined to a single gender. In some groups, there may be a conscious attempt to include typically developing peers both as role models and to serve, to some degree, as potential allies of the leaders (e.g., in social skills groups). Both the developmental level and chronological ages of the child or adolescent are relevant. A balance must be achieved that allows the group to function most efficiency. The group leader must provide a consistent, private, and physically appropriate setting. Sometimes, particularly for work with children, leaders of groups (and those doing individual psychotherapy) err on the side of "overfurnishing" offices and group rooms. Often, a more nuanced approach with, as needed, a smaller but relevant section of materials makes much more sense. For an adolescent group, this might include simple games or other activities; for children, some toys and other materials might also be available. For primary school children, activities such as games, Legos™, and other materials that facilitate interaction may be appropriate.

Typically, each group will last for a specific length of time (from 60 to 90 minutes), although in public school settings, shorter lengths of time are frequent. Depending on the context, the group may be time limited (meeting for X number of sessions or during the school year); in other cases, the group is ongoing. In the latter case, issues of departure of "graduating" members and entry of new members will arise. Typically, the leaders will provide a structure for the group that is conveyed initially and then reasonably adhered to throughout the life of the group. Depending on the nature of the group, for children, this usually includes some period of time for talking, for an activity (games, play, projects), snack time, and wrap up. The group leader(s) has an important role in monitoring the group and providing reminders of continuity from one meeting to the next. Sometimes a journal can be used to summarize the overall focus of a group meeting or can be used to document group rules and history. Periods of time can be adapted for various purposes (e.g., telling jokes at a snack period in social skills groups provides important opportunities for feedback from peers and adults). Group leaders should pay attention to potentially informative and communicative aspects of all undesired behaviors while simultaneously helping such behaviors not disrupt the group. Various techniques can be used to cope with behavioral difficulties, including changes in group activities or structure, verbal interpretation, limit setting, and so forth. Sometimes an individual is not able to tolerate the demands of being in a group; in such cases, removal of a group member should provide an opportunity for explanation as well as discussion.

The degree to which parents are involved can vary dramatically. For outpatient groups, parents may be physically present (having transported their child or several children). Sometimes parents can have their own group that meets at the same time. In any event, parents must be involved in making decisions about group treatment and their willingness to support such treatment. Depending on the specific clinical situation, periodic meetings or feedback to parents may help maintain the child's or adolescent's engagement. It is important that this does not violate the child's understanding about aspects of confidentiality or the group process.

In addition to providing a safe environment, the group leaders provide models for interpersonal relationships and for open and honest communication. Groups are typically led by two leaders, which thus gives the working dyad a chance to develop their own approached to effectively processing the wealth of clinical information and myriad process decisions encountered in the group. The leaders can and should disagree with each other at times, modeling a process by which such events are handled. By providing a degree of predictability and reliability, the leaders also set a tone for the group's activity. The group leaders also have a responsibility to manage whatever other relationships or issues are relevant to the group.

Support groups have been used extensively both in helping children and adolescents cope with chronic illness in their families and in fostering social skills for children on the autism spectrum. For children coping with illness in parents and family members, groups provide mutual support and opportunities to discuss issues that are difficult to discuss with the ill family member. Social skill groups for children and adolescents (and sometimes adults) with autism and related disorders are typically either time limited and focus on explicit teaching of specific social skills or are more open ended.

Time-limited groups have a much stronger didactic aspect and can be particularly useful for less able individuals with opportunities to practice social skills in a supportive context. Open-ended groups are more frequently used by more cognitive able individuals and focus on a broad range of issues and social functions. Such groups can include typically developing peers to provide diversity and peer models; the latter are given some, but minimal, preparation. An alternative approach includes students with other types of problems in the social skills group.

In weighing the potential benefits of group therapy, several issues should be considered, including the nature of the individual's difficulties, the degree to which a group experience may counter a tendency toward isolation or self-blame, or the degree to which group therapy may be more tolerable than individual or family therapy. Contraindications for group treatment include the potential for severe acting out or impulsive behaviors whose presence would consistently disrupt or pose a safety threat. Removal of a group member can be difficult for other members of the group, and careful consideration of membership is always indicated. In considering admission to a group, other considerations may also arise. In some cases, the nature of the clinical situation may suggest that individual treatment is more appropriate. As with other aspects of psychotherapy, research work documenting the efficacy of group therapy has become more rigorous in recent years. A series of studies has now demonstrated its benefits in a range of populations.

FAMILY THERAPY

The range of approaches to family therapy has increased dramatically over the past several decades. Concepts developed by early workers in the field had been adapted and combined with new approaches. In addition, new methods of service delivery, including home-based services (see Chapter 23), have advanced the field, particularly in the management of conduct and substance use disorders. Treatment approaches have become more flexible, and a substantial body of work on treatment efficacy now exists. As with other psychotherapeutic modalities, family therapy focuses on interpersonal relationships because these contribute to difficulties; family therapy differs from the individual and group treatment approaches in that the focus is on family relationships and not just a specific individual. This treatment recognizes the importance context of the family to the pathogenesis of specific problems and maladaptive processes as well as the positive and protective aspects nurturing family environments and attachments. Family therapy recognizes the complex interactions of family members within the family system and ways that these may both regulate interactions and lead to difficulties. Rather than focusing on a single person or his or her difficulty, the focus on family therapy is on family system change.

Family therapy can be used in many different contexts but particularly when familial contributions to chronic stress, repeated patterns of maladaptation, and interaction of family characteristics with specific areas of individual dysfunction arise. Relative contraindications include severe psychopathology in a family member and reluctance to engage in treatment. It is important that the family therapist be well trained in child development and psychopathology. Depending on the context, the focus may be on intergenerational issues, helping the family cope with a specific crisis. Family therapy may have a strong behavioral focus (e.g., in dealing with conduct disordered youth).

The various models of family therapy have different theoretical backgrounds and use different techniques (see Sholevar, 2007). For example, structural family therapy was originally developed for use in children and adolescents with eating disorders and acute-onset behavioral problems difficulties. Its focus was on issues of boundaries, autonomy, and independence with an emphasis on helping the family establish clear and flexible boundaries and develop more adaptive family functioning.

Psychodynamic family therapy has its theoretical base in psychodynamic understanding of family life with a focus on issues of attachment, object relations, and defense in response to unconscious conflicts. Behavior family therapy applies behavioral analytic principles to enhance family interaction and reciprocity and avoid reliance on less adaptive coercive family processes. There is an emphasis on enhanced communication and an explicit focus on problem solving. Increasingly, aspects of social learning theory and behavioral analytic principles have been used in the development of PMT (see Chapter 23) to help parents enhance prosocial behavior while reducing maladaptive behaviors. Another approach focuses on psychoeducation in providing patients and family members detailed information about major mental illnesses such as schizophrenia, depression, alcoholism, and anxiety disorders. Depending on the clinical context, it can be combined with other family therapy approaches after the clinical situation has stabilized and if additional intervention is needed.

Aspects of family therapy are now taught in both general psychiatric and child and adolescent training programs, and this has contributed to the increased use of this modality in younger patients. Approaches have been developed for a wide variety of psychiatric disorders. As with group therapy, consideration in family therapy should include provision of an appropriate environment with child-friendly materials available as appropriate. Family therapy has now been done with young children. Work in the area of ADHD has included parent training to reduce the child's impulsivity, foster attention, and encourage prosocial skills as well as supporting the child's self-concept. Multimodal Treatment Study of Children with ADHD provides 30 parent training sessions along with school visits and teacher-training. It can be used either with or without stimulant or other medication. Work on conduct disorder has also been extensive. Several approaches have been well studied. PMT focuses on helping parents interact proactively and more positively with their children while helping the child to focus, remain on task, solve problems, act prosocially with peers, and reduce impulsivity and aggression through cognitive processing. This approach can strengthen the positive parent-child bonds and the child's fragile self-esteem by reducing negative and counterproductive parental behavior and enhancing skillful and goal-directed intervention by parents; it also has benefit for siblings.

MST has also been widely used and targets youth who at high risk for outplacement from the home because of substance abuse or conduct problems (see Chapter 23). This home-based model of service delivery typically lasts about 5 months and has been noted to have many positive effects. With improved family functioning, reductions have been seen in rates of placement, substance abuse, and so forth. Other approaches have used family-based interventions in relation to depression as well as anxiety disorders. Historically, one of the first uses of family therapy in children and adolescents was in treatment of children with anorexia nervosa. In addition to the older family therapy treatment models of eating disorders, new approaches have used both psychoeducational and behavioral family therapy.

The body of research on family therapy research has increased dramatically in recent years. Studies have compared results of family therapy with other treatment approaches with encouraging results, particularly in the areas of conduct disorders and substance abuse. In a new and existing area of work Reiss and colleagues (2000) focus on the impact of shared and nonshared environments in assessing the contributions of genetic and environmental risk.

SUMMARY

Psychotherapy for treatment of behavioral and emotional disorders in children and adolescents has a long history. A large body of work has now confirmed that psychotherapy can be effective. Challenges remain in generalizing highly structured, research-based methods into more typical clinical treatment settings. The evidence for "treatment as usual" is not, unfortunately, particularly strong, but a growing body of work has established the effectiveness of several different structured treatment approaches.

Selected Readings

Bion, W. R. (1961). *Experiences in Groups and Other Papers*. New York: Basic Books.
Boettcher, M. A., & Piancentini, J. (2007). Cognitive and behavioral therapies. In A. Martin & F. Volkmar (Eds.), *Lewis's Child and Adolescent Psychiatry: A Comprehensive Textbook*, 4th edition, pp. 796–819. Philadelphia: Lippincott Williams & Wilkins.

Brent, D. A., Holder, D., Kolko, D., Birmaher, B., Baugher, M., Roth, C., Iyengar, S., & Johnson, B. A. (1997). A clinical psychotherapy trial for adolescent depression comparing cognitive, family, and supportive therapy. *Archives of General Psychiatry, 54,* 877–885.

Burlingame, G. M., Fuhriman, A. J., & Johnson, J. (2004). *Current Status and Future Directions of Group Therapy Research.* In J. L. De-Lucia-Waack, D. A. Gerrity, C. R. Kalodner, & M. T. Riva (Eds.), *Handbook of Group Counseling and Psychotherapy,* pp. 651–660. Thousand Oaks, CA: Sage Publications.

Casey, R. J., & Berman, J. S. (1985). The outcome of psychotherapy with children. *Psychological Bulletin, 98,* 388–400.

Chambless, D. L., & Hollon, S. D. (1998). Defining empirically supported therapies. *Journal of Consulting and Clinical Psychology, 66*(1), 7–18.

Chambless, D. L., & Ollendick, T. H. (2001). Empirically supported psychological interventions: Controversies and evidence. *Annual Review of Psychology, 52,* 685–716.

Chorpita, B. F. (2003). The frontier of evidence based practice. In A. E. Kazdin & J. R. Weisz (Eds.), *Evidence Based Psychotherapies for Children and Adolescents,* pp. 42–59. New York: Guilford.

Clarke, G. N., Debar, L., Lynch, F., Powell, J., Gale, J., O'Connor, E., Ludman, E., Bush, T., Lin, E. H., Von Korff, M., & Hertert, S. (2005). A randomized effectiveness trial of brief cognitive-behavioral therapy for depressed adolescents receiving anti-depressant medication. *Journal of the American Academy of Child Psychiatry, 44,* 888–898.

Cohen, J. (1992). A power primer. *Psychological Bulletin, 112,* 155–159.

Curtis, N. M., Ronan, K. R., & Borduin, C. M. (2004). Multisystemic treatment: A meta-analysis of outcome studies. *Journal of Family Psychology, 18,* 411–419.

Fonagy, P., Target, M., Cottrell, D., Phillips, J., & Kurtz, Z. (2005). *What works for whom? A Critical Review of Treatments for Children and Adolescents.* New York; Guilford Press.

Freud, A. (1946). *The Psycho-analytical Treatment of Children.* London: Imago Publishing.

Freud, S. (1955). Analysis of phobia in a five-year-old boy. In *Standard Editions of the Complete Psychological Works of Sigmund Freud,* Vol 10, pp. 3–149. London: Hogarth.

Haley, J. (1963). *Strategies of Psychotherapy.* New York: Grune & Stratton.

Henggeler, S. W., & Lee, T. (2003). In A. E. Kazdin, & J. R. Weisz (Eds.), *Multisystemic Treatment of Serious Clinical Problems.* New York: Guilford Press.

Henggeler, W. W., & Lee, T. (2003). Multisystemic treatment of serious clinical problems. In A. E. Kazdin & J. R. Weisz (eds.), *Evidence-based Psychotherapies for Children and Adolescents.* New York: Guilford Press.

Henggeler, S. W., Schoenwald, S. K., Borduin, C. M., Rowland, M. D., & Cunningham, P. B. (1998). *Multisystemic Treatment of Antisocial Behavior in Children and Adolescents.* New York: Guilford.

Hinshaw, S. P., Owens, E. B., Wells, K. C., Kraemer, H. C., Abikoff, H. B., Arnold, L. E., Conners, C. K., Elliott, G., Greenhill, L. L., Hechtman, L., Hoza, B., Jensen, P. S., March, J. S., Newcorn, J. H., Pelham, W. E., Swanson, J. M., Vitiello, B., & Wigal, T. (2000). Family processes and treatment outcomes in the MTA: Negative/ineffective parenting practices in relation to multimodal treatment. *Abnormal Child Psychology, 28,* 555–568.

Jones, M. C. (1924). A laboratory study of fear: The case of Peter. *Pedagogy Seminar, 31,* 308–315.

Kazdin, A. E. (2000). Developing a research agenda for child and adolescent psychotherapy. *Archives of General Psychiatry, 57,* 829–835.

Kazdin, A. E., Siegel, T. C., & Bass, D. (1992). Cognitive problem-solving skills training and parent management training in the treatment of antisocial behavior in children. *Journal of Consultative Clinical Psychology, 60,* 733–747.

Kazdin, A. E., & Weisz, J. R. (2003). *Evidence-Based Psychotherapies for Children and Adolescents.* New York: Guilford Press.

Klein, M. (1932). *The Psychoanalysis of Children.* London: Hogarth Press.

Krasny, L., Williams, B. J., Provencal, S., & Ozonoff, S. (2003). Social skills interventions for the autism spectrum: Essential ingredients and a model curriculum. *Child and Adolescent Psychiatric Clinics of North America, 12,* 107–122.

Minuchin, S. (1974). *Families and Family Therapy.* Cambridge, MA: Harvard University Press.

Moss, N. E., Racusin, G. R., & Moss-Racusin, C. (2007). Group therapy. In A. Martin & F. Volkmar (Eds.), *Lewis's Child and Adolescent Psychiatry: A Comprehensive Textbook,* 4th edition, pp. 842–854. Philadelphia: Lippincott Williams & Wilkins.

Mufson, L., & Young, J. F. (2007). Interpersonal psychotherapy. In A. Martin & F. Volkmar (Eds.), *Lewis's Child and Adolescent Psychiatry: A Comprehensive Textbook,* 4th edition, pp. 819–826. Philadelphia: Lippincott Williams & Wilkins.

Mufson, L., Dorta, K. P., Moreau, D., & Weisman, M. M. (2004). *Interpersonal Psychotherapy for Depressed Adolescents,* 2nd edition. New York: Guilford.

Muratori, F., Picchi, L., Bruni, G., Patarnello, M., & Romagnoli, G. (2003). A two-year follow-up of psychodynamic psychotherapy for internalizing disorders in children. *Journal of the American Academy of Child and Adolescent Psychiatry, 42*(3), 331–339.

Patterson, G. R. (1982). *A Social Learning Approach to Family Interventions: III. Coercive Family Process.* Eugene, OR: Castalia.

Reiss, D., Neiderhisser, J. M., Hetherington, E. M., & Plomin, R. (2000). *The Relationship Code, Deciphering Genetic and Social Influences on Adolescent Development.* Cambridge, MA: Harvard University Press.

Ritvo, R. Z., & Ritvo, S. (2007). Psychodynamic principles in practice. In A. Martin & F. Volkmar (Eds.), *Lewis's Child and Adolescent Psychiatry: A Comprehensive Textbook,* 4th edition, pp. 826–842. Philadelphia: Lippincott Williams & Wilkins.

Schectman, Z. (2004). Group counseling and psychotherapy with children and adolescents. In J. L. De-Lucia-Waack, D. A. Gerrity, C. R. Kalodner, & M. T. Riva (Eds.), *Handbook of Group Counseling and Psychotherapy,* pp. 429–444. Thousand Oaks, CA: Sage Publications.

Sholevar, G. P. (2007). Family therapy. In A. Martin & F. Volkmar (Eds.), *Lewis's Child and Adolescent Psychiatry: A Comprehensive Textbook*, 4th edition, pp. 854–864. Philadelphia: Lippincott Williams & Wilkins.

Weisz, J. R., Donenberg, G. R., Han, S. S., & Weiss, B. (1995). Bridging the gap between laboratory and clinic in child and adolescent psychotherapy. *Journal of Consulting Clinical Psychiatry, 63,* 688–701.

Weisz, J. R., Doss, A. J., & Hawley, K. M. (2005). Youth psychotherapy outcome research: A review and critique of the evidence base. *Annual Review of Psychology, 56,* 337–363.

Weisz, J. R., Weiss, B., & Donenberg, G. R. (1992). The lab versus the clinic: Effects of child and adolescent psychotherapy. *American Psychological Association, 47,* 1578–1585.

Weisz, J. R., Weiss, B., Han, S. S., Granger, D. A., & Morton, T. (1995). Effects of psychotherapy with children and adolescents revisited: A meta-analysis of treatment outcome studies. *Psychological Bulletin, 117,* 450–468.

Wells, K. B., Sherbourne, C., Schoenbaum, M., Duan, N., Meredith, L., Unutzer, J., Miranda, J., Carney, M. F., & Rubenstein, L. V. (2000). Impact of disseminating quality improvement programs for depression in managed primary care: A randomized controlled trial. *Journal of the American Medical Association, 283,* 212–220.

Weersing, V. R., & Dirks, M. A. (2007). Psychotherapy for children and adolescents: A critical review. In A. Martin & F. Volkmar (Eds.), *Lewis's Child and Adolescent Psychiatry: A Comprehensive Textbook*, 4th edition, pp. 789–796. Philadelphia: Lippincott Williams & Wilkins.

Weersing, V. R., & Weisz, J. R. (2002). Mechanisms of action in youth psychotherapy. *Journal of Child Psychology and Psychiatry, 43,* 3–29.

CHAPTER 23 ■ TREATMENT PROGRAMS: A CONTINUUM OF APPROACHES

Current approaches to delivery of mental health services to children and adolescents encompass a range of services from community-based clinics and private care providers to home-based services and, for those who need it, hospitalization and residential services. The range of services available today evolved over the past century in parallel with the many changes in demographics in the United States and the shift from a primarily agrarian society to an urbanized one. Indeed, some of the first attempts to provide community-based care arose in the context of providing treatment and rehabilitation to children involved in the juvenile justice system. This in turn was the stimulus for development of child guidance clinics through various care providers; these clinics were intended to provide a range of treatments, often at low cost, to children and their families. The organization of child psychiatry as a discipline and the increased interest of the federal government, beginning in the Kennedy administration, were also important in shaping the ways mental health services were delivered (Pumariega & Winters, 2007).

Provision of inpatient and residential treatment has its origin in development of institutions devoted to the care of children with chronic problems related to brain damage or mental retardation. The impact of psychoanalysis in the 1930s to 1960s also had an important impact given the tendency to view environmental factors as major in the pathogenesis of mental illness (i.e., it made theoretical sense to remove a child from a pathogenic environment with the residential setting presumed to help the child return to a path of normal development). Not surprisingly, this process was thought to be a long-term one, and lengths of stays were correspondingly prolonged.

Starting in the 1960s, the growth of experimental psychology began to have a major impact. The awareness that new behavioral methods could be used in patients with disorders such as autism or in other conditions (e.g., phobic disorders) had an important impact on treatment, and behavioral psychologists began to work actively in long-stay institutions. This approach had a number of advantages. It was explicit in terms of behaviors to be encouraged or discouraged through use of reinforcement or punishment. Both operant and classical conditioning procedures were used. The methods of applied behavior analysis were able to produce major behavior changes and were used to teach new skills such as anger management, assertiveness, anxiety reduction, and so forth (see Chapter 22).

The book *Unclaimed Children* (Knitzer, 1982) became a stimulus for establishing community-based services and was one of the factors that led to development of the Child and Adolescent Service System Program (CASSP) to provide community-based care (Stroul & Friedman, 1986). The CASSP helped in developing the system-of-care approach with the goal of providing a range of services and supports to children and their families. The CASSP program has now become one part of the Substance Abuse and Mental Health Services Administration (SAMSA), which funds a range of activities throughout the country.

Over the past 2 decades, an awareness of the importance of attempting, whenever possible, to treat children and adolescents in family and community settings and of the potential negative effects of long-stay institutions led to major shifts in provision of service with development of more comprehensive community and family- and home-based treatment approaches. Today, hospitalization is most frequently used only when problems are serious and pose a significant danger to the child or family or when problems are sufficiently complex that it becomes more efficient to conduct an inpatient assessment (Blader & Foley, 2007).

COMMUNITY-BASED SERVICES

Typically, the first-line providers of mental health care to children and adolescents are primary care providers. This is particularly true in areas with limited access to specialty services. The primary care setting has considerable potential for serving as the first line for screening, although usually, primary care providers have had little training in child mental health.

The availability of specialists is limited given issues of reimbursement and some aspects of the current system (e.g., provision of Medicaid carve-outs led to a separation of mental health and medical reimbursements, further complicating delivery of care). Fortunately, a few states, notably Vermont and Massachusetts, have facilitated access to child mental health consultation. In other states, there has been an emphasis on training primary care practitioners in use of specific screening methods and better use of mental health services. Other approaches (e.g., involving telemedicine) are also being explored.

Current approaches to integrated care emphasize the range of services children and families need. They emphasize child and family engagement in treatment and the need for flexibility in approach. For example, children and adolescents with circumscribed problems can often have their needs met effectively by time-limited or very specific service delivered by a single mental health provider in an office or clinic setting. Children with multiple and complex problems more typically are engaged for a longer period of time and often have service needs involving multiple systems and agencies. For these children, use of a multidisciplinary treatment can be particularly helpful.

The wraparound model of service provides a high individualized set of treatment and community supports designed for the particular child or adolescent. It aims to build on strengths and use community-based services as well as other supports (VanDenBerg & Grealish, 1996). Several studies have supported the usefulness of this approach in terms of improving functioning and decreasing problem behaviors as well as reducing placements outside the family.

There are many challenges in work with children and adolescents with more complex needs or life situations. The juvenile justice system exemplifies many of these challenges. Philosophically, there is a major divergence between a focus on rehabilitation and those who favor punishment. The desire to maintain public safety combined with the punitive approach has led to significant increases in the population served by the juvenile justice system. Although mandated to receive services, overcrowding, lack of access to service, and high rates of psychiatric needs have prompted a host of lawsuits. More than half of the youth in this system have serious emotional difficulties, and incarcerated juveniles include a disproportionate share of minority youth. Typically, these children and adolescents have not as frequently used mental health services before their entry into juvenile justice systems. High proportions of minority youth reflect the impact of psychosocial adversity and poverty and limitations of service access. Fortunately, there has been a recent tend to attempt an integration of mental health services within the juvenile justice system. As noted subsequently, alternative models of care, including multisystemic therapy (MST), have been shown to significantly reduce out-of-home placement.

Children being served by state child protective agencies and the child welfare system face other challenges. Children who have been removed from the care of their parents because of abuse or abandonment are at very high risk of mental health problems but have been significantly underserved in terms of mental health services. Given the significant risk posed by trauma and loss of parent contact, the high level of need is understandable (see Chapter 20). Although foster placements are frequently made, many children go through several such placements and may need residential treatment programs. Unfortunately, a lack of appropriate services in these programs leads to custodial care, a lack of emphasis on education and vocational training, and overreliance on medication.

Foster care presents its own problems. Even when, as often happens, children are returned to the care of their biological parents, there may be a lack of support for the child and family in the process of reunification. The various differences among the states in their approach to this problem are noteworthy. Both state and federal courts frequently become involved in attempts to reduce the use of residential treatments and foster care. For some families, involvement with child welfare is the only alternative when children are in need of costly mental health services (inpatient or residential treatment).

With the mandate for educating all children under Public Law 94-142, schools were forced to deal with children with serious learning, developmental, and emotional disorders in a more serious way. This in turn has led to controversies about funding.

Children with psychiatric and developmental disabilities often present with a range of needs, but in most cases, coordination with other providers and agencies is challenging. For example, children may be in the child welfare system, attending school, and have some involvement with the juvenile justice system simultaneously but with little or no coordination among service providers. Recent attempts to foster interagency systems of care through school-based services are of great potential interest in this regard. These clinics can potentially provide health and mental health services within schools, and several different models have now been implemented across the country (Pumariega & Winters, 2007).

The advent of more rigorously defined, manualized psychotherapy treatment models (see Chapter 22) has presented other challenges for community-based care. Although these models have a strong evidence base, they can be difficult to implement effectively in "real-world" (i.e., not university-based clinic) settings. Similar issues arise with drug treatments. As discussed in Chapter 21, a range of effective pharmacological treatments are now available and have an important role in the management of mental health problems in children and adolescents. Their effective use requires careful assessment and management, including monitoring of potential benefits and risks. Particularly in settings where various professionals are involved, medication should be one aspect of comprehensive treatment planning.

In some situations (e.g., management of attention-deficit/hyperactivity disorder in an outpatient setting), primary care providers may be comfortable doing most of the medication management, but for other problems, consultation with a specialist in the area is frequently needed. Depending on the situation, this may involve a more consultative model with the primary care provider working collaboratively with the specialist.

HOME-BASED SERVICES

Home-based programs, particularly if they are more intensive, provide an important alternative to hospitalizations. These services trace their beginning to the efforts of social workers in the early 1900s, who frequently made family visits to help needy families avoid child placement. The effort to development alternatives to detention for youth in the juvenile justice system was also an important stimulus for development of community- and home-based services. The importance psychoanalysis attributed to early experience and the increasing awareness of the adverse effects of institutional rearing on children's development added further impetus to the movement for treatments delivered in children's homes and communities. This movement received additional support in the Adoption Assistance and Child Welfare Act of 1980 (Public Law 96-272), which mandated states to provide supports for avoiding out-of-home placement. Various treatment models have been developed (see Rowland et al., 2007). Their focus, format, and use of various treatment models and procedures vary. Various terms may be used to refer to rather similar treatment programs (e.g., family preservation, intensive-in-home services, and home-based family therapy). They all share a major goal of avoiding removal of children from families. They also typically differ in several ways from more traditional, office-based treatment settings. Services are intensive, provided in home and community settings, and are provided at times convenient for the family. Although treatment is usually time limited, intensive support (including availability for crises and emergencies) is available. In contrast to more traditional models, the clinician typically works with a small case load at any point in time. Treatment approaches typically draw on multiple theoretical models. For example, the crisis intervention model provides brief (4 to 6 weeks) and concrete support. The home-based model has a somewhat expanded clinical orientation with more highly trained clinicians, typically has a duration of several months, and makes use of a broader range of clinical intervention strategies. In contrast, the family treatment model typically uses case manager (as opposed to therapists) for home-based service delivery with therapists available in an outpatient setting.

Research on outcomes of these programs has increased in sophistication over the years. Early research consisted mostly of program description and limited outcome data. Early enthusiasm was tempered as more sophisticated research approaches were used and important questions of the effectiveness of these program were raised, suggesting that the crisis intervention approach had relatively modest effects on averting out-of-home placements. Lindsey et al. (2002) summarized some of the reasons that early models were less effective, including lack of attention to important therapeutic issues, lack of flexibility in approach, degree of psychosocial stresses encountered, brevity of the intervention, and difficulties in targeting children most at risk. As a result of these concerns, new approaches to home-based intervention have been developed. These include Project 12 Ways and MST, both of which provide intensive home-based interventions in family and community settings. Project 12 Ways focuses on families in which issues of abuse or neglect place a child at risk for placement. Evaluation results have been promising. The MST approach has similarly been shown in a randomized clinical trial (RCT) to reduce the risk of placement for adolescents relative to physical abuse. The MST model has also been shown to be effective in work with youth at risk for placement because of juvenile justice or substance abuse issues, and its emphasis on ongoing staff training and quality assurance (to ensure treatment fidelity) is an important aspects of this approach. A series of research reports have demonstrated the efficacy of MST in reducing rates of re-arrest and out-of home placements with an average effect size (see Chapter 22) of 0.55. In this model, the therapist usually works with between four and six families for a period of 4 or 5 sessions with contacts with family and other important individuals (e.g., teachers, neighbors, peers) to the youth at risk. Problem behaviors are addressed through a range of treatment modalities (e.g., parent management training, behavioral or cognitive behavioral treatments, drug treatments).

Other treatment models include multidimensional treatment foster care (MTFC) and functional family therapy (FFT). Although not home based, both share a strong family focus. For example, in the MTFC approach for children in foster care, a set of highly trained foster parents are provided along with a full-time case manager and other therapists and supporters. The FFT approach provides a behavioral family therapy approach with emphasis on parent training and a focus on behaviors associated with delinquency.

The intensive in-home child and adolescent psychiatric service (IICAPS), provides intensive psychiatric home-based intervention for children and adolescents with serious psychiatric problems who are at risk for removal from the home. This manualized approach draws on findings from developmental psychopathology and earlier family work. Services are provided for a period of several (usually 4 to 6) months by a team that includes a clinician and mental health counselor with extensive training and supervision from a more senior clinician. Various services are provided, including treatment and service coordination and advocacy as well as assessment. Adherence to the basic IICAPS model (Woolston et al., 2006) is systematically addressed, and an Internet-based data system is used both to monitor the process and collect outcome information. This approach has been replicated in several sites, and outcome research is underway.

The Mental Health Services Program for Youth (MHSPY) is a Massachusetts-based program established in 1998 for children and adolescents with significant, chronic mental health issues and who are at risk of placement (Emmons, 2000). This model provides highly individualized and coordinated pediatric and mental health support along with social and family supports and educational services. The care planning team includes the family, care manager, and other providers. Care is provided on a longer term basis, and the system makes use of various care providers with the case manager having a major role in coordination of the available services. Ongoing staff training and periodic assessment are provided. Initial evaluation suggests a significantly reduced risk with lower hospitalization and placement rate and strong engagement of families.

INPATIENT AND PARTIAL HOSPITALIZATION

The decision to use inpatient or partial hospital treatments is particularly complicated for children and adolescents. Difficulties for the child include loss of autonomy and privacy as well as separation from important support systems of family and peers. As a result, the decision to seek hospitalization is usually one made as a last resort in situations when alternatives are limited and when the child's or adolescent's safety is a major concern. On the other hand, such crisis situations also provide important opportunities for change, both for the child and family. Clearly, children and adolescents with major mental health and developmental problems existed well before the advent of child psychiatric treatment programs. Most of our knowledge about such individuals comes from case reports. Maudsley, for example, reported on childhood "insanity" in the 1860s partly to document what was then seen as an interesting and relatively unusual clinical phenomenon.

The growth of the child mental health movement and interest in child development in this country in the first decades of the 20th century led to the establishment of child inpatient programs in the 1920s and 1930s that often served as custodial placements for children with significant brain damage. With the advent of modern child psychiatry, inpatient programs began to increase both in general and specialized psychiatric hospitals. A series of legal decisions established that parents had the right to compel care for minor children. Lengths of stay were usually extended, and admission and discharge standards were rather lax; this led to abuses in the system (e.g., for angry teenagers whose parents resorted to institutional care). This trend began to reverse as a result of the awareness of the potential for abuse and the impact of managed care, which began to impose much more stringent guidelines on admission. As a result, length of admission has dramatically decreased, although rates of admission or unchanged or actually increased, particularly if readmissions are included. Public policy makers also began to appreciate the disproportionate burden inpatient care placed on the system of care with reductions in opportunities for preventative and community-based programs. As a result, there has been a focus on the provision of a continuum of care ranging from outpatient to inpatient services. Additional services, including services within the home, respite services for parents, after-school programs, and partial hospitalization programs, have become more commonplace. Unfortunately, the availability of such services varies widely from one region to the next, and empirical research on many innovative treatments remains in its infancy.

As a result of this history and understandable concerns about the impact of hospitalization, the decision to hospitalize a child or adolescent is now regarded as desirable only after other options have not proven successful or when the safety of the child or others is at stake. Most hospitalizations are relatively short term with a few continuing to be for evaluative purposes (e.g., in response to a court order). In general, the preference is for evaluations to be performed on an outpatient basis whenever possible. Longer stay inpatient programs have become much less common and serve some of the most disabled individuals. However, even given all these caveats and difficulties, the ability to provide inpatient evaluation continues to serve an important function in the mental health care system. Indeed, rates of admission for children and adolescents have increased dramatically over the past decade, exceeding the increase in adult admissions.

In many ways, inpatient settings seemed ideal for such situations given the potential for much greater control and monitoring. Inpatient units often established token economies so that patients could work to earn desired privileges or rewards. Another advantage of the inpatient setting was the natural availability of a peer group to be used in providing feedback and developing adaptive and social skills. On the other hand, the intensity of the inpatient experiences also posed some problems for generalization of new learning to old settings (e.g., the home and school). Accordingly, an explicit focus on generalization and on family-focused treatment has become important. Various techniques are used in working with families, including parent management training for conduct problems and aspects of cognitive behavior therapy (see Chapter 22). One advantage of the inpatient setting is the opportunity for staff to model methods useful to parents. Support and education for families are now routine aspects of inpatient programs, a major shift from the time, not so many years ago, when families were viewed more negatively and not as allies in producing change.

Given the drastically shortened lengths of stay and the focus on rapid return of the child to the family and community, pharmacotherapy has played a much larger role in inpatient treatment programs. In 1980, fewer than half of child and adolescent inpatients were treated with psychotropic medications, but now such treatment is the rule. Part of this shift has likely resulted in the higher levels of severity now needed to prompt admission. Another likely reason is that medication management and adjustment may be an acceptable reason for insurance companies to approve longer hospital stays.

Typical reasons for admission to an inpatient setting include suicidal ideation or attempt or threats of aggression or actual aggression sufficient to cause serious concern on the part of the parents or school. Admission for diagnostic assessment purposes in the absence of these concerns is unlikely. Typically, the inpatient setting includes a secure, locked setting with 24-hour staffing and the ability to provide for the safety of the patient using seclusion or restraint if necessary. Most such programs are located either in free-standing psychiatric hospitals or within general hospital settings. Acute care has been arbitrarily defined as being for 30 days or less as a result of insurance policy; intermediate care (30 to 180 days) may require transfer to a longer term, often state-run, facility. Few programs provide services to preschool children; the usual age range is for children from 6 to 18 years. Some units specialize in prepubertal children; others specialize in adolescents. Some adult units begin admitting adolescents at around 16 years of age. Many state facilities have a mandate to serve the juvenile justice system with judges able to mandate inpatient assessments for specific time periods (usually 3 weeks). In 2003, more than 300,000 youth were evaluated in such settings (Blader & Foley, 2007). Some of these individuals go onto being placed in residential correctional facilities, where their massive mental health needs often go unmet. As with the adult correctional system, the juvenile correctional system has taken over some of the functions of the older long-stay residential institutions. Some inpatient program may specialize in highly selected populations (e.g., individuals with developmental disabilities or those with eating disorders).

Partial hospital programs are more intensive than outpatient programs but are somewhat less intensive than inpatient programs. Often, such programs either serve as an alternative to inpatient admission (e.g., for a child who can be maintained outside the full hospital setting) or as step-down, transitional programs after inpatient treatment. In many instances, the partial hospital program is provided within the inpatient unit, allowing for continuity of care after the more intensive inpatient stay. Some aspects of the administration of the partial hospital program are identical to the inpatient stay (e.g., for daily notes and for limited time duration). Accordingly, many day hospital programs do not have their own space and program. Many aspects of the program can be the same for both inpatient and partial hospital treatment, although typically, patient acuity is much lower in the latter. Day treatment programs usually have longer lengths of stay, and unlike inpatient and partial hospitalization, the school district more typically assumes the cost of the educational portion of the program; accordingly, the entire system of approval for such reimbursement must be undertaken with the school. These programs provide educational services with intensive levels of mental health support. The latter portion of the program is typically reimbursed by Medicaid or, in some cases, by other community or governmental funds. In contrast to the typical inpatient setting, partial and day hospital programs tend to be more open, and accordingly, such programs must be selective in their admission. Thus, children and adolescents who pose a danger to themselves or others or who have major substance abuse problems may not be well served in such settings.

Residential treatment programs represent a continuation of the older model of institutional care for children that existed a century ago (e.g., for orphans). The "cottage" model is often used in such settings with children living in small homes, often clustered together, with residential staff. Residential treatment programs vary somewhat in their orientation. Residential treatment facilities typically provide services for children and adolescents when a psychiatric impairment is primary, and residential treatment centers may provide services to children and adolescents who have experienced a range of psychosocial adversity (e.g., loss of a parent or parents unable to care for the child). In the latter situation, it is unfortunately the case that in many states parents are required to relinquish custody of their children, a practice that is not typically consistent with the best of interests of the child.

Admission to inpatient programs is typically driven by patient acuity. At the same time, depending on the situation and clinical context, some reasonable degree of selectivity is required. Children with severe developmental problems pose special problems, often requiring highly experienced treatment teams and one-on-one care. Through experience, staff running programs who are understandably tempted to make exceptions in such cases often discover the very significant problems in moving the child along to another placement or returning him or her to the previous one. Day and partial hospital programs as well as residential treatment programs have the ability to be more selective and focused in their admissions. Depending on the situation, particularly in less secure settings, there may be specific policies with regard to certain situations such as sexual acting out, fire setting, substance abuse, and so forth. Almost all admissions for psychiatric hospitalization are generally unplanned. Some hospitals have emergency departments (EDs) with provision for psychiatric assessment of children; others do not and refer to more specialized settings. Depending on the context, insurance concerns may loom large because authorization may be required. In contrast, admission to partial or day hospital programs or residential facilities is essentially always the product of a fairly complex admissions process.

Parents and youth typically prefer services that are close to home, although reputation is also a consideration. Schools are typically major referral sources to EDs as are families themselves. Other referrals come from community and state agencies, particularly those serving children in foster care. Depending on the context and situation, screening may be performed by one of several people such as a unit physician, social worker, or other member of the mental health team. The goal of screening is to ensure that hospitalization is appropriate, that required legal authorization is available, and that no major impediments to hospitalization exist. The decision of parents to hospitalize a child may be quite difficult, and they often understandably desire much information and to meet the unit staff or see the facility.

Insurance coverage must be checked to ensure that parents understand whether the hospitalization will be reimbursed (e.g., many insurance plans do not cover specific diagnostic groups unless other conditions are present). The preauthorization process entails ascertaining whether the insurance company will agree with the need for inpatient care and accept responsibility. Sometimes rejection by the reviewing agent leads to an immediate physician re-review. Given the complexities of the process, many hospitals now have staff who specialize in this work. For parents, the discovery of limited mental health coverage may be a shock as acute as the onset of the child's difficulties. The insurance company may only cover an admission to a facility some distance away from the parents and family. Situations in which there is clear danger to the child or lack of an alternative often result in approval for hospitalization. Typically, the preauthorization review will inquire as to the patient's diagnoses and the intended plan of treatment. It is usual for the initial approval to be for a short time to allow more extended evaluation. After this initial approval, a process of concurrent review will involve conversations between the managed care company's reviewer and inpatient staff regarding treatment planning and possibilities of discharge.

When possible, many units encourage families and children to visit the unit before admission. Practical issues can be reviewed (e.g., visiting hours, phone calls, school). Unit rules can be provided along with a description of any point system. The use of seclusion and restraints should be discussed along with the roles of members of the treatment team. Apart from emergency situations, it is typical for units to seek separate permission for the administration of psychotropic medications. Parents may be involved in support groups or parent training groups or discussions. It is essential that parents and children understand what realistically can and cannot be accomplished during a hospitalization. Because hospitalizations tend to be very short, the usual focus is on acute stabilization and planning for longer term intervention. Parents should be helped to understand what can and cannot be done in the limited time available. Often, the hospitalization provides an opportunity to examine issues such as school placement and academic supports. Parents should understand what is expected of them during their child's stay (e.g., visits, involvement in meetings).

Foster and Surrogate Care

Children in foster care are likely to be at increased risk for hospitalization. Although they may have a close and long relationship with their foster parents, it is usually the state agency's representative who must officially sign admission papers and consent to various procedures, including use of medications. Often, children in foster care have not had the rights of their biological parents terminated, leading to potential problems that sometimes require judicial resolution. In some situations, it becomes quite clear that the child cannot return to a previous foster home, so the process of seeking a new placement must be undertaken. Children in these situations are understandably confused, and their difficulties can be expressed in many ways on the inpatient unit.

Typically, children and adolescents who present for admission have long histories with many previous assessments and treatment recommendations. In these situations, it is also important that the evaluating professional understand what is different now and whether there has been a major change in the child's condition. An assessment of the acuity of the difficulties and their relationship to environmental stressors is important. Often, previous rating scales or checklists can be obtained, and given the brevity of current admissions, psychological testing is now usually selectively performed. It may be particularly helpful in document academic skill problems and learning difficulties. This should be a particular concern when school performance has decreased. Unfortunately, school problems are frequently attributed to psychiatric difficulties when, in fact, significant learning problems may more usually be seen as leading to behavior problems.

The patient's response to previous triala of medication should be explored Parents should be involved in this discussion as well as previous prescribers. Similarly, the efficacy of previous psychosocial treatments should be reviewed. In talking with the parents, it is also important to inquire as to any difficulties they have that may contribute to the child's problem (e.g., psychiatric history, substance use or abuse history).

Unfortunately, parent–child relationships frequently suffer when children exhibit significant psychopathology. Sometimes parents may be totally exasperated by the child and may see the inpatient admission as a happy solution to their difficulties. In other instances, parents will be strongly motivated to "hang in" even in the face of a relatively abusive relationship given their long history and attachment to the child. Brothers and sisters may play an important role in the child's life, and depending on context, their role may need to be considered in the long-term treatment plan. Similarly, the child's strengths and talents as well as areas of vulnerability need to be considered. For adolescents, an awareness of the peer group is also important (i.e., if the student has a substance abuse problem, is he or she returning to a setting that will encourage this behavior?).

Staff on the unit are in a unique position of being able to observe the child and interactions with family and other children on the unit. The ability to observe children throughout the day is also a potential asset. Sometimes after admission, there may be a "honeymoon" period during which the child seems largely asymptomatic before beginning to display more difficulties. This presents a problem given the shorter length of stays at present.

Access to medical care is important. Occasionally, a child will have a medical problem that contributes to or is independent from his or her psychiatric difficulties. It is important to attend to such issues and be aware of the potential for psychiatric problems resulting from or in association with other medical disease. Sometimes medical conditions can contribute to psychiatric difficulties. Access to appropriate pediatric consultation is particularly critical for free- psychiatric hospital and residential facilities. Typically, a standard set of laboratory tests is obtained on admission. Depending on the situation, levels of psychotropic medications should be obtained as should be any additional toxicology screens. It is important to keep in mind the potential for interaction of agents. Pregnancy tests are usually routine among women of childbearing age; this is particularly important given the potential for teratogenic effects of many drugs. Electroencephalography has a low yield and is rarely used in the absence of specific indications. Similarly, neuroimaging is indicated only when specific signs and symptoms are present (e.g., neurological symptoms, catatonia).

There is the potential for positive and negative learning from peers in all treatment settings. It is important that inpatient and residential programs attend to the peer milieu and sustain a climate that values therapeutic goals. Children with certain vulnerabilities (e.g., lower IQ or physical disabilities) may be particularly vulnerable even within inpatient programs, and it is important to monitor peer acceptance of such individuals. Members of various disciplines are typically involved in the many different activities entailed in inpatient, day or partial hospital, and residential settings. There may be discipline-specific treatments (e.g., speech-language therapy or occupational therapy), and it is important that all members of the group function as part of the treatment team.

Even in the best of circumstances, there is considerable potential for isolation of children from typically developing peers. Accordingly, almost all programs include trips into the community, and many RTCs provide children with more opportunities in the community than they would otherwise experience. Such activities provide important opportunities to practice, and generalize, adaptive skills. For psychiatrists, there is considerable pressure to evaluate appropriate pharmacological treatments. This is often a challenge given time and other constraints that do not allow adequate time for evaluation of drug treatments. Collaboration with outpatient providers both before and after hospitalization is accordingly essential. This is a particularly important issues because, unlike other branches of medicine, psychiatric inpatient programs tend to be facilities with closed staffs, so coordination with community providers is important when the attending psychiatrists are full-time hospital employees. Explicit treatment plans that use well-validated rating skills or other data can be particularly useful. Staff coordination and consistency are important. The inpatient unit provides a highly structured setting with a remarkable opportunity to truly implement a consistent treatment plan. Individual and family therapy can help the patient consolidate gains made and serve as an important monitoring function. Coordination of staff and adherence to the many regulatory and accrediting authorities require written procedures and policies. The use of level or point programs or token economies is extremely widespread. They have a number of advantages in that they can be readily adapted to the individual, they provide overall structure to the unit, and they provide quantitative information that can be included in treatment planning.

As with any good intervention program, consistency is important. The points, rewards, or privileges should be chosen so as to be motivating. This may take the form of special privileges or rewards. Policies should be designed to both short- and longer term goals. Educational services can range from an onsite school program to teachers who visit the unit for a few hours each day. Coordination with the school to which the student will return is essential.

Partial hospital and day hospital programs provide a number of advantages in terms of monitoring drug treatments. Often, there is more time to conduct adequate medication trials and more sources of information on which to evaluate efficacy. There is also the potential for observing the extent to which results of treatment generalize to home and community settings.

Residential treatment programs provide somewhat different challenges for mental health professionals. In these settings, the child psychiatrist usually has a consultative role. He or she may be involved with many different patients and staff members. The distance from the patient may pose problems compared with inpatient, day, or partial hospital settings. Often, the young people in the treatment program do not have the same level of severity or acuity of difficulties exhibited on inpatient units. On the other hand, the effects of psychosocial adversity may be much more apparent. Unfortunately, abuse and neglect are very common. A focus on supporting the child's adaptive attempts to cope with such adversity is essential. Depending on the situation, holidays and other times may be particularly stressful. Treatment programs specific to certain situations (e.g., substance abuse) understandably include disorder-specific interventions and program.

A series of financial issues confront clinicians in inpatient settings. These include utilization review and case review. Typically, prior review or authorization is done before admission. As part of case review, the treating clinician is typically asked for a comprehensive diagnostic assessment as well as a review of history and other relevant issues. Goals of treatment as well as the anticipated length of stay and procedures for monitoring progress are reviewed along with the patient's potential danger to him- or herself and others. Concurrent review involves a review of treatment progress and the need for continued hospitalization.

The Joint Commission (formerly the Joint Commission on Accreditation of Hospital Organizations [JCAHO]) provides guidance on issues of quality assistance, including steps designed to reduce medication errors. It is increasingly the case that psychiatric treatment programs are undertaking various steps to reduce levels of seclusion and restraint. This involves constant retraining of staff and monitoring of the use of as-needed medications.

SUMMARY

The prevalence of mental illness in children and adolescents in the United States is likely in the range of 15% to 20% with a substantial group, perhaps 5% or more, having serious difficulties. Unfortunately, most of these children receive insufficient or even no care. Fewer than 1% of children receive services in intensive treatment settings (inpatient or residential), and only about 5% receive services in outpatient clinics or community-based settings. This has happened even when the budgets for mental health services have increased dramatically. Much of the increase, however, reflects the use of the most expensive possible treatments (residential, inpatient) by a small group of children and adolescents. Concerns about lack of appropriateness and efficacy have appropriately been raised. For many children and adolescents, the transition into other systems of care, notably the juvenile justice system, means even further restrictions to access to appropriate mental health care.

Over the past decade, the role of child psychiatrists has been changing significantly with a move toward more comprehensive, integrated treatments, particularly for children whose problems are more challenging. This movement has not been without its problems—not least of all, funding. Other problems reflect difficulties of interdisciplinary work and the multiple agencies and providers often involved in more complex situations. The increased emphasis on involvement of the child or adolescent and his or her family in the treatment process has been important as has been an increased awareness of cultural and ethnic issues and potential community-based resources and interventions.

Psychiatric hospitalization of children and adolescents is an intervention of last resort. Various attempts have been made to reduce the frequency and duration of such interventions, but they continue to be needed when there are no alternatives. Increasingly, other services are available to provide family support or emergency respite care. These alternatives are variably available, unfortunately. Hospitalization and day treatment programs and residential facilities continue to be needed aspects of a comprehensive intervention program. The impact of currently pending insurance and health care reforms remains unclear.

Selected Readings

Alexander, J. F., & Parsons, B. V. (1982). *Functional Family Therapy: Principles and Procedures.* Carmel, CA: Brooks/Cole.

Azrin, N. H. (1977). A strategy for applied research: Learning based but outcome oriented. *American Psychology, 32,* 140–149.

Barker, P. (1974). *The Residential Psychiatric Treatment of Children.* London: Crosby, Lockwood, & Staples.

Bellack, A. S., Hersen, M., & Turner, S. M. (1976). Generalization effects of social skills training in chronic schizophrenics: An experimental analysis. *Behavioral Research Therapy, 14,* 391–398.

Blader, J. C., & Foley, C. A. (2007). Milieu-based treatment: Inpatient and partial hospitalization and residential treatment. In A. Martin & F. Volkmar (Eds.), *Lewis's Child and Adolescent Psychiatry: A Comprehensive Textbook,* 4th edition, pp. 865–877. Philadelphia: Lippincott Williams & Wilkins.

Blader, J. (2004). Symptom, family, and service predictors of children's psychiatric rehospitalization within one year of discharge. *Journal of the American Academy of Child and Adolescent Psychiatry, 43,* 440–451.

Blader, J. C., Abikoff, H., Foley, C., & Koplewicz, H. S. (1994). Children's behavioral adaptation early in psychiatric hospitalization. *Journal of Child Psychology and Psychiatry, 35,* 709–721.

Burchard, J. D., Bruns, J. D., & Burchard, S. N. (2002). The wrap around approach. In B. J. Burns & K. Hoagwood (Eds.), *Community Treatment for Youth: Evidence-Based Interventions for Severe Emotional and Behavioral Disorders.* New York: Oxford University Press.

Chamberlain, P. (2003). *Treating Chronic Juvenile Offenders: Advances Made Through the Oregon Multidimensional Treatment Foster Care Model.* Washington, DC: American Psychological Association.

Curtis, N. M., Ronan, K. R., & Borduin, C. M. (2004). Multisystemic treatment: A meta-analysis of outcome studies. *Journal of Family Psychology, 18,* 411–419.

Emmons, K. M. (2000). Health behaviors in a social context. In L. F. Berkman & I. Kawachi (Eds.), *Social Epidemiology,* pp. 242–266. New York: Oxford University Press.

Farmer, E. M., Dorsey, S., & Mustillo, S. A. (2004). Intensive home and community interventions. *Child and Adolescent Psychiatry Clinics of North America, 13,* 857–884.

Greene, R. W., Ablon, J. S., & Martin, A. (2006). Use of collaborative problem solving to reduce seclusion and restraint in child and adolescent inpatient units. *Psychiatric Service, 57,* 610–622.

Grimes, K. (2003). Collaboration with primary care: Sharing risks, goals, and outcomes in an integrated system of care. In A. J. Pumariega & N. C. Winters (Eds.), *Handbook of Child and Adolescent Systems of Care: The New Community Psychiatry,* pp. 14:316–331. New York: Jossey Bass.

Halliday-Boykins, C. A., Henggeler, S. W., Rowland, M. D., & DeLucia, C. (2004). Heterogeneity in youth symptom trajectories following psychiatric crisis: Predictors and placement outcomes. *Journal of Consulting Clinical Psychology, 72,* 993–1003.

Jones, K. W. (1999). *Taming the Troublesome Child: American Families, Child Guidance, and the Limits of Psychiatric Authority.* Cambridge, MA: Harvard University Press.

Knitzer, J. (1982). *Unclaimed Children: The Failure of Public Responsibility to Children and Adolescents in Need of Mental Health Services.* Washington, DC: Children's Defense Fund.

Lindsey, D., Martin, S., & Doh, J. (2002). The failure of intensive casework services to reduce foster care placements: An examination of family preservation studies. *Children and Youth Services Review, 24,* 743–775.

Lutzker, J. R., Frame, J. R., & Rice, J. M. (1982). Project 12-Ways: An ecobehavioral approach to the treatment and prevention of child abuse and neglect. *Education and Treatment of Children, 5,* 141–155.

Martin, A., & Leslie, D. (2003). Psychiatric inpatient, outpatient, and medication utilization and costs among privately insured youths, 1997–2000. *American Journal of Psychiatry, 160,* 757–764.

Marx, K., Benoit, M., & Kamradt, B. (2003). Foster children in the child welfare system. In A. J. Pumariega & N. C. Winters (Eds.), *Handbook of Child and Adolescent Systems of Care: The New Community Psychiatry,* pp. 332–352. San Francisco: Jossey Bass.

National Institutes of Mental Health Survey and Reports Branch. (1986, April). *Use of Inpatient Psychiatric Services by Children and Youth Under Age 18, United States, 1980* (Statistical Note No. 175). Bethesda, MD: U.S. Department of Health and Human Services.

Pumariega, A., & Winters, N. C. (2007). Community based treatment and services. In A. Martin & F. Volkmar (Eds.), *Lewis's Child and Adolescent Psychiatry: A Comprehensive Textbook,* 4th edition, pp. 887–911. Philadelphia: Lippincott Williams & Wilkins.

Rogers, K., Powell, E., Zima, B., & Pumariega, A. J. (2001). Who receives mental health services in the juvenile justice system. *Journal of Child and Family Studies, 10*(4), 485–494.

Rowland, M. D., Woolston, J., & Adnopoz, J. (2007). Intensive home based family preservation: Approaches including multisystemic therapy. In A. Martin & F. Volkmar (Eds.), *Lewis's Child and Adolescent Psychiatry: A Comprehensive Textbook,* 4th edition, pp. 887–886. Philadelphia: Lippincott Williams & Wilkins.

Schuerman, J. R., Rzepnicki, T. L., & Littell, J. H. (1994). *Putting Families First: An Experiment in Family Preservation.* Hawthorne, NY: Aldine De Gruyter.

Stroul, B., & Friedman, R. (1986). *A System of Care for Severely Emotionally Disturbed Children and Youth.* Washington, DC: Georgetown University Child Development Center, CASSP Technical Assistance Center.

Swenson, C. C., & Chaffin, M. (2006). Beyond psychotherapy: treating abused children by changing their social ecology. *Aggression and Violent Behavior, 11,* 120–137.

Teplin, L., Abram, K., McClelland, G., Dulcan, M., & Mericle, A. (2002). Psychiatric disorders in youth in juvenile detention. *Archives of General Psychiatry, 59,* 1133–1143.

VanDenBerg, J. E., & Grealish, E. M. (1996). Individualized services and supports through the wraparound process: Philosophy and procedures. *Journal of Child and Family Studies, 5,* 7–21.

Volkmar, F. R. & Wiesner, E. A. (2009). *A Practical Guide to Autism: What Every Parent, Family Member, and Teacher Needs to Know.* Hoboken, NJ: John Wiley and Sons.

Woolston, J., Adnopoz, J., & Berkowitz, S. (2006). *Intensive, In-Home Child and Adolescent Services (IICAPS): A New Intervention Paradigm for Children with Serious Emotional Disturbance.* New Haven, CT: Yale University Press.

CHAPTER 24 ■ PSYCHIATRIC EMERGENCIES

Psychiatric emergencies in children and adolescents become more common with age (but can occur with children of any age). Their urgency depends on the nature of the situation, available supports, and issues of safety for the child and others. Unfortunately, as with other aspects of medical care, psychiatric emergency services are frequently, but inappropriately, used to deal with problems more appropriate to less urgent settings, but given an absence of community resources, such problems may present in emergency department (ED) contexts. In other situations, the issues may be more ambiguous, with a long-standing problem escalating into an acute one. Referrals may come from many sources, including parents and family, schools, juvenile justice, community agencies, and so forth. Referrals from junior high and high schools are frequent except in the summer. Heightened sensitivities to violence have often led schools to adopt a policy of zero tolerance; these policies may require some sort of psychiatric assessment before the child returns to the school.

Psychiatric emergency referral has become more common in recent years, with more than 30 million visits nationally each year. Reasons for the increase remain unclear, although high rates of mental health problems include survey data suggesting high rates of suicidal thoughts and attempts in children and adolescents. Survey reports of violent behavior (either as victim or victimizer) show similar increases. Unfortunately, dwindling options for community-based care force more children and adolescents to ED settings when crises occur. Insurance coverage pressures force shorter lengths of stay when hospitalization is indicated with children and adolescents in and out of inpatient settings very quickly even while they remain at risk for difficulties. Finally, of course, the ED remains the place of last resort for the many uninsured children and adolescents who need acute mental health care.

Child psychiatric emergencies are characteristically times of great stress for all concerned. The sense of urgency is often complicated by anxiety about the outcome or ongoing conflict. Typically, many different factors are involved in precipitating the trip to the ED, and often a relevant place to begin is with the question, "Why now?" Clarifying the relationships of the various individuals centrally involved is another important priority. Children function in several different contexts, including the home and family, school, and community. A crisis can occur with any number of changes to these overlapping systems (e.g., school failure, parental discord, violence). Sometimes a sudden upsurge in level of severity of an ongoing problem can precipitate the crisis. Often, clarifying the questions of why now and who is involved become the first steps in thinking about a resolution of the crisis.

In understanding the nature of the emergency, the evaluator will typically have several important goals, including understanding the factor(s) that led to the referral (including interviewing all the relevant participants), developing a shared or working alliance with the child and family about goals for evaluation, obtaining a history of the child's current difficulties as well as longer-standing issues and problems and relevant support systems, and conducting a mental status examination focused both on issues of differential diagnosis and treatment but also with attention to the presence of suicidal or homicidal ideation, symptoms of psychosis or delirium, and so forth. Developing an emergency treatment plan and arriving at a disposition with due consideration for the safety of the child (and others) is the goal with follow-up and collaboration (e.g., with primary care providers) also important.

Given the intense pressures on a busy hospital ED, it is not surprising that often the focus in an emergency is the question of dangerousness and potential needs for hospitalization. This approach misses the potential therapeutic value of the ED visit and the opportunity it presents for significant benefit. In contrast to the somewhat more leisurely pace of typical assessments, the urgency of the ED situation typically leads to rapid clinical decisions and treatment formulation. This process can be severely hampered (e.g., by the absence of key adults or by limited community resources). The latter can be even more a problem when, as if often the case, the evaluation is conducted at night or on the weekend rather than regular business hours.

Given the pressures involved, the clinician must be efficient and well organized. With experience, clinicians rapidly develop a clear sense of the priority of problems and often begin to formulate their ideas about diagnosis and treatment as soon as the evaluation has begun.

The typical ED is a busy place with little privacy and many distractions. Depending on the situation, it can be very helpful if the clinician can locate a quieter and less stimulating area to use for interviewing the child and others. This area must, however, be safe, and the clinician should know that help is at hand should the need arise. Typically, an adult, rather than the child, will have be the source of the referral to the ED. Similar to other situations in child psychiatry (see Chapter 3), assessment often requires eliciting information from multiple sources, but in contrast to the usual outpatient situation, the adult bringing the child may not necessarily be the parent (e.g., a police officer, social service worker, or teacher might be involved). A lack of relevant information or conflicting sources of information can complicate the task of assessment. Practically speaking, the examiner copes and often ends up collecting information in a piecemeal fashion but with an overall understanding or overview of the most critically important issues to address. Clearly, whoever is present becomes a legitimate source of information (i.e., the child and whoever has transported him or her). If that individual (or individuals) is not the child's parent, interviews with him or her are a priority because often this person does not linger in the ED. In emergency situations, the clinician has considerable leeway in terms of assessment and emergency treatment, although parental contact is clearly indicated as quickly as possible. In many states, adolescents may be able to give consent when parents are not available, and the clinician should be aware of applicable state laws and guidelines (see Chapter 26).

The nature of the chief complaint may vary, sometimes markedly, depending on who serves as the informant. These discrepant views (also termed *informant variance*) simultaneously complicate the task of the clinician but also provide helpful information about the factors that led to the emergency evaluation. They can also serve as a starting point for intervention because they reflect major areas of discrepancy between the views of the child and important adults. Other variations arise depending on the setting or context within which the child or adolescent is observed and levels of demands or expectations places on him or her. The complaint, for example, that "Becky needs medication because of her behavior on the bus" suggests an important initial area of inquiry (i.e., "on the bus") that can tremendously streamline subsequent discussion!

As noted in Chapter 3, the various adult informants understandably provide somewhat different, often discrepant and sometimes contradictory, information relative to behavior but also their attributions of the child's intents, feelings, and motivations. Children who are both disturbed and disturbing (i.e., who present with high levels of externalizing behaviors) frequently are the focus of parental concern and complaint; on the other hand, a child who is disturbed but does not exhibit high levels of such behavior may have problems that are not readily observed by his or her parents or teachers. Parents may also have a selective bias in their recognition of family or personal factors contributing to difficulties in the child (e.g., marital conflict or violence in the home). Children with internalizing difficulties (the disturbed but not disturbing group) may, through denial or conscious avoidance, be less likely to complain either about their own feelings or problems or those of parents and other adults. The examiner should be alert to children who are vague or minimize their problems because often this results from an attempt on the child's part to protect the parent(s) or to maintain some family secret within the family (e.g., parental violence, illegal behavior, mental illness, substance abuse, or physical or sexual abuse). Evaluation in these cases is particularly difficult.

THE INTERVIEW OF THE CHILD OR ADOLESCENT

The child interview in emergency situations requires considerable focus. Given the nature of the setting, the examiner must cope (and help the patient cope) with intrinsic distress associated with the ED setting. Although not easy to do, every effort should be made to help the child feel as comfortable as possible. Unfortunately, by the time the child psychiatrist has arrived, the child often has been sufficiently stressed that he or she is angry, withdrawn, or overtly oppositional and antagonistic. In situations like this, the clinician can invoke the "constructive use of ignorance" and invite the child to provide a view of the events leading to the current situation.

The attitudes of the child and his or her parents and their ability to work with each other provide important information relative to potential discharge home with follow-up in outpatient settings. The child or adolescent's ability to reflect on his or her contributions to the current situation and the events leading up to the ED visit also become important in terms of disposition planning. Difficulties arise when children refuse to acknowledge their contributions to problems or when parents attempt to minimize the problem and attribute it to external sources and unreasonable expectations. On the other hand, the child or family who acknowledge the realities of the difficulties and seem motivated to change has a much greater likelihood to use outpatient treatment successfully.

The next sections of this chapter review three of the more important general areas of difficulty presenting in the ED: aggressive behavior, suicidal thoughts and behavior, and delirium and confusional states.

AGGRESSIVE BEHAVIOR

Aggressive and uncooperative patients present special problems for assessment in the ED. Oppositional and aggressive outbursts are a frequent cause of ED referrals, and the patient may be transported to the ED by law enforcement or emergency medical services. The child or adolescent, sometimes in physical restraints, may be agitated and belligerent and prone to act out. The child's threats and yelling may understandably disturb other patients and staff. Despite the pressure for a rapid solution or resolution (e.g., "shut him up"), the clinician should approach the aggressive child or adolescent patient in a thoughtful, calm, and deliberate fashion. Both in terms of doing an adequate assessment and contributing to the resolution of the crisis, the clinician should try, as much as possible, not to be caught up in the maelstrom but ally him- or herself with whatever capacity the child or adolescent has to remain in control. Unfortunately, the ED environment can contribute to irritability, anger, aggression, or defiant behaviors.

The clinician should be aware of the many causes of aggressive behavior and its association with many different conditions. To complicate the situation further, frequently oppositional defiant and more overly aggressive or violent behaviors have multiple origins and determinants and often a long history. In evaluating such behavior and developing a differential diagnosis, the clinician should be aware of the many factors that may contribute. Impulsive behavior and poor impulse control are frequent in various conditions, including attention-deficit disorders, hypomania, autism, and conduct disorder. Learning difficulties and cognitive delays and associated coping difficulties may also contribute to such behaviors. Exposure through observation or direct experience of aggression in violent families is as another risk as is psychosocial adversity more generally. Substance use or abuse can impair judgment; increase irritability; and

TABLE 24.1

AREAS FOR SYSTEMATIC ASSESSMENT IN EMERGENCY SETTINGS*

1. Impulsiveness vs. premeditation
2. Consistent or inconsistent with past behavior and personality or temperament
3. Degree of dangerousness (e.g., use of weapons) and risk of injury (to self or others)
4. Seriousness of behavior (intentionality, desired objective)
5. Role of disorganized or delusional behavior or thought disturbance
6. Degree of impaired judgment or consciousness
7. Degree to which behavior may result from a perceived threat
8. Child's ability to remember details and accept appropriate responsibility or express remorse (insight)

Adapted from Thomas, L., & King, R. (2007). Child and adolescent psychiatric emergencies. In A. Martin & F. Volkmar (Eds.), *Lewis's Child and Adolescent Psychiatry: A Comprehensive Textbook*, 4th edition, p. 904. Philadelphia: Lippincott Williams & Wilkins.

contribute to disinhibited, impulsive behaviors. Psychotic conditions of various types can similarly present with overt aggression (e.g., as the child or adolescent responds to a state of considerable confusion with paranoia or auditory [command] hallucinations). Aggression and apparent psychosis may also be seen as a feature of various medical conditions, including delirium, encephalitis, seizure disorder, and postconcussive states, as discussed later in the chapter. Taking a careful medical history is important, and the clinician should be particularly alert to the presence of such conditions.

The history should focus both on recent as well as past aggressive behavior (e.g., is this a new problem or one that emerges in the context of years of increasing difficulty?). A thorough history of the events leading up to the present problem is critical with attention to the precipitants of the aggressive outburst as well as the steps leading up to it. The perspectives of the patient and the various relevant adults often provide important information on these issues. When another person is involved as a victim, the actions of the victim, the setting of the event, and the broader context should be identified. Often, problems will have come about as an adult attempted to set a limit. In such cases, the context may clarify issues or factors that contributed to the child's response. Areas to be assessed are summarized in Table 24.1.

The safety of the child and others (including the clinician) is the first consideration in management. The clinician should feel comfortable in the setting with adequate support. In the absence of this, the clinician cannot be nearly as effective or helpful. Several steps can be taken to ensure that the patient is in sufficient control for a thorough assessment to be conducted. In approaching the patient and family, the clinician should be professional and respectful and avoid becoming angry or irritable. A stance of concern and professionalism is important. The clinician should not place her or himself in a situation in which backup is not available, and sensible precautions (e.g., sitting between the patient and the door) should occur as a matter of course. As in other areas of psychiatry, one's own inner sense will provide important clues (e.g., if a patient makes the clinician very anxious, there probably is a good reason). The waiting area and examination room should be free of safety hazards and objects that might be used in an aggressive outburst; as much as is reasonable, these areas should provide minimal stimulation (certainly compared with other parts of the ED) and have some privacy. At the same time, it should also be an area close enough to have help at hand, and there should be some potential for visual contact with other staff with use of appropriate codes or procedures for alerting staff if necessary. The possibility of seclusion and restraint should also be available if needed.

Clear expectations and firm but nonconfrontational limit setting may help de-escalate violent or potentially violent behavior. Communication of rules and expectations can be done to clarify what behavior is and is not considered acceptable. This should be provided both to the patient and family. Agitation and aggression related to confusion and disorganization make it particularly important that patients be monitored carefully. For such patients, avoiding an over-stimulating, disorganizing environment is important as is provision of another person (e.g., a family member) who can provide reassurance and orientating or organizing information. Although there is often a temptation to proceed directly to medication and sedation, it is important to have a clear sense of the nature of the difficulty (e.g., observing the patient for signs of other medical conditions, changes in levels of consciousness, and so forth; see below).

Pharmacological intervention may be needed if behavioral approaches are not successful; in such situations, consideration of sedation should involve an awareness of the severity of the symptoms; potential underlying causes of the difficulties; and the patient's medical status, history, and goals of the sedation. Various agents, but particularly the neuroleptics and benzodiazepines, are frequently used. The benzodiazepine lorazepam has a relatively short half-life (10 to 20 hours) and can be given orally (PO) or intramuscularly (IM). This agent has both sedative and anxiolytic properties, and as with other benzodiazepines, its effects can be reversed with the benzodiazepine antagonist flumazenil. In children, typical doses range from 1 to 2 mg (either PO or IM) hourly until the desired degree of sedation is achieved (see Thomas & King, 2007). Unfortunately, at times, the benzodiazepines can also result in a seemingly paradoxical disinhibition; this seems particularly likely in children and adolescents and can occur at a low dose. Haloperidol (Haldol™) is another frequently used agent. This high-potency neuroleptic has been shown to be more efficacious than lorazepam in addressing violent behavior in adults. Typically, doses are 2 to 5 mg either IM or PO with doses repeated hourly until the desired degree of sedation is achieved. Other neuroleptics can also be used, but the lower potency neuroleptics (e.g., chlorpromazine) may cause hypotension, may increase the seizure threshold, and have more anticholinergic side effects.

Occasionally, the antihistamine diphenhydramine (Benadryl™) is used in pediatric settings; this agent, which has soporific effects, is readily available and safely given either PO or IM, but as with the benzodiazepines, some children, particularly those with developmental difficulties or brain injuries, may be prone to behavioral disinhibition or increased agitation. Potential behavioral and medical effects of combinations of medication should also be considered (e.g., the combination of chlorpromazine and diphenhydramine can result in significant anticholinergic side effects, leading to further confusion and agitation and, occasionally, frank delirium).

The choice of a drug for rapid tranquilization should also be guided by the patient's medical history, current medications, and potential contraindications or drug interactions. For example, use of a neuroleptic might also prompt consideration of prophylactic administration of an agent such as diphenhydramine or benztropine (Cogentin™) to avoid acute dystonic side effects. The ED staff should monitor vital signs as well levels of consciousness and sedation and be alert for possible side effects. Newer atypical neuroleptics are now available, but experience with them has been limited, partly because of the lack of an injectable preparation. If possible, the child or adolescent can be given a choice of PO or IM administration; the latter may be needed for children who are less cooperative and has the advantage of a somewhat more active onset. As at any time in using a medication, the balance of risks versus benefits should be carefully considered.

The use of physical restraints is regulated by several sets of standards and should be reserved for situations when there is immediate danger to the patient or others. Restraints should be used only in such situations and only for as long as they are needed. Institutional policies for seclusion and restraint should be in place. These typically clarify indications for use, the role of key personnel, guidance on monitoring (e.g., to be sure vital signs are stable, that the airway is not restricted), and on periodic reassessment and removal. Such policies provide guidance on the ways orders can be written and the child monitored.

SUICIDAL BEHAVIOR IN CHILDREN AND ADOLESCENTS

Along with aggressive behavior, one of the most recent sources of ED referral is suicidal ideation and behavior. Prevention of suicide in children and adolescents has been increasingly recognized as an important public health problem in the United States and internationally (Pfeffer, 2007).

This awareness has been fostered by a number of well-publicized cases as well as recognition of the problem at the national level (e.g., the Surgeon General's Report). The sensitivity of parents, teachers, and primary care providers to this important topic has been substantially increased as a result. The Surgeon General's Report was built on a large body of work on suicide risk assessment and prevention that began the 1980s and then increased in the past 2 decades. This work has encompassed a range of topics, including suicidal behaviors (i.e., suicidal thoughts and acts) and important psychiatric and psychosocial correlates (e.g., with depression and general psychopathology). Researchers have identified a continuum of behaviors ranging in severity from nonsuicidal behavior to suicidal ideas, attempts, and actual suicide. As in other areas of child psychiatry, age and developmental factors are relevant, and sometimes complicating, considerations. Historically, the publication of Goethe's *The Sorrows of Young Werther* precipitated a wave of youth suicide. The topic was the focus on much interest, including to the Vienna Psychoanalytic Society in the first decade of the 20th century, when Freud emphasized the importance of conflict with significant others in suicide. Starting in the late 1960s and peaking in 1977, a rapid increase in rates of suicide in teenage and young men drew increased attention to the issue as did reports of "cluster cases." The result was increased demand for new and better approaches to suicide prevention. This effort stimulated further research as well as important attempts to achieve a consensus on the need for more consistent approaches to definition; database development; research approaches and work on education, treatment, and prevention of suicidal behavior.

In 2006, suicide was a leading cause of death for adolescents and young adults. Data from the National Institutes of Mental Health suggest rates of suicide ranging from 1.3 per 100,000 in children (10 to 14 years of age), 8.2 per 100,000 in adolescents (15 to 19 years of age), and 12.5 per 100,000 in young adults (20 to 24 years of age). Historically, suicide risk has been highest in white males of all ages followed by nonwhite males, white females, and nonwhite females. Over time, rates of suicide among black youths have increased, possibly related to greater degrees of assimilation into U.S. society. Native Americans have particularly high rates of suicide; loss of traditional cultural values, unemployment, and alcohol problems likely contribute to this risk. Firearms are a frequent means of suicide followed by hanging and poisoning.

Data on suicide attempts are based on the results of a nationally representative sample of high school students (no national registry exists). In this sample, about 20% of the students reported suicidal ideation, with higher rates (25%) in young women compared with (14%) young males. Young women were more likely than young men to attempt suicide, and about 3% of those who attempted suicide experienced a serious injury as a result. Males are more likely to use potentially more lethal means (accounting for higher rates in males). In preadolescents, about 1% of children had attempted suicide, and one-third of adolescents who had a psychiatric inpatient admission had a recent suicide attempt. A history of psychiatric hospitalization is associated with a substantially (ninefold) risk of suicide compared with a community-based sample.

Unfortunately, suicidal intent may be either very clear or very ambiguous. As a result, the attempt to evaluate the degree of intentionality is difficult, particularly in prepubertal children, who may exhibit overt suicidal behavior without clear-cut suicidal ideation or intent. In this group, changing conceptions of the meaning of life and death (see Chapter 2) pose a further complication (e.g., the child may not see death as an irreversible event). Conversely, some adolescents may make serious attempts (e.g., with ingestion of a potentially lethal dose of a medication) but not understand the seriousness of their attempts. As a result, clinicians should carefully consider the potential suicidality of any self-injurious act in children and adolescents; thus, both the overt seriousness of the act and the intent are important to understand.

Approaches to the Suicidal Child

Various factors contribute to suicidal ideation, and attempts and should be considered in the assessment of any child or adolescent. These include the presence of comorbid psychiatric problems (particularly depression but not *only* depression), stressful life events, and sociocultural

TABLE 24.2

MULTIAXIAL RISK FACTORS FOR YOUTH SUICIDE*

Epidemiological Characteristics
Age, Gender, Race/Ethnicity
Lethal Means for Suicidal Acts

Axis I: Primary Psychiatric Disorders
Presence of a Psychiatric Disorder
Comorbidity of Psychiatric Disorders
Mood Disorders, Disruptive, and Substance Abuse Disorders

Axis II: Developmental and Personality Disorders
Cluster B: Narcissistic, Borderline, and Antisocial Personality
 Disorders
Systems Related to Personality Disorders: Aggression,
 Impulsivity, Neuroticism

Axis III: Neurobiological Factors
Serotonin Neurotransmitter Function
Gene x Environment Interactions: the Serotonin Transporter
 Gene

Axis IV: Environmental Stress Factors
Family adversity: losses, violence, abuse, psychiatric disorders,
 suicidal behavior

Axis V: Psychosocial Functioning
Social Maladjustment
 Hopelessness, coping mechanisms
 Social support, cultural affiliation

Reprinted from Pfeffer, C. R. (2007). Suicidal behavior in children and adolescents: Causes and management. In A. Martin & F. Volkmar (Eds.), *Lewis's Child and Adolescent Psychiatry: A Comprehensive Textbook*, 4th edition, p. 531. Philadelphia: Lippincott Williams & Wilkins.

factors. A strong role of family and genetic factors has also increasingly been recognized. Accordingly, attention to the multiple potentially contributing factors is important. This includes the presence of signification psychiatric or developmental disorders, biological and environmental factors, and social adaptation and coping. Table 24.2 summarizes this framework.

Information derived from psychological autopsy studies has given us important information about youth suicide. In the majority of cases (about 90%), the child or adolescent has some psychiatric disorder; although the relative risk varies from study to study, it is clear that clinicians should be alert to the presence of possible suicidal thoughts in all youth who are evaluated. Frequently, some comorbid condition is present. A prior suicide attempt substantially increases the risk for suicide, suggesting that the clinician should inquire about such attempts and, in their presence, be particularly alert to the risk for suicide. Not surprisingly, many youth who complete suicide have a mood disorder; rates of depression vary from about 30% to 50% of cases. Bipolar disorder also contributes to an increased risk. Following mood disorder, substance abuse conditions are the next more frequent problems and are frequently seen in the presence of mood disorder as well. This risk factor is a stronger one among older adolescents (16 year of age or older). Other disorders, including anxiety disorders, eating disorders, and schizophrenia, are less frequently associated with suicide, although even in these conditions, there is some risk. The nature of gender differences has been clarified by results of psychological autopsy studies. In one study, a greater risk for males with prior suicide attempts and a greater risk for females in those with current major depressive disorder was observed.

For youth who commit suicide but without apparent psychiatric disorders, a history of previous attempts or suicidal ideation, access to firearms, and conduct issues have been observed. Studies of youth who attempt but do not complete suicide suggest rather a similar pattern of associations with psychiatric conditions and behavior and substance abuse problems.

In community samples, suicidal ideation is relatively common, with about 4% of males and nearly 9% of females reporting at least moderate levels. There is some suggestion that the seriousness and severity of the attempt can be related to the degree of associated mood problems and alcohol or substance abuse. For males, sexual orientation issues also contribute to increased risk. The presence of borderline and antisocial personality disorders is also a risk factor.

Studies of neurobiological risk factors in children and adolescents have been less common than in adults, in whom there is some suggestion of dysregulation in the serotonergic neurotransmitter system. Some suggestion of similar findings in adolescents has also been noted with lowered levels of serotonin (5-HIAA) in the cerebrospinal fluid of adolescents who had attempted suicide. Another line of work has suggested a possible association of suicidal ideation and the 102C allele in the 5-HT2A gene. Other work has suggested an interaction of the stress and 5-HIAA transporter gene and adolescent suicidal behavior. This suggests an important potential focus for suicide prevention research. Other lines of neurobiological work have focused on the hypothalamic–pituitary–adrenal axis and the stress response system. Other work has focused on sleep dysregulation, particularly in adolescents with major depressive disorder who attempt suicide.

Family factors can increase suicide risk. These include high levels of stress in the home, parents who have significant emotional problems or are abusive, and parents with a history of suicide attempts themselves. The latter increases risk among males about five fold and in females about threefold. Family histories of mood disorder, certain personality disorders, and substance abuse also increase risk. Abuse in the family is a strong risk factor. There is some suggestion that problems at birth may increase risk as do chronic medical problems such as diabetes.

Exposure to models of suicide (e.g., through the media) may result in clusters of cases. This seems particularly true when reports are more exaggerated and romanticized. An important implication is that suicide prevention strategies should be considered in a community when a child or adolescent commits suicide.

As part of the process of assessing suicidal potential, the clinician should evaluate the extent of social and environmental support. The presence of a sympathetic adult, supportive peers, and a supportive environment assist children and adolescents in coping adaptively; conversely, a poorly supportive social network only compounds the isolation, despair, and hopelessness of youth. In this regard, it is of interest that having dropped out of school increases suicide risk. Other factors that contribute to risk include poor coping ability with few resources for dealing with negative feeling as do less adaptive defenses mechanisms (e.g., of denial or reaction formation). The latter may contribute to risk-taking behavior. Cultural issues can be also important in terms of issues of support, cultural affiliation, and so on.

Assessment of Suicide Risk

The process of assessment should involve child or adolescent as well as interviews with parents. This assessment should include a systematic review of present (and past) suicidal acts or ideation as well as the presence of other risk factors, environmental and social stress and supports, history of impulsive behavior, family history, and so forth.

The presence of significant concern should prompt a plan for repeated assessment; if the child or adolescent appears to be a danger to him- or herself, psychiatric hospitalization is recommended. Factors to take into account include an assessment of risk based on the history and current evaluation, taking into account coping mechanisms, the presence of supports, the degree of suicidality, and levels of depression and impulse control. A lack of family support may be an important consideration in the need for hospitalization.

Several different rating scales for assessment of suicidal risk are available and readily administered. Other approaches can be used (e.g., human figure drawings may be helpful with younger children). These instruments supplement but do not replace a careful clinical assessment.

The assessment should take into account the degree of intended self-harm and the relative risk. The latter should include a review of relevant risk factors, including the nature and extent of psychiatric conditions present. The level of intent is an important consideration (e.g., the clinician should be very concerned even if a low lethality means of suicide was attempted if the intent was highly lethal, such as a child who takes 4 aspirin, thinking it will kill him). Conversely, even if the child's intent is apparently not to commit suicide but the means chosen are highly lethal, this is also of great concern. For younger children (and sometimes even older ones), exploration of the child's understanding of death may also be important (e.g., the child may believe that it is reversible or have the fantasy that she or he will be "around" to observe the suffering of a significant other who has rejected him or her). Suicidal thoughts in a child with psychotic symptoms are also a great concern as is access to highly lethal means (guns, poisons, drugs).

Hospitalization offers important advantages of providing a structured, contained environment with staff immediately available. Although not to be undertaken lightly, hospitalization is indicated in the presence of significant suicidal ideation. In cases in which risk is lower and when a more supportive family and psychosocial environment are available, other alternatives can include partial hospitalization and outpatient services.

A child or adolescent who has suicidal ideas should not be discharged from the ED without a clear and explicit discussion with the youth and family regarding the condition and agreement for participation in a treatment plan. This discussion can also include discussion about limiting access to lethal materials.

The ED evaluation can be helpful in beginning the treatment process. One part of the assessment should include consideration of the motivations underlying the suicidal ideas (e.g., breakup of a close relationship, anger at a parent, or overwhelming emotions). Treatment is typically multimodal. Various approaches have been developed, but unfortunately, controlled studies of their effectiveness are uncommon. Cognitive behavior therapy (CBT; see Chapter 22) has been shown to be more effective than supportive therapy or family therapy in dealing with depression, although its superiority in dealing with suicide is not clearly established.

Interpersonal psychotherapy has been shown to reduce depressive symptoms in adolescents, but efficacy with suicidal adolescents is not clearly established. Family involvement and support and improved communication can be helpful as can be thoughtful involvement of nonfamily supports (e.g., school personnel). Dialectical–behavioral therapy has been effective in suicidal adults and has promise in the treatment of adolescents. Family therapy may be helpful for many reasons but has had limited efficacy in suicidal youths who do not exhibit major depressive disorder.

Few studies have addressed the role of psychopharmacologic interventions. Some work in adults has found that lithium decreases the recurrence of suicide attempts in those with major depression or bipolar disorder. The use of this agent in children and adolescents requires particularly careful monitoring given its potential for lethality in high doses. One study, the Treatment of Adolescent Depression Study (TADS), addressed a medication (fluoxetine) alone, against placebo, combined with CBT, and against CBT alone in a study of adolescents with major depression but without high risk for suicide (the latter were excluded). The most effective treatment was the combined drug-CBT (71% improved) over medication alone (61%) over CBT alone (43%) and placebo (35%). It is noteworthy that in this study, adolescents using selective serotonin reuptake inhibitors (SSRIs), had a noteworthy increase in suicidal thinking and acts. As a result of the concern about increased suicidal ideation and attempts after a meta-analysis of clinical treatment trials, the U.S. Food and Drug Administration (FDA) mandated black box warnings for antidepressant medications given to children and adolescents. The FDA also recommended increased clinical monitoring of adverse effects. Special consideration also arises when giving medications that may lead to disinhibition (e.g., benzodiazepines) or impulsivity.

DELIRIUM

There has been a growing recognition of the importance of delusional states in children and adolescents. Part of this interest stems from our increased understanding of central nervous system (CNS) mechanisms in the pathogenesis of psychiatric conditions. Delirium can result from a range of difficulties and can be manifest in myriad ways. By definition, it is usually transient and typically is reversible, and it can have an acute or more subacute pattern of onset. Alterations in thinking, perception, mood disturbance, and various psychomotor features may be observed. Given the potential for delirium to progress, identification of delirium in children and adolescents presenting with apparent psychiatric problems is critical. Features of delirium are summarized in Table 24.3.

Various factors can predispose individuals to delirium, and children seem at higher risk if they are stressed; this presumably relates to their less mature CNS development. Other predisposing factors in children include a history of prior episodes, other cognitive difficulties, the presence of a CNS or sensory disorder, or conditions that result in greater blood-brain barrier permeability. Various medical conditions, drugs, and surgery are all potential risk factors. Indeed, hospitalization often provides a striking confluence of various factors that can result in delirium.

Anticholinergic drugs are particularly known to be associated with delirium. Careful monitoring is needed for children at risk, particularly in hospital settings, because the impression of regression (e.g., with hospitalization) on the part of staff may prevent early identification and treatment of delirium. Interestingly, some procedures known to be associated with delirium in adults (e.g., postcardiotomy) are less common in children. When possible, planned admission with preoperative interventions to help the child become familiar with the setting and cope more adaptively reduces perioperative management difficulties in children. In emergency situations, this is not always possible, and high levels of stress increase the likelihood that delirium will develop. Burn patients are at high risk for delirium. Some of the difficulties associated at times with hospitalization, such as sensory overload and sleep deprivation, contribute to risk. Medical factors, including thiamine deficiency (e.g., in oncology patients and those in intensive care units) and low serum albumin, can contribute to an increased risk, the latter because it results in more bioavailability of drugs in the bloodstream.

As Williams (2007) has noted, the many and varied etiologies of delirium make it more reasonable to think of delirium as a final common pathway leading to various, often fluctuating, symptoms. Table 24.4 summarizes these symptoms.

Work with adults suggests that some processes are more consistently impacted in delirium than others and may represent "core" features (e.g., attentional, cognitive, motor, and memory problems, as well as disorientation and a disturbed sleep-wake cycle). In this view, perceptual symptoms and features such as hallucination, delusions, and affective change are seen as secondary. There is some suggestion that motor activity levels vary somewhat depending on the cause (e.g., delirium associated with drug or alcohol conception is often associated with higher levels of activity, but metabolic factors more frequently result in low activity levels).

TABLE 24.3

FEATURES OF DELIRIUM

1. Change in level of consciousness (e.g., decreased focus, attention, lack of awareness)
2. Cognitive changes (can be expressed in language, communication, perception)
3. Relatively rapid onset (hours to days)
4. Fluctuation in levels of consciousness
5. Association with medical conditions, substance use (intoxication, withdrawal), or other problems may be noted in association with specific signs or symptoms, but the condition is not better accounted for by dementia.

TABLE 24.4

SIGNS AND SYMPTOMS OF DELIRIUM ("*PLASTRD*")

Psychosis
Perceptual disturbances (especially visual), including illusions, hallucinations, metamorphopsias
Delusions (usually paranoid and poorly formed)
Thought disorder (tangentiality, circumstantiality, loose associations)

Language Impairment
Word-finding difficulty, dysnomia, paraphasia
Dysgraphia
Altered semantic content
Severe forms can mimic expressive or receptive aphasia

Altered or Labile Affect
Any mood can occur, usually incongruent to context
Anger or increased irritability common
Hypoactive delirium often mislabeled as depression
Lability (rapid shifts) common
Unrelated to mood preceding delirium

Sleep–Wake Disturbance
Fragmented throughout 24-hour period
Reversal of normal cycle
Sleeplessness

Temporal Course
Acute or abrupt onset
Fluctuating severity of symptoms over 24-hour period
Usually reversible
Subclinical syndrome may precede or follow the episode (or both)

Reactivity Altered
Hyperactive
Hypoactive
Mixed

Diffuse Cognitive Deficits
Attention
Orientation (time, place, person)
Memory (short and long term; verbal and visual)
Visuoconstructional ability
Executive functions

Reprinted from Williams, D. T. (2007). Delirium and catatonia In A. Martin & F. Volkmar (Eds.), *Lewis's Child and Adolescent Psychiatry: A Comprehensive Textbook*, 4th edition, p. 649. Philadelphia: Lippincott Williams & Wilkins.
Adapted from Trzepacz, P. T., Meagher, D. J., & Wise, M. G. (2002). Neuropsychiatric aspects of delirium. In S. C. Yudofsky & R. E. Hales (Eds.), *The American Psychiatric Publishing Textbook of Neuropsychiatry and Clinical Neurosciences*, 4th ed, pp. 525–564. Washington, DC: American Psychiatric Publishing.

Delirium can be associated with significant morbidity and mortality. In their review of a large case series, Turkel and Tavare (2003) reported a mortality rate of 20%. The presence of delirium in a child or adolescent should prompt a thorough search for its etiology. Treatment can begin even as this search is underway. Some of the many potential etiologies of delirium are listed in Table 24.5.

In children and adolescents, the pattern of etiology is often somewhat different than in adults (e.g., illicit drugs use is a frequent cause as are hypoxia and head trauma).

Catatonia

Catatonia is occasionally seen in children and adolescents. Unlike delirium, it is defined on the basis of characteristic motor symptoms (rigid posture, stupor, mutism, fixed staring, and so forth). Similar to delirium, catatonia can be associated with diverse medical and psychiatric disorders, including schizophrenia; mood disorders; developmental disorders such as autism; and sundry medical conditions, including metabolic disorders and drug exposure or intoxication. Various medical complications can in turn result from catatonia and periods of prolonged immobility. As with delirium, various factors likely lead to the final clinical manifestations of catatonia, and various potential mechanisms have been identified (see Williams, 2007).

The diagnosis can be particularly challenging in children, although clinical signs are similar to those observed in adults. If an etiology is not clearly identified, carefully supervised administration of intravenous lorazepam may result in a positive response. The differential diagnosis includes mood disorder (bipolar disorder or depression), seizure disorder, autism or related conditions, and schizophrenia as well as exposure to psychoactive agents. Historical information from parents may help clarify the diagnosis. An electroencephalogram and neurological consultation may be indicated.

Unfortunately, delirium can be difficult to detect. This can result because the onset can be insidious and the presentation fluctuating. Hospital staff may not notice signs of delirium, particularly one not characterized by hyperactivity, and may misattribute unusual behavior to the child's "regression" or response to hospitalization.

Training regarding the ways in which delirium can present and the use of screening instruments should be encouraged. A host of other conditions are included in the differential diagnosis, including mood and anxiety disorders, schizophrenia and other psychoses, and so forth. Abrupt changes in mental status or in cognition or attention should prompt a thorough evaluation, including a careful history and clinical assessment (including cognitive assessment, laboratory testing, electroencephalography [EEG], and so forth). Various instruments for assessment of delirium have been developed for adults, and the Delirium Rating Scale has been evaluated in children and adolescents and found to be useful. This 10-item scale evaluates clinical features of delirium as well as their onset and relation to medical conditions. Although not usually needed, EEGs can be used if diagnosis is difficult and can also be followed over time to document progress.

Treatment includes a search for underlying cause as well as steps that can be taken to support the child or adolescent. These steps can include provision of a more supportive

TABLE 24.5

ETIOLOGIES OF DELIRIUM

Drug intoxication	Intracranial infection
Drug withdrawal	Systemic infection
Metabolic/endocrine disturbances	Cerebrovascular disorder
Traumatic brain injury	Organ insufficiency
Seizures	Other CNS etiologies
Neoplastic disease	Other systemic etiologies

(Adapted from Hales RE and Yudofsky SC: *The American Psychiatric Publishing Textbook of Neuropsychiatry and Clinical Neurosciences*, 3rd ed. Washington, DC: American Psychiatric Press, 2002.)

environment, psychosocial support, and pharmacological interventions. Although double-blind trials are lacking treatment haloperidol remains the most common pharmacological intervention with lower doses given PO or IM. With higher doses, electrocardiography is needed given the potential for QTC interval prolongation, and electrolytes should be carefully monitored to minimize the potential for cardiac toxicity. There is some suggestion that haloperidol's mechanism of action may relate to higher dopaminergic levels as one aspect of a final common pathway in the pathogenesis of delirium. Typically, the benzodiazepines are primarily used in delirium related to withdrawal from alcohol or sedative-hypnotics. Risks include excessive sedation and, in children, paradoxical agitation.

Modifications in the environment can include attention (from staff and family) to issues of providing orienting information (e.g., large clock and calendar, familiar objects and family members). Helping the child achieve a diurnal cycle (e.g., room with window, adjustment of lights down at night can help along with the presence of a parent). Parents should be given information to help them help the child orient (e.g., some basic understanding of the principles involved). Sometimes children with delirium are presented to psychiatrists because of unusual and fluctuating behavior.

Assessment of Risk and the Decision to Hospitalize

One of the most challenging tasks for the clinician in the ED is the assessment of potential risk (e.g., if the child returns home). Various guidelines have been developed, but considerable clinical judgment is required. In some situations, this decision is straightforward (e.g., the presence of a serious medical problem such as delirium, include intoxication, or serious ingestion or if a florid psychosis is present). More typically, the decision about disposition is more complicated. The history (from child and adults) along with the interview and mental status examination of the child should guide such decisions. Important considerations also include the factor(s) leading to the referral and the resources that the child or adolescent may be able to draw upon. One simple way of considering these issues is to ask oneself (and sometimes the parents or family) what is different after the clinical contact. This might include arrangements for follow-up, positive attempts at coping with crisis intervention management, arrangements for supports to be in place, and so forth. In some situations (e.g., when the risk of danger to the self or others is high and when the clinician has a strong sense of the lack of adequate supports), inpatient hospitalization may be needed (see Chapter 23). Similarly, a deteriorating course, often with an acute decomposition, is a strong argument for inpatient assessment as are escalating levels of dangerous behaviors regardless of whether suicidal intent is present (e.g., an individual with a severe eating disorder or with self-mutilating behaviors).

In assessing risk, it is important to be aware that the child's behavior in other settings (home or school) may be more informative of risk than the child's behavior in the ED setting. Conversely, some children who initially present as aggressive or violent may comfortably be discharged to supportive settings with a reasonable follow-up plan in place. Effective management and crisis intervention in the ED may result in at least a temporary solution and resolution for the child and family. Unfortunately, when hospitalization is indicated, considerable time and energy may be spent both in acquiring insurance approval and finding an often scarce inpatient bed. The clinician should be aware of all relevant laws and regulations relative to confidentiality issues, seclusion and restraint, involuntary hospitalization, the Health Insurance Portability and Accountability Act, and so forth (see Chapter 26).

Laws vary from state to state, and in some jurisdictions, parents have considerable leeway to hospitalize a child even without the child's assent.

Systems Issues

Provision of training in dealing with child behavioral health emergencies is a critical, but frequently overlooked, aspect of preparation of ED staff. Unfortunately, all too frequently, psychiatric patients, including children and adolescents, are viewed as a nuisance or "time drain," an attitude that interferes with effective treatment and mitigates against subsequent personal development of staff involved. Often, there is tremendous pressure to move the child or adolescent out of the ED. Sometimes this occurs because of understandable pressures, including a genuine desire to help; at other times, it stems from ambivalence toward psychiatric patients and their problems. It is important for child and adolescent psychiatrists and other mental health clinicians to be seen as valuable members of the ED team. To this end, regular meetings, ongoing discussions and inservice trainings, case review, and opportunities for interaction help foster more efficient use of ED time and facilitate patient management. Unfortunately, the 24/7 aspects of ED care often makes such contacts difficult to implement and to sustain such efforts. Periodic meetings with ED staff and between the primary care (pediatric and emergency medicine) physicians with the child psychiatrists is important. The involvement of professionals, including child psychiatric nurses, may help address some of the issues that inevitably arise. Considerations of location, physical environment, and patient and staff safety are some of the issues that can be reviewed. In addition to the difficulties intrinsic within the ED setting, coordination with other agencies outside this setting can be complex. But coordination is needed if treatment plans are to be reasonably well implemented and appropriate provision for follow-up care made. Unfortunately, ED visits, including with child psychiatrists, can become just another piece of a fragmented and poorly coordinated system of care. Somewhat intrinsic to the process (given the 24/7 nature of the ED), coordination with other agencies or care providers can be a challenge. One important role of child psychiatrists is to develop and foster better patterns of communication with and between relevant care providers. Follow-up with outpatient clinicians with appropriate consent will let the outpatient treater know that his or her patient was seen. Conversely, communication from outpatient clinicians or treatment settings before a child arrives at the ED is similarly helpful and increases the possibility of coordination in the child's care.

Recommendations for outpatient follow should, to the extent possible, include specific arrangements (time and name of clinician) for follow-up even before the child leaves the ED. In some situations, the child will be returning to a clinician familiar to him or her; in other cases, a new referral is made, and contact from the referring physician often expedites arrangements. Unfortunately, even when arrangements are made, follow-through on the part of patients and family may be less than ideal. Steps can be taken to increase the likelihood of follow-up, and an awareness of some of the practical challenges for patients and families is helpful. Consideration of cultural and other factors is also important.

SUMMARY AND FUTURE DIRECTIONS

A thoughtful and efficient approach to management of patients with psychiatric emergencies facilitates appropriate disposition in many cases. That being said, the lack of services, particularly the entire range of outpatient treatment services, often serves as a limiting factor. Pressure to control costs often leads to abbreviated inpatient stays during which the child often is at some distance from school and family members. Alternative paradigms and programs are clearly need to provide the kind of well-integrated "wrap-around" services in communities that can more effectively serve children and their families. Reforms in the health care system, particularly given the very poor reimbursement rates for most mental health services, may also contribute to a greater range and availability of community-based services (see Chapter 23).

Intrinsically, the crisis atmosphere of the ED visit presents challenges but also important opportunities to change. As much as possible, clinicians should attempt to use these opportunities productively.

Emergencies services function as the "front line" of the mental health system, particularly in times, such as the present, when appropriate community-based services are not readily available or easily accessed. The development of new models of care and changes in the health care system offer some promise for positive changes in the future.

Selected Readings

American Academy of Child and Adolescent Psychiatry. (1995). Practice parameters for the psychiatric assessment of children and adolescents. *Journal of the American Academy of Child & Adolescent Psychiatry, 34,* 1386–1402.

Apter, A., Gothelf, D., Offer, R., Ratzoni, G., Orbach, I., Tyano, S., & Pfeffer, C. R. (1997). Suicidal adolescents and ego defense mechanisms. *Journal of the American Academy of Child and Adolescent Psychiatry, 36*(11), 1520–1527.

Beautrais, A. L., Joyce, P. R., & Mulder, R. T. (1996). Risk factors for serious suicide attempts among youths aged 13 through 24 years. *Journal of the American Academy of Child and Adolescent Psychiatry, 35,* 1174–1182.

Berlin, I. N. (1987). Suicide among American Indian adolescents: An overview. *Suicide and Life-Threatening Behavior, 17,* 218–232.

Birmaher, B., Brent, D. A., Kolko, D., Baugher, M., Bridge, J., Holder, D., Iyengar, S., & Ulloa, R. E. (2000). Clinical outcome after short-term psychotherapy for adolescents with major depressive disorder. *Archives of General Psychiatry, 57,* 29–36.

Brent, D. A., Baugher, M., Birmaher, B., Kolko, D., & Bridge, J. (2000). Compliance with recommendations to remove firearms in families participating in a clinical trial for adolescent depression. *Journal of the American Academy of Child and Adolescent Psychiatry, 39,* 1220–1226.

Brent, D. A., Perper, J. A., Goldstein, C. E., Kolko, D. J., Allan, M. J., Allman, C. J., & Zelenak, J. P. (1988). Risk factors for adolescent suicide: A comparison of adolescent suicide victims with suicidal inpatients. *Archives of General Psychiatry, 45,* 581–588.

Centers for Disease Control and Prevention. (1992–2001). Methods of suicide among persons aged 10–19 years—United States. *MMWR Morbidity Weekly Report, 53,* 471–474.

Citrome, L., & Volavka, J. (1999). Violent patients in the emergency setting. *Psychiatric Clinics of North America, 22,* 789–801.

Dickson, L. R. (1991). Hypoalbuminemia in delirium. *Psychosomatics, 32,* 317–323.

Du, L., Bakish, D., Lapierre, Y. D., Ravindran, A. V., & Hrdina, P. D. (2000). Association of polymorphism of serotonin 2A receptor gene with suicidal ideation in major depressive disorder. *American Journal of Medical Genetics, 96,* 56–60.

Edelsohn, G. A., Braitman, L. E., Rabinovich, H., et al. (2003). Predictors of urgency in a pediatric psychiatric emergency service. *Journal of the American Academy of Child & Adolescent Psychiatry, 43*(10), 1197–1202.

Fortunati, F. G. Jr., & Zonana, H. V. (2003). Legal considerations in the child psychiatric emergency department. *Child & Adolescent Psychiatric Clinics of North America, 12*(4), 745–761.

Gould, M. S., Fisher, P., Parides, M., Flory, M., & Shaffer, D. (1996). Psychosocial risk factors of child and adolescent completed suicide. *Archives of General Psychiatry, 53,* 1155–1162.

Guerrero, A. P. (2003). General medical considerations in child and adolescent patients who present with psychiatric symptoms. *Child & Adolescent Psychiatric Clinics of North America, 12*(4), 613–628.

Harringtom, R., Kerfoot, M., Dyer, E., McNive, F., Gill, J., Harrington, V., Woodham, A., & Byford, S. (1998). Randomized trial of a home-based family intervention for children who have deliberately poisoned themselves. *Journal of the American Academy of Child and Adolescent Psychiatry, 37,* 512–518.

Heyneman, E. K. (2003). The aggressive child. *Child & Adolescent Psychiatric Clinics of North America, 12*(4), 667–677.

Inouye, S. K., Bogardus, S. T., Charpentier, P. A., Leo-Summers, L., Acampora, D., Holford, T. R., & Cooney, L. M. (1999). A multicomponent intervention to prevent delirium in hospitalized older patients. *New England Journal of Medicine, 340,* 669–676.

Institute of Medicine. (n.d.). *Hospital-Based Emergency Care: At the Breaking Point. The Future of Emergency Care.* Available at http://www.iom.edu/CMS/3809/16107/35007.aspx.

Katz, L. Y., Cox, B. J., Gunasekara, S., & Miller, A. L. (2004). Feasibility of dialectical behavior therapy for suicidal adolescent inpatients. *Journal of the American Academy of Child and Adolescent Psychiatry, 43,* 276–282.

King, R. A., Schwab-Stone, M., Peterson, B., & Thies, A. (2005). Psychiatric assessment of the infant, child, and adolescent. In H. I. Kaplan & V. A. Kaplan (Eds.), *Kaplan and Sadock's Comprehensive Textbook of Psychiatry,* Vol II, 8th edition, pp. 3044–3075. Baltimore: Williams and Wilkins.

Montgomery, E. A., Fenton, G. W., McClelland, R. J., MacFlynn, G., & Rutherford, W. H. (1991). Psychobiology of minor head injury. *Psychosomatic Medicine, 21,* 375–384.

Olfson, M., Gameroff, M. J., Marcus, S. C., et al. (2005). National trends in hospitalization of youth with intentional self-inflicted injuries. *American Journal of Psychiatry, 162,* 1328–1335.

Olfson, M., Gameroff, M. J., Marcus, S. C., Greenberg, T., & Shaffer, D. (2005). Emergency treatment of young people following deliberate self-harm. *Archives of General Psychiatry, 62*(10), 1122–1128.

Pfeffer, C. R. (1986). *The Suicidal Child.* New York: Guilford Press.

Pfeffer, C. R. (2007). Suicidal behavior in children and adolescents: Causes and management. In A. Martin & F. Volkmar (Eds.), *Lewis's Child and Adolescent Psychiatry: A Comprehensive Textbook,* 4th edition, pp. 529–537. Philadelphia: Lippincott Williams & Wilkins.

Pfeffer, C. R., McBride, P. A., Anderson, G. M., et al. (1998). Peripheral serotonin measures in prepubertal psychiatric inpatients and normal children: Associations with suicidal behavior and its risk factors. *Biological Psychiatry, 44,* 568–577.

Pfeffer, C. R., Newcorn, J., Kaplan, G, Mizruchi, M. S., & Plutchik, R. (1988). Suicidal behavior in adolescent psychiatric inpatients. *Journal of the American Academy of Child and Adolescent Psychiatry, 27,* 357–361.

Shaffer, D., Gould, M. S., Fisher, P. Trautman, D., Moreau, D., Kleinman, M., & Flory, M. (1996). Psychiatric diagnosis in child and adolescent suicide. *Archives of General Psychiatry, 53,* 339–348.

Stack, S. (2005). Suicide in the media: A quantitative review of studies based on nonfictional stories. *Suicide and Life-Threatening Behavior, 35,* 121–133.

Stoddard, F. J., & Wilens, T. E. (1995). Delirium. In M. S. Jellinek & D. B. Herzog (Eds.), *Psychiatric Aspects of General Hospital Pediatrics*, pp. 254–259. Chicago: Yearbook Medical Publishers.

Thakur, A., Jagadheesan, K., Dutta, S., & Sinna, V. K. (2003). Incidence of catatonia in children and adolescents in a paediatric psychiatric clinic. *Australian and New Zealand Journal of Psychiatry, 37*, 200–203.

Thomas, E., & King, R. A. (2005). Child and adolescent psychiatric emergencies. In A. Martin & F. Volkmar (Eds.), *Lewis's Child and Adolescent Psychiatry: A Comprehensive Textbook*, 4th edition, pp. 900–909. Philadelphia: Lippincott Williams & Wilkins.

Treatment for Adolescents with Depression Study (TADS)-Team-US. (2004). Fluoxetine, cognitive-behavioral therapy, and their combination for adolescents with depression: Treatment for Adolescents with Depression Study (TADS) randomized controlled trial. *Journal of the American Medical Association, 292*, 807–820.

Trzepacz, P. T. (1999). Update on the neuropathogenesis of delirium. *Dementia and Geriatric Cognitive Disorders, 10*, 330–334.

Trzepacz, P. T., Meagher, D. J., & Wise, M.G. (2002). Neuropsychiatric aspects of delirium. In S. C. Yudofsky & R.E. Hales (Eds.), *The American Psychiatric Publishing Textbook of Neuropsychiatry and Clinical Neurosciences*, 4th ed, pp. 525–564. Washington, DC: American Psychiatric Publishing.

Turkel, S. B., & Tavare, C. J. (2003). Delirium in children and adolescents. *Journal of Neuropsychiatry and Clinical Neuroscience, 15*, 431–435.

Turkel, S. B., Brazlow, K., Tavare, C. J., & Trzepacz, P. T. (2003). The delirium rating scale in children and adolescents. *Psychosomatics, 44*, 126–129.

U.S. Food and Drug Administration. (2004). Relationship between psychotropic drugs and pediatric suicidality. Available at http://www.fda.gov/ohrms/dockets/ac/04/briefing/2004-4065b1-10-TAB08-Hammads-Review.pdf.

U.S. Public Health Service. (1999). *The Surgeon General's Call to Action to Prevent Suicide*. Washington, DC: Author.

Velting, D. M., Shaffer, D., Gould, M. S., Garfinkel, R., Fisher, P., & Davies, M. (1998). Parent-victim agreement in adolescent suicide research. *Journal of the American Academy of Child & Adolescent Psychiatry, 37*, 1161–1166.

Williams, D. T. (2007). Delirium and catatonia. In A. Martin & F. Volkmar (Eds.), *Lewis's Child and Adolescent Psychiatry: A Comprehensive Textbook*, 4th edition, pp. 900–909. Philadelphia: Lippincott Williams & Wilkins.

Wing, L., & Shah, A. (2000). Catatonia in autistic spectrum disorders. *British Journal of Psychiatry, 176*, 357–362.

Zalsman, G., Netanel, R., Fischel, T., Freudenstein, O., Landau, E., Orbach, I., Weizman, A., Pfeffer, C. R., & Apter, A. (2000). Human figure drawings in the evaluation of severe adolescent suicidal behavior. *Journal of the American Academy of Child and Adolescent Psychiatry, 39*, 1024–1031.

CHAPTER 25 ■ CONSULTATION LIAISON: CONSULTATION IN PEDIATRICS

GENERAL PRINCIPLES AND MODELS OF CONSULTATION

Chronic medical illness increases the risk for psychiatric conditions in children and adolescents, with rates two- to fourfold those in the general population. Concomitant medical illness may color the presentation of behavioral difficulties. Further complications can arise given the significant stress experienced by parents and other family members (e.g., with higher rates of stress-related symptoms and even posttraumatic stress disorder [PTSD]). Consultation issues can arise in different contexts (e.g., outpatient or emergency settings) but most typically arise in the context of pediatric inpatient hospitalization. As described in Chapter 23, different models of care and options for treatment can arise, and an understanding of the nature of the differences between medical and psychiatric models of care is important.

A typical medical consultation in pediatrics can often be obtained quickly with a treatment plan rapidly in place, but in psychiatry, even when the initial assessment is expeditious, intervention may be a long-term process. Other issues include sensitivities to issues of confidentiality and privacy. An appreciation of both the biomedical and biopsychosocial approaches is helpful in providing effective consultation. Some appreciation of the nature of underlying medical conditions may be highly relevant (e.g., are symptoms a feature of the underlying disorder or might they be a manifestation of treatment?). In some circumstances, such as head trauma or central nervous system (CNS) radiation as part of cancer treatment, the potential brain contributions to behavioral difficulties may be easy to appreciate.

Medical procedures may be painful and stressful and are often associated with behavioral and emotional difficulties. Similarly, acute and chronic medical problems can represent different challenges for children and family members. Previous patterns of coping may be used with varying degrees of success. The reactions and behaviors of parents may also be important factors in relation to levels of distress in the child. Peer relationships may also be important (e.g., management of type I diabetes in which the availability of more supportive peers results in better control). The age and cognitive level of the child also have an impact on children's understanding of and responses to illness and medical procedures. Using Piaget's approach (see Chapter 2), Lewis (2002) noted the ways in which children's cognition color their responses to illness, physical functioning, and disease; this can inform intervention. Over time, children have an increased ability to understand cause and effect, but children in the phase of concrete operations (roughly early primary school) may see their illness as a punishment and may benefit from an explanation. In contrast, adolescents are capable of abstract thought and have a more adult understanding of pathophysiology, although in adolescents, a sense of invulnerability may complicate compliance with medical treatments.

Mental health professionals can provide a broad range of services with either a narrow or broad focus. Consultants must be aware of the context in which they are asked to consult and be familiar with the range of problems frequently encountered along with their potential treatments. For psychiatrists, a familiarity with issues of differential diagnosis and potential behavioral and psychiatric symptoms and complications associated with specific illnesses and treatments is important. In addition to work around a specific case, consultants are ideally involved on a longer term basis, providing suggestions for programmatic approaches designed to minimize stress, maximize coping, and facilitate outcomes.

Mental health professionals can draw on a number of treatments that have been used with support, to varying degrees, in the research literature. These include treatments for pain, encopresis, and obesity as well as interventions specific to disease such as sickle cell disease and other conditions. Methods from cognitive behavior therapy (CBT; see Chapter 22) have been adapted for procedure-related pain. These methods may also help ensure adherence to treatment for children with asthma, juvenile rheumatoid arthritis, and type 1 diabetes. A range of theories and model approaches exist for pediatric consultation (Table 25.1).

The Resource Consultation Model (also referred to as the Independent Functions Model) usually focuses on a specific diagnostic concern with a goal of obtaining diagnostic clarification, recommendations, and potential resources both for the medical team and family with usually no further involvement of the consultant. This is the approach similar to that of other specialists

TABLE 25.1

COMPARING AND CONTRASTING CONSULTATION MODELS WITH PEDIATRICS

Model	Consultee	Nature	Methods	Duration
Resource consultation	Patient	Contact with patient and pediatrician	Telephone, face-to-face; "curbside" consultation	Limited; as needed
Process—educative consultation	Pediatrician	Contact with pediatrician	Educational	Ongoing relationship with pediatrician
Collaborative team	Patient and treatment team (e.g., pediatrician; nursing staff)	Contact with patient and health care providers	Interdisciplinary and multidisciplinary approach; "shared caregiving"	Ongoing relationships with teams of health care providers
Family systems consultation	Patient, family, and staff	Contact with patient, family, and health care providers; entire system is unit of consultation	Joining with family; acknowledge strengths and competencies of family	Time limited
Multisystemic	Hospital and other systems	Contact with patient, family, health care providers, other systems (e.g., school settings)	Consultation with multiple care providers within and outside of the hospital setting	Proposed model; unknown

Reprinted from Campbell, J. M., & Cardona, L. (2007). The consultation and liaison process to pediatrics. In A. Martin & F. Volkmar (Eds.), *Lewis's Child and Adolescent Psychiatry: A Comprehensive Textbook*, 4th edition, p. 917. Philadelphia: Lippincott Williams & Wilkins.

who consult with the primary care provider. Although it has the potential to serve, over time, as a bridge to other more complex models of consultation, this model has limitations intrinsic to limited contact and a highly specific and narrow focus (e.g., it might not address relevant system issues). In contrast, the process (or educative) model may involve work primarily with the medical staff with, potentially, little or no actual contact with the patient. In this approach, the consultant provides relevant information to the primary provider. Broadly viewed, this model includes a range of educational activities and has the great potential advantage of "spreading the wealth" of information broadly. Limitations stem from the problems of variable knowledge base on the parts of the primary care providers and potential lack of specificity to the individual child's problems. In the collaborative team model, there is a sharing of responsibility and decision making and more intensive collaboration between the mental health consultant and medical personnel. If things go well, this model has the potential for influencing an entire system of care but it does, of course, intrinsically require a substantial commitment on the part of all concerned. Other approaches have attempted to take a broader systems perspective looking, for example, at how the family, school, and medical care system all interact to influence care. The family systems framework considers differences in family interaction and communication as well as disease management practices. Involving schools and the educational system may also be important. Some psychiatric and developmental problems have clear implications for school-based services, and children with medical conditions can also present issues relative to school reentry after illness or hospitalization. These issues are becoming increasingly common as children with serious medical illnesses are surviving more frequently and may present to schools with problems that impact their ability to profit from usual educational programs, as we discuss at the end of this chapter. Issues of school-based consultation are addressed subsequently in this chapter.

PEDIATRIC INPATIENT CONSULTATION

Various issues and problems may serve to elicit requests for consultation relative to inpatients in pediatric settings (Table 25.2). These requests can vary from consultation on aspects of

TABLE 25.2
FREQUENT CONSULTATION REQUESTS ACROSS THREE PEDIATRIC SETTINGS

Setting	Presenting Concerns (%)[1]	Primary Clinical Activities
Primary care	Heterogeneity of concerns: 1. Behavioral noncompliance (16.2) 2. Tantrums (12.8) 3. Aggression (8.1)	Assessment; parent guidance; psychotherapy
Inpatient ward	Heterogeneity of concerns: 1. Adjustment problems (14.9) 2. Noncompliance (13.3) 3. Depression or suicide (12.9) 4. Anxiety (6.6) 5. Pain management (6.6) 6. Parent coping (6.2)	Wide range of activities: assessment; time-limited psychotherapy; staff consultation; psychopharmacological consultation; parent guidance
Emergency department	1. Suicidal behaviors (47%) 2. Oppositional behavior (24%) 3. Threats of violence or aggression (17%)	Assessment, diagnosis, and disposition

[1]Percentages reported are from Carter et al. (2003) and Drotar, Spirito, and Stancin's (2003) review.
Reprinted from Campbell, J. M., & Cardona, L. (2007). The consultation and liaison process to pediatrics. In A. Martin & F. Volkmar (Eds.), *Lewis's Child and Adolescent Psychiatry: A Comprehensive Textbook*, 4th edition, p. 918. Philadelphia: Lippincott Williams & Wilkins.

management of behavioral difficulties, issues of differential diagnosis, adherence to treatment, and so forth. Some of the more frequent requests involve issues of depression and suicidal ideality, management of anxiety and psychiatric symptoms, and lack of adherence to treatment. Referral rates vary widely and may be more frequent in some service areas than others (e.g., hematology, oncology, and general pediatric services are common sources of referral). It is common for patients referred to psychiatric consultation to have longer lengths of stay, reflecting various factors. On the other hand, various factors may make referral less likely, and much of the available literature suggests that this is indeed the case.

Various guidelines for conducting a psychiatric consultation have been proposed (see Campbell and Cardona, 2007). Generally, the consultant seeks to define the specific, explicit question being asked; reviews the record; and talks with the staff before actually interviewing the patient, parents, or both. After this, there may be suggestions for additional tests or assessments and perhaps coordination with other agencies or providers (e.g., schools or mental health service providers). The consultant should be continuously aware of potential issues of coordination and communication (or lack thereof) because these impact the patient. There will usually be a feedback with specific recommendations. Depending on the context, services may be provided, and the consultant will wish to follow up on the assessment.

Clarification of the referral question is the first step in the process. The consultant should be aware of both the explicit and implicit issues raised at the time of referral (e.g., the explicit question might concern the child or may be more truly focused on the parents). As part of this process, the consultant can also elicit exactly what has been told to the child and family about the consultation and be sure that they have been adequately prepared for it. As part of the review of the medical record, the consultant should be particularly alert to issues of poor or miscommunication and fragmentation of care that can potentially play an important role; this becomes particularly important in more complicated situations in which multiple medical subspecialties are involved. The observations of nurses in the record or in discussion provide important information on the child's functioning and behavior. The consultant should be alert to potential behavioral or psychiatric effects of medications or medication combinations or the after effects of such agents (e.g., withdrawal symptoms). Often, the parents are interviewed before the child; as relevant, others "stake holders" (state child protective service agencies, foster parents, teachers, and others) may also provide important information. The consultant should aim to obtain a concise summary of the child's history with emphasis on special issues such as vulnerabilities or difficulties antedating the current hospitalization, family and social factors that may relate to the referral, community and financial resources, and so on.

The interview with the child typically includes a comprehensive mental status examination appropriate to the child's age and level of functioning (see Chapter 3). Observation of the child in the hospital setting can provide important information. At times, specific self-report inventories might be administered. If there are questions of potential CNS dysfunction or delirium, repeated interviews are essential to document baseline function and changes.

Depending on the situation, the consultant might ask for further procedures or tests (e.g., neuroimaging or electroencephalography [EEG]). Sometimes neuropsychological testing may be needed for children who have experienced CNS insults. The consultant has an important role in attempting to understand the relationships between the patient and family and other systems of care (educational, medical, or otherwise) that pose potential obstacles.

Even before the consultant places a formal summary of his or her assessment in the patient's record, it is important that the results be communicated to both the medical staff and to the patient and family. The consultant should conduct a direct discussion of the various factors that are contributing to current difficulties and attempt to foster a thoughtful discussion with both the medical staff and the family about these issues.

As noted in Chapters 21 to 23, a range of treatment procedures have been developed to help children and families coping with both acute and chronic illness. CBT methods can be used to help children deal with pain and anxiety around anticipated medical procedures. Other approaches can be used to target issues of treatment noncompliance within a family context. Depending on the context, psychopharmacological intervention may provide significant benefit (e.g., in management of anxiety, depression, or agitation). Although some interventions can be instituted within a hospital settings others may require helping families access community- and school-based services.

Many barriers to providing effective consultation services exist. These include a shortage of potential consultants, limited insurance reimbursement, and differences in models of service delivery in the pediatric and mental health systems. The pace of pediatric care moves much more quickly than that of mental health work, and an adequate psychiatric consultation can take several hours. Other issues have to do with resistance, on the part of families and medical professionals, to use of mental health services. The complex issues of confidentiality (see Chapter 26) can also be an issue. Pediatricians and primary care providers may complain about a lack of willingness to share results and recommendations; this is particularly unfortunate given the importance of primary care providers in providing comprehensive care. The consultant should attempt to keep the assessment and recommendations understandable, action oriented, and concise. Lewis (2002) has suggested that on larger inpatient services, the occasional, or frequent, presence of the consultant can reduce barriers to communication and facilitate improved service delivery. This is most practical in teaching hospital settings.

Pediatric Oncology

Around one in 6500 children and adolescents are diagnosed with cancer each year, and despite many advances in treatment, pediatric cancer remains the leading cause of disease-related death in children ages 1 to 14 years (Zebrack, 2007). Advances in treatment have increased long-term survival and, in many cases, recovery. With increased survival rates, the emphasis of intervention programs has, to a considerable extent, changed to include a more developmental and family-focused approach to care with greater attention to foster coping and dealing with stress-related symptoms and disorders Much of the available research literature focuses on children of middle school age with comparatively less on preschool and young school-age populations, reflecting, at least in some part, complexities related to assessment, consent, and so forth. The growing recognition of the importance of family and family factors reflects a greater awareness of the challenges pediatric cancer poses for parents and siblings. Similarly, the older literature, which emphasized only the stressful aspects of cancer, has come to a fuller appreciation of the range of outcomes, including positive outcomes, that may come with coping with pediatric cancer.

The time of initial diagnosis can be one of stress and confusion. It is helpful for the child to know, in developmentally appropriate ways, exactly what his or her condition is. Often, other information will have been gleaned from what they have overhead parents or staff members say, or information provided may be partial (often in the misguided attempt not to burden the child). This is also a time of stress for parents and siblings, whose needs should be attended to as well.

The many and sometimes painful procedures involved in cancer treatments pose other burdens. These can be compounded by isolation from peers, sometimes by isolation from family members, and the child's lack of participation in his or her usual daily activities.

As children begin to know other children undergoing treatment, they may also experience the death of friends and be reminded of the seriousness of their illness. Children and adolescents are frequently amenable to straightforward discussion of relevant issues with mental health professionals and others. Their ability to participate in discussion with medical staff may also help lessen their anxiety. In the absence of such information and involvement, children may (and often will) think the worst. They may develop symptoms of stress such as nausea and vomiting in anticipation of treatment. The latter may result from the associations of chemotherapy with specific environmental stimuli.

As with other chronic diseases, lack of adherence to treatments is frequent and can take many forms, ranging from overt treatment refusal and "forgetting" medications and appointments to uses of unproven, alternative treatments. Engaging the child and adolescent in the process through conversations and participation in decision making helps prevent these problems. Other issues may arise around cultural differences and beliefs; it is important for treating physicians and the team to understand how specific cultural issues might impact compliance with treatment.

Repeated school absence is often unavoidable, but lack of attendance creates several issues. It tends to isolate the child from peers, prevents the child from engaging in usual activities, and places the child at academic risk (sometimes further compounded by side effects of treatments). In some hospitals, the availability of a teacher may help the child maintain at least some continuity with homework. In other instances, the school district may be able to help provide services. Other problems may be encountered as the child returns to school;, changes in appearance or ability to participate in usual activities, issues of anxiety or depression, or even cognitive changes brought about by the chemotherapy may all have an impact. The child may be worried about being able to fit in with peers or feel embarrassed about his or her appearance. Having peers remain involved with the child through the hospitalization as much as possible will help the reentry process. Side effects of CNS treatments can impact various cognitive abilities, and attention; memory; and learning math, handwriting, and organization skills may be adversely impacted. These issues may be most dramatic in association with CNS irradiation and younger age (younger than 6 years).

Parents face many issues as they cope with the child's cancer. They must balance the needs of the child with the rest of the family. Siblings may feel (often accurately) that they are receiving less attention and may have their own issues in understanding the sibling's condition as they cope with feelings of anger, frustration, isolation, and sometimes resentment and jealousy. Even when things go well, the experience for siblings can be highly stressful. Siblings may seek to protect both their brother or sister and the parents. Sometimes, particularly when good lines of communication can remain open, siblings may ultimately view the experience as one that helped them grow closer to family members. Issues for parents include tensions around trying to maintain normative activities and parental role and coping with the stress of a child with cancer. Other problems can include overprotectiveness, long-term worries about the child's future, and so forth. Marital issues can arise and be compounded by stress and this can exacerbate preexisting problems.

The child, siblings, and parents may report various problems at the time of initial diagnosis and treatment. The data on these issues is somewhat mixed, presumably given individual differences, age of child, and differences in cancer and cancer treatment. Symptoms can include anxiety, depression, and regression in the child with cancer, and these difficulties may be related to the length of treatment. School reentry can be a further stress for the child. For some children, difficulties may be manifest somewhat later. Some studies have reported reasonably normative functioning after treatment, and symptoms often improve with time. There is some suggestion that for some children, the experience of surviving cancer may be associated with increased levels of maturity and emotional development.

As expected, parents experience various reactions. Feelings of initial shock, confusion, and denial may give way to anxiety, depression, grief, and anger. For some parents, issues of stress and anxiety persist even when the child does well, and there is some suggestion or increased risk for various problems, including PTSD, depression, anxiety, and marital difficulties. In many instances, parents are, however, able to cope well, although residual fears can remain. Studies of differences between fathers and mothers have produced mixed results, perhaps reflecting the effects of different stressors based on roles in the family. Fathers may have more difficulty talking about their experiences than mothers.

Problems in siblings include both internalizing and externalizing difficulties. These can also include posttraumatic stress symptoms, but many siblings do reasonably well. Adolescent siblings may be at somewhat higher risk for difficulties. There is some suggestion of a gender difference, with sisters reporting more physical complaints but with behavioral and social difficulties more common in brothers.

Several steps can be taken to help children cope as well as possible with the experience of cancer and its treatment. The differing "worlds" of normal life and cancer treatment pose obstacles for children, most of whom wish to resume a normal life as quickly as and as much as possible. Often, there is a wish not to be perceived as different. To this end, school attendance remains important. As much as possible, school attendance on a regular basis is helpful and prevents peer isolation and facilitates positive coping. Communication issues with schools can be a problem for parents who understandably can be very concerned about what information they need to provide. The child must decide if and how to share information with peers. For many children, participation in special oncology camps and activities can also be helpful.

Many children with pediatric cancer fall within the "other health impaired" category in qualifying for needed additional services. Parents should provide sufficient information about the child's illness and its treatment to help teachers and others provide appropriate educational services. Sometimes special resources are provided to school personnel through oncology programs, or a visit from a staff member to the school may be used.

Historically, it was often the case that children were told very little about their condition. Other care providers chose to wait for children to ask about their condition, and still others, particularly more recently, take a much more active stance relative to sharing information. The latter procedure has been recommended by the International Society of Pediatric Oncologists after a meeting with the parents and several studies suggesting better outcomes with more open communication about the cancer within the family.

Psychosocial outcomes depend on several factors. These include the child's age and developmental level and the degree to which the child is comfortable knowing about his or her illness. For some children, a degree of denial around medical procedures may be more adaptive, but for others, a straightforward, honest discussion of what is involved may reduce anxiety and fear. Open communication should be encouraged, and the questions of the child should be addressed in a supportive but honest way appropriate to the child's level of understanding. Sometimes a videotape will be made of the diagnostic conference held with the treating team and parents and child; this tape can then be taken home for review and discussion.

Children can have many ways of coping positively, including searching for more information, using humor and optimism, or denial and withdrawal. Factors that facilitate adjustment and coping include faith in the competence of the team; open communication; and supporting positive coping, along with emotional support and continued social supports for the child. Positive parent coping is associated with positive coping in the child.

For some children, the experience of childhood cancer becomes an opportunity for spiritual as well as emotional growth. This may be particularly true in families that have been involved in church and similar groups. Support of siblings can include support groups. Parents should be encouraged to use the resources available to them. For some, this may take the form of more formal psychotherapy, but for others, support from friends and parents of other children may be helpful and sufficient. In particular, parent support groups can be helpful (e.g., http://www.candlelighters.org). Over time, many parents of children who have survived cancer report positive aspects of the experience.

Pediatric Transplantation

There have been major advances in pediatric transplantation over the past decades with successful solid organ and bone marrow transplant procedures now frequent. The first of these procedures involved cardiac transplants in infants, which were beset but a host of problems. The introduction of the immunosuppressant cyclosporine in 1980 marked a major turning point and paved the way for improved outcome and quality of life. Similar advances have occurred in bone marrow transplantation, which had its origins in children. Transplantation procedures with children and adolescents have many similarities and a few differences from adults. Issues of suitability and preparation are relevant to all groups, but for youth, compliance issues, attention to developmental needs and status, and psychosocial issues can be more important. Over time, pediatricians, surgeons, and transplant specialists have become more interested in obtaining appropriate mental health supports for children and youth.

There are similarities and differences between transplant of bone marrow and solid organs. Children coping with these procedures are, depending on their cognitive level, acutely aware of their medical status and potential risk. Both they and their family are under very considerable stress, and the range of treatment options, with their associated risks and potential benefits,

Case Study: Side Effects of Immunosuppression

A 13-year-old boy with a history of autoimmune hepatitis and subsequent hepatic failure received a deceased donor liver transplant at age 12 years. Before his liver disease and surgery, he had the psychiatric diagnoses of attention-deficit/hyperactivity disorder and an atypical mood disorder, and he was treated with stimulant medications and atypical antipsychotics to prevent his often aggressive outbursts. Given the severity of his psychiatric disorder, his medication was continued throughout his perioperative course. However, after his transplant, he developed significant emotional lability that correlated with the addition of prednisone as a necessary part of his immunosuppressant regimen. This behavior was managed by increasing dosages of his atypical antipsychotic medications. Because atypical agents are hepatically metabolized, increased monitoring of his liver function tests was necessary to ensure that the added psychotropics were not further compromising his graft.

Reprinted from Schlozman, S. C., & Prager, L. (2007). The role of the child and adolescent psychiatrist on the pediatric transplant services. In A. Martin & F. Volkmar (Eds.), *Lewis's Child and Adolescent Psychiatry: A Comprehensive Textbook*, 4th edition, p. 940. Philadelphia: Lippincott Williams & Wilkins.

provide other challenges. Decisions can lead to a lifetime commitment to antirejection medications, which have short and longer term side effects. It is typical for families to have concern about future academic and reproductive success. The side effects associated with antirejection agents and with the corticosteroids can include agitation, mood problems, paranoid thinking, and cognitive changes. For children and adolescents with preexisting psychiatric problems, these may be exacerbated. Mental health consultants must be aware of the potential range of adverse effects. Potential problems can also arise because of drug interactions. Mental health consultants have an important role in assessing potential side effects, both in terms of risk and as these emerge.

There has been a growing awareness of the considerable distress involved in transplantation and risk for posttraumatic stress syndromes. It is important to look for stress-related symptoms in both patients and families because there is some suggestion that the degree to which parents feel traumatized correlates with the outcome (both medical and psychological) of patients. Adolescents face particular challenges given their urge for greater independence and this, combined with denial, can lead to noncompliance with treatment regimens. This is, unfortunately, the frequent cause of graft rejection.

Mental health consultants have an important role in facilitating clear and developmentally appropriate discussions with both the patient and family members. Parents face complex issues. The dilemma centers around tension between wanting children to grow and develop while simultaneously being vigilant for signs of rejection. In some cases, ongoing or new mental health issues complicate treatment. In general, psychotropic medications are used judiciously; it is important to be constantly aware of the potential for psychiatric or behavioral side effects. Careful monitoring and use of lower doses for treatment are good practice. The use of behavioral and psychotherapeutic interventions can be helpful.

Transplantation associated with cancer is associated with an even greater psychological burden. This and the potential negative effects of isolation add to the risk in bone marrow transplantation. For solid organ transplants, the range of conditions encountered is now considerable more varied. The mental health consultant should have a good understanding of the medical and surgical issues associated with the specific disease process and the potential risks and benefits of the transplant. Often, the consultant is asked to participate in the evaluation for children who are being considered for transplantation. This provides an opportunity to know the patient and family before the transplant, to do a comprehensive assessment, and to educate patient and family regarding the risks and benefits. This also sets the stage for allowing the mental health consultant to coordinate and assist the family in working with the transplant team. Procedures for conducting the initial assessment vary but should be cognizant of the child's age and level of functioning. Often, psychologists or social workers conduct some psychological and psychosocial assessments. Centers also often have their own unique procedures for screening, and in some cases, histories of substance abuse, active psychosis, or suicidal ideation are viewed as exclusionary criteria.

Contact before the transplant can also have important educative function and can sometimes be therapeutic. Concerns include the presence of significant psychiatric conditions as noted above and any developmental or learning problems that might complicate obtaining informed consent. Any history of psychological treatments or medications should be noted along with any history of substance abuse (the latter is much more likely in adolescents). The assessment can also explore aspects of the child's relationship with parents, availability of supports, motivations for and expectations of the transplant, and so forth. Assessment of the understanding of the child and parents to the requirements for treatment after the transplant is important.

Procedures involved in the transplant can be traumatic. In some cases, a prolonged period of waiting may precede abrupt availability of a donor organ. Before this happens, it is wise to prepare the child and family for what will happen and develop a "game plan" for coping after an organ becomes available. After the transplant, other issues can arise. The child or adolescent may experience anxiety and stress-related symptoms as well as significant mental status changes. Preparation can help parents recognize signs of complications. For the mental health consultant, an important aspect of the work is developing a consultative relationship with the treatment team. Many different professionals (physicians, nurses, social workers, teachers, child life specialists, physical therapists, and others) can be involved in the child's care. Many issues can arise as team members develop long-term relationships with children and families. These can be particularly acute when children are not deemed suitable for transplantation because of advanced disease or history of noncompliance.

In some situations, living organ donation is an option (e.g., for kidney, lung, and liver transplants). In such situations, the potential donor must have a comprehensive assessment and assessment of capacities for informed consent. This is particularly important if the living donor is biologically related and some degree of implicit coercion is potentially involved. These issues can also be complicated when a parent is offering to serve as a donor. Living organ donors should understand what is involved and be realistically aware of possible outcomes. Advances in immunosuppression have significantly improved transplant outcomes, but these agents by themselves, or in interaction with other agents, can have significant neuropsychiatric side effects. Issues of drug metabolism are somewhat different in children than in adults given children's faster rates of hepatic metabolism. Some agents specifically impact drug metabolism, and others potentially increase the risk for graft rejection. Table 25.3 summarizes some of the common side effect profiles. Psychiatric complications can also arise in graft versus host disease, which is sometimes seen in bone marrow transplantation. This can present as delirium and encephalopathy.

Patients involved in transplantation typically have long-term relationships with the transplant team. In the ideal situation, this has to do with long-term maintenance, but for some patients, an additional transplant is needed, with attendant distress and anxiety. The mental health consultant has a long-term role in monitoring adjustment.

Pediatric Epilepsy

Recurrent seizures (epilepsy) place children at significantly increased risk for mental health problems even when compared with other chronic conditions. For many children and their families, the psychiatric difficulties are often even more problematic than the seizures themselves. Conversely, the risk for developing seizures is increased in some psychiatric disorders such as autism, attention-deficit/hyperactivity disorder, and major depressive disorder. Although some

TABLE 25.3

POTENTIAL PSYCHIATRIC SIDE EFFECTS OF IMMUNOSUPPRESSANT AGENTS

Immunosuppressant Agent	Description	Potential Psychiatric Side Effects	Laboratory Findings
Cyclosporin Neoral; Sandimmune	Polypeptide fungal product	Delirium, auditory hallucinations, visual hallucinations, other psychotic symptoms	Side effects more prominent at high serum values and tend to resolve as serum levels decrease, SSRIs may increase levels; carbamazepine may decrease levels; herbal agents such as Saint Johns Wort may decrease levels; question of increased sensitivity to neuropsychiatric side effects among bone marrow transplant recipients
Tacrolimus Prograf	Also called FK506 or 5FK; macrolide antibiotic	Delirium, auditory and visual hallucinations, other psychotic symptoms, seizures, akinetic mutism	Side effects more prominent at high serum values and tend to resolve as serum levels decrease; MRI may reveal white matter changes in toxic patients
Mycophenolate mofetil CellCept	Suppresses T- and B-cell proliferation as adjunct immunosuppressant or for patients who cannot tolerate cyclosporine or tacrolimus	Anxiety, depression, sedation	
Muromonab-CD3 OKT3	Given immediately after surgery to prevent rejection, monoclonal antibody that suppresses CD3 T-cell function	Aseptic meningitis, hallucinations during administration	
Corticosteroids	Mainstay of most transplant regimens; usually started high and tapered over weeks to months, although many patients remain on small doses indefinitely	Increased appetite, anxiety, depression, hypomania, mania, paranoia	Often dose related and resolve with lowered dose

MRI, magnetic resonance imaging; SSRI, selective serotonin reuptake inhibitor.
Reprinted from Schlozman, S. C., & Prager, L. (2007). The role of the child and adolescent psychiatrist on the pediatric transplant services. In A. Martin & F. Volkmar (Eds.), *Lewis's Child and Adolescent Psychiatry: A Comprehensive Textbook*, 4th edition, p. 944. Philadelphia: Lippincott Williams & Wilkins.

TABLE 25.4

CAUSES OF SEIZURES

High fever[1] ■ Systemic infection ■ Hyperthermia	Metabolic derangements ■ Hypoglycemia ■ Electrolyte disturbance
Congenital disorders ■ Cerebral palsy ■ Tuberous sclerosis ■ Phenylketonuria	Anoxia ■ Hanging ■ Carbon monoxide poisoning ■ Cardiac disorders
CNS infections ■ Meningitis ■ Encephalitis	Substances ■ Lead toxicity ■ Medications ■ Cocaine
Structural damage ■ Head trauma ■ Intracranial bleed ■ Neoplasm	Inflammatory disorders ■ Multiple sclerosis ■ Lupus

[1] Most common in children.
CNS, central nervous system.
Reprinted from Rao, J., Poncin, Y. B., & Gonzales-Heydrich, J. (2007). Epilepsy. In A. Martin & F. Volkmar (Eds.), *Lewis's Child and Adolescent Psychiatry: A Comprehensive Textbook*, 4th edition, p. 959. Philadelphia: Lippincott Williams & Wilkins.

medicines frequently used for psychiatric difficulties can lower the seizure threshold, other medicines, sometimes given for seizures, can also be used for psychiatric problems (e.g., as mood stabilizers; see Chapter 21). A seizure arises from abnormal electrical activity in the brain and can have behavioral or sensory aspects (or both). Various factors may predispose children to seizures (e.g., high fever, brain infection). Typically, the term *epilepsy* is used when seizures are recurrent. Between the seizures (the "interictal period"), the brain problems associated with the seizures can continue and thus have associated behavioral and psychological impact. Common causes of seizures are listed in Table 25.4. Epilepsy has been noted since ancient times, and Hippocrates first observed the association with depression ("melancholia").

Seizures are relatively frequent clinical phenomena; typically, about 150,000 children and adolescents in the United States will have a seizure every year. Most of these are febrile seizures in younger children. Unprovoked seizures are less common but develop in up to seven in 10,000 children a year with rates similar in the United States and other countries. In most cases, the etiology is unclear. Fortunately, most children with epilepsy go into remission (at least 5 seizure-free years). This is less common if developmental or other neurological problems are present. Unfortunately, a significant number (about one in 10 pediatric patients) will continue to have intractable epilepsy.

In the past, epilepsy was thought of as a mental health problem, and only in the past decade did it come to be recognized as a brain disturbance. On the other hand, the frequent association with psychiatric issues and the complex issues of disentangling these problems apart from each other contributed to the early confusion. Psychiatric issues can arise in relation to the child's perception of self, the effects of the seizures, or side effects of medications given to control the seizures. Developmental skills can be impacted (e.g., both cognitive and adaptive skills), with resultant problems in learning and, potentially, further worsening of self-esteem. Child psychiatrists and mental health workers can have an important role in treating, and hopefully minimizing, the psychiatric repercussions of epilepsy.

Clinical Presentation and Seizure Types

Seizures can present in myriad ways. These can be obvious or subtle. Tonic-clinic seizures are difficult to miss, but brief staring spells or altered sensations or less dramatic changes in consciousness may take some time before being noticed. Seizures are typically brief (seconds to a few minutes). Postictal effects can include confusion, headache, and so forth. Various factors may prompt evaluation for possible seizures. Most evaluations begin with the clinical suspicion that a child is having some form of seizure activity. These can range from the dramatic, such as outright tonic-clonic activity, to the subtle, such as brief staring spells. Other common presentations include unusual sensations, repetitive movements, automatic behaviors, and altered consciousness. Often, seizures are followed by headache or fatigue. A detailed history is particularly important, often as important as the EEG, which is not always abnormal between seizures. Unfortunately, the child's or adolescent's memory of the event may be compromised, so additional sources of information are usually needed. Areas to explore in the history include the onset of the seizure, nature of any abnormal movements, loss of bladder control, any damage the patient might have sustained as a result of the seizure, the length of the seizure, and the length of the recovery time. Inquiry with the patient may yield important information on the aura, including any sensations or premonitions of the seizure. The history and examination will also clarify what additional workup is needed. Typically, an EEG is done unless there is some obvious feature such as high fever in a small child or focal neurological finding in an adolescent that might suggest other tests that have priority. The sophistication of the EEG has increased dramatically over the past decades. Typical EEGs are based on the international 10- to 20-electrode placements from nose to back of head. Typically, at the beginning of the recording, the technician will ask the child to close his or her eyes (or put a hand over the eyes of the younger child) to elicit the alpha rhythm, which is the predominant pattern during wakefulness. Subsequent opening of the eyes will then be associated with other rhythms, including the beta and theta rhythms as the alpha rhythm is attenuated. Stimuli designed to elicit seizure activity are administered during the EEG (e.g., hyperventilation, photic stimulation).

Classification of seizure types has evolved over the years. Early terms, often derived from French neurological terminology ("petit mal," "grand mal") have been replaced with the International League Against Epilepsy Classification system (1989), which is now most commonly used (Table 25.5). This approach to classification is based on whether the seizure is localization related or generalized and on its etiology. In idiopathic epilepsy, no associated neurologic signs, symptoms, or structural brain changes are noted; these seizures are thought to have a genetic basis and are usually related to age. In infants, febrile seizures, infection, after effects of ischemia, and metabolic problems are the most likely causes of seizures. In adolescents, trauma, tumors, brain infection, and sometimes congenital abnormalities are observed. In infants, generalized seizures are most frequently seen, but in older children, partial seizures come to predominate.

Differentiation of epileptic seizures from nonepileptic events can be complex. Video EEG monitoring is often helpful. Absence seizures can sometimes present as attentional problems. Sometimes somatoform disorders (particularly conversion disorder) can present as an apparent seizure. Sometimes an individual child will exhibit seizures along with other paroxysmal behaviors, making differentiation difficult. Table 25.6 summarizes some of the behaviors frequently mistaken for seizure activity. Paroxysmal events that can be taken to suggest seizures include syncopal episodes and hypoglycemia.

Nonepileptic Seizures

In cases of nonepileptoform seizures, dissociative states (see Chapter 17) associated with psychological trauma and mood disorders can be present. Sometimes patients with seizures also exhibit nonepileptic ones. Observation of the seizure may suggest that it is nonepileptic in nature. Video-monitored EEGs are helpful in establishing EEG correlates of unusual behavior, although even here some seizures, particularly in the front lobe, may present without clear EEG correlates. If the apparent seizure is not associated with a postictal state, it may be nonepileptic. Similarly, clinical observation may reveal movements or features not likely to be epileptic. If these problems are addressed quickly through psychiatric intervention, they are less likely to persist.

TABLE 25.5

INTERNATIONAL LEAGUE AGAINST EPILEPSY CLASSIFICATION, 1989

Localization-related epilepsy and syndromes
1. Idiopathic
   a) Benign childhood epilepsy with centrotemporal spikes
   b) Childhood epilepsy with occipital paroxysms
   c) Primary reading epilepsy
2. Symptomatic
   a) Chronic progressive epilepsia partialis continua of childhood
   b) Reflex seizures, startle seizures
   c) Temporal lobe epilepsies
   d) Frontal lobe epilepsies
   e) Parietal lobe epilepsies
   f) Occipital lobe epilepsies
3. Cryptogenic

Generalized epilepsies and syndromes
1. Idiopathic
   a) Benign neonatal familial convulsions.
   b) Benign neonatal convulsions
   c) Benign myoclonic epilepsy in infancy
   d) Childhood absence epilepsy
   e) Juvenile absence epilepsy
   f) Juvenile myoclonic epilepsy
   g) Epilepsy with grand mal seizures on awakening
2. Cryptogenic or symptomatic
   a) West syndrome
   b) Lennox-Gastaut syndrome
   c) Epilepsy with myoclonic-astatic seizures
   d) Epilepsy with myoclonic absences

Symptomatic
1. Nonspecific etiology
   a) Early myoclonic encephalopathy
   b) Early infantile epileptic encephalopathy with suppression burst

Undetermined epilepsies and syndromes
1. With both generalized and focal features
   a) Neonatal seizures
   b) Severe myoclonic epilepsy in infancy
   c) Epilepsy with continuous spike waves during slow-wave sleep
   d) Acquired epileptic aphasia (Landau-Kleffner)
2. Without generalized or focal features

Special syndromes
1. Febrile seizures
2. Isolated seizures or status epilepticus
3. Seizures precipitated by a metabolic or toxic event

Reprinted from Rao, J., Poncin, Y. B., & Gonzales-Heydrich, J. (2007). Epilepsy. In A. Martin & F. Volkmar (Eds.), *Lewis's Child and Adolescent Psychiatry: A Comprehensive Textbook*, 4th edition, p. 961 Philadelphia: Lippincott Williams & Wilkins.

TABLE 25.6

BEHAVIORS THAT CAN BE MISTAKEN FOR SEIZURE ACTIVITY

Behavior of Psychiatric or Undefined Origin	Clinical Manifestations
Nonepileptic seizure	May appear very much like a true seizure, but there is no epileptiform activity on EEG. Duration greater than 10 minutes, the lack of a postictal state, and motor movements incongruent with seizure activity are clues.
Breath-holding	Crying followed by cessation of breathing. Within seconds, cyanosis occurs followed by a loss of consciousness and falling. Quick return to consciousness. No neurological damage. Triggered by fear, frustration, or minor injury.
Staring	May need to rule out epilepsy depending on clinical presentation
Cyclic vomiting	Repeated, spontaneous vomiting lasting days followed by asymptomatic periods; may have an EEG correlate
Stereotyped movements	Tics or other stereotypies
Violent attacks	Violence associated with epilepsy is nondirected thrashing; if violence is organized, this does not suggest epilepsy
Shuddering	Shakes and shudders; no loss of consciousness; lasts seconds.
Jitteriness	Jittering movements in infants; stopped by holding down the arms
Head drops	Can be mistaken for infantile spasms, but no EEG correlate
Behavior Associated with Defined Syndromes	
Syncope	
1. Sandifer. Seen in children with GER 2. Chiari malformations 3. Cardiac conditions	1. Intermittent contractions of the neck with flexion and syncope 2. Syncope from increased ICP; torticollis, ataxia, opisthotonus, nystagmus. 3. Lightheadedness, palpitations, pallor; may need EEG with ECG strip running to clarify etiology
Cataplexy (e.g., of narcolepsy)	Atonia; partial or full loss of tone
Paroxysmal movement disorders (e.g., channelopathies, dysfunction of ion channels)	Hard to differentiate at times but no loss of consciousness
Episodic ataxia types 1 and 2	Brief attacks of cerebellar ataxia; type 2 also involves eye movement difficulties
Paroxysmal kinesigenic dyskinesia	Choreathetosis or dystonia lasting seconds to minutes; triggered by things such as getting up from a chair or out of a car
Paroxysmal exercise-induced dyskinesia	Dystonia occurs 10 to 15 minutes after starting exercise
Benign paroxysmal upgaze of childhood	Spells, lasting hours or days, of intermittent upgaze deviation associated with ataxia; language delay is often present
Benign paroxysmal torticollis	Starts in infancy with attacks of torticollis lasting minutes or hours

ECG, electrocardiography; EEG, electroencephalography; GER, gastroesophageal reflux; ICP, intracranial pressure.
Reprinted from Rao, J., Poncin, Y. B., & Gonzales-Heydrich, J. (2007). Epilepsy. In A. Martin & F. Volkmar (Eds.), *Lewis's Child and Adolescent Psychiatry: A Comprehensive Textbook*, 4th edition, p. 962. Philadelphia: Lippincott Williams & Wilkins.

Psychiatric and Developmental Conditions Associated with Epilepsy

Intellectual disability (mental retardation) is strongly associated with epilepsy. In children with intellectual disability, rates of epilepsy range from 20% to 40% and thus are significantly elevated relative to the general population prevalence rate of about 1%. Conversely, about 40% of children who exhibit epilepsy also exhibit intellectual deficiency. The severity of cognitive deficits is associated with an earlier seizure onset. Complexities for differential diagnosis and management are posed by the frequency of unusual motor manifestations in more cognitively challenged individuals. Other difficulties include unusual behavioral manifestations associated with specific syndromes (e.g., hyperventilation, self-injurious behaviors).

Specific epilepsy syndromes that can cause significant cognitive delay include infantile spasms, Lennox-Gastaut syndrome, and the various epileptic encephalopathies. In the syndrome of acquired aphasia with epilepsy (Landau-Kleffner syndrome), characteristic EEG activity is associated with loss of language skills as well as various behavioral manifestations. Autistic disorder (see Chapter 4) is frequently associated with epilepsy with estimates of rates varying from 5% to 20% with one peak of onset early in life and another in adolescence. Various seizure types are observed.

In the classic Isle of Wright Study, nearly one-third of children with idiopathic seizures also exhibited psychiatric problems. Recent work has confirmed these findings. Some of these difficulties relate to the additional risk posed by any chronic illness; others seem more specific to epilepsy. Frequent mental health problems in children with epilepsy include mood or anxiety disorders (about one-third of cases). Unfortunately, this additional diagnosis is frequently missed. The origins of the mood or anxiety problems have both psychosocial and potentially more syndrome-specific aspects. High rates of suicidal thoughts and behavior are observed in children and adolescents with epilepsy. Psychotic thinking in relationship to epilepsy has been well studied. Pre-, post-, and interictal psychotic symptoms may be observed; these may be noted during the seizure as well, although the interictal symptoms usually prompt psychiatric referral. Epidemiological data from child samples are limited, but adult studies suggest a significant increase in the frequency of psychotic symptoms in the interictal period. Some of the symptoms of ADHD (see Chapter 8), particularly those related to inattention, can mimic epilepsy syndromes, and some data have suggested that children with otherwise uncomplicated ADHD have epileptiform discharges even without seizures being observed. Conversely, in children with epilepsy, there is an increased risk for ADHD symptoms. Rates of oppositional defiant disorder and conduct disorder are also increased (about 20% to 25% of cases).

One body of work has investigated the potential for epilepsy to adversely impact learning and cognitive functions. This is a complicated area given differences in age of onset, type of seizure, and so forth, but in general, studies find epilepsy to be associated with lower IQ scores. Complicating the area further, chronic drug treatment may, particularly if not well monitored, be associated with further decreases in IQ. Academic achievement can also suffer, with higher rates of grade repetition or special education services use. The severity and type of epilepsy can be important factors along with the age of onset and degree of seizure control. About one-third of children with epilepsy have problems in reading, math, or writing. It may be that seizures with onset in the brain hemisphere associated with language dominance may be frequently associated with reading and language-related difficulties.

Further complications for children, particularly adolescents, with epilepsy are increased rates of family difficulties and perception of stigma on the part of peers. Not surprisingly, children with epilepsy often have issues with self-esteem. The severity of seizures and female gender are predictors of greater difficultly, although socioeconomic, family, and cultural factors also play important roles. For adolescents, driving restrictions may have a negative impact on peer relations and self-esteem. Laws vary, but typically, a seizure-free period of 3 to 12 months is required before driving can be resumed.

Pharmacological Interventions

Drug treatment issues can arise in several contexts, including in treatment of epilepsy, treatment of psychiatric conditions observed in addition to epilepsy, and potential drug interaction

TABLE 25.7

COMMON ANTIEPILEPTIC DRUGS AND THEIR MECHANISMS OF ACTION

Drug	Site of Action	Clearance	Indications
Carbamazepine	Blocks Na^+ channel	>95% hepatic	Partial seizures
Ethosuximide	Blocks Ca^{2+} channels	80% hepatic; 20% renal	Childhood absence
Felbamate	Blocks NMDA receptor; modulates Na^+ channel conductance	50% hepatic; 50% renal	Lennox-Gastaut syndrome; focal seizures
Gabapentin	Modulates Ca^{2+} channel	100% renal	Partial seizures; as an add on
Lamotrigine	Blocks Na^+ channels; attenuates Ca^{2+} channels	85% hepatic	Lennox-Gastaut syndrome; partial seizures
Levetiraceteam	Under investigation	Body water; needs to be renally dosed	Partial seizures; complex partial status
Oxcarbazepine	Blocks Na^+ channels; increases K^+ channel conductance; attenuates Ca^{2+} channels	45% renal; 45% hepatic	Partial and generalized seizures
Phenobarbital	Increases GABAa receptor activity; decreases glutamate excitability; decreases Na^+, K^+, and Ca^{2+} conductance	75% hepatic; 25% renal	Partial and generalized seizures
Phenytoin	Blocks Na^+ channels; some Ca^{2+} and Cl^- action	>90% hepatic	Partial and generalized; frontal lobe seizures
Topiramate	Blocks Na^+ channels; modulates GABAa, NMDA, and AMPA	30%–50% hepatic; 50%–70% renal	Partial and generalized seizures
Valproate	May affect GABA glutaminergic activity; decreases Ca^{2+} and K^+ conductance thresholds	>95% hepatic	Childhood absence; JME; idiopathic generalized, and add on for partial
Zonisamide	Inhibits glutamate excitation; blocks NA^+, K^+, Ca^{2+} channels	>90% hepatic	Idiopathic generalized and partial

AMPA, α-amino-3-hydroxyl-5-methyl-4-isoxazole-propionate; GABA, γ-aminobutyric acid; JME, juvenile myoclonic epilepsy; NMDA, N-methyl-D-aspartic acid.
Reprinted from Rao, J., Poncin, Y. B., & Gonzales-Heydrich, J. (2007). Epilepsy. In A. Martin & F. Volkmar (Eds.), *Lewis's Child and Adolescent Psychiatry: A Comprehensive Textbook*, 4th edition, p. 965. Philadelphia: Lippincott Williams & Wilkins.

and the risk of lowering the seizure threshold. Given the potential for side effects and depending on the clinical context, it is not common to begin antiepileptic drug (AED) treatment after an isolated seizure. Much more commonly, AEDs are administered if seizures recur or if there are very specific risk factors suggesting they may return. Some of the common AEDs are listed in Table 25.7. The choice of an AED should take into account the type of seizure, potential side effects, and potential for drug interaction. It is usual to start with a single agent and then, if it is not effective, move to a drug with different mechanism of action. Usually, the initial AED would be continued until the second achieved a therapeutic dose; at that point, a taper off the initial drug would be attempted because treatment with a single agent is preferred. Sometimes this is not possible and, unfortunately, use of more than one drug increases the likelihood of adverse effects. These agents impact multiple psychological processes, including attention and processing speed. From the mental health side, the AEDs are of great interest because many have cognitive and behavioral effects; some of these effects are desirable (e.g., for mood stabilization or lessening anxiety) but others are not (e.g., cognitive dulling or behavioral disinhibition or agitation). Lack of good data on side effects and the complexities of using the drugs in children with epilepsy mean that our understanding of the effects of AED on thinking and cognitive processing remains somewhat limited. This group of drugs is of particular interest to psychiatry for three reasons: (1) many have cognitive and behavioral adverse effects, (2) many have desirable psychotropic effects such as mood stabilization and decreased anxiety, and (3) both these sets of effects could provide clues into the pathophysiology of psychiatric disorders. Side effect profiles vary with agent (see Rao et al., 2007, for an additional discussion).

Treatment of psychiatric disorders in children with epilepsy should include a broad view of the various areas of the child's life and functioning. Behavioral, psychotherapeutic (for the child, family, or both), and educational interventions should all be used as appropriate. In considering drug treatment for comorbid psychiatric difficulties, the potential risks and benefits should be carefully considered, including the potential for lowering the seizure threshold or for the drug to have other adverse effects. Research on this topic is limited. Often, the apparent risk of a psychoactive medication for lowering the seizure threshold is more theoretical than real, and particularly when the situation is urgent, the potential benefit may be worth the relatively small risk. In other cases (e.g., with methylphenidate), there is clearly an increased risk for exacerbating seizures. There can be various drug interactions between psychotropic agents and the AEDs; potential interactions should be carefully considered. Issues in relation to specific psychoactive medications are summarized in Table 25.8. It is important that clinicians treating children with seizures be alert to the presence of psychiatric problems in this patient population.

Life-Limiting Illness, Palliative Care, and Bereavement

In the past, childhood death was relatively common, but over the past century and a half, advances in public health and immunization and the development of antibiotics have led to a dramatic decrease in childhood mortality. In the United States, about 50,000 children die each year, with perhaps 10 times that number experiencing some life-limiting illness. There has been an increased recognition of the need to support children and families facing end-of-life issues, including pain, anxiety, depression, and other problems. The modern hospice movement has achieved greater prominence, although only recently has hospice care been extended to children.

Pediatric palliative care encompasses a range of issues, including pain management, other medical issues, psychosocial issues, spiritual issues, planning for care needs, and practical matters such as where and how services are best delivered. Care for the family after the loss of the child is also part of this process. Life-limiting illness represents a growing phenomenon, with advances in care prolonging lives in patients with illnesses that were previously terminal in childhood or adolescence (e.g., cystic fibrosis). Advances in chemotherapy, transplantation, and other areas are significantly extending life for many children and adolescents.

Both health and mental health care professionals should be aware of the importance of developmental factors in children's understanding of death. This topic has been well studied by Piaget and others. Major issues include understanding irreversibility and finality, universality (inevitability), and causality. Some data suggest that an understanding of irreversibility, nonfunctionality, and universality typically occurs between 5 and 7 years of age. Infants and younger children can and do respond to issues of loss and bereavement. For infants, these issues become more acute as object and person permanence is more fully established (see Chapter 2). For younger children, death is usually experienced as disappearance or separation, although even toddlers begin to have some understanding of death as a concept. Cultural variations, religious beliefs, and other factors interact with developmental issues in forming and informing

TABLE 25.8

RECOMMENDATIONS FOR COMMONLY USED PSYCHOTROPICS IN CHILDREN WITH SEIZURE DISORDERS

Medication or Class	Recommendations (Low Seizure Risk ≠ Absent Risk)	Key Drug–Drug Interactions with AEDs
First-generation antipsychotics	■ Use not advised for chlorpromazine and loxapine ■ Use others judiciously ■ Haloperidol has among the lowest risk	Carbamazepine, phenobarbital, phenytoin, and perhaps oxcarbazepine may reduce levels through CYP 450 3A4 induction
Second-generation antipsychotics	■ Use not advised for clozapine ■ Seizure risk low for others	Risperidone, quetiapine, aripiprazole, and ziprasidone may be reduced by above AEDs through CYP 450 3A4 inhibition
SSRIs and SNRIs	■ Seizure risk low ■ Venlafaxine may have increased risk over others	Fluoxetine and fluvoxamine may increase carbamazepine levels through CYP 450 3A4 inhibition
Trazodone	Seizure risk low	Substrate of CYP 450 3A4; above AEDs may reduce
α-Agonists	Seizure risk low	No known drug interactions with AEDs
Bupropion	Use not advised	Phenytoin and phenobarbital may reduce levels through CYP 450 2B6 induction
Atomoxetine	Seizure risk unclear; use judiciously	No known drug interactions with AEDs
Lithium	Use judiciously; considered proconvulsant	Neurotoxicity with carbamazepine and phenytoin
Stimulants	FDA contraindicates when comorbid seizures are present, but data suggest can be used judiciously	No known drug interactions with AEDs
TCAs or tetracyclic antidepressants	■ Use not advised for clomipramine, amoxapine, and loxapine ■ Use others judiciously	Valproate may increase and carbamazepine may decrease TCA levels
Benzodiazepines	Anticonvulsant but proconvulsant if suddenly discontinued	Alprazolam, diazepam midazolam, and triazolam are substrates of CYP 450 3A4

AED, antiepileptic drug; FDA, Food and Drug Administration; SNRI, serotonin–norepinephrine reuptake inhibitor; SSRI, selective serotonin reuptake inhibitor; TCA, tricyclic antidepressant; CYP 450 3A4, Cytochrome P450 3A4.

Adapted and reprinted from Rao, J., Poncin, Y. B., & Gonzales-Heydrich, J. (2007). Epilepsy. In A. Martin & F. Volkmar (Eds.), *Lewis's Child and Adolescent Psychiatry: A Comprehensive Textbook*, 4th edition, p. 969. Philadelphia: Lippincott Williams & Wilkins.

the ways children understand death and dying. During adolescence, growing cognitive abilities and the acquisition of what Piaget has termed *formal operations* brings new perspectives. For adolescents, struggles with autonomy and independence run directly counter to aspects of end-of-life care and can result in significant psychiatric morbidity. Multidisciplinary pediatric palliative care teams have increasingly used the available literature on this topic to tailor their approaches to intervention.

Management of Pain and Other Symptoms

The work of Eland and others began to document a now well-known tendency to under-treat pain in children, with significant consequences for both medical and psychological care. Subsequent work showed that even preterm infants undergoing surgery without sufficient anesthesia exhibited increased stress, morbidity, and mortality. Despite the recognition of the need for appropriate and adequate pain management, this continues to be a challenging area. Studies in pediatric oncology patients show that in fewer than one-third of cases did parents feel that pain treatment was successful in the final month of life. Further complicating these issues in children, pain can be experienced in ways that closely mimic "psychiatric" symptoms.

The developmentally appropriate assessment of pain management is an essential feature of effective practice. Many issues, including age, intellectual level, personality, prior experience, nature of the pain, coping strategies, cultural issues, and likely outcome color this process. It is reasonably clear that by about age 2 years, most children can begin to identify being in pain and its location, and by age 4 years, they can start to give ratings of pain. By age 8 years or so, a 10-point visual scale is widely used. Before that time, less complex methods include cartoon faces exhibiting various pain intensity levels or photographs of faces. Despite the availability of these procedures, formal documentation remains less frequent than it should be.

Several different strategies can be used in pain management. Pharmacologically, nonopioid pain relievers (e.g., acetaminophen) are used for mild pain. For mild to moderate pain, as with adults, the nonsteroidal antiinflammatory agents and the opiate codeine can be used with or without an adjuvant with more potent opiates used for moderate to severe pain. Acetylsalicylic acid (Aspirin) is usually avoided given potential problems in bleeding, and the agonist and antagonist opioids are avoided because of ceiling effects. Other opioids such as meperidine (Demerol) can accumulate to become toxic with extended use. Although the literature on the topic of pediatric analgesic pharmacotherapy is growing, it is important to be cautious in the interpretation of the research given the factors that limit this literature. Other issues arise given the age-related changes in drug pharmacokinetics and pharmacodynamics. The mechanism giving rise to the pain also is important; nociceptive pain (from tissue damage but reflecting an intact nervous system) should be distinguished from neuropathic pain (resulting from nerve tissue damage). Neuropathic pain is more likely to require adjuvant pharmacotherapy. Clinicians should be alert to drug interactions and potential side effects. Various other agents have been used in adults (e.g., the tricyclics and certain of the anticonvulsants such as gabapentin and pregabalin), but their use in children is not established.

Psychological and behavioral approaches can also be used with significant benefit in the treatment of pain. It is important to keep in mind that every medical intervention involving a person has some potential psychological aspects. Empirical evidence is particularly strong relative to psychological and behavioral interventions for medical procedures and headache. Simply having the parent present reduces distress. Behavioral techniques such as progressive relaxation and other interventions derived from CBT (see Chapter 22) include guided imagery, distraction, and deep breathing. Involvement of the parent can be helpful in this regard (i.e., the parent can help the child in implementing the strategy, giving the child support while simultaneously helping the parent feel effective). Hypnosis can also be used sometimes with success even in relatively young children.

Good clinical practice for pain management includes explicit acknowledgement of the pain and the importance of monitoring and measuring it over time, the use of developmentally appropriate methods and language, and the presence of parents. At the end of life, other issues such as nausea, shortness of breath, and somnolence should also be addressed. For children with life-limiting illnesses, various interventions can be considered. One study explored the use of the selective serotonin reuptake inhibitors for depression and anxiety in pediatric oncology patients. Almost all the participants in this open-label study showed improvement in ratings of depression, and half improved anxiety. Children with life-limiting illness face various challenges, including discomfort, repeated hospitalizations, and so forth. They may experience behavioral regression as well.

Appropriate honesty in dealing with health issues is important. Parents, and sometimes medical care providers, may be uncomfortable with this, but children perceive and sometimes misinterpret the anxiety of the adults and join with their parents in denying the reality of their situation often as a way of helping the parents. In such situations, the child is unable to communicate his or her concerns and receive appropriate support. The actual conversation(s) about the seriousness of illness can be ongoing with information provided in a developmentally appropriate and progressive way. Goals include helping the child have as optimal a life as possible and supporting normative developmental engagement (with family, friends, and others). Developmental issues may impact the child's understanding, so with younger children, a sense of personal responsibility may be present. Potential mistaken interpretations can be avoided if children are asked to repeat back what they have been told. Occasionally, a child will ask directly if he or she is going to die. The clinician should consider the context and motivations before giving an answer (e.g., is the child in pain? Is the child concerned about issues of abandonment?) As much as possible, giving the child an active role is helpful. It is possible that older children and adolescents may wish to be involved in decision making, including decisions about life-prolonging treatments.

Various risk factors are associated with more complex mourning in adults (e.g., unexpected, particularly traumatic death, death of child, preventable death, and so forth increase risk). Lack of social supports is another relevant issue. Anticipatory grieving can help parents deal with the child's death. If this process is in operation, it is important that parents (or medical staff) not disengage (and thus isolate) the child. Parents may become overly protective in response to wishes that the process would reach its end. Sometimes denial of the gravity of the situation occurs. Parents should be involved with the health care team, as sometimes should be the child, in decision making. This does not abrogate the responsibility of health care providers. When additional treatment is futile and the child is maintained on life support, members of the health care team should discuss the situation and timing for ending life support.

After a child's death, parental mortality from both "natural" (disease related) and "unnatural" (accidents and suicide) is higher than for parents who had not experienced the loss of a child. Although not a psychiatric disorder per se, the term *bereavement* is recognized as a potential focus of clinical attention. Both parents and siblings can require support and clinical attention. The impact of a sibling's death on older children and adolescents is probably particularly insufficiently recognized. Religious resources may also be important. The palliative care team has a responsibility for active follow up with the family.

Children who lose a parent or sibling have an increased risk for psychiatric morbidity. For children losing a parent, risk factors include loss in earlier childhood (younger than age 5 years) or early adolescence and the loss of mothers for prepubertal girls and fathers for adolescent boys. Risk is increased by premorbid difficulties, sudden death, and conflicted relationships with the deceased parent. Lack of appropriate parental, environmental, and community supports is also a risk factor. Finally, death resulting from homicide or suicide adds to the risk. Various intervention models have been developed.

Health care providers also exhibit difficulties in dealing with a child's death and dying or in dealing with a grieving parent. Anxiety and discomfort can lead to withdrawal and isolation with a negative impact on care. Health care providers go into the field because of their desire to fight illness and prolong life. Accordingly, any death of a patient can be stressful, and this is amplified for children and in situations in which providers come to have longer term relationships with the child and family. It is appropriate for health care providers to be aware of these challenges and their own potential needs for support. A number of training models have been proposed and are now mandated as part of residency programs.

MENTAL HEALTH ISSUES IN PRIMARY CARE

The integration of mental health resources and treatments into primary pediatric care settings presents many opportunities and challenges. Most children in the United States have at least one visit with a primary care provider each year. Typically, this provider serves as a resource and potentially a gatekeeper in facilitating access to service. The significance of mental health problems is underscored by various recent epidemiological studies suggesting high rates of mental health problems in children, with probably 20% of children having significant problems. These problems take a significant toll on school success and may impact peer and family relationships. The public health significance of these problems is underscored by work suggesting that about half of all mental health disorders have an onset by age 14 years and 75% by age 24 years.

Unfortunately, the historic divisions between medical and psychiatric service systems have tended to fragment service delivery and complicate provision of effective, integrated care. This unfortunate dichotomy is now greatly compounded by issues of insurance reimbursement and the organization (or lack thereof) of health care. These issues become further complicated for some disorders specifically covered within the mandates of schools for providing service under the Individuals with Disabilities Education Act (see Chapter 26).

Although there are major conceptual distinctions between "physical" and "mental" disorders, in reality, it is commonly the case that psychiatric conditions present with physical problems and that patients with physical problems have associated psychiatric disabilities. Psychiatric conditions also have important associated medical risks (e.g., for accidents and injuries, suicide, violence, substance abuse, and teen pregnancy, among others). Improved medical care and increased access to care also means that chronic physical illness is a growing problem. Some disorders such as epilepsy and head trauma carry substantially increased risk for subsequent mental health problems. Conversely, the association of depression with a chronic condition such as diabetes may be associated with significant risk for other problems. Sadly, despite the awareness of the effective interventions, most children and adolescents do not receive treatment, and even those who do do not necessarily received treatments considered best practice, evidence-based interventions. Primary care providers provide clinical management for most psychosocial problems and account for majority of use of psychoactive medications. This is true for various conditions ranging from depression, anxiety, and mood problems to ADHD. Fortunately, there have now been some attempts on the part of the American Academy of Pediatrics to produce guidelines for management. The emerging field of developmental-behavioral pediatrics arose from concerns about the need for more sustained and effective training of pediatricians. This approach has focused on common behavioral and developmental problems, and the subspecialty has been officially recognized and now includes a period of fellowship training.

There is some suggestion that identification of mental health and psychosocial problems in primary settings has begun to increase. This does not, unfortunately, always result in effective management. In most cases, children and adolescents receive limited mental health services, if any. In addition, pediatric primary care providers generally feel more comfortable in the management of some disorders, such as ADHD, but not others, such as depression. There are many obstacles for providing mental health service, including lack of access, social stigma, the shortage of child and adolescent psychiatrists, and reimbursement and administrative issues. Even when these services are recommended, compliance is sporadic, with apparently fewer than half of these referred ever actually receiving specialized services. Various steps have been taken to address these problems, including changes in training, new models of information dissemination and continuing medical education, and new methods of service delivery. These include development of approaches like the *chronic care model* to more effectively integrate mental health services into primary medical settings. Challenges become even more dramatic when the focus of attention shifts to rural health care settings; in such settings, the development of collaborative models of care is particularly important and can make use of long-distance collaborative relationships with mental health staff (e.g., advanced practice nurses and social workers, who can be involved in the "front line" of care).

ISSUES IN SCHOOL CONSULTATION

Mental health consultation services in schools are highly desirable. Children with mental health problems often have problems in schools, school absence rates are high, and various services and supports are available. The range of services that can be delivered in schools is varied, ranging from direct treatment to more consultative and indirect services (e.g., in which a consultant might make a referral to community-based providers or resources). Although about 8 million children and adolescents are thought to need mental health services in schools, fewer than 25% actually receive needed services.

School-based services developed for several reasons. These included the influx of refugees at the end of World War II; mandates at the federal level for services associated with both the civil rights and children's rights movements; the growing recognition of mental health, behavioral, and substance problems over the past decades; and the reduced use of psychiatric hospitalization as a result of insurance and other pressures. Recent legislation, including the No Child Left Behind Act, has also called for intervention.

Various models of school-based consultation have been recognized. Mental health consultation is often indirect and focuses on a particular student and his or her problems to expand knowledge of the school staff in approaches to dealing with similar problems. The student may not necessarily actually be seen. In this context, the school usually pays for the consultation, and responsibilities for follow-up with any recommendations made are left to the school. In contrast, the behavioral consultation model is much more focused on the specific behaviors of students and teachers and typically uses a series of progressive steps (identification, analysis, implementation of an intervention, and evaluation). Typically, the focus is on a behavioral difficulty. The consultant may adopt the framework of the *collaborative problem-solving* described by Greene and Ablon (2006), which considers that students may lack appropriate behaviors to use, so that they revert to less adaptive (e.g., aggressive) responses in problem situations. In contrast to these two approaches, the organizational consultation approach is more concerned with the school as a whole rather than individual students. Here the focus is often on improving communication (e.g., between teachers and administrators, organization issues, and so forth). The difficulties of the individual student may be used as examples for study of how more systemic issues can impact students. For example, the Comer School Development Program provides a comprehensive approach focusing on school restructuring and changing school climate to improve student achievement and motivation in low-achieving schools.

As noted in Chapter 26, schools have come under an increasing range of mandates for services. As a result, demands on staff have increased, and it is important that consultants are realistic about recommendations. As with any consultation, the consultant should be aware of the potential complexities of the organization, the multiple levels of need, and the potential for sometimes even small gains to have a major impact. A wide range of professionals work in school settings, including teachers, teacher aides and assistants, school psychologist, social workers, nurses, guidance counselors, speech pathologists, occupational and physical therapists, and administrators. Consultation issues may also change somewhat in dealing with private, parochial, or charter schools. It is important for the consultant to have a clear sense of the school and the purpose of the consultation. Visiting the school can provide considerable information on issues as varied as the building, classroom, school personnel, support services, and overall atmosphere (see Bostic et al., 2007, for a detailed discussion). Students in special education or those with Section 504 Plans because of a disability present special issues (see Chapter 26).

Unfortunately, the unmet mental health needs in schools are substantial. Although many children (about 20%) are identified as having significant difficulties, fewer than one in five of these actually receive treatment. Unfortunately, minority status and lack of insurance are frequent challenges. About 25% of schools do not even have guidance counselors, and more than half do not have social workers, but these schools are still being asked to address the significant mental health problems of students. Increased recognition of the risks of bullying (both to the bullied and bullies) have lent increased importance to these issues. Other frequent problems include violence, sexual acting out and sexual harassment, substance abuse, school disciplinary problems, and discrimination issues. The advent of after-school programs, sometimes poorly staffed and organized, creates other challenges.

About one in 10 U.S. schools has a school-based mental health center that provides direct access to services. These are most common in a few states and sometimes selected areas within states. A number of models now exist, and some have strong track records of providing mental health services in school settings. Benefits of onsite service include higher achievement, improved attendance, and lower rates of behavioral problems. Some programs now offer expanded services and explicit links and referral arrangements to other agencies. Prevention and early intervention models have been used for high-risk as well as a broader range of children in schools. These models coordinate and integrate family, community, and school services. Various prevention and intervention programs are increasingly available for various purposes (see Bostic et al., 2007, for a review).

Advances in technology have also impacted provision of consultation services in schools and other settings. Sometimes these provide services of child psychiatrists to areas or populations with limited access to serves. At other times, they help schools plan for intervention in students with disabilities. Although offering many potential advantages, other issues, including confidentiality and billing, can pose obstacles to implementation.

SUMMARY

Although many advances have been made, barriers to the provision of effective consultation continue to exist. These include the limited number of child psychiatrists, tensions between medical (or school) and psychiatric models of care, insurance and time pressures, and difficulties in communication. In some respects, the availability of a consultant who is at least a periodic presence goes a considerable way in dealing with some of these issues. Challenges remain in integrating good mental health principles in pediatric and educational care, but the range of effective models and solid research has increased dramatically. Mandates for coverage, health care reform, the increased use of technology, and the use of electronic medical records all have at least the potential for fostering advances in the coming decade.

Selected Readings

American Academy of Pediatrics, Committee on Quality Improvement. (2001). Clinical practice guidelines: Treatment of the school-aged child with attention-deficit/hyperactivity disorder. *Pediatrics, 108*, 1033–1044.

Berg, A. T., Shinnar, S., Levy, S. R., Testa, F. M., Smith-Rapaport, S., & Beckerman, B. (2001). Early development of intractable epilepsy in children: A prospective study. *Neurology, 56*(11), 1445–1452.

Bostic, J., Stein, B., & Schwab-Stone, J. (2007). Schools. In A. Martin & F. Volkmar (Eds.), *Lewis's Child and Adolescent Psychiatry: A Comprehensive Textbook*, 4th edition, pp. 981–998. Philadelphia: Lippincott Williams & Wilkins.

Brophy, P., & Kazak, A. E. (1994). Schooling. In F. L. Johnson & E. L. O'Donnell (Eds.), *The Candlelighters Guide to Bone Marrow Transplants in Children*, pp. 68–73. Bethesda, MD: Candlelighters Childhood Cancer Foundation.

Brunquell, P., McKeever, M., & Russman, B. S. (1990). Differentiation of epileptic from nonepileptic head drops in children. *Epilepsia, 31*(4), 401–405.

Campbell, J. M., & Cardona, L. (2007). The consultation and liaison process to pediatrics. In A. Martin & F. Volkmar (Eds.), *Lewis's Child and Adolescent Psychiatry: A Comprehensive Textbook*, 4th edition, pp. 912–920. Philadelphia: Lippincott Williams & Wilkins.

Cardona, L. (1994). Behavioral approaches to pain and anxiety in the pediatric patient. *Child and Adolescent Psychiatric Clinics of North America, 3*, 449–464.

Carter, B. D., Kronenberger, W. G., Baker, J., Grimes, L. M., Crabtree, V. M., Smith, C., & McGraw, K. (2003). Inpatient pediatric consultation-liaison: A case-controlled study. *Journal of Pediatric Psychology, 28*, 423–432.

Cavusoglu, H. (2001). Depression in children with cancer. *International Pediatric Nursing, 16*(5), 380–385.

Christ, G., Bonanno, G., Malkinson, R., & Rubin, S. (2003). Bereavement experiences after the death of a child. In M. Field & R. Behrman (Eds.), *When Children Die: Improving Palliative and End-of-Life Care for Children and their Families*, pp. 553–579. Washington, DC: National Academies Press.

Comer, J. P., & Woodruff, D .W. (1998). Mental health in schools. *Child Adolescent Psychiatry Clinics of North America, 7*(3), 499–513, viii.

Costello, E. J., Burns, B. J., Costello, A. J., Edelbrock, C., Dulcan, M., & Brent, D. (1988). Service utilization and psychiatric diagnosis in pediatric primary care: The role of the gatekeeper. *Pediatrics, 82*, 435–441.

Drotar, D., Spirito, A., Stancin, T. (2003). Professional roles and practice patterns. In M. C. Roberts (Ed.), *Handbook of Pediatric Psychology*, 3rd edition, pp. 50–68. New York: Guilford Press.

Eland, J. M., & Anderson, J. E. (1977). The experience of pain in children. In A. Jacox (Ed.), *Pain: a Sourcebook for Nurses and Other Health Professionals* (pp. 453–473). Boston: Little Brown.

Erchul, W. P., & Martens, B. K. (1997). *School Consultation: Conceptual and Empirical Bases of Practice*. New York: Plenum.

Glazer, J. B., & Schonfield, D. J. (2007). Life limiting Illness, Palliative care, and bereavement. In A. Martin & F. Volkmar (Eds.), *Lewis's Child and Adolescent Psychiatry: A Comprehensive Textbook*, 4th edition, pp. 917–980. Philadelphia: Lippincott Williams & Wilkins.

Gothelf, D., Rubinstein, M., Shemesh, E., Miller, O., Farbstein, I., Klein, A., Weizman, A., Apter, A., & Yaniv, I. (2005). Pilot study: Fluvoxamine treatment for depression and anxiety in children and adolescents with cancer. *Journal of the American Academy of Child and Adolescent Psychiatry, 44,* 1258–1262.

Greene, R. W., & Ablon, J. S. (2006). *Treating Explosive Kids: The Collaborative Problem-Solving Approach*. New York: Guilford.

Hesdorffer, D. C., Ludvigsson, P., Olafsson, E., Gudmundsson, G., Kjartansson, O., & Hauser, W. A. (2004). ADHD as a risk factor for incident unprovoked seizures and epilepsy in children. *Archive of General Psychiatry, 61*(7), 731–736.

Himelstein, M. D., Bruce, P., Hilden, M. D., Joanne, M., Morstad-Boldt, M. S., & Weissman, A. (2004). Pediatric palliative care. *The New England Journal of Medicine, 350,* 1752–1762.

Jennings, J., Pearson, G., & Harris, M. (2000). Implementing and maintaining school-based mental health services in a large, urban school district. *Journal of School Health, 70*(5), 201–205.

Kanner, A. M. (2003). Depression in epilepsy: Prevalence, clinical semiology, pathogenic mechanisms, and treatment. *Biological Psychiatry, 54*(3), 388–398.

Kelleher, K. J., McInerny, T. K., Gardner, W. P., Childs, G. E., & Wasserman, R. C. (2000). Increasing identification of psychosocial problems: 1979–1996. *Pediatrics, 105*(6), 1313–1321.

Kessler, R. C., Berglund, P., Demler, O., Jin, R., & Walters, E. (2005). Lifetime prevalence and age-of onset distributions of DSM-IV disorders in the National Comorbidity Survey Replication. *Archives of General Psychiatry, 62,* 593–602.

Kestenbaum, C. J. (2000). How shall we treat the children in the 21st century? *Journal of the American Academy of Child and Adolescent Psychiatry, 39*(1), 1–10.

Kriechman, A., Salvador, M., & Adelsheim, S. (2010). Expanding the vision: The strengths-based, community-oriented child and adolescent psychiatrist working in schools. *Child & Adolescent Psychiatric Clinics of North America, 19*(1), 149–162.

Lauria, M. M. (2001). Common issues and challenges for families dealing with childhood cancer. In M. M. Lauria, E. J. Clark, J. F. Hermann, & N. M. Stearns (Eds.), *Social Work in Oncology: Supporting Survivors, Families, and Caregivers*, pp. 117–142. Atlanta: American Cancer Society.

Levinson, J. L., & Olbrisch, M. E. (2000). Psychosocial screening and selections of candidates for organ transplantation. In P. T. Trepacz & A. F. DiMartini (Eds.), *The Transplant Patient*, pp. 27–28. Cambridge, UK: Cambridge University Press.

Lewis, M. (2002). The consultation process in child and adolescent psychiatric consultation-liaison in pediatrics. In A. Martin & F. Volkmar (Eds.), *Child and Adolescent Psychiatry: A Comprehensive Textbook*, 3rd edition, pp. 1111–1115. Philadelphia: Lippincott Williams & Wilkins.

Li, J., Precht, D., Mortensen, P., & Olsen, J. (2003). Mortality in parents after death of a child in Denmark: A nationwide follow-up study. *Lancet, 361,* 363–367.

McGrath, P. J., Dick, B., & Unruh, A. M. (2003). Psychologic and behavioral treatment of pain in children and adolescents. In N. L. Schechter, C. B. Berde, & M. Yaster (Eds.), *Pain in Infants, Children and Adolescents*, pp. 303–316. Philadelphia: Lippincott, Williams & Wilkins.

McLaren, J., & Bryson, S. E. (1987). Review of recent epidemiological studies of mental retardation: prevalence, associated disorders, and etiology. *American Journal of Mental Retardation, 92*(3), 243–254.

Mintzer, L. L., Stuber, M. L., Seacord, D., Castaneda, M., Mesrkhani, V., & Glover, D. (2005). Traumatic stress symptoms in adolescent organ transplant recipients. *Pediatrics, 115*(6), 1640–1644.

Olson, A. L., Kelleher, K. J., Kemper, K. J., Zuckerman, B. S., Hammond, C. S., & Dietrich, A. J. (2001). Primary care pediatricians' roles and perceived responsibilities in the identification and management of depression in children and adolescents. *Pediatrics, 2,* 91–98.

Pendley, J. S., Kasmen, L. J., Miller, D. L., Donze, J., Swenson, C., & Reeves, G. (2002). Peer and family support in children and adolescents with Type I diabetes. *Journal of Pediatric Psychology, 27,* 429–438.

Rando, T. (1993). *Treatment of Complicated Mourning*. Champaign, IL: Research Press.

Rao, J., Poncin, Y. B., & Gonzales-Heydrich, J. (2007). Epilepsy. In A. Martin & F. Volkmar (Eds.), *Lewis's Child and Adolescent Psychiatry: A Comprehensive Textbook*, 4th edition, pp. 958–970. Philadelphia: Lippincott Williams & Wilkins.

Ringeisen, H., Oliver, K. A., & Menvielle, E. (2002). Recognition and treatment of mental disorders in children. *Pediatric Drugs, 4,* 697–703.

Rushton, J., Bruckman, D., & Kelleher, K. J. (2002). Primary care referral of children with psychosocial problems. *Archives of Pediatric and Adolescent Medicine, 156,* 592–598.

Sarvet, B. D., & Wegner, L. (2010). Developing effective child psychiatry collaboration with primary care: Leadership and management strategies. *Child & Adolescent Psychiatric Clinics of North America, 19*(1), 139–148.

Sawyer, M., Antoniou, G., Rice, M., & Baghurst, P. (2000). Childhood cancer: A 4-year prospective study of the psychological adjustment of children and parents. *Journal of Pediatric Hematology/Oncology, 22*(3), 214–220.

Schechter, N. L., Berde, C. B., & Yaster, M. (2003). Pain in infants, children, and adolescents: An overview. In N. L. Schechter, C. B. Berde, & M. Yaster (Eds.), *Pain in Infants, Children, and Adolescents*, pp. 3–18. Philadelphia: Lippincott, Williams & Wilkins.

Schlozman, S. C., & Prager, L. (2007). The role of the child and adolescent psychiatrist on the pediatric transplant service. In A. Martin & F. Volkmar (Eds.), *Lewis's Child and Adolescent Psychiatry: A Comprehensive Textbook*, 4th edition, pp. 939–945. Philadelphia: Lippincott Williams & Wilkins.

Schonfeld, D. J., & Campo, J. V. (2007). Integrating behavioral services into pediatric care settings: principles and methods. In A. Martin & F. Volkmar (Eds.), *Lewis's Child and Adolescent Psychiatry: A Comprehensive Textbook*, 4th edition, pp. 921–927. Philadelphia: Lippincott Williams & Wilkins.

Smilansky, S. (1987). *On Death: Helping Children Understand and Cope*. New York: Peter Lang.

Speece, M., & Brent, S. (1984). Children's understanding of death: A review of three components of a death concept. *Child Development, 55,* 1671–1686.

Stuber, M. L., Kazack, A. E., Meeske, K., Barakat, L., Guthrie, D., Garnier, H., Pynoos, R., & Meadows, A. (1997). Predictors of posttraumatic stress symptoms in childhood cancer survivors. *Pediatrics, 100,* 958–964.

Swick, S. D., & Rauch, P. K. (2006). Children facing the death of a parent: The experiences of a parent guidance program at the Massachusetts General Hospital Cancer Center. *Child and Adolescent Psychiatric Clinics of North America, 15*(3), 779–794.

U.S. Public Health Service Report of the Surgeon General's Conference on Children's Mental Health (2000). *A National Action Agenda*. Washington, DC: Department of Health and Human Services.

Weigers, M. E., Chesler, M. A., Zebrack, B. J., & Goldman, S. (1998). Self-reported worries among long-term survivors of childhood cancer and their peers. *Journal of Psychosocial Oncology, 16*(2), 1–24.

Zebrack, B. J. (2007). Cancer. In A. Martin & F. Volkmar (Eds.), *Lewis's Child and Adolescent Psychiatry: A Comprehensive Textbook*, 4th edition, p. 9. Philadelphia: Lippincott Williams & Wilkins.

CHAPTER 26 ■ CHILD PSYCHIATRY AND THE LAW

This chapter provides an overview of the interface of child and adolescent psychiatry and the law. These issues arise in many different ways and range from offering testimony; assisting the court in evaluations or custody disputes; in adoption; in helping secure school services; and occasionally, in the context of malpractice. It is important that clinicians have some understanding of the ways in which the legal system works and the myriad of often significantly differing state and local laws as well as federal laws and guidelines. It can be a source of frustration to clinicians and others that even if the law seems straightforward, the legal system may be complex to deal with. Given the nature of the court system, many mental health professionals try, as much as possible, to avoid it—although not always successfully. On the other hand, others may have a practice that includes considerable amounts of forensic work and find this rewarding.

Many aspects of court procedures may be frustrating or confusing, and their adversarial nature is a further complication. Adding to this complexity is the nature of the justice system in the United States with dual federal and state legal systems, each with its own processes for appeal. In both systems, both criminal and civil cases are tried within the general court. In addition, there are various specialized courts (e.g., the juvenile courts), and often specialized courts are the ones involving testimony from mental health experts. This has become increasingly true over the past decade as the emphasis with the juvenile justice system has shifted away from an earlier emphasis on rehabilitation.

PARTICIPATION IN THE JUDICIAL PROCESS

Child and adolescent psychiatrists are frequently asked to give testimony and may be served with subpoenas (Table 26.1), which compel their cooperation either to produce records or other materials or to appear in court or elsewhere to give testimony. Being "served" with a subpoena does not mean that the professional has done something wrong; rather, it means that a lawyer for one party or the other believes that the clinician may have some information relevant to their case. For mental health professionals working for a state or private organizations, notification should be immediately given to the relevant legal representative or to the private practitioner's attorney. It is particularly important that the mental health provider understand the rules of confidentiality and privacy because some health-related information can remain protected and confidential. In such situations, the patient may be willing to grant a release

TABLE 26.1

DEFINITIONS OF LEGAL TERMS

Confidentiality: Secrecy; the state of having the dissemination of certain information restricted.

Cross-examination: The questioning of a witness at a trial or hearing by the party opposed to the party who called the witness to testify. The purpose of cross-examination is to discredit a witness before the fact finder in any of several ways, as by bringing out contradictions and improbabilities in earlier testimony, by suggesting doubts to the witness, or by trapping the witness into admissions that weaken the testimony. The cross-examiner is allowed to ask leading questions but is traditionally limited to matters covered on direct examination and to credibility issues.

Defendant: A person sued in a civil proceeding or accused in a criminal proceeding.

Deposition: A witness's out-of-court testimony that is reduced to writing (usually by a court reporter) for later use in court for discovery purposes.

Direct examination: The first questioning of a witness in a trial or other proceedings, conducted by the party who called the witness to testify.

Expert witness: A witness qualified by knowledge, skill, experience, training, or education to provide a scientific, technical, or other specialized opinion about the evidence or a fact issue.

Fact witness: A witness who may testify only to information that is based on firsthand knowledge.

Guardian ad litem: A caretaker, usually a lawyer, appointed by the court to appear in a lawsuit on behalf of an incompetent or minor party.

Plaintiff: The party who brings a civil suit in a court of law.

Preponderance of evidence: The greater weight of the evidence; superior evidentiary weight that, although not sufficient to free the mind wholly from all reasonable doubt, is still sufficient to incline a fair and impartial mind to one side of the issue rather than the other. It is also referred to as *preponderance of proof* or *balance of probability*.

Privilege: A special legal right, exemption, or immunity granted to a person or class of persons; an exception to a duty.

Reasonable doubt: The doubt that prevents one from being firmly convinced of a defendant's guilt or the belief that there is a real possibility that a defendant is not guilty.

Redirect examination: A second examination after cross-examination, the scope ordinarily being limited to matters covered during cross-examination.

Subpoena: A writ commanding a person to appear before a court or other tribunal, subject to a penalty for failing to comply.

Subpoena duces tecum: A subpoena ordering the witness to appear and to bring specified documents or records.

Voir dire: A preliminary examination to determine the qualifications of a prospective witness or evidence.

Adapted and reprinted from Sharma, S., & Thomas, C.R. (2007). The child and adolescent psychiatrist in court. In A. Martin & F. Volkmar (Eds.), *Lewis's Child and Adolescent Psychiatry: A Comprehensive Textbook*, 4th edition, p. 1000. Philadelphia: Lippincott Williams & Wilkins.

of the information or the court may order it, but there are some situations (e.g., if there are claims of malpractice) when special rules may apply.

Similarly, the response to requests for medical records may differ for individuals in private practice and those working for organizations where a central repository of such records exists. In some situations, the patient or parents may request that the child psychiatrist be involved, although it is important that the professional clearly understands the nature of the request (e.g., relative to providing facts or serving as an expert witness). When clinical contact is ongoing, there are other issues to be considered relative to the impact of any involvements or testimony on the treatment.

Some familiarity with the court and court procedures is helpful. Depending on the nature of the proceeding, an appearance in court may be involved, and this might be open or closed, or the request may involve a deposition (i.e., sworn testimony taken in an attorney's office). Dress and demeanor should be appropriate. Even though a specific time may be arranged, it is frequently the case that court proceedings run late or that changes in schedule occur. A court reporter will typically transcribe or audio record testimony that become part of the official court record. Often, the testimony begins with a request for the professional to list past training and other qualifications. In instances in which the psychiatrist is present as a fact witness, there is no reimbursement nor can an insurance company be billed for this time. Time spent as an expert witness is, however, typically reimbursed.

It is important for the mental health professional to realize that both (and sometimes even more) sides will have an opportunity to ask questions. The order of questioning may vary depending on the context. Typically, after the "direct" testimony (questions from the first lawyer), there will be cross-examination by the other attorney (or attorneys) and then a chance for additional ("redirect") questions from the original attorney followed by another round from the opposing attorney. At the end of the testimony, the judge will indicate that the witness is excused. In some situations (e.g., family or juvenile court), the judge may take a more active role in the questioning process.

In providing testimony, the mental health professional should think about the question and provide a direct and straightforward response delivered clearly. The tendency of psychiatrists (and other professionals called as witnesses) is to provide overly elaborate answers based in part on the psychiatrist's knowledge of the case. This tendency should be resisted. It is best to firmly give a simple and responsive answer. If something is complex, one can try to explain it but should keep in mind that attorneys (on all sides) will be thinking about potential implications of literally everything that is said. Conversely, the attorney is usually careful to ask questions when he or she already knows the answer. If the question is unclear, ask for it to be rephrased. If the psychiatrist is not able to answer a question, he or she should just say so. If the question is one that can be addressed based on medical record, it is perfectly appropriate to ask to see the record (or other documentation). It is also possible to indicate uncertainty in an answer or to indicate no relevant knowledge of the answer. If called to testify on certain facts (i.e., as a fact-based witness, it is important that the psychiatrist *not* stray into becoming an expert witness); this is particularly complex when the patient remains in ongoing treatment.

At times, the various attorneys will raise objections; these are of various types, but from the point of view of the witness, it is important to stop speaking and wait for the judge to make a decision and give direction. Often, questions are asked in very specific ways. If the meaning is unclear, the witness should ask for clarification. The lawyer may ask if the psychiatrist can answer a question within a reasonable degree of "medical certainty." This concept usually means more likely than not but can be a source of confusion for those who constantly cope with uncertainty as they revise diagnoses and treatment plans. Intrinsically, the legal system is divisive, and lawyers may use a number of tactics in questioning in the hope of helping bolster their case. For example, the lawyer may offer up a summary of earlier testimony; often, this is cast in a certain way, and the witness is well advised to carefully listen and correct any errors or misrepresentations. Similarly, witnesses should be careful about rather vague and general questions that may precede a much more specific and loaded one. When being asked about earlier testimony, it is always possible to ask to have a previous answer repeated. Similarly, when asked about medical records, it is also quite reasonable to ask to review the specific material in question.

The demeanor of the witness is important. Often, the process of being a witness is the source of considerable anxiety and fatigue. It is just at such times that the witness will provide a less well-formulated answer. If testimony has been going on for some time, it is reasonable to ask the judge if a short break may be taken.

Depositions are an important aspect of the legal system. They are conducted as part of what the attorneys call the "discovery" phase and help the attorneys involved plan their strategy for trial. They also provide the attorneys (on all sides) a chance to observe a witness. The deposition is a legal proceeding, and testimony obtained becomes part of the court record and can be reviewed or presented at the time of a trial. It is possible for the witness being deposed to have his or her own attorney present, although this is usually not needed. If there is a question of personal liability or legal action, then legal counsel should be present. Sometimes depositions are videotaped. During a deposition, a judge is not present. Attorneys make objections, but the witness will still be asked to answer the question (the judge can later decide on the objection). The witness will be given a copy of the deposition to review.

SERVING AS AN EXPERT WITNESS

Child and adolescent psychiatrists sometimes serve as expert witness (e.g., in cases within the juvenile justice system, custody cases, and sometimes suits related to educational services). In this role, the court expects the professional to offer specific information relevant to the case based on his or her new knowledge and experience. In the role of expert, the professional is given somewhat more leeway (e.g., in expressing professional opinions, not just simple facts). Occasionally, a psychiatrist is appointed by the court and issues a report to the judge rather than to a specific attorney (although the other attorneys, if any, will typically have access to it). In working as an expert witness, it is important for all concerned to understand the role of the mental health professional. Standards of proof differ in civil versus criminal proceedings. In juvenile court, the standard of proof is similar to that in an adult criminal court (i.e., beyond a reasonable doubt), but in civil or family court, the standard is a preponderance of the evidence. In serving as an expert witness, it is critical to avoid conflicts of interest (e.g., serving both as an expert witness and treating physician raises issues). The specific requirements for what constitutes a medical expert vary from state to state as, to some extent, do other court procedures.

In dealing with requests to serve as an expert witness, it is important that the mental health professional have a clear understanding of what is being asked. Often, this is reasonable, but sometimes it is not. A clear understanding and agreement on what is be asked will also clarify some aspects of the procedures involved. For example, an evaluation in relation to a custody dispute will typically involve meetings with the parents and child (separately and together), and, if relevant, other important adults in the child's life. In taking a case, the potential expert witness should be clear that the issues involved fall within his or her areas of expertise (sometimes other issues will, of course, emerge). The initial discussion should also be done so as to reveal any potential conflicts of interest that might exist and gives a chance for the expert to provide a fee schedule, typically an hourly rate, and have an initial review of the basic aspects of the case with the attorney. Given the nature of these assessments and the considerable time they often require, it can be perfectly reasonable to decline an invitation to serve as an expert witness. In some cases, the expert and attorney may agree on an initial record review, after which a decision is made regarding additional work.

A forensic evaluation has similarities and some important differences from routine clinical evaluations. The issues may have less to do with current diagnosis and treatment than with past status (e.g., mental disorders present at the time a crime was committed). Similarly, in a custody assessment, issues will have to do no only with the child but also with the child's relationship to the parents and parental capacities to parent. It is particularly important in forensic evaluations that all those involved be clear about the purpose and nature of the evaluation (e.g., a parent should understand that anything she or he says might end up in a report to the court or might be repeated if the psychiatrist testifies in court). Depending on the context, ancillary sources of information (e.g., school records) may be helpful.

It is not the job of the expert to ferret out records or materials; rather, the court or attorneys involved should request relevant records and be informed if it becomes clear that some records have not been provided. Depending on the context, the expert may ask that other consultations be arranged (e.g., psychological testing might be requested to evaluate psychotic thinking, learning difficulties, or intellectual functioning).

Before writing the report, it is often helpful to discuss preliminary findings with the retaining attorney or the judge even before a final report is submitted. This gives them the opportunity to clarify any questions that have not been answered. Such conversations should not, of course, change the report (unless new facts come to light based on these discussions). Composition of the report should parallel, in many ways, the approach to providing testimony as a witness. The report should be clear; easy to read; and free, as much as possible, of jargon. Usually, it will include a discussion of the background of the case and the questions the psychiatrist is asked to address. A list of interviews conducted, any special procedures or testing, and results of record review should precede a summary of opinions. Direct quotations can be helpful. The report should be professional in its tone and not inflammatory or pejorative. The rational for any specific recommendations should be clear, and the expert should be prepared to defend his or her recommendations in court. The court procedures and advice presented earlier on testifying apply to expert testimony as well. Attorneys retaining expert witnesses will most likely want to go over the material that will be presented in court and the questions that are likely to come up. Depositions are frequently used, and the experts will receive a transcript of the deposition for authentication and correction (e.g., of any medical terms). If followed by later courtroom testimony, statements made in the deposition may be used to challenge the consistency of expert opinion by answers that the expert has made in court.

The process of establishing qualifications may be detailed if the child and adolescent psychiatrist is appearing for one side of the case, especially if opposing experts might testify. The opposing attorney may try to undermine the value of any subsequent opinion offered by indicating during establishment of qualifications that the child and adolescent psychiatrist is inexperienced, or less so, than the opposing side's expert. The volume of forensic work done by the child and adolescent psychiatrist might be raised not only to challenge his or her experience but also to demonstrate if that is the primary work activity and that the expert is merely a "hired gun."

The process and the advice for handling of direct, cross, redirect and recross examination in expert testimony are essentially the same as with fact witnesses. In addition to the qualifications of expertise, the testimony of a child and adolescent psychiatrist is expected to meet the general acceptance rule or Frye Test, named after the case of *Frye v. United States*, which holds that a medical test, procedure, or disorder has been generally accepted in the scientific community. For example, describing that person has a particular syndrome is unlikely to be considered unless it is included in the *Diagnostic and Statistical Manual of the American Psychiatric Association* (DSM-IV). A new standard for scientific opinion in federal cases was set by the U.S. Supreme Court's ruling in *Daubert v. Merrill Dow Pharmaceuticals, Inc.*, which determined that the judge is the one to determine if the offered evidence is scientifically valid and if it will assist the court in understanding or determining facts relevant to the case. In addition, this assessment by the judge of expert opinion must be made before it is presented in court before a jury. Sometimes opposing attorneys will object to expert testimony as "hearsay," as evidence based on the statements or experience of those other than the expert witness. Such evidence is permitted for expert witnesses because the use of others' statements and experience gathered as part of clinical evaluation is a recognized practice in formulating psychiatric opinions. Opposing attorneys may also ask if the child and adolescent psychiatrist accepts or recognizes another professional as an expert in the field or a particular study, paper, or book as authoritative. This is usually done to present information that may conflict or appear to contradict the evidence presented by the expert witness. It is important to maintain objectivity throughout testimony and avoid the appearance of personal bias. The expert is not a patient advocate in such situations but presents psychiatric opinion and the data on which it is based.

CHILD CUSTODY

Legal conceptualizations of children and childhood have evolved significantly over time. This evolution has reflected many factors, including a desire for encouraging education, changing conceptualizations of the nature of childhood and expectations relative to parent rights and child labor, and advances in extending rights to various groups in the population. Historically, children were viewed within the legal system as "chattels" (property) and, similar to women, had few specific rights. Fathers typically were assumed to "rule" the family and make major decisions for family members. These notions started to change as women began to demand and receive additional rights and as child development research began to emphasize the important role of parent–child (including mother–child) relationships for healthy development. Courts began to recognize the principle of "best interests of the child" in decision making regarding child custody.

The increasing frequency and acceptance of divorce has raised other issues, with current trends suggesting that about 50% of marriages will end in divorce. Other issues arise given the frequency of single-parent household, particularly for children growing up in poverty. Parental separation and divorce increase the risk for children and adolescents to have various problems, probably doubling this risk relative to intact families. The effects may be seen over both the short and long term. After parental separation, children may exhibit a range of reactions, including anxiety, distress, anger, and sorrow. The nature of difficulties exhibited varies depends on the age and developmental level of the child so that, for example, younger children may have sleep problems or exhibit anxiety but older children or adolescents may experience distress, and academic performance may suffer. Relationships may also be impacted. Issues for adolescents are particularly complex given that the tasks of adolescence include separation from their own family of origin and development of new relationships. Behavioral difficulties can take the form of more externalizing problems (e.g., in conduct and behavioral difficulties) or internalizing ones (e.g., anxiety or mood problems). Complicating issues of psychological adjustment, there may be stresses related to ongoing parental struggles or disputes and to changes in financial circumstances. Mitigating factors include stable relationships with one parent and the presence of a support network (e.g., of peers or other family members). Fortunately, in most cases, children cope effectively with the situation.

Increasingly, the rights of both parents have been emphasized in terms of the need for continued contact with minor children. In most states, the principle of the child's best interest is now well accepted, although in practice, judges have considerable discretion. Mental health professionals often have been used to clarify what is in the child's best interest, particularly if the child is young or unable to clearly articulate his or her preferences or if special circumstances (e.g., alleged vulnerabilities in parents or child) make the situation more complex.

In custody disputes, several potential outcomes are possible (e.g., one parent or the other might be awarded custody or custody could be awarded jointly). If one parent is the sole custodial parent, she or he can make all relevant decisions regarding the child. This parent might have physical custody of the child as well, although court-ordered rights of visitation with the other parent might also be imposed. In joint custody, both parents participate in decision making and typically share physical custody of the child. Work in the area of child custody requires skilled clinicians to have an understanding of child development, family functioning, and mental health issues and problems. The consultant must also be aware of the specific applicable laws. In some states, specific additional or ongoing training is required.

The consultant should be particularly careful to respect ethical and professional boundaries (e.g., it is important that the consultant not assume the role of therapist). In initial discussions with all the parties involved, including the child or children, the consultant should carefully explain his or her role and the special nature of the professional contact (e.g., usual confidentiality rules do not apply in the sense that anything that is said may appear in a written report or be noted in testimony to the court).

Referrals should usually come from the court with the agreement of the various attorneys involved and a clear description of the nature of the question(s) to be addressed. Data may be provided or requested from various sources, and a series of clinical interviews is usually conducted, typically with each of the parents and the child or children. Depending on the situation, interviews might be done in the home. Information collected usually includes a review of the history of the child and family, the factors leading to divorce, the psychosocial history of the parents, vulnerabilities in them and the child, areas of strength, and so forth. In some situations, additional consultations (e.g., psychological testing) may be requested.

Interview of the child should be done as appropriate to the developmental level of the child with careful attention to evidence of attachments and relationships with the parents. Exploration of the parent's views of the child and of the home environment and observation of the parent–child interaction are all relevant. Collateral sources of information (e.g., from pediatricians, schools, and so forth) may also inform the process.

A final written summary typically includes a review of the background of the consultation, including the specific questions of interest to the court and a summary of the sources of information used by the evaluator. Usually, the next section of the report provides a narrative description of the process of the assessment and summaries of interviews and observations, and the final section includes recommendations and conclusions. After the report has been submitted, conferences with the various parties or a deposition may be requested.

Various special issues or situations may arise in custody assessment (e.g., the rights of grandparents or stepparents to visitation, issues of reunification of children with parents who have been abusive or neglectful). Issues increasingly arise from new approaches to reproductive technologies (e.g., the woman carrying the child to term may not be the biological mother). Courts frequently turn to mental health consultants in these situations. Often, the preference of courts is to honor biological relationships, but clear evidence of the child's best interest may outweigh such considerations. Visitation of grandparents has been an area of active legislation and litigation in recent years. Most states now give some form of visitation right to grandparents, but the U.S. Supreme Court has placed some limitations on such rights.

Increasingly, fathers seek custody, and the past presumption that mothers should automatically be custodial parents, particularly of infants and young children, has given way to views that seek to minimize anxiety over separation and continue to foster parent–child relationships and attachments. As a result, frequent visitation and joint custody arrangements are encouraged. In such situations, consistency should be a goal, with regular and predictable transitions rather than unpredictable and irregular ones. When the parents have had a bitter divorce, joint custody arrangements and visitations can continue to serve as a source of continued conflict, sometimes to the detriment of the child's development. Issues of gay and lesbian parents have also assumed increasing prominence in recent years. Available data suggest that children developing in families with such parents are not at increased risk. Various states have differing views on these matters, as reflected both in legal precedents and legislation. For the evaluator, issues of the child's best interest and relationships should remain guiding principles. For some parents, desperation after adverse legal decisions leads to parental kidnapping. These situations are fraught with risks for the child, and consultants should be familiar with relevant state and federal laws in the area.

Alleged sexual or other types of abuse occur with some frequency as part of disputes regarding children's custody. These issues can be extremely difficult to sort out and require a thoughtful approach on the part of a highly experienced clinician. In such situations, several steps may be taken to avoid potential bias and effects of coaching or indoctrination (e.g., use of open-ended rather than leading questions). In other situations, allegations may center around a parent being unfit based on the presence of some specific mental health problem (e.g., schizophrenia). In general, having a disorder of any kind is rather less relevant than the demonstrated ability of the parent to serve as parent and the impact, if any, of the parent's difficulties on the relationship with the child.

The highly mobile nature of U.S. society means that increasingly, divorced parents live at some distance from each other. In most states, there is recognition that parents may need to move, although specific issues may arise that lead to a revisitation of custodial or visitation issues. These can be some of the most difficult and challenging cases for the courts. Typically, the needs and developmental level of the child, the preference of the child (if he or she is capable of expressing one), the need for the move, the ability for parents to work collaboratively even at a distance, and existing custodial arrangements are all factors to be considered.

Special considerations arise when one parent has a history of violent behavior or such behavior is alleged on the part of the divorcing spouse. A history of domestic violence is one of the factors increasingly recognized by courts in determining child placement. In some states, there is a "rebuttal presumption" of allowing sole or joint custody if a parent has been violent. In these cases, careful assessment is also indicated to be sure that the allegations of violence, the nature of the violent behavior and level of danger involved, and the risk to the child are evaluated and verified.

Given the considerable financial burden of extended court proceedings and the divisive nature of such processes, interest has centered on alternative approaches to resolution of divorce and child care issues. Alternative resolution techniques attempt to provide less confrontation and divisive approaches to these problems by providing information and helping parents seek mutually satisfactory approaches to resolving disputes. Several states have now explicitly fostered this approach (e.g., mandating either private or court-appointed mediation before a trial is scheduled). An awareness of the potential negative effects of chronic marital conflict, including after divorce, has led to development of various intervention programs. These aim to minimize negative effects of conflict and the adversarial process and help parents cope and parent more effectively.

ADOPTION

Adoption represents a specialized custody issue, albeit one not always involving mental health professionals. Adoption has been practiced since ancient times. In Rome, the practice included adoption of adults as well as children if, for example, an heir was needed. In the United States, informal adoption preceded the first laws on the topic. It arose in the context of parents taking care of orphaned babies, in apprenticeship of children, and in the practice of sending homeless children from large cities to work on farms. Legal formalization of adoption is a much more recent historical phenomenon in this country with statues now present both at the state and federal levels. There have been major changes in adoption over recent decades with adoption of infants born to unwed mothers being much more common in the past and adoption of foreign-born infants and children now much more frequent. Less formal adoption procedures (e.g., with arrangements made privately by lawyers and physicians) have given way to much more formalized systems.

The move towards support for permanency planning for children who had been abused or neglected had a further impact with new incentives for foster parents. Another law, the Adoption Promotion Act, provided incentives for adoption of older children. Changes have also occurred in patterns of international adoption with the earliest waves of adoptees, in the 1950s, from Korea and Southeast Asia to, more recently, a range of other countries, including China, India, South American, Africa, and Eastern Europe.

Around 120,000 children a year are adopted, many as infants and young children. Depending on the circumstances, biological parents, particularly mothers, may maintain some contact with the child and adoptive family (open adoption). One of the challenges, particularly for children who are international adoptees and who have spent varying periods of time in orphanages or foster care, are the developmental and other problems sometimes observed. Orphanages vary widely in quality. Some children are placed because of difficulties in the parent that may be transmitted to some degree to the child (e.g., alcohol exposure or substance abuse during the pregnancy or difficulties with impulsive behavior in the mother that may have longer lasting impact on the child). For children adopted internationally, there may be little or no information on biological parents and similarly scant exposure to cultures of origin.

Most frequently, children, and their families do well after adoption. In general, most clinicians favor talking to the children from early on about adoption and whatever they know of the child's origins. As children become older, they frequently become more interested in their families of origin. They may ask their adoptive parents about the adoption, and parents should generally be open and honest about what they know. As with children of divorce, there is some potential for children to experience adoption in a self-referential way (i.e., that it was somehow their fault that the birth parents could not care for them). Fantasies about these issues may include notions that the child was unwanted because of his or her gender or because of concerns that he or she was somehow "damaged goods." A major complication can arise if children, as is often the case, wish to protect their adoptive parents from these worries and concerns. Adolescence, in particular, may present some challenges given the normative developmental task of the individual in leaving the psychological parents. Adolescent concerns and fantasies may prove challenging for the adoptive parents, particularly when this takes the form of searching for the biological parents. This can be the source of distress and sadness because it may be experienced as rejection even when this is not in fact intended.

Adoptive parents face some unique challenges, including anxiety and concerns relative to delay in the actual adoption process often compounded by preexisting issues relative to difficulties in fertility. Other challenges emerge as the adopted child becomes older and may contribute to seeking clinical consultation and referral. Historically, and even at present, children who are adopted are more likely to present for clinical evaluation, both in outpatient and inpatient settings. In itself, adoption is of relatively low risk, although, as a group, there are somewhat higher rates of externalizing problems, particularly in adolescents. There is also some suggestion of increased risk for mood and anxiety problems. On the other hand, if rates of referral or psychopathology are compared with those of children returned to families in which they had been abused or neglected, it is clear that adoptive children fare better, and indeed for most adopted children, it is clear that adoption is a benefit and one usually associated with a good outcome.

Children adopted from other countries may show delays in both development and in growth. This seems particularly the case when the child has been reared in an institutional (orphanage) setting rather than in family-based foster care. These delays may be in multiple areas and can also be associated with various medical problems, albeit usually minor ones. Younger age at placement is associated with a better outcome. There is some suggestion that international adoptees may be at somewhat higher risk for mental health problems, including mood and behavior problems, although again most children do very well. Various factors may be associated with higher risk, including a longer time in orphanage care, male gender, and placement with single parents. The potential impact of subtle, or not so subtle, bias based on appearance may also contribute. Clearly, children who have been extremely deprived may be at greatest risk for difficulties.

Adoption of children within the child welfare system has been an important and controversial topic for many years. In the past, overtly expressed policy favored reunification of child and parent(s), but this has now shifted to encourage early foster placement to ensure stability. Unfortunately, it is clear that adoptive children are more likely to have problems if they have been placed at an older age. Mental health clinicians, of course, tend to have contact only with situations in which the adoptive child is not doing well. Occasionally, clinicians see situations in which the adoption is not completed.

THE INTERFACE OF EDUCATIONAL SYSTEMS AND THE LAW

Over the past several decades, the role of child psychiatrists, psychologists, and other professionals in the identification of children who present to schools with special educational needs has expanded considerably. Child psychiatrists and other mental health professionals are often asked to provide consultation or recommendations relative to disorders or disabilities that may impact the child's ability to profit from his or her educational program. These accommodations can range from very small to much larger (e.g., modifications in home work or test taking with extra time for support from other members of the school staff regarding speech-communication intervention, social skills training, special classes, and so on).

Several different laws are relevant to this process. These laws apply in somewhat different situations to students with different levels of disability. The Americans with Disabilities Act (ADA) passed in 1973 applies to children as well as adolescents and adults. It specifically forbids denial of educational services to students who exhibit disabilities and prohibits discrimination against such students. Parents can request an evaluation to document the presence of a disability and identify the accommodations that can be made to help the student. Unlike the process under the Individuals with Disabilities Education Act (IDEA) (see below), which results in a detailed educational plan (Table 26.2), review for accommodations within the ADA typically results in what is called a 504 Plan (504 refers to the section of the act that relates specifically to schools and mandates provision of a "free appropriate public education"

TABLE 26.2

SCHOOL SERVICE PLANS FOR STUDENTS WITH PSYCHIATRIC DISORDERS

Type of School Service Plan	District Service Plan	504 Plan	Individualized Educational Plan
Purpose	To respond quickly to mild changes in the student's life that impact learning; the focus is on mild or brief circumstances that may impact learning	To ensure that all students have equal opportunity to learn even if they have a disability; the focus is on the student's opportunities compared with other students in that school	To remediate symptoms of a student's disability; student's unique needs are the focus
Criteria to receive this plan	Student has a symptom or disorder that impacts learning	Student has an impairment that limits a major life activity but may not require specialized instruction	Student has a disability that interferes with educational progress and that requires specialized instruction
Who develops this plan	Teacher and administrator, usually with parental input	Teacher, administrator (often the school's designated "504 Coordinator") school counselor and usually parent and student (if appropriate)	Educational team, including staff certified in special education; may include evaluations by school psychologist or social worker; parent may bring friends, advocates, own evaluators to be part of team
What is usually provided	Changes within classroom to enable student to perform better	Changes within classroom or school building to enable student to complete curriculum expectations	Changes within classroom setting(s) to provide student different instruction; may substantially alter what is required of student
Example of what is provided	Student is allowed to sit closer to teacher during instruction; student is met by familiar staff to decrease anxiety	Student is allowed more time to complete tests; student may be provided device to hear better	Student may leave regular language arts class and receive specialized reading program; student may be exempted from course requirements
Which staff deliver services	Usually regular education staff	Usually regular education staff	Staff with specialized training (special education teachers, speech therapists, occupational therapists, and so on)
Where the student receives services	Regular classroom	Regular classroom with regular peers "to the maximum extent appropriate"	Wide ranging, from regular education classrooms (inclusion) to pullout for special education classrooms, to offsite day school programs, to 24-hour a /day residential schools

(continued)

TABLE 26.2

CONTINUED

Type of School Service Plan	District Service Plan	504 Plan	Individualized Educational Plan
Review of the plan	As needed	Plan reviewed at least every year	Plan is reviewed at least every year, and every 3 years, the student is retested to see if he or she still qualifies
Disciplinary actions	Usually not applicable	If "manifestation hearing" indicates student's impairment or disability caused misbehavior, then student cannot be suspended or expelled; school is not required to provide FAPE for suspended or expelled students	If "manifestation hearing" indicates student's disability caused misbehavior, then student cannot be suspended or expelled; if student is suspended or expelled, school must still provide FAPE
Appeal recourses	None provided	School may alter 504 Plan immediately if circumstances indicate need; "notice" may be provided verbally; family may appeal to the OCR if they perceive the school is discriminating against child because of a disability	School must provide "prior written notice" before changes in educational plan or placement are made; family may appeal decisions or plan to local and then state departments of education

FAPE, free appropriate public education.
Reprinted from Bostic, J. Q., Stein, B., & Scwab-Stone, M. (2007). Schools. In A. Martin & F. Volkmar (Eds.), *Lewis's Child and Adolescent Psychiatry: A Comprehensive Textbook*, 4th edition (p. 986). Philadelphia: Lippincott Williams & Wilkins.

[FAPE] in the "least restrictive environment" [LRE]). Unlike the IDEA process, 504 services can be used for individuals with a wide range of difficulties, and accommodations are usually carried out while maintaining the student in the regular educational setting. Regardless of the specific diagnostic label, it is important to understand that the intention is the identification of problems or disabilities that interfere with the student's ability to learn.

For students who need more extensive services, a different law usually applies. Originally passed in 1975, Public Law 94-142 marked a very major shift in services provided within school settings. Before that time, only a small number of children with severe disabilities received services within public school. Parents would be turned away and often told to look at other (e.g., residential or institutional) settings for children with significant disabilities. Of children with autism, for example, maybe only 20% received public school services (Volkmar & Wiesner, 2009). The passage of The Education for All Handicapped Children Act mandated school services for all children. This law has been modified over time and is most recently revised as the IDEA. As a result of this law, schools are required to provide FAPE to students whose difficulties require special instruction and services. Several conditions are specifically listed as disabilities, including autism, intellectual deficiency, sensory impairments such as deafness or blindness, emotional disturbance, multiple disabilities, speech-language disorders, learning disabilities, traumatic brain injury, orthopedic impairments and "other" health impairment (the last typically includes attention-deficit/hyperactivity disorder). *Emotional disturbance* is defined as a persistent and serious condition that negatively affects educational performance. In addition, the student must need specialized instruction (i.e., if a child has a condition but does not need such instruction, he or she would not qualify). Typically, special instruction is required if the child does not make progress effectively in school; this progress may include academic progress but also social-interpersonal progress. Often, when children are not technically eligible under IDEA, they still may be eligible for some accommodations under the ADA Act (i.e., they may have 504 Plans to provide reasonable accommodations of their needs).

The process of establishing eligibility under IDEA is more involved than that needed for a 504 Plan. As opposed to the section 504 Plan the Individualized Education Program (IEP) allows for important modifications of the program that do not necessarily require the student to meet the same academic requirements as other students in the classroom. The IEP development process typically includes an assessment conducted by a multidisciplinary team of professionals and often includes an evaluation of cognition, language-communication, academics, social-emotional skills, overall health status, and screening for sensory and motor difficulties. Testing by school professionals may be used to document abilities and problems. General medical or psychiatric assessments may also be needed. Goals of this process include establishing the presence of at least one (or sometimes more than one) disability, the degree to which the child is or is not making satisfactory progress, and the degree to which this results from the disability and whether special instruction or related services are need to help the child be able to use the school program. When eligibility has already been established, reevaluation may be used to document whether the disability continues to impact the child and whether special services are still needed. Parents must be involved in this process; if they are not in agreement with the results, they can request an independent assessment (although the school is *not* required to necessarily agree with it).

Any number of relevant modifications can be considered in putting the IEP together, including educational or academic goals along with accommodations and modifications, participation in special educational or other programs or in the mainstream (sometimes with support), behavioral interventions and accommodations, extended school services, transition planning, modifications of the curriculum, and special services (occupational, speech-language, or physical therapy or counseling) along with school health services and even transportation (see Bostic et al., 2007). Specific interventions can be made relative to specific psychiatric symptoms, such as helping anxious students anticipate transitions and times of anxiety, structuring the classroom and providing organizational supports for students with attentional or learning issues, making relevant modifications for children with mood disorders, and providing social skills interventions to students on the autism spectrum. Some of the key concepts, terms, and rights and protections under IDEA are provided in Table 26.3. Under IDEA, services can be provided up to the twenty-second birthday of a student. This law gives states incentives (i.e., funding) to ensure their participation. For older individuals (e.g., those in college or in technical school after age 21 years) IDEA does not apply, but other laws, such as the ADA, may apply. The age of the child is also relevant for younger children because requirements for early intervention (before age 3 years) differ from those for public schools.

A number of special situations can arise. For example, if a student is dangerous or threatening or is involved in substance abuse at school, an emergency IEP meeting can be held and alternative placement put into place. Special rules relate to student suspension with provision for rapid response to emergent situations as well as continued provision of due process protections. If, for example, a problem behavior is determined to be the result of a disability, the school must continue to provide services (e.g., a child with Tourette's disorder whose tics seemed to disrupt the class could not be suspended if the behavior [tics] is a manifestation of his or her disability). Protections also extend to children in whom a disability is suspected but an evaluation process has not yet been completed.

The IDEA provides extensive procedural protections to parents of children with disabilities, including "the right to participate in the development of the IEP, the right to independent evaluations, the right to inspect educational records," and "the opportunity to present complaints

TABLE 26.3

EDUCATIONAL LAW: KEY CONCEPTS AND TERMS

ADA: Americans with Disabilities Act
FAPE: Free appropriate public education
504 Plan: A plan developed to accommodate the special needs of children with disabilities
IDEA: The Individuals with Disabilities Education Act; an act of Congress giving specific rights to children with disabilities for educational services
IEP: Individualized Education Program
IFSP: Individualized Family Service Plan; a plan similar to the IEP but for younger children (younger than age 3 years)
LRE: Least restrictive environment
PL-94-142: The original (1975) law passed by Congress mandating school services to children with disabilities

Rights and Safeguards Under IDEA
Consent of parents: Parents must give consent for an evaluation to be done or if reevaluation is done; schools have the right to seek such an evaluation if parents do not consent but must go through due process procedures or mediation to do so.
Due process: Parents or the school can initiate a due process hearing to resolve disputes at any stage in the process (from evaluation, planning and placement, and review). Parents must be informed of their rights and the possibilities for free or low-cost legal representation. The due process hearing is similar to a regular court hearing (but less formal), and parents or the school may be represented by attorneys. An entire appeals process is also available.
Mediation: Rather than going through due process, parents and schools can use the more informal mediation process to resolve disputes.
Notice requirements: The school must give written notice to parents of proposed changes (e.g., in placement or program) and of the parents' rights (e.g., to voice complaints or contest a planned change).
Stay put: The stay put provision means that if a child is in a program and there is a dispute about moving the child to another program, this cannot be done until a placement decision is reached, that is, the school cannot unilaterally remove a child from a program (parents, of course, can). Practically, this usually means that when a dispute is under way, the child stays where he or she is until the dispute is resolved.

Adapted with permission from Volkmar, F. R., & Wiesner, L. A. (2009). *A Practical Guide to Autism: What Every Parent, Family Member, and Teacher Needs to Know* (pp. 88, 96). Hoboken, NJ: John Wiley and Sons.

with respect to any matter relating to the identification, evaluation, or educational placement of the child, or the provision of a free appropriate public education to such child." Such a proceeding, referred to as a due process hearing, requires a neutral adjudicator, a right to counsel at the parent's expense, and the right to present evidence and cross-examine witnesses. If dissatisfied, either party has a right to judicial review in the appropriate state or federal court. With a growing number of students doing well in more mainstream settings, more students with some developmental and psychiatric vulnerabilities are entering school and college programs. It is important for them and their parents to realize that mandates for service under IDEA do *not* apply to college settings where ADA mandates do. Several excellent resources with detailed information on educational advocacy, rights, and entitlements are provided in the Selected Readings.

MALPRACTICE, LIABILITY, AND CONFIDENTIALITY

Both state and, to some extent, federal laws regulate medical practice. Allegations of misconduct can be raised at the level of the state medical licensing board or through litigation on allegations of malpractice. The current system is somewhat arbitrary and haphazard in nature.

However, relative to many other specialties, child psychiatrists are rather less likely to be investigated or sued, although when such investigations occur, they are sources of great anxiety and distress to those involved. For child psychiatrists, only a small minority of claims result in any payment. However, even investigations by medical licensing boards can be highly intrusive and problematic. For a claim of malpractice to be sustained, it typically must be the case that the physician had a duty of reasonable care of a patient but was derelict in some way relative to a reasonable standard (usually of the typical practitioner in the community). As a result, the patient has to show some degree of damage that can be compensated and must demonstrate that it was a direct result of a failure to adhere to a reasonable standard of care. Although these issues are often relatively straightforward, gray areas are also observed. For example, does free advice imply a doctor–patient relationship (it potentially can). Thus, it is particularly important, in this day of rapid information exchange and ready access to Internet resources, to carefully consider implied relationships, and, typically, an explicit statement about the need for patients (and parents) to obtain advice from practitioners specifically familiar with them should be made.

These issues have increasingly arisen relative to advice about psychopharmacology. They are probably particularly likely to emerge when a psychiatrist is responsible for medication management but some other professional (e.g., a social worker or psychologist) is engaged in psychotherapy with the individual. In these instances, a written explanation of roles and responsibilities can be helpful.

Other issues arise after treatment is terminated. Typically, the physician owes only the obligation of confidentiality (i.e., a right to follow-up treatment or consultation is not required). In considering termination, it is important for physicians to be aware of the potential for being seen as abandoning patients (i.e., the patient must have reasonable notice if treatment is to be terminated, and the physician should assist in arrangements for subsequent care if this is indicated). It may be helpful to have an explicit, documented discussion of factors that can lead to termination of the professional relationship from the outset (e.g., treatment noncompliance).

Inadequate or improper diagnostic assessments can also lead to liability (e.g., failure to detect psychosis or suicidality), although lawsuits of this type are relatively uncommon. Similarly, inappropriate treatment can be alleged, but it may be difficult to prove except in certain circumstances (e.g., sexual exploitation of the patient). Liability issues can also arise around medication use and problems in any of several different ways. In one case, for example, a patient who had been treated for a period of time with psychotherapy sued after being transferred to a different setting and being treated, successfully, with medications. Errors can also arise when a medication is given based on an incorrect diagnosis, when a contraindication to administration was present but missed, or when medications are used inappropriately.

There are several other areas of potential liability for child psychiatrists. The actions of employees or supervisees are a potential liability (this is technically termed *vicarious liability*). In addition, supervisors can also be held liable for inadequate supervision. Consultations and second opinions represent another area of potential liability. Typically, as long as no doctor–patient relationship is formed (e.g., if there has been no written report or medication prescription or order), the physician has a duty only to the consulting doctor. Even if an evaluation is conducted at the request of a third party, there can be some potential for liability, although this is a gray area. It is important to inform and document the person being evaluated about the nature of the contact.

In instances of malpractice, the issue is often not so much whether an error was made but whether the error was below the standard of care (i.e., in general, clinicians are on safe ground if they exercise reasonable judgment and a reasonable standard of care). This means, for example, that physicians cannot be held liable for a bad outcome as long as they adhered to a reasonable standard of care in treatment; the latter can, of course, be the topic of much debate, particularly in some areas in psychiatry in which a clear consensus has not always developed. There have been some attempts at the national level to develop such standards.

Malpractice claims can arise based either on some deliberately wrong or incorrect conduct or, more frequently, through negligence. It is important that clinicians realize that for minors, the statute of limitations relative to malpractice suits does not begin until the child has reached

TABLE 26.4

COMMON ISSUES IN MALPRACTICE LITIGATION

Area of Practice	Example Plaintiff Allegation
Dangerousness	
Suicide	Weak suicide assessment documentation (e.g., "SI-")
Homicide	No violence risk assessment in chart
Failure to protect from danger	Inpatient sexually assaulted by another inpatient
Failure to protect third parties	Dangerous patient escapes from hospital and family not notified
Protecting and releasing information	Confidential information released without authorization
Treatment	
Failure to obtain informed consent	Possible side effects not discussed
Psychotherapy	Implanted memories of sexual abuse
Sex with patient	Therapist had sex with patient
Medication	Girl with bipolar disorder treated with sodium divalproex for 8 months gives birth to baby with birth defects, and there is no documentation of pregnancy status when medication is started
Ending treatment	
Negligent discharge	Patient discharged while still suicidal
Abandonment	Therapist terminated treatment without referral when patient failed to pay bill

Reprinted from Ash, P., & Nurcombe, B. (2007). Malpractice and professional liability. In A. Martin & F. Volkmar (Eds.), *Lewis's Child and Adolescent Psychiatry: A Comprehensive Textbook*, 4th edition, p. 1022. Philadelphia: Lippincott Williams & Wilkins.

legal adulthood. A series of relevant legal issues and principles apply in this area (see Ash & Nurcombe, 2007). There can also be important variations in the law from state to state. Among the many complexities for child psychiatrists are the young age of the patients, who often cannot consent to treatment without the parents' involvement. Parents are themselves often involved in treatment, raising further complications. Table 26.4 summarizes some of the areas in which malpractice is more frequently alleged.

Assessment of Dangerousness and Violence

The area of assessment of dangerousness, to self or others, represents a major area of potential malpractice liability for all mental health professionals. A series of legal decisions have led to major exceptions in usual confidentiality laws as these apply to threats and assessment of dangerousness. In malpractice cases arising in these contexts, major issues have to do with whether the danger could reasonably be foreseen and if the clinician took appropriate steps to protect the patient or a potential victim. Similarly, the high rates of suicidal thoughts in adolescents present major challenges for clinicians (see Chapter 24). Documentation of a careful and thoughtful assessment and adherence to a reasonable standard of care is important in these cases. The assessment of suicide risk should be done thoughtfully with documentation of factors that provide risk as well as potential protection. In inpatient settings or situations in which the psychiatrist has oversight of others, clear documentation is also needed. Continued documentation is needed when a patient is in a longer term treatment relationship. Even if a decision is reasonable, supporting documentation is important. Consideration of family involvement is important in considering precautions relative to youth suicide. Discussion with parents can be used to help them monitor the child' condition or need for hospitalization.

The issue of warning third parties (i.e., relative to potential dangerousness of patients) arises as a result of the Tarasoff decision in 1974. Before that time, the clinician could be held liable by the patient but not by a third party. When it first heard the case, the California Supreme Court found that the "duty to warn" was indicated. Because of serious concerns about the potential for reducing confidentiality, the court revised this in a subsequent decision, clarifying that there was duty to protect (i.e., rather than warn) if a serious danger of violence existed for a foreseeable potential victim. The issue of what constituted reasonable care in this regard was left unresolved. After this decision, both state lawmakers and courts have struggled with the myriad of complex issues created by the Tarasoff decision. Unfortunately, requirements vary from state to state, with many states agreeing there is a duty to warn and others not requiring warning, and in a few states, the issue remains ambiguous. Fortunately, this issue is a relatively uncommon one in children and adolescents. In the rare cases when this issue arises, the clinician should evaluate the seriousness of the threat and involve parents, taking appropriate precautions (e.g., hospitalization) if the risk is significant. In some situations (e.g., when an adolescent has eloped from a hospital program), informing the police may be appropriate. These are complicated issues, and consultation with colleagues as well as legal counsel (e.g., of the hospital) is often helpful (Table 26.5).

Violence within inpatient settings can also represent legal liability. Other patients should be protected from violent patients with thoughtful assessment and documentation of appropriate procedures to ensure safety. Similarly, issues of sexual abuse can arise in inpatient and residential treatment settings. Sexual activity among school-aged children in inpatient settings is one of the more frequent causes of litigation. Cases can be complex because details may be presented to one patient's clinician but not the others. Consideration of inappropriate sexual behavior should also be part of inpatient or residential treatment center planning, although monitoring, particularly in the latter setting, can be difficult if the residents have free access to grounds and community activities. Sometimes difficulties arise in such settings (e.g., a patient may commit suicide or commit a crime while out on a pass). In such situations, a reasonable standard of care will be the main focus of legal inquiry. Courts do recognize the challenges involved in rehabilitation and the need to take sensible risk. The increasing pressure for shorter length of stays in inpatient settings does, unfortunately, likely increase risks, a source of concern relative for the liability of professionals involved.

Within inpatient settings, seclusion and restraint issues often present some of the greatest potential for physical injury to patients. It is important that staff be trained in the use of appropriate management techniques, the emphasis be on positive programming rather than punitive use of seclusion, careful monitoring of the patient be maintained, and overall procedures to review and minimize seclusion and restraining be in place (see Martin et al., 2009). Hospitals can also be held liable if an employee engages in inappropriate sexual behavior or violence with a patient.

Confidentiality Issues

Concerns around issues of confidentiality have always been a major concern in psychiatry and become even more complex in child psychiatry because consultation and collaboration with parents and, often, others is frequent. Good clinical judgment is needed to weigh issues of the child's desire for privacy relative to parental rights to know (and release) information relative to their child's care. Some variation exists among states in terms of what information can or cannot be withheld from parents and guardians. For example, parents clearly should be informed if their child is engaging in potentially dangerous behavior. In most cases, a discussion of confidentiality issues should be held very early in treatment to clarify exactly what information is shared and in what circumstances. Privilege (e.g., from having to testify) has been established by law or court decision in many states. The U.S. Supreme Court has held that a mental health privilege applies in the federal court system.

TABLE 26.5

AREAS FOR ASSESSMENT OF RISK OF VIOLENCE TO OTHERS

Past history of violent threats or actions
Nature of threat
  Direct threat
  Has potential victim has bullied or provoked patient?
  Plan for harming the victim
  Access to lethal weapons?
  Leakage of preoccupation with violence in journals, Web surfing, and writings
  Taking steps toward action, such as following or stalking victim, obtaining a weapon,
    rehearsing an attack
  Threat communicated to others, especially peers

Past history
  History of being abused
  History of alcohol or drug abuse

Demographic factors
  Late adolescent
  Male
  Disadvantaged ethnic groups with a cultural tradition of masculine defensiveness

Psychological factors
  Copes with anxiety or hostility by externalizing or projecting it in the form of impulsive,
    explosive actions; suspicious vigilance; or frank persecutory delusions
  Command hallucinations that instruct the patient to take violent action or that threaten
    violence to the patient or his or her family
  Inner controls against violent actions subjectively or objectively reduced
  Strong inner urge to be violent

Social environment
  Family psychopathology in the form of rejection, neglect, physical or sexual abuse, or family
    violence
  Parental mental or physical health impaired
  Intelligence below average
  Impairment of the sensorium
  Alcohol or substance abuse
  Repeatedly victimized or scapegoated at school

Therapeutic alliance
  Has the patient lost or terminated a therapeutic relationship?
  Is he or she competent and motivated to enter into one?

Protective factors
  Younger, female, white, religious, middle class
  No access to lethal means
  If there has been a threat of violence, a threat without a plan or an identified victim
  Secure family without major psychopathology
  Positive relationship with a therapist

Reprinted from Ash, P., & Nurcombe, B. (2007). Malpractice and professional liability. In A. Martin & F. Volkmar (Eds.), *Lewis's Child and Adolescent Psychiatry: A Comprehensive Textbook*, 4th edition, p. 1030. Philadelphia: Lippincott Williams & Wilkins.

Even if the clinician receives a subpoena, he or she may not necessarily be compelled to testify about confidential information unless authorization from the patient is provided or if, for example, the judge orders the clinician to do so. The latter might occur in a situation in which the mental health issues are relevant to a lawsuit or criminal action. The passage of the Health Insurance Portability and Accountability Act (HIPAA) of 1996 resulted in a new set of regulation that became effective in 2003. The privacy rule established by these regulations sets a federal standard relative to protected health information (states can provide for higher levels of protection). The implications of these regulations are complex, and important aspects remain to be resolved. However, it is clear that violations can result in prosecution. Patients (or parents) must be given a Notice of Privacy Practices during their first appointment. In addition, HIPPA specifically gives patients rights to see their records (with rare exceptions). HIPPA also restricts access from third parties (e.g., insurance companies) to information that is the "minimum necessary." Within psychiatry, the latter usually includes identifying information, a treatment plan, diagnosis, and dates when services were provided but does not allow more extensive access to material. As part of the process, a new form of medical record, the psychotherapy note, has been established and can be kept apart and might even be destroyed by the clinician (except under certain circumstances). These notes are only released when the patient consents (e.g., concerns about HIPPA can also arise relative to unprotected e-mail communications).

Confidentiality issues also can arise regarding reporting of potential child abuse or neglect. All states mandate reporting if a reasonable suspicion is present. The laws that mandate reporting also provide legal protections for clinicians who, in good faith, report potential abusive activities. Gray areas and ambiguities can arise (e.g., around allegations made in custody cases), and consultation with legal counsel may be helpful.

Children have special protection as research subjects under federal law, typically including assent from the child as well as consent from the parents. Additional protections to research subjects are provided by HIPPA as well. As in work with adult psychiatric patients, it is good practice to have clear communication with patients (and parents as appropriate), with good documentation and sensible treatment programs grounded as much as possible in evidence-based medicine and conforming, at a minimum, to the community standard of care.

Failures to provide proper treatment can arise in many ways. These may include failures to obtain informed consent or to provide information sufficient in that process. Consent cannot always be obtained in emergency situations, although even then attempts should be made if possible (e.g., to obtain consent from parents or others). In many states, it is possible for adolescents to give consent to (e.g., emancipated minors) or for evaluation of certain problems (e.g., sexually transmitted diseases). Given variations from state to state, clinicians must be aware of the current laws in their own jurisdictions. Inappropriate admission to a mental health hospital (e.g., without adequate evaluation or monitoring) can also result in liability for the physician.

Termination and "Abandonment"

Liability can also arise when patients are "abandoned" (i.e., when treatment is terminated abruptly and unilaterally without appropriate arrangements for transfer of care or when appropriate coverage and accessibility is not provided). Termination can be done unilaterally in some circumstances, although usually with adequate notice, provision of alternative treaters, and a follow-up (certified) letter to document the discussion and the reasons why treatment is being terminated. Liability is also potentially the result of inappropriate disclosure (e.g., of patient names in research reports).

SUMMARY

Child and adolescent psychiatrists and other mental health professionals have had an increasing role in various legal proceedings. Involvement may range from serving as a "fact" witness to serving as an expert witness or consultant to the court, in helping mediate a custody dispute, or providing an opinion about needed accommodations to address a developmental or psychiatric problem in a school. It is vital that professionals remain aware of changes in the law and are aware of new laws and decisions that may impact their care of children and families. Having some awareness of the judicial process facilitates this effort.

Changes in practices of custody and custody dispute resolution have been an active area for involvement of mental health professionals over the past several decades. Considerable progress has been made in considering children's needs (rather than only adults' needs) in this process, and advances have been made in terms of facilitating, as much as possible, the continued involvement of both parents in the child's life. As with other aspects of forensics, it is important that professionals remain current with laws and practices in their jurisdictions.

Adoption touches many lives. Many adults joyfully become parents through adoption, and for most children, adoption has a positive outcome, contributes to positive psychological adjustment, and is clearly protective; for a minority, adoption may be associated with emotional and behavioral problems and psychiatric disorders. Children at particular risk include those adopted later in life, those adopted after early adverse experiences, and those at particular genetic risk. Clinicians working with adopted children and their families should be aware of the complexity and variability of the circumstances in which adoption takes place, as well as the meaning of the process for all the individuals involved.

Complaints of malpractice are, fortunately, relatively infrequent in work with children and adolescents but do sometimes arise. These can take the form of lawsuits (e.g., relative to patients who have been harmed) or direct complaints to state licensing boards. Such complaints are and should be taken seriously. The process of being sued for malpractice is not a happy one. Physicians should be careful to adhere to good standards of professional practice and should be aware of relevant laws and responsibilities. One of the complexities of work with child and adolescents has to do with issues of confidentiality, particularly when, as is frequent, parents are also understandably involved in some way in the treatment.

Selected Readings

American Academy of Child and Adolescent Psychiatry. (1997). Practice parameters for child custody evaluations. *Journal of the American Academy of Child and Adolescent Psychiatry, 36,* 57S–67S.

Ash, P., & Nurcombe, B. (2007). Malpractice and professional liability. In A. Martin & F. Volkmar (Eds.), *Lewis's Child and Adolescent Psychiatry: A Comprehensive Textbook,* 4th edition. Philadelphia: Lippincott Williams & Wilkins.

Bernet, W. (1998). The child and adolescent psychiatrist and the law. In *Handbook of Child and Adolescent Psychiatry,* pp. 438–468. New York: Wiley.

Billick, S. B., & Ciric, S. J. (2003). Role of the psychiatric evaluator in child custody disputes. In *Principles and Practice of Forensic Psychiatry,* 2nd ed, pp. 331–347. London: Arnold.

Borland, M., O'Hara, G., & Triseliotis, J. (1991). Placement outcomes for children with special needs. *Adoption and Fostering, 15,* 18–28.

Borum, R., Fein, R., Vossekuil, B., & Berglund, J. (1999). Threat assessment: Defining an approach for evaluating risk of targeted violence. *Behavioral Science Law, 17,* 323–337.

Bostic, J. Q., Stein, B., & Scwab-Stone, M. (2007). Schools. In A. Martin & F. Volkmar (Eds.), *Lewis's Child and Adolescent Psychiatry: A Comprehensive Textbook,* 4th edition. Philadelphia: Lippincott Williams & Wilkins.

Brown, J. M. A. (2007). Adoption. In A. Martin & F. Volkmar (Eds.), *Lewis's Child and Adolescent Psychiatry: A Comprehensive Textbook,* 4th edition. Philadelphia: Lippincott Williams & Wilkins.

Goldstein, J., Solnit, A. J., Goldstein, S., & Freud, A. (1996). *In the Best Interest of the Child.* New York: Free Press.

Hannibal, M. E. (2002). *Good Parenting Through Your Divorce.* New York: Marlow and Co.

Hetherington, M. E., & Kelly, J. (2002). *For Better or for Worse.* New York: W.W. Norton C. Company.

Hodges, J., & Tizard, B. (1989). Social and family relationships of ex-institutional adolescents. *Journal of Child Psychology & Psychiatry, 30,* 77–97.

Howe, D. (1997). Parent reported problems in 211 adopted children: Some risk and protective factors. *Journal of Child Psychology & Psychiatry, 38,* 401–411.

Kelly, J. B., & Emery, R. (2003). Children's adjustment following divorce: Risk and resilience perspectives. *Family Relations, 52,* 352–262.

Kuo, A. D., & Sikorski, J. B. (2007). Divorce and child custody. In A. Martin & F. Volkmar (Eds.), *Lewis's Child and Adolescent Psychiatry: A Comprehensive Textbook,* 4th edition. Philadelphia: Lippincott Williams & Wilkins.

Martin, A., Krieg, H., Esposito, F., Stubbe, D., & Cardona, L. (2009). Reduction of restraint and seclusion through collaborative problem solving: A five-year prospective inpatient study. *Psychiatric Services, 60*(3), 406.

Maughan, B., & Pickles, A. (1990). Adopted and illegitimate children grown up. In L. Robins & M. Rutter (Eds.), *Straight and Devious Pathways from Childhood to Adulthood*. New York: Cambridge University Press.

O'Connor, S. (2004). *Orphan Trains: The Story of Charles Loring Brace and the Children He Saved and Failed*. Chicago: University of Chicago Press.

Recupero, P. R. (2005). E-mail and the psychiatrist-patient relationship. *Journal of the American Academy of Psychiatry Law, 33,* 465–475.

Reed, J. (2004). Cybermedicine: Defying and redefining patient standards of care. *Indiana Law Review, 37,* 845–877.

Rutter, M. (1998). Developmental catch-up, and deficit, following adoption after severe global early privation. *Journal of Child Psychology & Psychiatry, 39,* 465–476.

Schetky, D. (2002). History of child and adolescent forensic psychiatry. In *Principles and Practice of Child and Adolescent Forensic Psychiatry*, pp. 3–14. Washington, DC: American Psychiatric Publishing.

Sharma, S., & Thomas, C. R. (2007). The child and adolescent psychiatrist in court. In A. Martin & F. Volkmar (Eds.), *Lewis's Child and Adolescent Psychiatry: A Comprehensive Textbook*, 4th edition. Philadelphia: Lippincott Williams & Wilkins.

Simon, R. I. (2004). *Assessing and Managing Suicide Risk: Guidelines for Clinically Based Risk Management*. Washington, DC: American Psychiatric Publications.

Skolnick, A. (1998). Solomon's children: The new biologism, psychological Parenthood, attachment theory, and the best interests standard. In *All Our Families*. New York: Oxford University Press.

Tesler, P. (2001). *Collaborative Law: Achieving Effective Resolution in Divorce Without Litigation*. Washington, DC: American Bar Association.

Tizard, B. (1991). Intercountry adoption: A review of the evidence. *Journal of Child Psychology & Psychiatry, 32,* 743–756.

Volkmar, F. R., & Wiesner, L. A. (2009). *A Practical Guide to Autism: What Every Parent, Family Member, and Teacher Needs to Know*. Hoboken, NJ: John Wiley and Sons.

Wallerstein, J. S., Lewis, J. M., & Blakeslee, S. (2000). *The Unexpected Legacy of Divorce*. New York: Hyperion.

Zeanah, C. H., Larrieu, J. A., Heller, S. S., Valliere, J., Hinshaw-Fuselier, S., Aoki, Y., & Drilling, M. (2001). Evaluation of a preventive intervention for maltreated infants and toddlers in foster care. *Journal of the American Academy of Child and Adolescent Psychiatry, 40,* 214–221.

Note: Page number followed by *f* and *t* indicates figure and table respectively.